Introduction to
Social Cognition
The Essential Questions and Ideas

Gordon B. Moskowitz

THE GUILFORD PRESS
New York   London

Copyright © 2024 The Guilford Press
A Division of Guilford Publications, Inc.
370 Seventh Avenue, Suite 1200, New York, NY 10001
www.guilford.com

Printed in the United States of America

This book is printed on acid-free paper.

Last digit is print number: 9   8   7   6   5   4   3   2   1

Library of Congress Cataloging-in-Publication Data

Names: Moskowitz, Gordon B., author.
Title: Introduction to social cognition : the essential questions and ideas
   / Gordon B. Moskowitz.
Description: New York : The Guilford Press, [2024] | Includes
   bibliographical references and index. |
Identifiers: LCCN 2024002702 | ISBN 9781462554546 (paperback ; alk. paper)
   | ISBN 9781462554553 (cloth ; alk. paper)
Subjects: LCSH: Social perception. | BISAC: PSYCHOLOGY / Personality |
   PSYCHOLOGY / Social Psychology
Classification: LCC BF323.S63 M668 2024 | DDC 302/.12—dc23/eng/20240217
LC record available at *https://lccn.loc.gov/2024002702*

To my family—my wife, Cindy Gooch, and my sons, Ben and Isaac

Thank you to the mentors who supported me
through the various stages of my life in psychology—
Shelly Chaiken, John Bargh, Tory Higgins, Peter Gollwitzer, and John Darley

Thank you to my friends and collaborators
who made my research career so much fun—
Mike Naccarato, Peter Deschamps, Jeff Stone, Bob Roman,
Irmak Olcaysoy Okten, Joe Vitriol, Kai Sassenberg, Peizhong Li, Ruud Custers,
Erica Schneid, Heidi Grant, Ute Bayer, Adam Galinsky, Carlos Rivero,
Naomi Rothman, Melissa Ferguson, Emily Balcetis, Jim Uleman, Eun Rhee,
Roger Giner-Sorolla, Len Newman, Ian Skurnik, Dominic Packer, Penny Visser,
Felicia Pratto, and my social cognition/PMIG family of Jackie Chen,
Kerri Johnson, Ap Dijksterhuis, Neil Macrae, Henk Aarts, Don Carlston,
Eliot Smith, Rachael Smallman, Pam Smith, Keith Maddox, Cami Johnson,
John Jost, Elizabeth Haines, Dave Hamilton, Steve Stroessner, and Jeff Sherman

And thank you to my "brothers"
—Paul Rizzo, Brett Moskowitz, Neil Hertzman, and Stephen Bilkis

About the Author

Gordon B. Moskowitz, PhD, is Professor in the Department of Psychology at Lehigh University. He has served as Director of Lehigh's Cognitive Science Program and Chair of the Department of Psychology. He served two terms on the executive committee of the Society of Experimental Social Psychology, has hosted the Society's conference twice, and annually co-organizes the preeminent social cognition conference, the Person Memory Interest Group. He has held editorial positions for *Social and Personality Psychology Compass*, as well as for the *Journal of Experimental Social Psychology*, and sits on the editorial board for *Motivation Science* and the *Journal of Personality and Social Psychology*. Dr. Moskowitz conducts research at the intersection of motivation, implicit bias, and social cognition. His work spans the topics of proactive control, impression formation, stereotyping, minority influence, bias reduction interventions, perspective taking, egalitarianism, self-regulation, impression updating, ambivalence, and backlash. His research program more recently has examined bias in the practice of medicine and the reduction of disparities in health and health care.

Preface

This book provides an introduction to, and broad overview of, the field of social cognition. It is intended for newcomers to this discipline and for use as a text in undergraduate courses on social cognition. Other books on this topic have placed an emphasis on speaking to people who are already somewhat advanced in their study of psychology—such as professors in adjacent domains of social psychology or graduate students in social cognition. These approaches assume a level of prior knowledge that is not expected here. The approach here is to introduce a relative novice to the discipline to the (1) major questions of the discipline, (2) methods used to explore the questions, and (3) theories that detail *how* knowledge is produced.

Given this approach, the book is organized around chapters that identify broad research questions that have defined the field. For example, research on attribution theories reviewed in Chapter 7 addresses the question of how we make meaning and assign cause/blame. Research on implicit bias reviewed in Chapter 11 addresses the question of why we stereotype so easily, even if we have no overt dislike for a group. Research on the updating of first impressions reviewed in Chapter 13 explores the question of when we change our first impressions, and Chapters 5 and 6 explore the question of why first impressions have such an oversized influence on how we think and act. The remaining chapters address questions such as "Can bias be produced simply as a result of the cognitive processes we use, without one trying to distort the information?" "Is prejudice controllable, and if so, how?" "How do our goals and motives shape the way we reason about the world?" "What are the structures that serve as the lens through which we see the world, and why do they operate without our ability to see their influence?" "How can we be both rational and deep thinkers while at the same time be thinkers who rely on their 'gut' and produce judgments spontaneously and with seemingly little thought?" "When are we resistant to information that challenges our beliefs and when do we dismiss that which is inconsistent with what we already know, and when do we instead embrace that which disconfirms our beliefs?" "Are there two systems for thinking—a fast one and a slow one—and why does this matter?"

This organizational scheme differs from other books on social cognition that approach the topic with either chapters focused on individual responses (such as attitudes, judgment, decision making, etc.) or chapters on specific cognitive processes (such as perception, attention, memory, and causal reasoning). By appealing to understanding broad questions at the heart of human behavior, this book hopes to center the reader on how scientific experiments can inform us about everyday matters. And, as mentioned above, it shifts the focus from the advanced reader that other books have targeted to those newer to psychology.

Why this approach at this point in time? Social cognition has finally bubbled up to everyday discourse. Questions surrounding implicit bias have been front and center during Presidential debates in the last decade and in Supreme Court justice confirmation hearings. Ideological polarization and the spread of misinformation have become essential topics of the modern era. Popular press books such as *Blink: The Power of Thinking Without Thinking* by Malcolm Gladwell, *Mindset: The New Psychology of Success* by Carol S. Dweck, *Thinking, Fast and Slow* by Daniel Kahneman, *Biased: Uncovering the Hidden Prejudice That Shapes What We See, Think, and Do* by Jennifer L. Eberhardt, *Clearer, Closer, Better: How Successful People See the World* by Emily Balcetis, *Predictably Irrational: The Hidden Forces that Shape Our Decisions* by Dan Ariely, and *Think Again: The Power of Knowing What you Don't Know* by Adam Grant (to name just a few) have shown a public interest in many specific subfields of social cognition. And college curricula are seeing an increase in courses dedicated to social cognition. The time seems right for a book aimed at broadly addressing the central questions of this hub science that can speak to a wide range of people, from family members to policymakers, and everyone in between. In the undergraduate classroom, the book can be used for a large lecture course where multiple-choice tests are used or in a seminar course focused on discussion. For the latter type of class, each chapter of the book can be paired with a journal article reviewed in that chapter so the class can dive deeply into the methods and analysis. A set of thought questions can be provided to help students organize the chapter and to provide their instructors with weekly essays to grade. To help students in any type of class, each chapter identifies specific key terms. When a term is first discussed at length it is bolded and its definition is pulled out in a box. When these central terms later appear in other chapters, they are italicized. Example terms include "prejudice," "motivated reasoning," "attitude," "fundamental attribution error," "mindset," "propositional reasoning," "automaticity," "availability heuristic," "process dissociation," "naïve realism," "schema," "implementation intentions," "priming," "minimal group," and "implicit stereotyping."

THE DECISION TO WRITE THIS TEXTBOOK

Why me? This is a question I have asked myself all too often. My passion for this discipline has been fueled by the age in which I live. I was born in the 1960s just after the baby boom. As an early member of Generation X, I was raised in a culture of civil rights laws being passed, the women's movement taking shape, and the ideological entrenchment that has deepened in the United States in the post-Watergate years. Overt bias has waxed and waned, implicit bias grown, and motivated reasoning has allowed the economic gap to widen. It has been hard not to think about how and why the social forces that shape our society impact the individuals and the structures within it. Before I knew the term existed, I was always a student of social cognition. But as I entered college, my life would change. As an undergraduate I was exposed to one of the great teachers of social psychology: Don Taylor of McGill University. An unusual number of people working in the discipline today were introduced to the field in his course, one that, as far back as the late 1970s, emphasized a social-cognitive approach to social psychology. I was drawn in as a 17-year-old during his very first lecture in my first semester at college. I was fortunate to stumble into the circle of such an amazing teacher. Next, at age 21, I again found myself fortunate: I had joined a graduate training program at New York University, which over my time there had become the global center for social cognition. A unique collection of young scientists, all working on this somewhat new discipline, were gathered in an amazing location that drew scholars from around the world to visit and contribute to the milieu. All of our faculty (Bargh, Chaiken, Higgins, Ruble, Trope, Uleman) have won recognition by various organizations for career contributions to the field. After graduate school I again was fortunate to find myself working as a postdoctoral scholar with the world's leading researcher blending the study of motivation with social cognition: Peter Gollwitzer. This academic journey took me from Montreal to Manhattan to Munich, having uniquely positioned me to be at the cutting edge of the field's development, paired with its most impressive scholars. This allowed a final stroke of fortune, being hired at Princeton University. When I eventually was transitioning from being an assistant professor at Princeton to an associate professor at Lehigh, I found myself without a lab, without a graduate student, and facing a period of 2–3 years to establish those things at Lehigh. I took that time to reflect (as we often do during times of transition) on where the field had gone from the early 1970s to the turn of the century. I chose to use that time to (aside from start a family) write a book on social cognition, one meant for graduate students and other experts, as a way to provide a sort of closure, for me, on an era.

I did not anticipate writing another book. However, during the COVID-19 pandemic my lab was shut down and I again found myself in a period of transition. While not imminent, retirement was now closer than my "rookie season," and younger faculty in our department would need the limited resources to do research more than I would over the next few years. During the pandemic I was invited to write several sprawling reviews on vastly different topics. One was a history of social cognition. One was a review of attribution models. One was a review of how and when first impressions are updated. One was a review of procedures to control and mitigate stereotypes and prejudice. I agreed to write all four to keep busy during the pandemic. Along with having just written these enormous overviews that seemed to span the entire discipline, I had also been asked to coedit a book on impression formation and co-organize an annual social cognition conference. In these tasks I found myself surrounded by an exciting group of young scholars, which motivated me to again share the field's innovations. This transition period seemed like another good moment to take stock, especially since my own activities had broadened to be more field spanning. Writing a new book seemed like a good way to redirect my energy, particularly given the recent interest in the popular press in our discipline and a lack of textbooks aimed at nonexperts.

Despite knowing the enormous time costs of writing an overview of a discipline alone, I wanted to get it done quickly. I decided to embark on the adventure without a coauthor, despite having a collaborator with whom I wanted to work. But distance, the pandemic, and my desire to work quickly led me to pursue it alone, hopeful that Irmak Olcaysoy Okten will work with me on future (if there be any) iterations of this book. I wrote an initial 1,000-page draft in a fevered 4 months in the fall of 2021, and in the 18 months from January 2022 to June 2023 I went through three revisions of that draft. In under 2 years, with little sleep, I produced this book and managed to not totally alienate my wife and children, whose support enabled me to take this on.

Note to Students

Many years ago I was on a job interview in a distant town. If I got the job it would mean moving, and if not, I would likely never be in this place again. I was being interviewed to become part of a two-person unit and the other person, who held the power to determine if I got the job, took me to lunch as part of the interview process. My host ordered a dish that I despise. Over the course of our lunch he kept talking about how great his meal was, until finally he looked at me square in the face and said, "This is so good, you really need to try this."

Did this stranger really want me to try his food during my job interview? He knew I'd never be in this town again, so his meaning couldn't have been "You need to try this the next time you are here." Or perhaps he knew I was getting the job, and would indeed be in this town again, and what he really meant was "After you move here, you should return and try this dish." Should I have been brazen enough to assume I had the job and that he meant to order it the next time? Perhaps this was a power play and he was telling me what to do. Should I have been subservient enough to just do what he asked of me, given that he was being so persistent about it? Maybe he didn't mean it at all and it was just a turn of phrase. I had two choices—eat the food or decline the invitation. But my choice would depend on the result of my thinking about what he meant and my understanding of what his goals were.

In the one second I had to make my choice there seemed to be two reasons I should choose to eat the food I despised. First, his persistence could have been interpreted as a demand, and I would then need to appease his demand in order to foster his having a positive opinion of me. If I wanted the job, I needed to do what he said. Second, his persistence could have meant he was overly enthusiastic about his food, and that he was sending a clear and unambiguous signal that he wanted to share the experience. If true, then to not eat the food off his plate would have been rude. In that same one second there also seemed to be two reasons to choose *not to* eat the food. First, continuing on the last theme, his over-enthusiasm about the food might not have been an invitation to take his request literally, but rather to see it as a figure of speech that indicated he was enjoying it so much. In which case it would have been rude of me to actually eat food off his plate and to take away the very thing he was enjoying. Finally, I could have inferred that he was making a demand of me, but I could have chosen to use that demand from him as an opportunity to assert my independence and difference of opinion on the matter despite his effusiveness. I could have been clear that I did not care about impressing a potential employer, and that I found his eggplant dish disgusting. When someone says, "This is so good, you really need to try this," how do we make meaning and decide what to do?

I reached over, took a taste of his eggplant, and lied: "This is delicious." Years later, I learned that he told people, "This rude guy actually took food off my plate during a job interview." I had "read" him incorrectly! And he had "read" me wrong by labeling me rude.

We face moments like this hundreds of times every day, where we must understand the situation around us and prepare to act appropriately. We need to understand what type of behavior the person has enacted or what meaning they are communicating through the things they are saying. Next, we must infer (based on our understanding) what they are saying about themselves and what they are asking of us. We need to make inferences about what others' goals are in our current situation along with inferences about what type of person they are. Once armed with an understanding of what they did and why they did it, we next need to decide how to act and what the appropriate range of responses are. We need to run counterfactual simulations that determine the consequences of doing action "A" versus action "B." Finally, we need to anticipate how the person, with whatever characteristics and goals we impute to them, will react to us based on the action we select. And we do all this within a second. This is the cognitive challenge that meets us all day long, with every social exchange. It is a foundational aspect of the human experience. We must make sense of the world around us and decide how to respond, and we do this constantly.

In my story, the inferences made and actions chosen were consequential since a job was in the balance. However, all interactions, all day long, every day, have this same flavor of needing to create meaning from the words and actions we perceive, consequential or not. We cannot see into the hearts and minds of others to know what their intent is and what they truly mean, so we must "read their minds" as best we can. We do so by picking out elements to attend to from the actions and words we observe. We categorize what we observe and make inferences about what it means. From that meaning comes an understanding of why others say and do what we have observed. We plan how to act in response. We reason about the consequences of how we act for how others will impute meaning to us. This is the essence of being human.

Thus, understanding other people—from detecting their presence, to focusing attention on them, to labeling them, to making inferences about what they are like and likely to do, to remembering them—is one of the most frequent and important activities in which humans engage. In the brief 150-year history of psychological science, this all-consuming cognitive activity has gone by several names. The beginnings of this field of study in psychology are typically traced to Fritz Heider, who in the title of his seminal book, *The Psychology of Interpersonal Relations*, described this domain of inquiry with the term "interpersonal relations," explaining that it

> denotes relations between a few, usually between two, people. How one person thinks and feels about another person, how he perceives him and what he does to him, what he expects him to do or think, how he reacts to the actions of the other. (Heider, 1958, p. 1)

An older term, "epistemology," is the study of the origin and nature of knowledge, and one concern of this book is with the origin and nature of a specific type of knowledge—that formed about people. *Person perception* is now the more common term used to refer to this examination of the processes concerned with how we come to "know" and understand what other people are like (e.g., Schneider, Hastorf, & Ellsworth, 1979). Each new interaction with a person brings new stimuli we need to examine, comprehend, and understand through processes of attribution. An *attribution* is the end result of a process of classifying and explaining behavior in order to arrive at a decision regarding its reason or cause. Today, all of these concerns are the domain of the broader field of inquiry, in that its concern moves beyond how we understand people to also include our understanding of social situations and social influence, known as *social cognition*.

SOCIAL COGNITION AS A HUB DISCIPLINE

Undoubtedly, the author of any book you read, or the professor of any course you take, is passionate about their topic and feel it is crucial. The physicist, chemist, or mathematician surely feel that laws of nature are on the line, and our ability not only to exist in the natural order, but to manipulate it and thus innovate, is tantamount. As social animals, humans can only survive and thrive by knowing others. As such, psychologists see their concern of inquiry as tantamount. In academic circles it is often common to hear psychology described as a "hub science." As I wrote for the psychology department web page at Lehigh University:

> Psychology is often described as a "hub" discipline because it stands at a crossroads of many disciplines and facilitates traffic between the natural sciences, the social sciences, the humanities, education, and policy. . . It provides links to *Health, Medicine, Biology, Political Science, Global Studies, Computational Modeling, Cognitive Science, Gender and Sexuality Studies, Africana Studies, Marketing, Management, Anthropology, Philosophy, Behavioral Neuroscience, Law, Education, Journalism, Communications, Sociology, and Economics.*

And social cognition scholars see their discipline as at the heart of psychology, the hub of the hub so to speak. It sits at a level of explanation above the micro-level understanding of the biology of the brain and below the macro-level descriptions of group behavior, providing theories of the processes through which an individual's thought and behavior is produced. Only through knowing how people come to see the world can psychology help to explain the ability to empathize with others, our susceptibility to misinformation, our tendency to stereotype, our ability to update attitudes, our capacity to make decisions quickly and with limited information, our ability to reason about the causes for events, our feeling patronized (rather than supported) when others attempt to help us cope with stress in a time of need, how we set and best achieve goals, when we conform versus dissent, and the endless list of activities that define being human.

REALITY AND BIAS

Social cognition is a tricky topic to ask others to learn about because we all have access to our own cognition and believe that we know fully well what shapes how and what we think. We believe that our thinking is rational and deliberate, that it is aimed at producing the *best possible* judgments and decisions. We do not experience others as hard to read, but that we form impressions of them easily, and we feel that these impressions must be accurate. We often feel confident that we see things perfectly. The challenge of social cognition as a field of study is that it needs to overcome this sense that people hold regarding their mental makeup. The truth is that we are not always rational or interested in the best decisions possible. Thinking is also motivated; it is aimed at producing the conclusions we *desire*. It can be biased, often without us realizing. It can rely on shortcuts that do not adhere to the rational model described above. It happens without our conscious monitoring. It may involve, as in the story above, selecting from many possible meanings and deciding on one from among them in a manner that suits our needs, which may not align with what is most accurate. It may involve distorting what we attend to and what we believe we see/hear, as when we identify with a political affiliation and are asked to evaluate if a politician in whom we have invested energy and trust is worthy of that investment. It may involve ignoring evidence altogether, such as that which suggests a mentor has engaged in research fraud or data manipulation to create a newsworthy scientific finding. Of course, the conclusions we desire in the moment, such as seeing a mentor as trustworthy, may cause one irreparable harm in the long term, if biased. For example, if seeing the mentor as trustworthy leads to fame in the coming months, it can then later lead to the destruction of one's reputation if one had been motivated to miss the red flags of fraud that then cause the mentor's fall from grace.

Do we see what is there, or do we see what we want to be there? I can recall being in graduate school when George H. W. Bush, the 41st President of the United States (and father of the 43rd President, George W. Bush) was running for President against Bill Clinton and conveyed the following message that supposedly distinguished him from his opponent: "I never attended Oxford University" (his reference was to the fact that Clinton, as a student, had attended Oxford as a Rhodes Scholar, and later Yale Law School). Bush's motivation for this statement seemed to be to capitalize on an anti-intellectualism/elitism he assumed was dominant in the electorate. Bush realized that perception was what mattered most, and he wanted to create the perception of himself (in others) as a man of the people. Clinton was to be labeled, in this war of person perception, as the Ivy League, ivory tower, leftist intellectual who could not relate to the people. Never mind that Bush himself (and his son George W., another so-called "man of the people") graduated from Yale University, one of the most elite academic institutions in the world, or that the Bush family comes from extreme wealth (while Clinton was a child of a broken home and depressed financial means, who made it to the elite institutions based on sheer academic achievement). The handlers for the 41st president knew what social cognition research shows us all too clearly—the way in which we interpret other people is often irrelevant to the facts about those people and more directly related to *what we are prepared to see in them and desire to see in them*. By playing to our motives, our beliefs and attitudes can be swayed.

This is not to say that reality does not matter. But as we shall discuss throughout this book, meaning is made not solely by objective facts, but by the goals, attitudes, expectations, values, and norms held by the perceiver. In this book we examine precisely how these various social forces shape our implicit and explicit cognition, often in ways we cannot detect. The central questions of social cognition focus on how the structures and processes of our mind are used in producing our understanding of the social stimuli that bombard our senses. How are cognitive processes such as perception, attention, categorization, memory, inference, and judgment guided by social forces? And how is our understanding of social objects produced by these same cognitive processes, mostly operating outside of our awareness and without our conscious intent? Why does bias seem to arise so naturally from such processing, and seem so difficult to change?

Acknowledgments

I was lucky to find the discipline of social cognition that matched the interests that had followed me throughout my life. I was even luckier to be mentored by the many students and teachers who share my passion for it. But I am especially grateful to my peers, the generation of people with whom I have moved through the field. At the risk of forgetting someone, I want to recognize "my generation"—the people who received their PhD's within 4 years of me and whose work continues to inspire me some 30 years on: Jeff Stone, Jeff Sherman, Steve Stroessner, Felicia Pratto, Len Newman, Roger Giner-Sorolla, Eva Pomerantz, Eun Rhee, Serena Chen, Orit Tykocinski, Gerd Bohner, Veronika Brandstaetter, Steve Neuberg, Jacquie Vorauer, Miguel Brendl, Markus Brauer, Henk Aarts, Ap Dijksterhuis, Neil Macrae, Sabine Otten, Irene Blair, Duane Wegener, John Jost, Neal Roese, Margo Monteith, Michael Morris, Rick Robbins, Dacher Keltner, Oliver John, Alex Todorov, Lorella Lepore, Monica Biernat, Steve Spencer, Kerry Kawakami, Alan Lambert, Bill von Hippel, Buju Dasgupta, Allen McConnell, Terri Vescio, Andrew Elliot, Todd Nelson, Steve Fein, Linda Skitka, Laurie Rudman, Bernd Wittenbrink, Nick Haslam, Kees van den Bos, Keith Markman, Bertram Malle, Sonja Lyubomirsky, Verónica Benet-Martínez, Naomi Ellemers, Daniel Wigboldus, Janet Ruscher, Sandra Murray, Stephen Wright, Curtis Hardin, Brett Pelham, Megan Thompson, Denise Sekaquaptewa, Michele Gelfand, and Michael Zárate. While there is an embarrassing lack of racial and ethnic diversity in this cohort, an examination of the decade of scholars who followed us (our first students) does reveal a tremendous change in the discipline along that dimension. Hopefully this book will inspire more people to join the exploration of social cognition.

Contents

CHAPTER 1

Thinking Is for Action (Purposeful), So We Make Meaning from Chaos

Social cognition is a domain of inquiry within the scientific discipline social psychology. The focus of each is on the fact that social forces guide human thinking, emotion, and action. People are not driven solely as a function of internal forces, such as their personality or needs. There are myriad ways, both obvious and subtle, that one's psychological state is additionally shaped by external forces—pressures out in the social world. Most notably by other people. By describing humans as "social animals" possessing a "social psychology" and living in "social networks," social scientists are acknowledging that environments (and the people in them) play an important role in what we think, feel, and do. **Social psychology** represents the study of how individual persons (with their somewhat static personalities and needs) meet and interact with the social world (and its ever-shifting pressures). Social psychology is concerned with examining the power of the social situation to impel even vastly different individuals to respond in similar ways. The social and environmental forces that impact people include:

> **Social psychology:** The study of how social situations impel even vastly different individuals to respond similarly. People are not driven solely by internal forces, such as personality and needs. External forces in the environment (most notably pressures exerted by other people) play an important role in what we think, feel, and do.

1. The identity groups we join that shape our sense of who we are, with whom we belong (political affiliations, sports teams, summer camps, school memberships, occupations, art/music affiliations, military units, etc.).
2. The culture in which we live both globally (as humans) and more locally (as nations, regions, cities, villages, schools, and workplaces) that dictate the rules to which we all adhere for living in a shared society. These rules are dictated through norms (our perceptions of what our local culture both prescribes as acceptable to do, and describes as what other people typically do).
3. The laws and mores of our nations and religious groups that provide ideology and morality as guides for how to live.
4. The families we inherit and the friendships we cultivate.

5. The media we consume that disseminates not just "facts" but shares what others accept as true and good, or false and bad (attitudinal influence).

6. The institutional structures (e.g., health care systems, police, courts, financial institutions, education systems) through which order is enforced, and a shared system of justice is communicated.

Interaction of the person and the situation: Each individual is not passive in response to the situations that can shape how they act and think. Rather they meet that situation with a mental apparatus that makes meaning from what is transpiring, and use existing knowledge, attitudes, and goals to construct a construal of events and appropriate responses.

Social pressure from all of these sources is ubiquitous and powerfully felt. It permeates all we think, feel, and do. Even when we do not see it or take the time to note it consciously. In this way, social psychology describes an **interaction of the person and the situation**—each individual has their own unique mental makeup that allows them to respond distinctively, yet that person's individuality is met by strong situational forces that may overpower that distinctiveness. While people can use their existing knowledge, attitudes, and goals to construct how they construe the people and events they observe, and develop appropriate responses as a result, at times that construal is shaped by the norms, stereotypes, and rules that meet people from out in the social world.

In its concern with how social forces impact us, social psychology saw a tremendous period of growth during and after the second world war. Scholars who escaped the Nazi genocide turned their scientific eyes toward studying how people (in that case, Germans) could be pressured by social forces to either commit acts of atrocity, or to support such acts, or to stand by silently without objection. Why do we conform, even to what seems like a malevolent authoritarian regime? What is the nature of prejudice and what function do stereotypes serve? The field expanded to ask other questions such as:

How do we rationalize bad behavior and distort the way we see the world to maintain a sense of ourselves as good and positive?

What is the nature of the power wielded over us by identity and norms?

Why do we feel pressure, anxiety, and stress when experiencing the gaze of others?

When do attitudes and beliefs change to leave us succumbing to the persuasive power of rhetoric?

What type of persuasive messages are most influential?

How is our behavior shaped by our attitudes (and what is an attitude, and how does it differ from a goal, a norm, or a value)?

Why is inconsistency in our own beliefs/behavior, or even in the actions of others, so unpalatable?

How do we create a coherent sense of knowing and a sense of "feeling in control" from the seeming chaos of living among a sea of other people whose intentions and dispositions we cannot see directly?

How do we "know" what others are like when we cannot read their minds?

Why are we ready to blame, and what function is served by pointing fingers?

Why do we fail to reach our goals, and how does commitment, grit, efficacy, and planning contribute to achieving goals?

How do we change habits and control unwanted thoughts?

In its answers to these questions, social psychology places human cognition in a central role. When a person interacts with their social world, that person must first understand the nature of what they are encountering. The world outside our own mind is an unknown, and it comes at us fast in every waking second. To live in a social world is a constant barrage of needing to categorize who and what we see. From those categorizations we need to form inferences about what other people want (why they act as they do) or what is expected in the situation we have entered. With those inferences we must anticipate what people will likely do next, or what will transpire in our current situation. From those inferences and expectations we must create plans to act accordingly. All the while we must juggle those concerns with our understanding of our own beliefs, attitudes, and goals. Without such cognition, we would experience chaos and confusion from the bombardment of stimulation that meets our senses. Social psychology has always been concerned with cognition. How we construe the social world, make plans based on our interpretation of others' intent and goals for interaction, and make decisions by filling in gaps caused by having limited information and being in ambiguous situations, has always been at the heart of social psychology. However, the term *social cognition* refers to more than the fact that humans rely on cognition to navigate through the world. It is not simply that we need to categorize, infer, and predict in order to survive in a complex world. What is social cognition?

SOCIAL COGNITION DEFINED

In 1984 a three-book volume provided a first overview of social cognition research, at that point a decade old. In the first chapter of this *Handbook of Social Cognition*, a definition of the field was provided by Tom Ostrom. He described it as the study of "how people perceive and judge other people and the question of how social factors affect perception, memory, and thinking. That is, social cognition is involved when either the dependent variables or the independent variables in cognitive research pertain to persons" (p. 5). He further described *social cognition* as a "struggle to understand the interdependence between cognition and social behavior" (p. 2). Aligning with Ostrom, our definition allows social cognition to encompass both how cognitive processes and structures determine the manner in which we "know" the social world (the social force is the dependent variable), as well as how our social nature shapes our (low-level) cognitive processes and structures (the social force is the independent variable).

We define **social cognition** as concerned with investigating the cognitive *processes*, and the *structures* that support these processes, that give rise to how humans create understanding and meaning from the social stimuli they encounter. It encompasses how we perceive, attend to, categorize, form inferences about, reason about, react affectively to, and make judgments about stimuli. Such low-level cognition is both shaped by social forces, while at the same time is used to form knowledge about those social forces. It is concerned simultaneously with *how* cognition allows for social objects to be "known" (even if such cognitive processes are invisible to the perceiver employing them) and *how* such cognition itself is guided by social forces (culture, motivation, values, shared beliefs, norms), even if those social forces are not physically present or not easily seen. Social cognition is focused on *how* we come to have attitudes, beliefs, goals, emotions, and judgments that serve as the foundation for the sense we make of our world. While certainly concerned with the fact that we "make meaning" in a way that is biased by social pressures, it is additionally concerned with more than illustrating the bias but understanding the mechanisms of the mind through which meaning is produced. However, this definition begs for

> **Social cognition:** The study of the cognitive structures and processes used to create meaning. It is simultaneously concerned with *how* cognition allows social objects to be "known" (even if that cognition occurs unconsciously) and *how* cognition is guided by social forces (even if those social forces are not physically present or seen).

three further definitions. What are cognitive processes? What are cognitive structures? What is meant when we use terms such as "low-level cognition" and invisible processes?

Cognitive processes: Sets of cognitive operations that manipulate and transform stimulation into meaning. They include processes at both the low level (perception, attention, learning, categorization, inference, memory encoding, memory retrieval, and language) and high level (judgments, reasoning, decision making, attributions, deliberating, intentions, attitudes, action plans, and emotions).

Cognitive processes are the mechanisms used by the mind to transform stimulation into meaning, and they include cognition that occurs at both the low level (perception, attention, learning, categorization, inference, memory encoding, memory retrieval, and language) and high level (judgments, reasoning, decision making, attributions, deliberating, intentions, attitudes, action plans, and emotions). These cognitive processes are themselves actually systems or sets of cognitive operations that manipulate information in the service of the process. Let us briefly consider four examples:

1. Memory encoding involves, among other operations, the creation of associations that attach new learning to existing knowledge.
2. Memory retrieval, among other operations, involves the spreading of activation and inhibition among these associations.
3. Attitudes involve, among other operations, the automatic experience of positive or negative affect when encountering a person or thing.
4. Judgment, among other operations, engages comparisons among stimuli to assess their relative standing (and the type of judgment made changes as the type of comparison being used changes).

Cognitive structures: The systems by which the mind constrains and shapes the making of meaning. This can refer to specific structures in the brain or to abstract representations stored in memory such as schemas and theories.

The **cognitive structures** that support cognitive processing can be thought of at the neuroscientific level (such as the brain regions and chemical and biological factors that constrain processing). The structures can also be thought of at the representational level, where the structures are described as nodes in memory where social forces such as morals, ideology, shared beliefs, schemas, scripts, traits, stereotypes, exemplars, values, mindsets, orientations, culture, and so on are internalized and constrain how processing is carried out.

Everything we know is represented in the mind, and how we conceive of the structure of that representation determines how we think about any given piece of knowledge. For example, consider knowledge I have of two of my oldest friends (from summer camp)—Stephen Bilkis and Paul Rizzo. Paul now owns one of the most famous bars and music clubs in New York City (The Bitter End) and is a champion for up-and-coming artists. Stephen is a well-known lawyer in New York whose focus on criminal defense and on personal injury has made him a champion of the less fortunate. These descriptions bring in a vast amount of knowledge—summer camp, bar, music, injustice, alcohol, injury, "champion," New York, hardworking, loyal, smart, funny—some of which is inherently associated (bar–alcohol), others connected only because Paul and Stephen are associated with each other (summer camp–loyal). How is all of this knowledge represented and structured in my mind? How does the way it is structured affect the way I think about these friends? How do I know that when Stephen and bar are referenced, that the bar in question is the New York State legal licensing board? Yet when Paul is mentioned, the meaning of bar shifts to something different? Do I have a "node" in memory for Stephen that is associated with abstract qualities (as in Figure 1.1A), or do I associate Stephen with specific behaviors and then need to construct

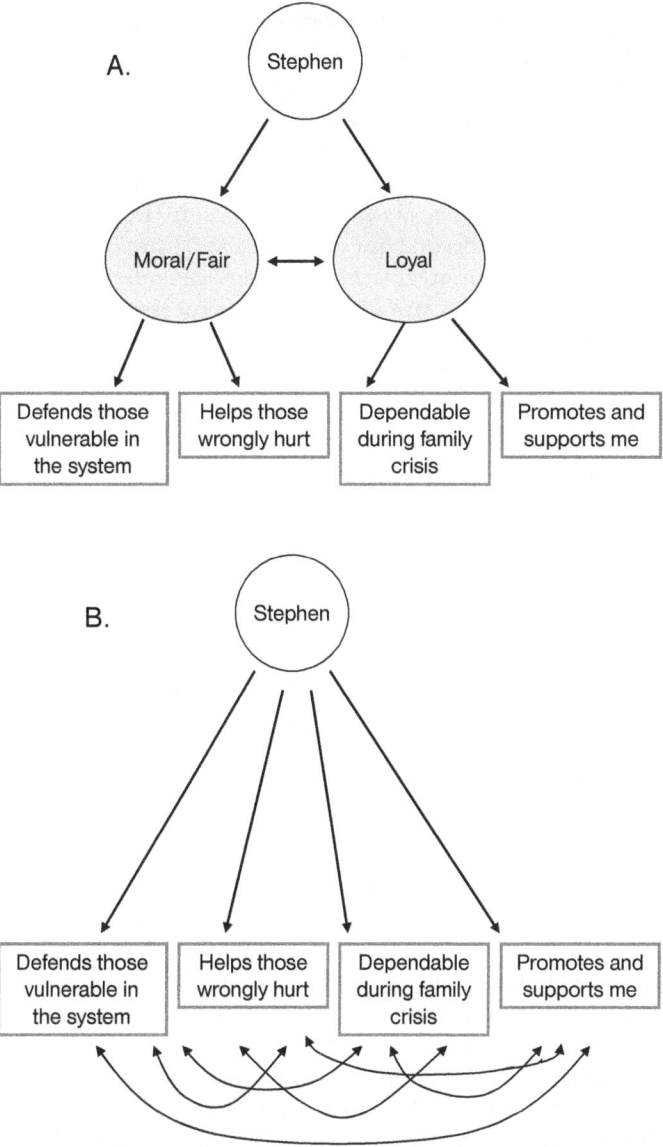

FIGURE 1.1. Two possible cognitive structures.

a judgment of his more abstract "qualities" from those specific behaviors whenever a judg-ment is needed (as in Figure 1.1B). As we see later in the book, many organizations of such a structure, aside from these two, can be imagined.

Finally, what is meant when we use terms such as *low levels of cognition* and *invisible pro-cesses*? Conscious thought emerges only after perception brings stimuli to our senses, atten-tion filters out that stimulation for further processing, categorization applies structure to the stimulation by placing it within a grouping of related constructs, and inferences about what it means to belong to the category add meaning. These, and other acts of thinking, proceed outside of conscious awareness (are invisible), and deliver conscious experience to us in a way that merely feels immediate. Phenomenally, we often just experience the "know-ing" without seeing the incredible amount of mental work that has gone on behind the scenes. Thoughts pop into consciousness as if they are absolute truths, and not the product of the mind's many processing stages. If we were to try to introspect and describe how we "know," we would get it wrong since many of the processes are at too low a level to be seen. Perception, categorization, attention, and many types of inference are "invisible" processes. They (1) happen extremely fast (they are *efficient*), (2) are difficult to see (we *lack awareness* they are even happening), (3) are beyond our *conscious control* (they continue even if we wanted to stop them), and (4) and are initiated without our *conscious intent* (they happen without us willing them, triggered simply by a stimulus). When a process has these four features it is called an **automatic process**.

Automatic process: Cognitive processing is not as conscious and controllable as we surmise. Complicated processing happens without our awareness or consciously willing it, at incredibly fast speeds, and is unable to be stopped even if we tried. Automatic processes have all these features; they are efficient, uncontrollable, outside awareness, not consciously initiated.

Much of social cognition has its concern with understanding these, often impossible to see with the naked eye, processes and structures. Unlike other fields of study that attempt to unlock the secrets of a once-hidden concept (gravity, DNA, electrical currents, elements, etc.), social cognition, when it began, (1) lacked the tools needed to study it (at least physicists had math) and (2) faced the obstacle presented by people's own intuitions about their cognition. Researchers initially had to ask people to reflect on their own thought processes and report back what they could detect. Asking people how they "know what they know" reveals people to be reliant upon false and inaccurate understanding of where their own knowledge comes from (Nisbett & Wilson, 1977). Tools needed to be developed to study how people think that moved beyond self-report. Additionally, unlike other fields of study that attempt to unlock the secrets of a once-hidden concept, the study of thinking is trivialized by people who themselves can (without the help of scientists) think. Personal experience with thinking renders us purported experts in a way that experience with gravity or photosynthesis does not make us feel expert in physics, calculus, chemistry, or biology. While the concept of gravity offered by physicists asks us to trust an explanation that invokes things we cannot see, it does not ask us to challenge our own naïve explanations in a way that social cognition does when explaining our own thought processes. These are challenges that the discipline of social cognition continues to grapple with.

Finally, in defining social cognition it becomes necessary to be precise about how our cognition is in fact social. There are three distinct ways that cognition is social. The first is that the object being studied is social in nature. One early definition of social cognition focused on the simple notion that it examines the cognition we have about social beings. As opposed to objects and places, it concerns how we think about people (individuals and groups). I would modify this statement. Cognition is indeed social because the thing being studied is social in nature. But I would argue that all things we can study are in fact social

Shared reality: People and things only have meaning in the context of what our culture tells us. Groups, from dyads to entire cultures, provide people with meaning by specifying mutually agreed-upon understanding of people and things in the world. We live in social networks that define everything we see.

in nature. It is not just people as targets of our cognition that are social but all objects, animals, and places are inherently social. They are inherently social because they only have meaning through a **shared reality**, a mutually agreed-upon understanding with other people. All that we know is defined within a network of shared meaning. At the most abstract level, all we know about any object is socially defined, only having meaning within one's culture, and within the system of meanings society imposes on it (e.g., Hardin & Conley,

2001). Thus, one aspect of cognition as being "social" relates to this fact: Any and all meaning is derived from our connection with other people. An object, such as a right angle, only has meaning and its properties understood because of the system of meaning the prevailing society or culture imposes upon it. Our culture has taught us to use and to see value in right angles. Other shapes or objects might be oblivious to us. What is an ashtray in a culture where smoking does not exist? A bagel is only a bagel because of shared knowledge (as I learned the hard way when living in southern Germany in the 1990s, where bagels did not exist). Later in this chapter we review research showing that optical illusions common in one culture are not experienced by people raised in a separate culture. Distortions in perception are caused by socially defined ways of seeing objects. Humans exist in social groups that specify how to make meaning from the stimuli our cognitive system processes. More than examining the cognition we have concerning social beings, it examines the social determinants of cognition.

A second reason that cognition is social is that humans have needs beyond the physical and biological needs that drive us to eat, drink, and reproduce. We have social needs to join groups. From social needs arise motives and goals that are capable of influencing our cognitive processes—that is, social groups specify morals, values, beliefs, attitudes, goals, and norms that subtly shape how we think, and what we think about (what we choose to allow to enter through our attentional filters). For example, I was struck in 1994 when living in Europe that many people saw a song written and performed to address famine relief as a clear signal of American arrogance, whereas Americans saw it solely as an effort to express a shared humanity. The song was "We Are the World." In one culture this clearly meant that Americans saw themselves as the world, with all others "insignificant pawns." In another culture, this meant that all people are the same, wherever you are from, and that we need to treat one another with equal kindness and generosity. The shared beliefs and assumptions within a culture and the motives instilled in individuals through their social identities determine what meaning is made. Later in this chapter we spend an entire section reviewing the idea that social forces—our values, beliefs, attitudes, emotions, norms, motives, goals, and identity—and culturally bound morals—have consequences (a top-down influence) on our thinking. Cognition is social because we interpret all that we see through a social lens, even at the lowest levels of cognition.

A third reason that cognition is social is that it prepares us for interacting with the social world. Our cognition tells us what to expect from people, places, and things, and additionally tells us what is appropriate to do in response to those expectations. It arms us with a set of assumptions and plans that allow us to navigate each novel encounter, allowing us to draw on similar experiences so we do not feel continually in the dark or any sense of control over what to do. We turn to this social component of our cognition in the next section.

THINKING IS FOR ACTION

Over 100 years ago, William James (1890/1950) stated that "thinking is first and last and always for the sake of my doing" (p. 333). This declaration that thinking is purposeful presents a pragmatist approach to social cognition. Gordon Allport (1954) reiterated this simple rule: "Thinking is basically an endeavor to anticipate reality. By thinking we try to foresee consequences and plan actions that will avoid whatever threatens us and will bring our hopes and dreams to pass" (p. 157). James provides a simple example regarding a piece of paper. As a writer, James tells us that he conceives of paper as a surface on which to inscribe words. Most of us are not writers, yet our first thought regarding "paper" is the same as James'. Next, he then asks us to imagine a change in purpose. Imagine that he needs to start a fire and no other materials are close by. His thinking about paper shifts entirely and immediately, and with this comes a shift in his action plans. Not only is his paper now reflected upon solely as combustible material but the more typical category (inscription item), and the associated inferences to that category, are inhibited and put out of mind. His thoughts have nothing to do with writing and only to do with burning. How we think is shaped by what we plan to do; thinking is a tool to prepare us to act.

Thinking about paper is one thing, but let us apply this same logic to thinking about people. Taylor (1981) provided a thought experiment about the stereotyping of Black men. She argued that in almost any context, people have the goal of responding using race and gender as guides. Taylor asked us to imagine our thoughts upon seeing or meeting a Black fireman (such as at the grocery store). She argued that most of us end up responding to the person in ways that align with cultural stereotypes of Black men (just as when we see paper we think of writing). Our culture has taught us to use race when identifying people because it provides a large amount of expectations about what that person is like and how we might expect an interaction to unfold. Stereotypes allow us to go beyond what is known and to plan how to respond. However, when the same man is encountered at a fire—where he is heroically fighting a dangerous blaze—a totally different thought process should ensue where expectations about firemen are far more likely to shape how we think. Just as needing to start a fire changes how we think of paper, needing to stop a fire changes how we think of the same Black fireman. Now thoughts of heroism and saving people from danger should emerge instead, and stereotypes about Black men should be inhibited. Taylor proposed this as a thought experiment, yet Moskowitz and Li (2011) illustrated (with an experiment) that inhibition of stereotypes actually does happen *with such a subtle shift in goals* (as reviewed in Chapter 12). Our goals in a situation, the action we need to prepare for when encountering a person, drives cognition (even stopping stereotyping).

It does not take a dramatic shift in goals—needing to start a fire, needing to stop a fire—to cause such changes in thinking. James's point was that preparing for action is the guide for cognition, and even subtle shifts in our action plans can have dramatic changes in what we think. Cognition is never unbiased and impartial; the goal associated with potential action toward/with the object or person in our immediate environment determines how the object or person is classified. These classifications make one partial (biased) toward thinking about the object or person in line with those goals. A person can go from a threat (a stereotype of Black men) to a hero (a stereotype of firemen) in the blink of an eye, with presumably no more difficulty than seeing a piece of paper as something to write on or as something to burn. This might suggest that it is quite easy to *not stereotype* since it merely requires a simple change in goals. We return to this point later (Chapter 12). For now, our focus is on the purposeful nature of cognition more generally.

Harvey (1963) provided an excellent summary of what we mean when we say **thinking is for action**:

Thinking is for action: Cognition helps us prepare to act. Even if we ultimately choose not to act, thinking helps us prepare appropriate ways to respond to the people around us (even if this means not responding in the moment).

To cope adequately with the environment, even to survive in it, seems to necessitate the ability to read it or define it in some degree of veridicality at least. To satisfy even the simpler motives requires that the organism be able to see relevant means–ends relationships, that is, to be able to "know" what objects or stimuli are motive relevant and to be capable of delineating and engaging appropriate courses of action for their attainment. (p. 3)

The pragmatic nature of cognition adopted by James reflects an intellectual tradition that has gestated over the last century (plus), especially at Harvard University. The Harvard pragmatists include (chronologically) the philosopher Charles Pierce (1877), William James (1890/1950, 1907), Walter Lippmann (1922), Gordon Allport (1954), Jerome Bruner (1957), Ned Jones (e.g., Jones & Davis, 1965), Shelley Taylor (1978), Susan Fiske (1980), and Dan Gilbert (1998).

Meaning, Expectations, and Predictability

Implicit in the statement "thinking is for action" is another core assumption—to know how to act is to *know what to expect and predict* from an object or person with whom we will be interacting. Bruner (1957) stated that

> the results of categorization are representational in nature: they represent with varying degrees of **predictive veridicality** [emphasis added] the nature of the physical world in which the organism operates. By predictive veridicality I mean simply that perceptual categorization of an object or event permits one to "go beyond" the properties of the object or event perceived to a prediction of other properties of the object not yet tested. (p. 129)

Predictive veridicality: Our social cognition not only helps us prepare action, but it does so by allowing us to predict what people are like and what they will do. We hold these predictions to be veridical assessments of other people, even if made quickly and invisibly.

Thus, thinking is in the service of action because it provides reliable (veridical) expectations (prediction) about what a person is like, and likely to do, and what is an appropriate response. Further, predictions (that promote appropriate action) only emerge because thinking provides *meaning* about what a person is doing (and from **meaning making** one can infer or predict what other qualities are likely). The meaning we imbue in objects and people—the traits, goals, attitudes, emotions, and categories of action we believe we see in others as a function of our cognition about their behavior and statements—provides us with expectations for what they are like and likely to do, and for what to do toward/with them. It is the meaning we arrive at that allows us to make predictions about what to expect from others, what to prepare to do ourselves, and what predictions to make about the consequences our chosen course of action will yield. To prepare appropriate action requires knowing what is appropriate in a given setting, with given goals, with a particular person. Thinking imbues such meaning, and with it predictability, that allows for appropriate action. As Heider (1944) stated: "If we are convinced that the pain we feel at the dentist's had its ultimate source in the malevolence of a person instead of in the poor health of our teeth, we would react to it quite differently" (p. 367).

Meaning making: The complex world that bombards our senses would be difficult to respond to without a cognitive system that categorizes what we see, understands the qualities and behaviors associated with being in that category, and informs us about what we know about people and things based on those associations.

If meaning is something that prepares us to act appropriately, two next questions emerge that are central to the field of social cognition. The first is why is it that we seem to take shortcuts when creating meaning? People do not always strive to be as accurate as possible or dedicate as much effort as they possibly can when reaching their conclusions. Why not be perfect? The second question is what goal are we trying to reach when producing knowledge to prepare us to act? If not seeking perfection and 100% accuracy through cognition, what are we seeking?

Limited Capacity *(Why is it that we seem to take shortcuts when creating meaning?)*

Cognitive psychologists and philosophers have long noted that humans seem to have a limitation regarding the amount of information they can process at any moment in time. The cognitive psychologist George Miller declared in 1956 that seven was a "magic number." Miller argued that we resolve the limited capacity of our mental apparatus by chunking information into manageable units, and that seven was the amount of units we can process simultaneously. What comprises a unit can vary from person to person, such that a term such as *Implicit Association Test* (IAT) might be three units of information (three distinct words) to most people, but a person practiced with using this test might simply perceive one

> **Limited capacity:** The human ability to process information is constrained. We possess an ability to process huge amounts of sensory information outside conscious awareness, but more effortful processes such as reasoning, deliberating, and judgment are bounded by the amount of information that can be held in consciousness at any given moment.
>
> **Cognitive load:** When the information-processing system is in a state where its ability to operate is constrained by the stimuli having overburdened the system (due to the amount or complexity of information received or the speed with which the information is received).

unit (IAT) and thus have greater capacity for processing additional items. Bruner, Goodnow, and Austin (1956) described it as paradoxical that humans have such great capacity to finely discern among similar and complex things (we can differentiate among 50 shades of grey), yet have such **limited capacity** regarding how much we can entertain at once (we cannot multiply 32 × 3.5 while simultaneously rehearsing a phone number). Making complex judgments about stimuli, or performing multiple cognitive tasks at the same time, can usurp this limited processing capacity. Once one reaches the limits of the system (due to too much information, complex stimuli, information speeds that are too fast to handle, multitasking, etc.), performance deficits can result from capacity being unavailable (e.g., Gilbert, 1989). Cognition is constrained by the problem of having a limited capacity that is taxed. We often experience the system as taxed due to this state of one's limited capacity having been exceeded, or being in a state of **cognitive load**.

This limitation becomes especially problematic when we consider the amount of information people are bombarded with all the time. Walter Lippmann (1922) has a somewhat famous quote in the social sciences that summarizes a dilemma that faces humanity: our senses, and our limited capacity mental system, are met by the "great blooming, buzzing confusion of the outer world" (p. 55). The stimulus world is characterized by millions of items bombarding us from moment to moment, and without imposing structure on it, our experience of the world would be chaotic and meaningless. Lippmann introduced the word "stereotype" to our lexicon by describing it as a way that we impose such meaning and unity on the chaos of the stimulus world—we attend to only that "which we have picked out in the form stereotyped for us" (p. 55). James (1907/1991) expressed this idea by saying we impose meaning because experience is "a motley which we have to unify by our wits" (p. 76). Allport (1954) summarized this perspective: "outer reality is in itself chaotic—full of too many potential meanings" (p. 169). Stop reading for a moment and consider the hundreds of noises and images you had been filtering out of your experience while reading—the humming of computers and appliances, the tweeting of birds, the cars and sirens on the street outside, the heating, ventilating, and air-conditioning (HVAC) system, the roar of the wind or ocean or thunder, and so on. There is too much information to transcribe all of it accurately. And even if we focus on a subset of that information, our system is constrained by processing limitations that make deep, systematic, and full accountings of each piece of information impossible. Thus, the answer to the first question of why we cannot simply be accurate when creating meaning is because of our limited capacity. Let us turn to the second question of how we create meaning under such limits.

The Sufficiency Principle *(What goal are we trying to reach when producing knowledge?)*

We resolve the complementary problems of stimulus overload and limited capacity by using our overloaded mental system to create structure out of the chaos. Lippman (1922) called this stereotyping. Allport (1954) said we "have to *simplify* in order to live; we need stability in our perceptions. . . . We like nothing left dangling" (p. 170). Thus, we cannot process fully because our capacity to process is limited, yet we are left in chaos if we do not somehow impose meaning. To resolve this dilemma, we develop cognitive tools to prevent us from being overwhelmed by the complexity of our environment. While we may not be able to always think as deeply as we like to, we think using shortcuts to produce what are sufficiently good judgments, beliefs, decisions, and so on (e.g., Chaiken, 1980). Simon (1956) called this **satisficing**. Chaiken, Liberman, and Eagly (1989) referred to social cognition as following a **sufficiency principle**, where meaning is attained not by thinking as deeply and accurately as possible but by any knowledge that can struc-

> **Sufficiency principle (Satisficing):** We think deeply enough to produce sufficiently good judgments, beliefs, and decisions. Intense scrutiny of information (being accurate) is forsaken for judgments, decisions, and behaviors that are "good enough." Over their lifetime people learn that intense scrutiny and effort are not needed to respond in a sufficient and functional manner.

ture the situation in a way that allows for making sufficient (good enough) predictions about what to expect. The sufficiency principle promotes this pragmatic view that thinking exists for a practical purpose: to produce meaning in a manner that allows us to act appropriately. This is often accomplished without knowledge being perfectly rooted in experience or obtaining the complete facts about an object or person we are interacting with. Instead, people are willing to rely on theories about the data rather than rely on a close inspection of the data. An Instagram post or TikTok video might be sufficient. If sufficient knowledge (that which allows for useful inferences and appropriate action) is able to be produced without exhaustive effort or vast experience with the person/object being perceived, then the perceiver will be satisfied to feel as if they "know" enough without a thorough appraisal being conducted. Our past experience and knowledge about categories of people and things—our beliefs, attitudes, and norms of the groups with which we identify—provides such meaning.

In fact, many scholars believe that humans develop a default strategy of relying on such shortcuts, of not thinking deeply, because over their lifetime they learn that such effort is often unable to be exerted (the bombardment of stimuli is too vast) and that shortcuts typically produce judgments and behavior that are good enough. Bruner et al. (1956) argued that we "group the objects and events and people around us into classes and respond to them in terms of their class membership rather than their uniqueness" (p. 1). Allport (1954) called this **the principle of least effort**, and early social cognition scholars saw this as an important principle to demonstrate. Can we show that even when given the opportunity to think more deeply, we seem to prefer more efficient and less effortful modes of thinking, relying on categories and stereotypes? Does less effort produce sufficient judgments? How can we detect if the use of less effortful thinking is the default way of processing? By examining if such

> **The principle of least effort:** Humans develop a default strategy of relying on cognitive shortcuts (like grouping people into categories and treating all category members identically), especially when they are unable to exert greater effort. We produce evaluations, judgments, and actions without thinking deeply, but by following heuristics and overly relying on prior knowledge.

processing is found to occur even when there are no specific motivating circumstances to engage in this processing mode. Such processing should merely require the presence of the appropriate cues in the environment to trigger its use.

Petty, Cacioppo, and Schuman (1983) provide an illustration of people using "least effort" as a default strategy. Their research examined why people are persuaded by celebrities who endorse a product in a commercial. The logic was that rather than evaluate the details about the product, seeing a celebrity leads people to rely on simple rules of impression formation such as "famous people are trustworthy" or "attractive people know a lot about dietary and cosmetic products." Petty et al. had research participants read about a razor that was being endorsed either by a sports star or an unknown person. There are two potential sources of influence in such a situation. One can read the text of the endorsement carefully and evaluate the product based on its merits, or one can superficially evaluate the product and rely on the word of the endorser. If the former strategy is being used, people should find the product equally good regardless of whether the celebrity or the regular guy is the person endorsing it. If people rely on heuristics, the celebrity should be much more persuasive at selling the product than the regular guy, even if the text of their sales pitch is the same. The results revealed that rather than using the text to guide impressions, one uses a heuristic about the person delivering the text. Instead of evaluating products (and other people) in detail, scrutinizing the relevant qualities, we rely on simple and easy rules that do not require such an analysis.

Thousands of experiments have illustrated the importance of such less effortful thinking, and we review many throughout this book. However, it is important to note that this principle of least effort does not doom us to never thinking carefully or deeply. It simply argues that such thinking is often sufficient. However, when motivated for our judgments to be better, we can shift our processing to be more effortful. This too is an important element of social cognition. What we feel to be sufficient can shift, and with it, the nature of our thinking. We dedicate much time in this book to this idea as well. Let us review one example here.

Maheswaran and Chaiken (1991) examined this by looking at how consumers respond to advertising messages. Participants in their experiment were asked to read about and evaluate a new product. Let's call it "product X." The participants first received information about how product X had performed in prior consumer tests, with participants being told that a sample of consumers that had been previously surveyed liked product X very much. This should trigger a heuristic to agree with the vast number of others who like product X. Thus, the participants in this experiment should now be ready to evaluate the product fairly positively, regardless of what the information they are provided with about the product actually says. However, there was one proposed catch to this logic. If it turns out the information that describes the product is clearly negative, this would undermine one's confidence in the heuristic. Most people like the product, yet the information one receives about it is highly incongruent with this fact. This unexpected information, that is inconsistent with what one's heuristic suggested, motivates one to want to know more. Contrast this with what should happen when participants receive clearly positive information about product X. In this case, they have an expectation that the product will be good, and a superficial assessment of the information provided (minimal processing effort) should inform one that this is correct without needing to really read carefully. People should have no need to exert effort in evaluating the product relative to the people in the other group.

Maheswaran and Chaiken (1991) examined these hypotheses by manipulating whether participants received information about product X that was consistent or inconsistent with their first impression. The information was said to have been provided by a product-testing agency's report that compared product *X* with competing brands. People receiving a positive report on product *X* should feel free to exert relatively little processing effort when doing their evaluation of the product. People receiving a negative report on product *X* should be exerting greater processing effort (since it is unexpectedly incongruent with their initial impression). How can we detect whether people exert little versus much processing effort? The report had detailed information about the product's performance along several test dimensions, as well as general summary statements about the product's quality. The experiment's logic hinges on the idea that if people process effortfully, they will pay attention to the details in the report, thinking about product *X*'s performance on these specific dimensions. Less effort processing will instead lead to a superficial assessment only of information summarizing product *X*'s overall quality.

The results provided support for the notion that when one's judgment no longer feels sufficient, more effortful processing is triggered. First, people who received the unexpectedly negative report about product *X* reported having significantly less confidence in their rating of product *X* than people who saw a report that coincided well with the consensus information. Second, when people were asked how much confidence they *desired* to have, people who received the unexpectedly negative report about product *X* and people who saw a report that coincided well with the consensus information both expressed similar amounts of desired confidence. Combining these two points, the groups had equal amounts of confidence they desired to have in their judgment, and one group (the people with confirmed expectancies) had an actual level of confidence that was sufficient in that it did not differ from the confidence they desired. The other group, however, desired a level of confidence they lacked (because of the inconsistency between the report and the consensus of the people surveyed). Finally, the most important question of the experiment addressed what type of information processing was used. As predicted, people who lacked sufficient confidence in their judgment engaged in more thinking about the qualities and attributes of the products being evaluated. They gave more attention to and thought more explicitly about the details of the report than people who had sufficient confidence. They are also better able to remember these details when unexpectedly asked to try to recall the details of the report at the end of the experiment. By default, people who were *not surprised* processed less.

Are There Specific Types of Meaning We Prefer to Make?

We shall see throughout this book that certain types of assessments seem to be dominant when we try to understand other people. One type of assessment that predominates is an evaluation of whether the person is positive or negative. A second powerful quality we use to understand others is to assess their warmth or trustworthiness. Finally, a third powerful quality to make sense of others is an assessment of their competence or skill. Of course, our lexicon is filled with words that describe hundreds of qualities we can apply to people, and that we do apply. The argument is simply that these three seem to have a most-favored status and serve as an initial way of categorizing people, around which more information is incorporated as the impression grows.

Starting with Asch (1946), research has shown that assessments of a person's warmth-coldness are central to how we create meaning. Asch showed that the qualities of warm and cold play an organizing role around which other information learned about a person coheres. Other qualities shift in meaning as a function of whether a person is said to be warm or cold. When Asch replaced warm with cold in a list of qualities shown to participants, the emerging impression shifted dramatically. This also occurred when warm versus cold was not included in the list, but participants spontaneously inferred it. Those who insert warmth themselves see the person described by the list of qualities dramatically differently from those who spontaneously inserted cold. In separate investigations over the years, an assessment of a person's warmth versus coldness emerges as a primary way we first make meaning about a person. For example, Willis and Todorov (2006) show that during face perception, people make judgments about traits communicating a person's warmth (such as their trustworthiness) faster than other traits.

Fiske, Cuddy, and Glick (2007; see also Cuddy, Fiske, & Glick, 2008) provided data on stereotypes across a wide set of nations (and hence a broad swath of stereotyped groups) that revealed two primary dimensions people used when stereotyping others: warmth and competence. They argue that these two qualities alone account for most of the variance (82%) in how perceivers evaluate another person's behavior. In their **stereotype content model**, Fiske et al. (2007) argue that similar forms of inaccurate stereotyping emerge in different cultures due to the same patterns of false beliefs used to characterize that particular culture's stigmatized groups. Across societies, economic/political/religious forces and power dynamics create stereotypes, but the content of those stereotypes all rely on assessing people on the dimensions of warmth (also referred to as trust) and competence. Warmth is an assessment of whether a person or their group intends to help or to harm me or my group. Some groups are seen as warm and trustworthy, potentially helpful; others as cold or untrustworthy, potentially harmful. Competence is essentially an assessment of whether a person or their group has the ability and skill to achieve their intended actions. Are they capable and efficacious or unskilled and ineffectual?

> **Stereotype content model:** Across societies, economic/political/religious forces and power dynamics create stereotypes, the content of which emerges from assessing people using two underlying dimensions—competence and warmth (also called trust/cooperation). Similar inaccurate stereotypes describe different cultures' stigmatized groups due to the propensity to assess people using competence and warmth.

Fiske et al. (2007) argue that because "warmth and competence are reliably universal dimensions of social judgment across stimuli, cultures and time" (p. 82), the combinations of these two dimensions produce distinct categories of types of groups and types of inaccurate stereotypes that we see repeated across cultures. For example, a group that is categorized as high in warmth and low in competence is viewed, across cultures, through the lens of a stereotype that dictates that the dominant group needs to care for them and oversee them. They are seen as having low status and are ineffectual, yet well-meaning and likable. This type of "paternalism" or "colonialism" constrains the opportunities afforded to such group members, while disrespecting them as unthreatening and worthy of pity. These impressions are significant because they direct action—paternalistic responses such as supervision, active caregiving, social isolation, and neglect will result. In American culture this describes stereotypes toward older adults, women, gay men, and people who are differently abled. This category of stereotyping can be contrasted with groups that are both low in warmth and low in competence that are viewed, across cultures, as threats, criminals, potentially violent, and intellectually challenged. They elicit stereotypes of contempt, disgust, danger, and dehumanization. In American culture this describes stereotypes toward the poor, African Americans, and immigrants. They are seen through the lens of a stereotype that dictates that the dominant group needs to guard against and control the violent tendencies of the stereotyped group. High competence and low warmth is viewed, across cultures, through the lens of a stereotype that dictates that such groups are successful, but potentially untrustworthy and manipulative. This type of envy or jealousy leads to a rather unsympathetic view of such groups that makes one wary of being exploited by them and wishing for their failure. These impressions are significant because they too direct action, perhaps actively taking steps to promote their failure—envious responses such as workplace sabotage, jealousy and active harm in the form of backlash—and in health care it can manifest as less active intervention or an unnecessary invasive procedure. In American culture this describes stereotypes toward Jewish people, Asian Americans, Black professionals, female professionals, and the wealthy. The high warmth and high competence pairing is usually reserved for the dominant groups in the culture that sit atop the social hierarchy.

Thus, not only do cultures teach us these different forms of negative stereotypes about groups, they teach us ways to react to these stereotypes—passive reactions versus active reactions. For example, Fiske et al. (2007) describe the low competence and low warmth category being reacted to with passive harm via neglecting and demeaning people from the group, whereas they can also be met with active harm through reactions that involve attacking or fighting people from these groups. For example, in health care a passive reaction might appear as inferior treatment or medication neglect, and an active reaction might involve unnecessarily aggressive treatments such as amputations in patients with diabetes. Different forms of passive and active responses exist for each warmth–competence pairing, with an excellent review by Dovidio and Fiske (2012).

Judd, James-Hawkins, Yzerbyt, and Kashima (2005) state that a perusal of literature findings suggests that when it comes to making trait judgments of an individual, the dimensions of warmth and competence are often positively related. Yet, when it comes to making group judgments that invoke social stereotypes, these two dimensions are often negatively related. A person is usually seen as both warm and competent, yet groups are viewed as incompetent if they are warm, and as competent if they are cold. They sought to experimentally explore this by providing research participants with a description of novel groups that were described as either high or low on one of the dimensions (such as Group X is high in competence). They then asked participants to make judgments about the group on the other dimension (such as how warm is this group). They found a negative relationship between the two dimensions when people are asked to judge an unknown and novel group: Competent groups are judged to be lower in warmth than less competent groups, and a group high in warmth is seen as less competent than a group low in warmth. This might suggest that in the natural world, the strongest stereotypes evolve around the groups that are high competence–low warmth and low competence–high warmth. Though an interesting possibility, the data of Judd et al. do not explore this.

Fiske et al. (2007) further argue that from among these two pervasive trait judgments, the assessment of warmth is more primary than an assessment of competence: "people are more sensitive to warmth information than to competence information" (p. 79). Why is warmth such an influential quality to assess when trying to assign meaning to the behavior we observe? Some scholars have argued that warmth is merely a proxy for positivity more generally—that this is purely an affective response. The argument is that for reasons that are linked to our survival, it is urgent to make an assessment of whether a person (or any stimulus) is positive or negative so that we know whether to approach or avoid it. Chen and Bargh (1999) stated that "automatic evaluation results directly in behavioral predispositions toward the stimulus, such that positive evaluations produce immediate approach tendencies, and negative evaluations produce immediate avoidance tendencies" (p. 215). Asch (1946) had considered this possibility as to why warmth is such a dominant quality we perceive in others, but argued instead that the assessment we make does more than shine a positive or negative light on the person, but imbues it with specific semantic meaning. It is the specific quality of being warm (and synonyms such as "kind," "nice," "good") that people use to assess others, not the more general assessment of whether they are positive or negative. This is not to disagree with the quote from Chen and Bargh but to argue simply that even if people value making quick assessments of whether a stimulus is positive or negative, this is a separate phenomenon from the pervasive use of the trait "warm." Inferring that a person is warm tells us not only if that person is positive or negative, but what their intentions are. It provides an immediate assessment of whether the individual (or group) intends to be a friend or a potential foe/threat. Seeing warmth in a person is useful in that it communicates a constellation of specific qualities such as helpfulness, friendliness, and trustworthiness.

It is for this reason that Williams and Bargh (2008) argue that competence is the next fastest assessment made, rising to the top two of the most universally observed ways people make meaning. If warmth allows us to know whether people intend to harm or help us, we next need to know whether people have the capacity or efficacy to act on those intentions. Do they have the competence to harm us or help us? As Fiske et al. (2007) put it:

> warmth and competence are reliably universal dimensions of social judgment across stimuli, cultures and time. The consistency with which these dimensions appear might reflect the answers to two basic survival questions: first, and crucially, does the other person or group intend to harm or help me (or us)? Secondarily, does the other have the ability to enact those intentions? (p. 83)

In essence, these assessments are made to allow one to know how to act toward group members. In yet another (more recent) approach to explore the most common qualities humans use when judging and describing other humans, Lin, Keles, and Adolphs (2021) used a novel approach of applying machine learning algorithms and statistical procedures to develop and sample from a set of facial stimuli and trait words. The research participants made judgments of 100 faces using 100 identified trait words, and those judgments were quantified to disclose the most common traits people use to characterize faces. What they found is that, once again, warmth and competence emerged as among the most important psychological dimensions used to characterize faces (as well as two additional dimensions that were most frequently used—femininity and youth, which corroborates other research showing gender, age, and race to be important categories).

THE ACTIVE CONSTRUCTION OF KNOWLEDGE: SEEING THROUGH A SOCIAL LENS

We have already asserted that part of what makes social cognition "social" is the assumption that there are social determinants of cognition—we interpret all that we see through a social lens, even at the lowest levels of cognition. Humans are not like antenna that simply receive signals from the world. To "know" a person or thing requires far more than simply transcribing the events and features observed. This view is hardly new to social cognition. For example, Kant (1781/1990) argued that what people already know determines what they see and how they come to understand that which they experience: "Without the sensuous faculty no object would be given to us, and without the understanding no object would be thought" (p. 45). This **top-down processing** as a way of knowing, where existing knowledge is used to interpret the facts, is a contrasting view to that of empiricism, which holds that experience alone—and the facts transcribed from that experience—shape what we know to be true. Locke (1690/1961) presumed that the mind starts out like a piece of white paper—"void of all characters, without any ideas: How comes it to be furnished?" The one-word answer was through "experience." Knowledge of coldness comes through experiencing the way in which an object labeled as cold to the touch affects the sense of touch. Hume (1748/1961) described the process through which knowledge gained through sensation is combined to produce more complex knowledge through a process of association. Thinking and attaining meaning, from this perspective, is "built" through **bottom-up processing**, with stimulus information driving what is perceived, categorized, and encoded.

It is undoubtedly true that there can be inherent meaning in the things we experience; the actions of others and the qualities of things we observe can impress a singular meaning upon us. There is power in data, and stimuli afford a particular way to respond. Yet despite these truths, the social-cognitive approach has focused on a complementary point. In social cognition, there is the recognition that social forces infiltrate the process of knowing even when the data are seemingly clear and supposedly dictate how we understand what we have experienced. Rather than focus solely on how knowledge is built from the "bottom up," social cognition additionally focuses on how meaning is made from the top down. A perceiver's values, goals, and expectations meet the data received by the senses, and rather than merely transcribing those signals, absorbs them into existing knowledge, filtered through the social forces that imbue meaning on that stimulation.

> **Top-down processing:** A view of how knowledge is produced that sees meaning being *made* through new experiences passing through the filter of one's prior knowledge and attitudes. As such, meaning is assimilated into and shaped by an existing structure, helping one to impose a coherent meaning onto current stimuli.
>
> **Bottom-up processing:** A view of how knowledge is produced that sees meaning being made by perceiving a stimulus's inherent qualities and linking them in memory. With each new experience with the stimulus, new associations form and a more complex sense of knowing the stimulus builds on the foundation of the initial experience.

James (1890/1950) argued for the strong role that prior knowledge plays in how we understand what we experience. In a denouncement of empiricism, James stated:

> These writers are bent on showing how the higher faculties of the mind are pure products of experience . . . [they] regard the creature as absolutely passive clay upon which experience rains down. The clay will be impressed most deeply where the drops fall thickest, and so the final shape of the mind is moulded. . . . These writers have, then, utterly ignored the glaring fact that subjective interest may, by laying its weighty index finger on particular items of experience, so accent them as to give to the least frequent associations far more power to shape our thought than the most frequent ones possess. (p. 403)

From this view, expectations and wants shape what we believe is true even more than what the data suggest. Demonstrating this to be true with experiments was first pursued in the 1930s by scholars such as Frederic Bartlett (1932; who introduced the *schema* concept) and Jerome Bruner. Even basic perceptual processes are not immune from top-down influences. Representational structures provide expectations and desires that drive what we perceive, categorize, and encode. As Melnikoff and Bargh (2023) put it:

> High-level concepts are used to issue predictions about low-level sensory input, which are compared to the actual input to infer the state of the world. . . . [This] suggests that automatic processes need not be simple, bottom-up mappings from stimulus to response, but can be sophisticated, top-down processes. (p. 185)

The New Look in Cognition

Perhaps the seeds of social cognition as a field of inquiry were planted by research on perception and attention of Jerome Bruner and his colleagues. From the late 1930s into the 1950s, they presented work labeled as providing a "**New Look**" to understanding cognition. What was new was a fusion of the study of social influences with a study of the stages of cognitive processing, turning a scientific eye on showing that processes once held to be unmediated

New look: An approach to understanding cognition from the 1930s through 1950s focused on how an individual's motives alter perception and attention. What was "new" was a fusion of the study of social influences on specific stages of cognitive processing, showing that low-level processes thought to be unmediated were, in fact, mediated.

were in fact mediated. For example, Bruner and Goodman (1947) proposed that the value of a stimulus would distort the perception of it. A valued object will be accentuated and appear to be larger than it really is. Bruner and Goodman illustrated this by asking participants to hold a circular object in their hand and to draw it using a circular patch of light they controlled with a knob. The object they were asked to hold was manipulated in the experiment. It could either be a *coin* or a *disc* that had no value but that was the same size as the coin. The results revealed that, even though the objects were being held in the hand and could be directly assessed to be the same size, perception of an object was distorted if it had value. Coins were perceived to be larger relative to discs of the same size. This distortion in perception of the coins was even greater for poor participants (who needed money more) relative to wealthy participants.

Across a large body of experiments, Bruner and colleagues showed a variety of ways in which low-level processing is influenced by social forces. They show that people can perceive self-relevant items faster than other items. People can inhibit the perception of threatening items. Items of value were perceived as not only larger (as just detailed) but closer than items of lesser value. We review this work in depth later in this book. For now, it is hoped that you can see that perception is not solely a function of the features of the object being perceived. Even low-level cognition is distorted by what the perceiver needs or wants.

The Gestalt Tradition

The earliest support for a top-down nature of cognition came from the German Gestalt psychologists such as Max Wertheimer, Kurt Koffka, and Wolfgang Köhler. A fundamental focus of Gestalt theorizing is that the parts of a stimulus array interact to make up a structure, and those interacting parts are dynamic in that they influence one another. Understanding of the structure is not achieved by examining the individual elements but by examining the nature of the relationship between the parts and the emerging properties that the dynamic system imposes on the elements (**holism**). The whole is more than the sum of the parts is a lesson first delivered by Gestalt psychology. Consider the Ebbinghaus

Holism: The whole is more than the sum of the parts in a stimulus array, which dynamically interact to influence one another in comprising a representational structure. Understanding is not achieved by examining the individual elements but by examining the nature of the relationship between the parts and their emergent meaning.

illusion (see Figure 1.2), where the perceived size of the inner circle of each set is altered by the size of its surrounding circles. Despite the two inner circles being identical, they look different due to the contrast with the immediate context. Thus, the same image is perceived differently based on the whole of the context in which the image is seen. Many modern examples of such optical illusions exist, some of the most fascinating being those where the color we "see" is different based on the shifting context that surrounds an object (even though its actual color is unchanged).

Gestalt psychologists further argued that we seek meaning from stimulus environments through a removal of doubt and ambiguity (**closure**). To do so we perceive and structure information in a clear and unambiguous way. Even if the stimulus is not clear and unambiguous, we see simplicity and regularity in it to the degree the stimulus will allow (*Prägnanz*). To remove ambiguity and uncertainty we go beyond the information given, or fill in the gaps and produce regularity and meaning. For example, a triangle that is obstructed so that one of the angles is not visible will still be perceived as a triangle. It was

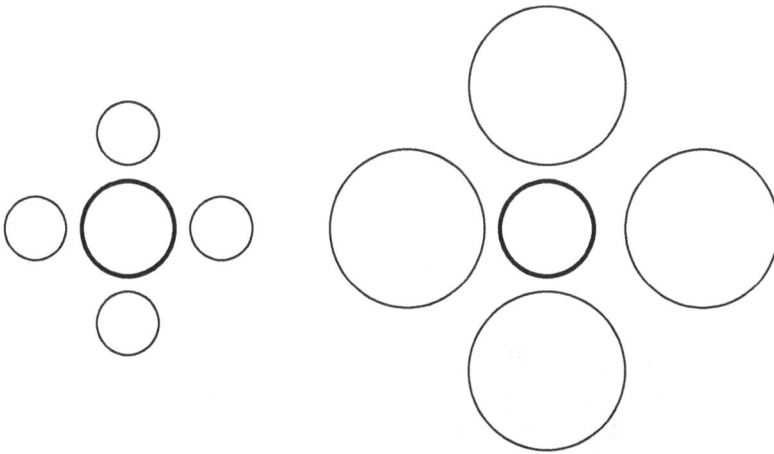

FIGURE 1.2. The Ebbinghaus illusion.

the social psychologist Fritz Heider (1944) who believed that these principles that explain how we perceive triangles and circles would impact how we perceive people as well: "processes of organization in the perceptual field" are "applied profitably to the perception of other persons and their behavior" (p. 358). As with the Ebbinghaus circles, we judge people in a context, contrasting their behavior against standards. As with an obstructed triangle, we categorize a person based on a partial view and make inferences that go beyond what is provided based on those categories.

> **Closure:** Humans seek meaning from, and a sense of understanding of, stimuli. Even at the perceptual level, our system strives to see structure and meaning rather than uncertainty or ambiguity. Uncertainty and doubt are aversive (to varying degrees, as an individual difference), and its removal constitutes closure and removes the aversiveness.

Gestalt theorizing also tells us that some aspects of the stimulus field jump out and capture the eye to shape what is clearly seen, while the rest of the situation fades into the background. They called these different aspects of the stimulus field **figure and ground**. The perceptual system supplies information to our experience to give it meaning (figural components are observed, understood, and separated from the background). What is seen as figural is not absolute, but dependent on where one happens to focus attention. Situations specify appropriate ways to act, and what is figural is determined by the context specifying and limiting what is appropriate. Imagine you walk into a funeral and a woman is laughing hysterically.

> **Figure and ground:** The elements of a stimulus array can either jump out and grab attention or recede into the background and serve as a context. The ground elements serve as a context, while the figural elements are salient or leap out at the perceiver.

This person will leap out against the background and capture attention. But take the same person and same behavior, and change the background, such as putting her dockside (at a boat party) not graveside (at a funeral), and perhaps she would no longer be seen as figural; you might not notice her at all. Figure 1.3 illustrates the relationship between the background context ("ground") and what leaps out from the context ("figure") as providing emergent meaning when considered as a whole unit. On the left, we see that with one "ground" we see an old woman. With another she is young. On the right we see a horse if we focus first at the top of the picture, but a seal if we focus on the bottom part first.

Foundational figures of social psychology—Kurt Lewin, Solomon Asch, Fritz Heider, Muzafer Sherif—emerged from this Gestalt tradition, and their theorizing in social

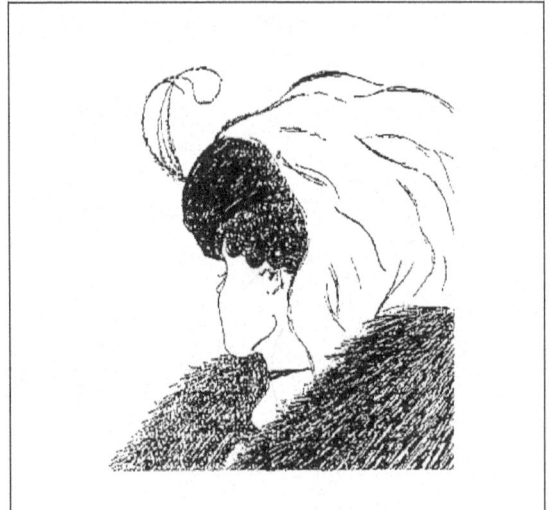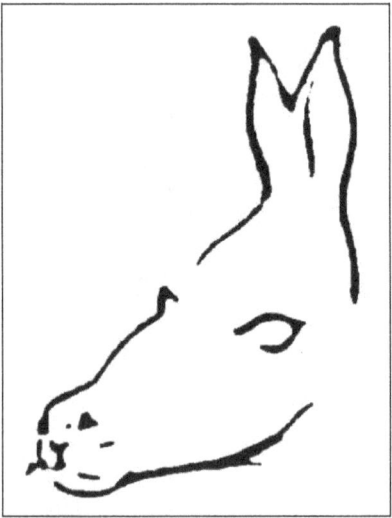

FIGURE 1.3. What is figural can vary, and changes in what is figural bring changes in closure.

psychology from the 1930s and 1940s helped spur the cognitive revolution in social psychology in the 1970s. For example, Sherif (1936) argued that one's internal representation of one's culture emphasizes some aspects of the perceptual field over others. Thus, people from different cultures could perceive the same stimulus differently:

> In the course of the life history of the individual and as a consequence of his contact with the social world around him, the social norms, customs, values, etc., become interiorized in him. These interiorized social norms enter as frames of reference among other factors in situations to which they are related, and thus dominate or modify the person's experience. (pp. 43–44)

In this way, culture creates a readiness to organize stimulus information in specific ways during perception. Where a member of one culture might hear beautiful music, a member of another culture might lack the cultural experience to piece together the sound into a meaningful unit, and might perceive sheer noise. The perceptual building blocks are identical, but perceptual experience is guided in a top-down fashion by the organizational meaning provided by culture (e.g., Markus & Kitayama, 1991).

Asch's (1946) experiments on forming impressions of personality similarly reflect the Gestalt perspective. Asch explored how a set of traits, taken as a collective, provide an emergent meaning. Rather than thinking of a person as a list of disjointed qualities, the set is merged into a whole and a coherent narrative of what the person is like emerges. The judgment of some subset of traits or behaviors leads to the formation of a general impression that unifies and explains the rest of the information learned about the person. And, as mentioned earlier, some traits are figural and jump out—such as warmth—and play a stronger role in organizing the other qualities we have learned about the person. One trait known to be possessed by a person imposes itself on how we evaluate other behaviors and traits that are also attributed to that person. In his textbook entitled *Social Psychology*, Asch (1952) stated,

> Although phenomenally we see objects directly, with no process intervening, objectively the process is mediated. [We cannot maintain] that the perceived object is a photographic reflection

of the real object. We have to say that the object in the environment and our experience of it are two distinct, though related, events. (p. 47)

Our experience is that we perceive bottom-up, our reality is that we perceive top-down (mediated).

People see what they want to see, what they are ready to see, in a way that goes beyond the set of information that is observed. It is remarkable to read a sampling of the impressions formed by Asch's (1946) participants. From a list of six traits describing a person they produce complex and comprehensive narratives of what such a person is like. Asch argued that such narratives emerge because one quality is more central than the others (what he called a **central trait**), and it organizes all the other information around it in a way that makes it all cohere. As mentioned earlier, qualities such as warmth and competence seem to have this power. Asch also discussed how this organization around a central trait might occur. One possibility is a **halo effect**, where the process reflects an affective response. The positivity (or negativity) of the central trait might, like a halo, surround the individual and illuminate the entire person with positivity; each individual characteristic is biased by the valence associated with the general impression. Yet, Asch was a firm believer that impressions are shaped by more than just an affective halo. He believed there was a specific semantic response in which central traits have a specific meaning that is then used as an organizing principle around which meaning is imposed on the other qualities observed. Thus, it is not just the affect of the impression that changes from these top-down influences, but the specific qualities thought to be possessed by the person. As with the Ebbinghaus illusion, a trait—such as smart— is seen very differently when in the context of the central trait "warm" versus the context of the central trait "cold." If paired with warm the trait "smart" is seen as helpful and mentoring, but as deceitful and plotting if paired with "cold."

Central trait: A quality of a person that is useful for making sense of other qualities and that organizes the other information around it in a way that makes it all cohere. Qualities such as warmth and competence seem to have this power, although many traits can serve this role, depending on the context.

Halo effect: When the positivity or negativity of an impression surround the individual being judged and illuminate their entire character, like a halo. Each characteristic is then biased by this general impression. For example, the person judged to be attractive is then also seen as courteous, kind, forgiving, moral, generous, helpful, etc.

The impact of Gestalt theorizing is also seen in the work of another founding figure to social psychology: Fritz Heider. In 1921, a 25-year-old Heider arrived at the Psychological Institute of the University of Berlin, where Heider audited courses taught by the Gestalt psychologists Wolfgang Köhler and Max Wertheimer. If the impact of Gestalt psychology was not ingrained during this period, in 1930 Heider took a sabbatical leave to work with Kurt Koffka at Smith College. Heider's (1958) book adopted the Gestalt perspective. It posits that each time we see a behavior (or any new event in our environment), a change to our context has been produced. The unexplained action triggers a state of doubt, or lacking closure, and a pursuit of meaning is initiated. The cognitive system is no longer in equilibrium, and equilibrium can only be attained by reducing uncertainty and doubt. How does the person do this? Through making an attribution for the event. Thus, the pursuit of meaning central to social cognition emerged from Heider's view of it as similar to a drive—a drive to reduce what Gestalt theorists would call a state of disequlibrium (lacking closure). Heider (1944) stated:

A great many studies have been made of the processes of organization in the perceptual field. It is the thesis of this paper that the principles involved in these studies can be applied profitably to the perception of other persons and their behavior, and that one of the features of the organization of the social field is the attribution of a change to a perceptual unit. (p. 358)

The Rise of Social Cognition: Old Ideas Turned Revolutionary

The field of social cognition emerged in the 1970s, spurred by young scholars and doctoral students of that era who grew frustrated with social psychological approaches that merely illustrated that social forces influenced thinking (as we have seen in the Gestalt tradition) without providing an explanation of *how*. Thus, their concern with the social forces that impact how we think, feel, and act was an old one. What was (and continues to be) revolutionary was the idea that we could examine *how* these top-down influences occur, even their influence over low levels of cognitive processing. In 1970 it was a novel insight to apply the new(ish) methodologies of cognitive psychology to study social psychological phenomena such as reasoning, stereotyping, decision making, judgment, impression formation, and person perception. They saw self-report as a limited tool for uncovering the hidden mind, and had immense creativity in the development of ways to detect the processes and structures that shape thinking about the social world.

Since developing novel methods was essential to the advancement of social cognition, this has led some people to misconstrue the entire discipline as merely a methodology used by some subset of social psychologists. Yet while developing important and creative tools for studying psychological processes is an outgrowth of social cognition, it is not its purpose. Like any instance in which people pave a new path, some amount of developing new tools was essential. Following the lead of Bruner (and the so-called New Look), who had done this type of research in the 1930s–1950s, social cognition began when scholars took on the task of studying *the processes and mechanisms* through which top-down influences are exerted. This required using methods developed by the cognitive revolution in psychology that took hold in the 1950s.

One group of young scholars (Ebbe Ebbesen, Dave Hamilton, Reid Hastie, Tom Ostrom, Bob Wyer) might be pointed to as the pioneers of the discipline. This group happened to all be attending the same conference in 1974, and over several days found themselves—late into the night—debating their shared and idiosyncratic passion for using cognitive methodologies to study social psychology. Several of these pioneering figures are still active and mentoring students and younger colleagues. When the conference ended, they vowed to meet annually to continue these vigorous discussions and to share ideas. In the first year they expanded their group to include the graduate student Don Carlston. The group has expanded further with each passing year. This tradition of meeting annually to discuss social cognition started by these pioneers has taken place for 50 years and counting. Today this meeting is seen as a home for social cognition researchers across the globe and meets for 3 days every October. I am proud to say that organizing this event has fallen to me and Dr. Jaqueline Chen, who dedicate a chunk of our year to fostering this intellectual tradition. The field has grown into a thriving collection of global scholars numbering in the thousands, with an International Social Cognition Network (ISCON; *www.ucl.ac.uk/~ucjtrc1/ ISCON*) that also hosts a conference every February.

Of course, the group of six scholars mentioned above were not alone in their interest in the cognitive processes through which social knowledge is produced. During the 1970s, scattered across the United States, a series of graduate students worked on doctoral dissertations that pushed along the emerging discipline (e.g., John Bargh, Nancy Cantor, Don Carlston, Shelly Chaiken, Jennifer Crocker, Russ Fazio, Susan Fiske, Peter Gollwitzer, Arie Kruglanski, Patricia Linville, Brenda Major, Hazel Markus, Rich Petty, Eliot Smith, Claude Steele, Robin Vallacher, and Tim Wilson). These students were supported not only by the pioneers named above but also by young mentors who were working as professors. Such mentors include Marilynn Brewer, Tory Higgins, Charles Judd, Ellen Langer, Dick Nisbett,

Mick Rothbart, Jim Sherman, Shelly Taylor, Dan Wegner, Bob Zajonc, and Leslie Zebrowitz. Some young professors of this era, such as Jim Uleman and Tony Greenwald, shifted research focus entirely to join in the revolution.

WHAT MAKES COGNITION *SOCIAL*?

The "social" component in the term *social cognition* refers to both the dependent variable (when people are the target of our cognition) and the independent variable (when people are exerting an influence on cognition). As an independent variable, the social force exerted by people can occur when people are physically present, such as when we feel one type of social pressure when at work, and another when around our significant other's parents, and another when in a bar. We change how we think and act to fit with the people with whom we are interacting, since different people specify different goals we hope to meet, different expectations to live up to, different stereotypes that define what we think is correct, and different norms for what is typical and appropriate. However, social forces are exerted even when others are not physically present, but when those people are representationally present. If one's mother is 1,000 miles away, her influence exists in the form of internalized standards and morals. When alone on a mountain hike, one's culture still shapes how one thinks by specifying norms and rules. Different situations speak to different goals and pressures that are felt even if the people who dish out the consequences are not currently in the room (fidelity does not require your partner to be standing next to you). Cognition, therefore, can still be social even if people are not the target of study. There can be social cognition about objects and places, where a social force influences how we think about those objects and places. How does thinking about people differ from objects?

People versus Objects

As mentioned earlier, we describe all cognition as *social* because nonhuman objects still only have meaning when embedded in a social system that provides that meaning. Indeed, the mental operations that govern how we think about people and objects are often identical. For example, with both people and objects stimulus information first hits the perceptual apparatus; attention is focused on elements of the physical features presented; and the stimulus is quickly, often unconsciously, categorized. Further, there is a drive for the stimulus to be understood, to transcribe the sensations into meaning, so that we can prepare how to respond.

This does not mean we should fail to make a distinction about the processing of objects versus people; we have expectations and goals toward people that are quite unique. Unlike objects, people have minds of their own! While it is true that their behavior may be random, it usually reflects a person's goals, needs, and willed activity. Unlike the movement of objects, the movement of a person can reflect an intention. Thus, a unique feature of our thinking about people is our understanding that the psychological state of others is separate from our own, and thus we develop the belief early on (what Wellman, 1990, called a **theory of mind**) that there is a relationship between a person's behavior and that person's psychological state. Even the lack of behavior can be perceived to be caused

> **Theory of mind:** The theory that people are different from objects because people have goals and intentions, whereas objects move because they are acted upon by other forces. It is the realization that comes with a child's development that other people have their own internal beliefs, desires, and goals which we cannot directly see. It is an understanding that these mental states can be different from one's own and shape how others act.

by intentions that we would not infer in objects. Jones and Davis (1965) saw deducing the intentions of others from observing their behavior to be among the most fundamental processes of social cognition.

Additionally, because people exert the will to produce their action, and because their goals can change from moment to moment, perceivers need to approach cognition relating to people with an eye toward anticipating the goals and needs of the person in order to predict the person's next step and plan appropriately. This inference of will does not exist with object perception. Finally, unlike objects, the people we perceive are returning the favor. A person is not only aware we are perceiving them and perhaps evaluating them but is also perceiving and evaluating us. This creates a confounding variable that does not exist with objects—what people say and do might reflect their anticipation of *our* wants and goals rather than reflect their own will and goals. Others may try to influence or appease us, and act in ways that reflect their anticipation of our desires, rather than their own. With this understanding that cognition can be social because other people exert an influence on our cognition, we next focus on types of influence. What types of social forces exert a top-down influence on the way in which we think?

Culture

Perhaps the most obvious social force is the culture we live within. Cultures specify norms, mores, standards, and mindsets that reflect the values and practices of the culture. But culture does more then set the rules, or spell out 10 commandments. Culture infiltrates ways of thinking and ways of making meaning. For example, an entire literature has arisen examining differences in cognition that result from being raised in Western versus Eastern cultures (e.g., J. G. Miller, 1984; Newman & Marsden, 2023). Morris and Peng (1994) argued that individualistic cultures (such as the United States and much of Europe) saturate people with messages about personal accountability and the role of one's personal abilities and disposition to produce outcomes. Collectivistic cultures were said to provide its members with messages that highlight interpersonal dependence, connectedness, and the role of other people in helping to shape outcomes. These respective mindsets have come to be known as **individualism** and **collectivism**.

Individualism: A cultural mindset or philosophy that emphasizes the role of personal ability in action and success, stressing individual agency, accountability, and responsibility.

Collectivism: A cultural mindset or philosophy that emphasizes the role of social support and social networks in shaping one's action and success, stressing shared dependence and mutual responsibility.

To illustrate the impact of these cultural forces they had participants watch cartoon displays of fish in "social settings," such as a group of fish being approached by a single fish and then the group exiting. Participants from the United States viewed the actions in such displays as the result of an individual fish as the cause, and participants from China viewed the actions in such displays as the result of the group of fish as the cause. In two other studies they switched from explaining movement of animals to explanations for human behavior, such as homicide. Across two experiments, they revealed that there was a tendency for American participants to emphasize dispositional reasons internal to the accused murderer as the cause for the homicide. Chinese participants, in contrast, saw factors external to the disposition of the accused murderer as more relevant (their background and social conditions). In this work, one culture's emphasis on personal agency and individualism leads to a style of sense making that places relatively greater emphasis on the traits and culpability of the individual. The same behavior was seen by a member of the other culture, with its relatively greater emphasis on collectivism, as more likely to be derived from social pressures and interpersonal networks of relationships that compel people to act.

Others have made this point that perceptual experience is shaped by culture with cross-cultural studies, examining how people of different cultures react to perceptual illusions. For example, the Mueller–Lyer illusion (see Figure 1.4) shows an influence of context on how we perceive lines. For many people reading this book Figure 1.4 will seemingly show lines of two different lengths. The lines are, however, the same length. It is one's perceptual experience that is being distorted by a perceiver's top-down influences that is creating the illusion of a difference.

There are several explanations regarding what top-down theory from one's culture could cause the Mueller–Lyer illusion. For example, some people propose a "**carpentered world hypothesis**" in which living in a society with angled buildings and rectangular-shaped homes creates a distortion in how lines are perceived. We expect rooms to be rectangular, and when they are not (as with an Ames room, where the construction is trapezoidal) we perceptually impose that structure anyway and this causes perceptual illusions. Despite there being no one accepted explanation for the Mueller–Lyer illusion, the perceptual bias exists. Further proof of there being a top-down influence is the fact there are people from some cultures who do not see the illusion at all. The lines appear to them to be of equal length (e.g., Segall, Campbell, & Herskovit, 1963). Once again, the reason for the cultural difference is unclear. But what is clear is that the illusion occurs for some groups of people and not for others. This argues for an organizing influence on the perceptual process from a social force, in this case, culture.

> **Carpentered world hypothesis:** An illusion in how lines and angles are perceived that exists among people raised in cultures with angled buildings and rectangular-shaped homes. A lifetime of exposure to such images leads to a perceptual "expectation" that straight lines and right angles exist, leading us to see them even when they are not there.

Another literature exists on more local cultures and the norms that exist within more concrete social groups (such as political groups, gangs, occupations, etc.) that serve to shape cognitive processing. Even a group of people who come together for a psychology experiment can create a local culture with norms that shape how people see something as basic as the movement of light in a dark room (illustrated in a classic old study by Sherif from 1936). As Van Bavel and Packer review in their 2021 book, one's group identity affects basic perceptual experience such as what we taste and smell. And as Jost reviews in his book from 2021, political ideology motivates people to justify and rationalize the structures that maintain inequality through subtle processes that shape how we explain and understand the standing held by different groups within a social hierarchy. Even basic processes that determine whether we see a behavior as driven by a person's trait or by a pressure in their current situation are determined by group-based ideology.

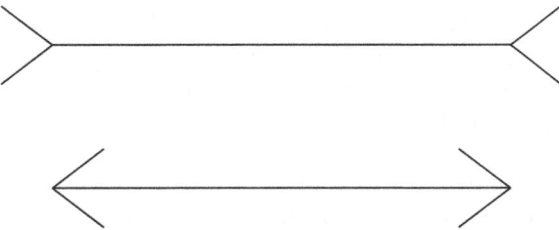

FIGURE 1.4. The Mueller–Lyer illusion.

Social Needs

Another set of top-down forces that shape cognition are those that represent the needs that permeate across all aspects of cognitive and social life. Psychological theory has historically assumed that beyond biological needs that drive human behavior (needs to survive, to reproduce, etc.), there are three socially defined motivational principles that operate as needs—that is, although a person would not immediately die if denied these needs, they nonetheless drive our mental life, with great despair and confusion arising if these psychological needs were to be denied. They are (1) a need for social connection, or affiliation needs; (2) a need for positive self-regard, or self-esteem needs; and (3) a need to have understanding and meaning that allow us to prepare for action, or epistemic needs. The three psychological needs at times overlap (e.g., Hardin & Conley, 2001; Hogg, 2007), such as when belonging to a social group (affiliation need) provides a sense of shared meaning that helps to reduce uncertainty in the world (epistemic need). Or when an affiliation need leads one to join a group of like-minded others that provides corroboration and support for one's worldview and gives one a positive sense of identity (esteem need). All motivations and goals that humans pursue are derived from these needs.

Epistemic Needs

An **epistemic need** is the need to identify/label, understand, and be able to make predictions about people and objects. It is a need to find meaning and derive a sense of understanding from the uncertainty of the complex stimulus world, because meaning allows us to feel a sense of control and predictability over our environment rather than being held hostage to random forces (e.g., Heider, 1944). Heider stated that "some authors talk of a general tendency towards causal explanation, a 'causal drive'" (p. 359). Why has this cognitive activity been elevated to the status of a basic need? Almost every thought and action we undertake during the course of our waking moments is aimed at either avoiding aversive stimuli or approaching pleasurable ones. But how do we know what is dangerous and painful in order to avoid it? What alerts us as to which stimuli will bring us pleasure and should be approached? This information is delivered by our cognitive system's pursuit of meaning. If I am lost while walking in Central Park at night, whether or not I approach a stranger depends on how I label that person and the inferences I draw from having categorized that person. Is it a man or a woman? Does the person seem physically imposing and dangerous? Is it likely the person is armed? Will the person speak my language? Will the person see me as a threat? These questions get answered quickly, as the mental apparatus races to provide information about whether a situation poses an opportunity for help or harm. Let us say the person is categorized as a woman, the clothes identify her as a jogger. Her status as a jogger suggests she knows her way around the park. The revealing nature of her sportswear suggests she is not carrying a gun. The relative physical sizes of each of us implies she poses no physical threat. All this information is provided in milliseconds, without me deciding to form an impression. But armed with an impression I can reduce my fear of being lost in a potentially dangerous place by approaching the woman. And the wise person will take into account that the woman also has epistemic needs, and will herself be wary of being approached, in a park, by a more physically imposing stranger. Making meaning provides for us inferences about what to expect, allows us to make predictions about consequences (is pain or pleasure likely), and prepares us for behavior so that we are ready

> **Epistemic need:** The need to identify/label, understand, and be able to make predictions about the people and objects in our world. It is a need to have meaning.

to respond appropriately. A last function it provides for us is to allow us to feel in control. Feelings of control are essential to well-being and avoiding depression (e.g., Lerner & Miller, 1978; Seligman, 1975). Without it, the world would feel random and dangerous, where one would never be able to predict what threats lurk around the corner. As epistemic needs increase, so too does the value on control and prediction.

To illustrate this, Hamilton, Katz, and Leirer (1980a, 1980b) created heightened epistemic needs in half of the participants by asking them to judge people from reading about their behaviors. For the other half of the participants they were simply asked to read and memorize the behaviors. The information they were asked to process was not very rich in terms of social power; the behaviors were extremely low in the social information they communicated. The participants read a series of sentence predicates such as "rented an apartment near where he works," "played ball with his dog in the park," "went to a movie with friends Saturday night." As might be expected, when epistemic needs were low, people did not form any particular impression from these behaviors. What was the impact of having heightened epistemic needs? The perceiver now tried to find meaning from these pallid behaviors, making predictions about what the person who performed each behavior was like (making a trait judgment). They formed a more complex and interconnected mental representation of the information that improved memory for the behaviors. Ironically (since they were asked to memorize the items), people with low epistemic needs had worse memory for the items than people with high epistemic needs (who formed impressions). Keep in mind that these findings are not meant to imply that people only form impressions when asked. To the contrary, it has been argued that epistemic needs are, by default, strong enough to lead us to infer traits and make meaning without being asked (e.g., Moskowitz, 1993a). What this research does show is that even when the information we are presented with is incredibly uninformative (it used sentence predicates *that did not even mention the names of actual people*), we can still manage to create meaning from it when our epistemic needs are heightened enough.

Epistemic needs arise out of the fact that people do not wish to feel as if they are subject to random and haphazard forces that are beyond their control. This feeling that our destiny is ours to make is promoted by processing that allows us to feel that what happens to us is a product of what we would like to happen to us. We feel control, particularly over the good outcomes. This feeling of control works somewhat more liberally when judging others, since others tend to be seen as responsible for what happens to them regardless of whether the outcome is good or bad. In fact, seeing others as having control over their bad outcomes also promotes a feeling of our own personal control. It allows us to feel as if we can prevent bad events from infecting our future since we will not make the same bad (and controllable) choices that others must have made (e.g., Lerner & Miller, 1978). Without such a sense, the world would be in anarchy. As perceivers we prefer to see justice and fairness in the consequences other people face for their actions, a pattern of reasoning about the causes for events that Lerner (1965) called the **just-world hypothesis**. Outcomes being labeled as "deserved" allow one to believe the world is a controllable and predictable place, which can make one feel a sense of security over their own futures. Random acts of violence, innocent people who suffer and die, and criminals being rewarded rather than punished are events that suggest the world is unfair and unpredictable; a place where the self cannot be protected from harm. Just desserts suggest personal control. Such a sense of control allows people to invest in long-term goals, which would be foolish to pursue if a causal link between outcomes and effort was not maintained (e.g., Hafer, 2000).

Just-world hypothesis: A theory that the world is generally knowable and controllable, and thus outcomes are deserved, since people should have known and been able to control them. It is a tendency to see the world as just, where people have control and get what they deserve.

Sadly, one result of our epistemic needs creating a heightened desire for control is that people will blame victims. They reason that if bad outcomes are assumed to be just and deserving, then such consequences must arise from bad actions (or from bad people), which makes the person, even if the victim of a terrible crime, blameworthy. For example, Lerner (1965) found that when research participants had been randomly selected to receive electric shocks, other research participants who learned of this fact denigrated these individuals. As if receiving shock is not bad enough, they must suffer the injustice of being seen as responsible for this negative event simply so that others may maintain the belief that the world is just. Hafer (2000) showed a similar denigration of victims, with the victim blaming being especially pronounced when need for control was high. Need for control was created by having some research participants contemplate their long-term goals (which requires predictions and assumptions about having control over one's future outcomes), while others simply contemplated current classes and extracurricular activities. All of the participants then watched a video where a female student discussed having contracted a sexually transmitted infection and a variety of the accompanying symptoms with a counselor. Half of the participants learned that the infection was the result of an accident, when a condom broke while the woman was having sex. Half of the participants learned that it occurred because she had failed to use a condom at all when having sex. The question of interest is how much blame participants place on the woman, especially when she is the innocent victim of an accidental negative event. The results revealed that when participants contemplated their long-term goals prior to the video, the innocent victim was derogated to a greater extent than when goals had not been contemplated. This difference in how much a victim is derogated did not emerge when the woman was clearly responsible for her outcome (failing to use a condom at all). People not only disliked the innocent victim more when contemplating their own long-term goals, they also found her to be more blameworthy and responsible for her fate. People even dissociated themselves from the victim, being more likely to say "she is nothing like me."

The Need for Positive Esteem

People have a need to experience a positive sense of esteem and identity. Taylor and Brown (1988) argue that a variety of cognitive strategies are used to promote self-esteem and to create unrealistically positive views of the self. These strategies are reviewed in Chapters 5 and 9 where they are described when reviewing the term "*Motivated Reasoning*." We review a few examples here to illustrate the power of self-esteem in meaning making, starting with how defensively people respond to negative feedback.

Consider how people respond to simple information about the self. Miller (1976) asked research participants to take a test that supposedly measured how "perceptive" they were. The participants then received feedback about their test performance (they believed this feedback was real, though in reality it was provided to participants randomly). Some people were told they scored poorly (the results suggested they were relatively socially awkward and clueless), others were told they scored well (the results suggested they were relatively high-functioning socially). How do people make sense of themselves in light of this feedback, especially if they believe the test used to measure their perceptiveness was a well-established one? When the results provided negative feedback, this was damaging to their positive expectations (perhaps even threatening), and as a response the participants rationalized away the test result as due to bad luck on the test. This defensive reaction is even stronger among people who cared about their social competency deeply. In contrast, when positive feedback was received, the research participants believed they had learned valuable new information about themselves and their personal abilities. This result shows that when judging the self, the way we make sense of our qualities and actions is filtered through the lens of a need to enhance and protect self-esteem. Expectations that we will receive positive information about the self is strong, as is the desire to hear positive things, and these desires and expectations determine how receptive we are to new information, such as feedback from others about how positive or negative we are.

In a similar experiment, Sicoly and Ross (1977) gave research participants false feedback that led them to think they either succeeded or failed at a task. The participants next judged how much responsibility they felt they deserved for their performance on the task. The findings replicated those above, where participants saw success as due to their own personal abilities, but saw failure as due to something irrelevant to them (explain it away). This bolsters self-esteem by protecting it from negative feedback. However, this experiment added a new twist. Participants also received feedback from a third party who was supposedly observing the participant (actually another student who worked for the experimenters and provided false feedback). Some of the participants learned that the observer saw them as responsible, others learned that the observer saw them as not responsible. What do the participants think about the observers? When the observer states that the participant is responsible for a success, then the participant judges the observer to be accurate. However, when the observer states that the participant is responsible for a failure, the participant responds in a defensive way to protect self-esteem. Rather than accept threatening feedback from others, they instead dismiss the threat by challenging the reliability of the others; the observer is labeled as biased and inaccurate, and the validity of the test is questioned (it is flawed and untrustworthy). Vitriol and Moskowitz (2021) show that such defensiveness is even stronger when the feedback that threatens the self is in a domain important to the self-concept.

Negative feedback is especially threatening to self-esteem because it comes unexpectedly. Norms of interpersonal communication (e.g., Grice, 1975) prevent people from providing one another with negative feedback. Even if feedback is not entirely positive, it is then "sugarcoated" to not seem as bad (Rosen & Tesser, 1970). It is also the case that people create bubbles of positivity. They choose friends with similar views, they select media outlets that reinforce opinions and keep dissenting views away, they form online echo chambers to reinforce their beliefs, and follow people on Twitter who share their identity (e.g., Barberá, Jost, Nagler, Tucker, & Bonneau, 2015; Cinelli, Morales, Galeazzi, Quattrociocchi, & Starnini, 2021; Mosleh, Martel, Eckles, & Rand, 2021; Pariser, 2011; Pennycook & Rand, 2021; van der Linden, 2022). This is why any job that involves delivering accurate feedback (such as being a mentor) is difficult; one is critical when others are not, and one bumps up against others who expect praise and affirmation from a life spent in such a self-esteem bubble. Thus, people respond defensively to negative feedback when it shatters that bubble ("my mentor is a jerk!").

In modern times, "identity politics" and "tribalism" are terms with currency, and their importance ties directly to the fact that humans have *a need for positive identity*, a substantial portion of which is drawn from the groups with which we are associated (see Brewer, 1991; Tajfel & Turner, 1979). One person can derive identity from all of the following social groups: Americans, Jews, music lovers, Yankee fans, hikers, McGill graduates, Lehigh Valley residents, baseball/softball players, New Yorkers, academics, authors, homeowners, Beatle devotees, Liberals, cat lovers, fathers, summer camp alumni, brothers, Ivy leaguer, social psychologists, and so on. The groups we identify with serve to set our most important standards that we use when evaluating our abilities (e.g., Higgins, 1989) so that we derive pleasure when we meet those socially defined standards (and experience negative emotions when we do not live up to these self-guides). Thus, a good deal of our experience of self-esteem is linked to social comparisons made among groups—how we and our group members perform relative to others.

Perhaps the most famous illustration of the need for positive esteem is shown by **"minimal group"** studies in which people are randomly assigned to meaningless groups based on a trivial and pointless feature of their personality that they happen to share with others. This is described in more detail in Chapter 9. However, for the current discussion it is sufficient to say that people show an instinct to value such a random group over other randomly determined groups to which they do not belong. Tajfel, Billig, Bundy, and Flament (1971) showed that research participants show favoritism to others who share this (otherwise meaningless) identity. Of course, such favoritism is more extreme when the groups have

> **Minimal group:** A group to which one is assigned that has no meaningful basis for membership. It is based on either random assignment or agreement on something trivial (such as guessing the number of beans in a jar). Yet even these trivial or minimal groups create an identity that one is motivated to support.

meaning, and self-esteem is often achieved by denigrating groups to which we do not belong, or whom we see as competitors and rivals. In 1992, during the period I lived in New York City, David Dinkins was elected as the first African American mayor in the city's history. His opponent made the unprecedented claim that the election was fraudulent and the outcome should be overturned. Many of the voters who supported Dinkins's opponent came to believe that fraud was real, and they inspected the evidence of the election outcomes in a manner that led them to see the outcome as biased. They protected their self-esteem, and the threat to it caused by the loss to not only a Democrat, but the first Black mayor, by denigrating that mayor and the election that delivered him. "They cheated and stole the election" they cried. Despite no evidence, they were using elaborate cognitive processes to ignore some findings, and to exaggerate others, in order to reach the conclusion that protected their identity. To avoid such threats, we often strategically decide who to compare ourselves against, so that we seek to compare ourselves to groups of inferior others, safe in the knowledge we will come off positively in the comparison (e.g., Lambert & Klineberg, 1967).

Taylor and Brown (1988) alert us to the fact that promoting self-esteem is at times functional in that warding off negative self-views can promote stronger mental health. They highlight a set of **positive illusions** (unrealistic positive views of the self) that derive from the human need to have a positive identity and to feel positively about the self. They argue that rather than being a panacea, accuracy in how one views the self can contribute to depression, while positive illusions are important for maintaining well-being. This can filter down to low-level processing, such as seeing positive information more readily, or interpreting ambiguous information in a way that aligns itself with positive outcomes for the self. For example, Balcetis and Dunning (2006) had participants view the ambiguous

> **Positive illusions:** A need to experience a positive sense of esteem and identity creates unrealistic positive views of the self. This can filter down to low-level processing, such as more readily seeing positive information, or interpreting ambiguous information in a way that aligns itself with positive outcomes for the self.

drawing in Figure 1.3 that could be seen either as a horse's head or a seal's body. If positive outcomes for the self were created earlier in the experiment with the general category "farm animals," the drawing was more often interpreted as a horse. However, if negative outcomes for the self were associated with "farm animals" the drawing was more often seen as a seal. What we "see" aligns with self-esteem goals.

The Need for Social Connection

A popular introductory-level textbook in social psychology (e.g., Aronson, 1988) reminds us that humans, by their very nature, are a "social animal"—we need one another to survive. Not merely because the physical dangers and pleasures of the world are, respectively, best avoided and attained through the help of others (it is impossible to reproduce, for organisms like humans anyway, without the help of others; it is more difficult to defend oneself from harm if one is alone than if protected by a group or army; it is easier to get nourishment if some of us are hunting and others are gathering).

Additionally, humans have an emotional need to "belong" to something outside themselves, to commiserate and share experiences with others, to feel wanted/loved by a group such as a family, colleagues, a team, and so on (e.g., Baumeister & Leary, 1995). Humans **need to affiliate** with other people, not just for physical survival (which requires the ability to predict others' intentions and actions for purposes of coordination, as well as to develop trust for purposes of shared support) but for feeling connected with others via culture, norms, kinship, social support, and community. We have a need to feel as if one is approved of, loved, and belongs to a group of others that is larger than the self. This need to develop, affirm, and protect social relationships affects even basic information processing since individual thought is a product of social activity, directed by the norms of the culture we are linked to and the social bonds we seek to maintain (see Hardin & Conley, 2001, for a review of how affiliation needs connect with epistemic needs).

> **Need to affiliate:** A need to "belong" to something outside the self, to commiserate and share experiences with others, and to feel wanted/loved by a group. This promotes not just physical survival (which requires coordination and trust with others for shared support), but identification with others through culture, norms, kinship, social support, and community.

To deny the needs for love, identity, and community would be to remove oneself from human existence. Objects (like a rock) can exist void of these characteristics, but to be human requires a pursuit of the psychological need to affiliate, to deliver a sense of love and community that can only be attained through being linked to others (and that often delivers the unwanted negative consequences of this pursuit, such as loss of love, negative identity, and ostracism). The need to affiliate propels the search for meaning so that we may know who to approach and who to avoid when seeking love, identity, and community.

NAÏVE REALISM

As argued in this chapter, human perception and judgment is biased by social and contextual forces that shape how we see. Most people are easily convinced that their perception of objects can be distorted and biased. One need merely show them the Mueller–Lyer lines from Figure 1.4. Or ask them to do a thought experiment. Think of a time you saw a giant yellow moon creeping in your window, or a huge sun setting (my earliest memory is of a seemingly gargantuan sun on the horizon down the street where my great-grandparents lived in Brooklyn). Now consider the facts. Are the lines in Figure 1.4 different lengths? Has the size of the sun varied from moment to moment? No. Your perceptual system has distorted the image. We readily accept that objects, rigid and immutable objects, are perceived in a biased way. Our cognitive system allows us to see an object we know to be of one constant size (the sun) as changing in size, and it also allows us to preserve the constancy even if it appears to be changing (a ball that rolls closer to you does not seem to be larger, although the image on the retina suggests it is). This is unbothersome.

Now consider the personal qualities of people. They are far more ambiguous and subjective than judgments of the size of an object (like the moon, sun, or a ball). Surely, if one can accept that one is biased in how they see something as stable as objects, one can accept that one is obviously biased in how they see the personal qualities of other people. An assumption that we have perfect insight into a person's "essence" from observing their behavior (that they have characteristics that are simply revealed to us) might be deemed to be inappropriate given how biased we are when thinking about objects. Unfortunately, no. Our willingness to accept that we are sometimes anything less than rational, that we produce impressions that are not tied explicitly to the data provided, seems to be thrown out the window when it comes to perceiving people. This is what is called **naïve realism**. Ichheiser (1943) captured this point eloquently:

Naïve realism: A belief that we see what is real, even when believing other people are biased. It is a sense that our perceptual experience is valid; what we think about the qualities of other people is based on what they do and say, and not biased by what we think and feel.

The psychologically naive, unreflective person lives in the belief that he experiences and observes other people in an objective, unbiased way . . . not aware of the fact that certain processes [of misinterpretation] are at work within himself, which distort and falsify his experience of other people even on the level of immediate observation. It remains concealed from him that what he considers as "facts" is permeated by—and partly the result of . . . unconscious but nevertheless systematically proceeding misinterpretations. (pp. 145–146)

Most of us like to believe that there are inherent qualities about the people and things we come into contact with, and, through our experience with them, the properties and essential features that make up the "essence" of the observed person/thing are simply revealed to us. We have a blind spot when it comes to seeing that part of our cognitive experience is determined not by the properties of the object or person we have observed but by the social forces at work in the context where the observation occurs. Even if we know other people are biased, even if we know our perception of objects is biased, we naïvely believe that what we see in other people is real.[1]

Phenomenal Immediacy

Why are we perceivers naïve to the possibility of bias when judging other people? There are two prominent reasons. First, our knowledge is what we use to guide our behavior (thinking is for action), so we feel that it would obviously be ill-advised to do anything other than react to what would be considered factual properties and qualities. To acknowledge bias would be to acknowledge that we act inappropriately. And since we do typically act successfully (we are not usually called out for being wrong), this suggests to us that we typically are correctly receiving the signals that the stimuli are sending us and that the knowledge we possess comes from fact. Why accept we are routinely biased if we routinely seem to be acting appropriately!

Second, our psychological experience of the world is typically one of **phenomenal immediacy**. Our perception and meaning making happens so quickly, without us being able to see our role in how it develops, that our knowledge of a stimulus just feels as if it "pops into the head" as if it is just something true revealed to us by the stimulus—that is, our experience seems to us to be that we simply receive the sensations that stimuli provide to us. Thus, a bagel has certain essential features that tell us "this object is a bagel" and also tell us what we can do with it. We know what it is and what it does, because it tells us. This sense of phenomenal immediacy hides from us the true nature of cognition. It does not feel like social forces are at play or that what we think is in the service of our action plans. These forces remain invisible to us, creating a false or naïve sense of realism that what we perceive and know is an unbiased reflection of the outer world. When we have the sense that a politician is a liar, or that our grandfather is a respectable man, this knowledge seems to us to be facts dictated to us by the qualities of the people in question. It seems to us as if our role is to observe what they have done, and the essential knowledge about them is revealed to us by their words and deeds.

> **Phenomenal immediacy:** Our perception and meaning making happens so quickly, without us seeing our role in how it develops, that our knowledge of a stimulus just feels as if it "pops into the head," as if it is just something true revealed to us by the stimulus. Our experience is that stimuli are received, transcribed, and known with such immediacy that our knowing must be due solely to the properties of the stimulus, not our processing.

Is that a horse or a seal? Is the woman young or old? These seem like judgments that should be unambiguous and clear, dictated to us by the features we observe. Yet as Balcetis and Dunning (2006) showed us, perception is not so clear-cut. Whether we see a horse depends on our goals relating to farm animals. Yet we often fail to see how easily our perceptual experience is altered. And judgments of the qualities of people are far more complex than perceiving whether an animal is a horse, or an object is constant in size. Thus, with such judgments we are even more likely to feel that people are, simply, what their actions are telling us they are, failing to realize that we are instead seeing what we want to see (e.g., Dunning & Balcetis, 2013). Prior to conscious knowing is the constant whir of what was defined above as *automatic processes*. Because such thinking is invisible and not open to our conscious inspection, we do not see when it is directed from the top-down. Phenomenally, what we experience is an immediate impression that feels so fast as to be unvarnished.

Let us consider two examples where bias is hard to see because it infiltrates the lowest levels of cognition, and the judgment simply feels immediate. Using visual attention as the low-level process under investigation, Chiao, Heck, Nakayama, and Ambady (2006) conducted an experiment that illustrated how one's identity guided attention. In their case they were interested in exploring the influence of racial identity, and they specifically chose to study individuals who had multiple racial identities. Participants who identified as biracial were perfect for showing how attention shifts with identity because they can have one of their two identities made salient. Chiao and colleagues could look to see if what their participants pay attention to in a visual display changes as their identity changes. To manipulate identity, the participants were asked to write an essay about one of their parents, with some people writing about their White parent (thus triggering their own White identity) and some writing about their Black parent (thus triggering their own Black identity). With one of these identities made salient in this way, they next performed a visual attention task. The task asked them to observe a group of faces and to identify whether there was one face in the set that was of a different race from the others. They repeated this task multiple times, with some of the times the faces being of all the same race, and other times there being one that was not the same race as the others. For example, a set of faces might have seven faces of Black people and one face of a White person. At other times the set might have five faces of White people and one face of a Black person. And so on. All people were particularly adept at identifying a Black person's face among a set of White people. But *their speed of identific*ation was especially fast when one's identity as a Black person had been triggered. Racial identity determines which faces one is able to identify most quickly by lowering the threshold of visual attention to make faces that align with one's identity easier to detect. Chaio et al. conclude:

Biracials primed with their White identity showed a visual search advantage of similar magnitude to White [people], whereas biracials primed with their Black identity had a greater visual
search advantage, similar to that of Black [people]. These findings demonstrate that visual perception is malleable to top-down influences. (p. 391)

Despite this response clearly being biased by the participant's own racial identity, they
see no bias. The response feels immediate and uninfluenced. They are naïve to their biased
attention.

A similar illustration can be made using perception rather than attention (e.g.,
Niedenthal, Halberstadt, & Setterlund, 1997). Clinical research has shown that items that
people fear loom larger in their perceptual experience. For example, people with a spider
phobia perceive the speed of a spider moving toward them as faster when compared to
people without such a fear (Riskind, Moore, & Bowley, 1995). Similarly, people who were
afraid of spiders saw a spider as relatively closer to them as compared with people who were
not afraid of spiders (Cole, Balcetis, & Dunning, 2013). It is not just spiders. Does a broad
social force such as one's identity group have a similar effect? Will groups of people who are
perceived as threats to our identity group seem larger in number, or closer to us, or moving toward us more quickly, or lingering longer? Xiao and Van Bavel (2012) examined this
question by looking at identification with a sports team and also looking at identification
with one's country. For example, it was found that people who strongly identify as Americans, and who belong to groups in American society that stress immigration as a threat
to America, perceive Mexico and Mexican people as closer and as larger. When compared
against Americans with less of an identification to their American identity, or Americans
less threatened by immigration, they found that (1) Mexican immigrants coming across the
border into the United States were perceived to be doing so in larger numbers, and (2) Mexican cities were perceived to be closer to the United States than reality dictated. A similar
distortion is found with identification with a team. For example, fans of the New York Yankees were approached at Yankee stadium before a game against the hated Boston Red Sox.
They were asked to perceive the distance (by placing pins on a map provided for them) from
Yankee stadium to the stadium in Boston and the stadium of another baseball team that is
less hated (the Baltimore Orioles). At the time of the study the Yankees were in first place,
Boston in second, and the Orioles woeful in last place. They found that for people without
any relevant identity (fans of teams that were neither Yankees nor Red Sox) there was no
bias in their perception of the distance from New York to Boston or New York to Baltimore.
However, for people who identified as fans of the Yankees, they incorrectly perceived the stadium in Boston as closer to New York compared to their perception of the distance between
New York and Baltimore (in reality Boston is 20 miles farther away).

The Threat Created When Naïve Realism Is Pointed Out

When discussing self-esteem needs above, we noted that people are defensive about receiving negative feedback. And feedback that one is biased can most certainly be interpreted
as a threat. Indeed, at this point, there are likely objections growing in some readers that
bias is not as pervasive as described here, and they are not naïve regarding what they think
and feel. After all, our ability to not only think, but to think deeply, and to *reflect* on our
thinking, is what signifies being human. We all can inspect and examine our own thinking. Thinking is one thing all people have experience with, and that experience tells us
that our knowledge is not "made." When we feel as if we know something, we can trust
that it is useful and true since we have confidence in what we think by being able to point

to our ability to reflect on and verify our thinking. To argue that thinking is biased, or that our knowledge is misinformed or shaped, seems to be an affront since it suggests that we are naïve about something we easily and often reflect on (and when we reflect, an influence is hardly ever detected). Descartes famously said, "I think, therefore I am." Therefore, to suggest that thinking is biased is to suggest that I am biased. Most people see this as defying their own experience. Through self-examination we can see we are *not* biased. To argue otherwise would mean that we are wrong about something deeply personal; this is a threat.

This security and confidence people have in the sanctity of their thinking is what makes psychology a difficult area of study. People feel as if their mind is an open book, fully explored over the course of a lifetime, with little need for scientific investigation except for those instances in which the mind appears to "malfunction." It is for this reason that most people think of psychology as the study of psychopathology, or equate psychology with "abnormal" or clinical psychology. Even in modern times, with advances in neuroscientific methods, many still see these advances as providing a clearer window into pathology to better understand conditions such as Parkinson's disease, aphasia, depression, addiction, brain lesions, and so on. But much of psychology is about the study of everyday thinking—the so-called normal state of cognition and emotion. And our own naïve understanding of our own thinking clouds what we are willing to accept about typical cognitive processes. While we have the ability to engage in reflection, and to think about our own thinking, this does not mean we can accurately see how the mind is working. As we review in Chapter 3, when Nisbett and Wilson (1977) asked people to describe how they "know what they know" in order to study the accuracy of self-reflection, they found that people simply have a false and inaccurate understanding of how their own knowledge is produced. They have a blind spot for seeing their own biases (e.g., Pronin, 2007, 2008; Scopelliti et al., 2015).

The social cognition revolution challenged this naïve understanding of their own thinking held by most people. Yes, we all can think deeply and can think with great powers of reasoning. Yes, we can reflect on our own thinking and inspect it for flaws. However, people know very little about their own thinking, so reflection yields inaccurate assessments. This is unpleasant to learn, violates our own experience, so it is often taken as a threat.

CONCLUSIONS

Social cognition is the study of the processes involved in perceiving one another and the social environment, how we come to know and feel about the world. It has its focus on the nature of the processes, the structures that support these processes, and the influences from social forces exerted at every stage of cognition. It is the study of *how* people make sense of the social world through their low- and high-level cognitive processing, biased as it is by the culture, values, ideology, goals, beliefs, and other representational structures that constrain and guide how those processes occur. It is the study of how meaning is "made," and how that meaning is shaped by biases introduced by us being social animals embedded in social groups. What separates social cognition as a discipline from the sister disciplines from whence its name derives (social psychology and cognitive psychology) is not a distinction in the type of stimuli studied but in the type of questions asked. It blends questions about processing mechanisms that underlie cognitive psychology with questions about the influence of social forces from social psychology.

Social cognition may best be understood as the result of a collision between two powerful forces of the 20th century. One of these forces is the American pragmatist tradition with its emphasis on how thinking has a purpose. The other is the European Gestalt psychology tradition that emphasized how meaning is produced from the context in which stimuli are embedded. This merger provided a way to think about the construction of meaning that allowed for social context to be seen as a powerful organizing force around which processing is structured. The same act, such as telling a joke, can be perceived entirely differently if told at a party or during an animal-rights protest. The meaning shifts from funny to insensitive and stupid as the context and social goals shift. These forces determine what others think of you, changing the most basic ways in which they process your behavior and the inferences they make about you.

By allowing for an understanding of how we think, and how thinking can be less transparent than we believe, social cognition provides a road map to helping control or reverse the ills that (undetected) flaws in our thinking can inflict on society. Many of the century's greatest social problems—stereotyping, prejudice, discrimination, misinformation—have roots in cognition. The ability to see one group of people as less human than another, or the ability to see the ideological systems of another group as entirely flawed and immoral, only emerges because of the social lenses through which the very understanding of the people and events in our world are filtered and meaning about them is delivered. These meanings are delivered so effortlessly, so easily, that we believe them to be inherent truths about the world and not meanings we have built in a top-down way. This makes us incalcitrant about our convictions. Solutions to such ills are going to be harder to find if they do not incorporate the psychology at the root. While social cognition is grounded in low-level processing, it touches all we know and all we do.

From this opening chapter we see two central themes of this book emerge. The first is that humans have a need to belong to social groups to bring them a sense of identity and esteem, and from those "identity groups" they derive a sense of what is appropriate (normative) and a sense of self-worth. The second is that humans have a need to understand the world around them and to see meaning in the environment so that they know what is appropriate to do and say and feel in that moment. Often that meaning is inherent and clear from the social situation, but often the meaning is projected onto the situation by the person through the use of their personal preferences to "make sense" out of ambiguity. We see a certain symbiosis in these two themes. To survive it is imperative to know how to act, and what to do, and to see meaning in and understand the events and people around you. However, to exact such meaning we might need to rely on the norms, goals, prior beliefs, stereotypes, attitudes, and values of the very people and groups we are attempting to understand. We need to have an understanding of the situation to know how to act appropriately with other people, but we need to belong to groups of other people to have the foundational knowledge to tell us what is appropriate and to "make sense" when it is not inherently clear.

This discussion of the distortion of cognition by social forces is not to suggest there is no "truth," or that all cognition is flawed and error prone. It is simply to say that thinking is merely one basic feature of being human. Another is that we are social animals that are interdependent on one another for survival. Social forces define and shape every aspect of our humanity, including our thinking. We can know precisely how many immigrants come to the United States from Mexico each year. Yet, our perception of how many immigrants arrive over the Mexican border each year need not be tethered to the actual number. It can be seen as a drip or a caravan. Even if tethered to the actual number, the threat experienced in relation to that number may depend on who is President. If it is my person, I may see immigration as being dealt with; if it is the other side's person I may see the same number as a problem indicative of larger mismanagement.

The notion that we need thinking to imbue meaning on people and objects reveals that as perceivers we must be careful to note that meaning is not purely inherent in any given person or object or situation. It is constructed, or built, from the evidence that is available meeting our perceptual apparatus. We must constantly "check ourselves" to be aware of how our point of view is partly determining what we know to be true. One reason this occurs is out of necessity—information comes at us in such large amounts, at such a fast pace, that a structure needs to be imposed on it to make sense of it (what we earlier called a problem of limited capacity and cognitive load). Another reason this occurs is out of efficiency—even if not overburdened by perceptual overload, we still have a lifetime of experience to ease the process of "sense making." Our goals, our culture, our prior experience not only make low-level processing easier but infuse it with prior learning that allows us to "know" a stimulus without elaborate reflection (what we earlier called satisficing); we even go beyond the information given to know things not yet seen.

When the data/stimuli are strong, such distortion is often weak. The stimulus affords a particular meaning and dictates a particular way to respond to it. But such information, even that which is abundantly clear, is still filtered through our low-level cognition, which invisibly alters what we experience, aligning it with the social forces that we bring to the perceptual experience. A person highly motivated to see a stimulus as otherwise is able to use their cognitive apparatus to do so. As with the election of Mayor Dinkins described above, there was no evidence for fraud. The stimulus was clear. Yet those who desired to see Dinkins lose confidently believed they saw it.

While many social situations are quite clear in the social pressure that is being exerted (such as when an authority figure demands you to act), or in the behavior that is being observed (such as when someone assaults another person violently, or highly regulated voting procedures are impeccably implemented), many other situations are far less clear. Social pressures are often difficult to detect (such as when a person conforms to what their parents would want them to do, even when their parents are not present). And much of the information we receive from our social world is by nature ambiguous and uncertain. Was that an insult or a compliment? Did our keynote speaker just endorse violence or merely vocalize disapproval with the status quo? Was I selected ahead of another person (for a job, admission to college, a bank loan, etc.) because of superior performance or because of a bias in the selection process? When the data/stimuli are weaker in this way, where ambiguity exists, the opportunity for distortion from social forces, for top-down processing, is greater. The opportunity for error is greater. What we know is that even when these types of ambiguity exist, we perceivers still manage to see clearly and confidently. This is because the social groups to which we belong—our culture, our political identity, our religious upbringing, and so on—will minimize the uncertainty and force a particular way of seeing the social event so that it seems as if it was never ambiguous at all. For example, to the person whose social groups have always held a privileged status in society, the ambiguity inherent in why they have been selected for a job over another person is not experienced. They unambiguously see their inherent worth and superior performance. From ambiguity, they see clarity, and hence they can confidently feel they know how to act. Social forces will shape the type of clarity that emerges from ambiguity.

NOTE

1. Such naïveté makes us especially susceptible to manipulation and propaganda. So much of the behavior we observe in others is ambiguous and leaves itself open to interpretation, yet

we fail to see that we are interpreting through a lens of what our culture or needs or influencers would have us believe. Thus, even when we are manipulated into thinking we see one thing, we remain steadfast that we have not been manipulated. This is bad enough when the behavior of others is ambiguous and our judgment is being biased, but this is even worse when the manipulation is to the behavior itself. In modern times the behavior we observe can be falsified through deep fakes, where people appear to do or say things that never actually happened. If we fail to see a biased view of another person when their behavior is ambiguous, this naivete is only magnified when we are tricked to think a person is doing something unambiguous.

CHAPTER 2

We Create Internal Mental Representations of External Reality

When I moved to Munich to work as a research scientist following graduate school in New York, I did not speak the language or have any experience with the culture. Yet I had no problem navigating from the airport to my apartment arranged for me by the Max Planck Institute. In my first weeks there, I had no difficulty using subways and buses to get around the city, shopping for food, going to restaurants, or knowing the norms about how to behave at work. The knowledge and experience gathered over a lifetime in two cultures (New York and Montreal) was able to be translated to the new culture and allowed me to know how to predict what to expect and how to act appropriately. In 2 years there, my past experience got me into trouble only once. That was at 7 A.M. on a Sunday morning when riding in an entirely empty subway train. A police officer informed me that I was in the incorrect empty car (I learned from the officer that there were first-class subway cars, and for sitting in first class without a first-class ticket I received a fine). I had a faulty mental representation of German "subways." However, my mental representation for police officers was correct. He ticketed me despite the fact that I was not trying to sneak into first class to escape crowded and unpleasant conditions elsewhere on the train; every other car was also empty. Intentions are the domain of courts, laws are the domain of officers, and I broke one (unintentionally). The question for this chapter concerns how we know about categories such as officers, subways, grocery stores, restaurants, and how to act at work. This chapter examines how the information we have learned is organized and represented in the mind.

The first point to be made is that we build knowledge through experience and learning. As infants, our experiences with the outside world and early learning are represented in the mind to serve as the foundation for more complex ideas. Much of that early learning is from bodily states and sensation. We develop more complex knowledge through **associations** that are formed among the information learned through experience. Associations start as links that connect two constructs (such as physical warmth and safety). An association is about how separate pieces of related information are stored and linked in memory. Eventually, the association that

> **Associations:** Links among information learned and stored in memory. These links connect two constructs with varying degrees of strength.

develops among items links them in complex chains of associated constructs—what is known as an **associative network**. Thus, one piece of represented knowledge, such as information about professional athletes, is linked to associated features such as competitiveness, persistence, strength, intelligence, intensity, health consciousness, agility, and wealth (see Figure 2.1). Wealth then might be associated closely with features such as nice cars, charity, philanthropy, expensive homes, gold and diamond jewelry, tax evasion, and job creation. In such a network, two closely associated links (such as fast and agile) will trigger each other easily, but even more distally related items (such as fast and wealthy) can trigger each other as activation spreads along the network. These links can vary in strength. Stronger associations exist for more closely related constructs (such as fast and agile, bread and butter, doctor and nurse) than for more remotely related constructs (such as fast and wealthy, bread and soup, doctor and debt).

> **Associative network:** Any construct is associated with multiple other constructs, with the entire set of related constructs being interlinked in a network.

Spreading activation is the idea that when one item in an associative network is retrieved from memory, it brings the related information to bear as well. While close associates may be triggered more strongly and quickly, even more distal associations will be activated. Activation and spreading activation is perhaps best thought of as a process of retrieval from memory. Once one item is retrieved (such as interpersonal warmth), other items associated with it (such as notions of trustworthiness or helpfulness) are retrieved or activated, as well (e.g., Collins & Loftus, 1975). Much of the early history of social cognition was concerned with examining how mental systems represent the external world by combining information into associated networks. When we associate disparate pieces of information, how do these associations cluster and take shape, and how does the nature of the representation impact thinking? Will activation spread along an associative network, and how does the increased prevalence of those items then impact how new information is understood, absorbed, and integrated? Is the existing representation altered and updated?

> **Spreading activation:** Due to their connection in a network, two associated constructs trigger one another as well as other constructs linked in the network. When one item in an associative network is retrieved from memory, it brings related information to bear as well. One need not consciously experience this triggering of constructs.

This chapter explores the different types of representational structures that organize our vast network of knowledge. It is important to state at the start that we are not

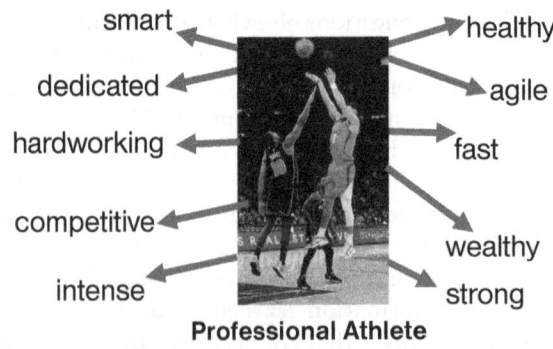

Professional Athlete

FIGURE 2.1. Associations among a category (athlete) and features that can form a network.

approaching these issues the way a neuroscientist might. In fact, to date, neuroscience has not taught us how the physical workings of the brain produce our knowledge or the conscious experience of knowing. It is certainly not being argued that the way the mind knows about "athletes" is through a little picture of a basketball player being connected through physical links in a net, as depicted in Figure 2.1. This is a metaphor of one way the organization of knowledge can be conceptualized (regardless of the yet unknown realities of how the mind physically links information). Without direct access to the actual brain processes, social cognition aims to use behavioral measures to gain insight into how we organize information, since it is believed that the nature of the organization constrains how we think and what we infer. Throughout the chapter we explore different types of organization, with the term "**schema**" being used to refer to the broad notion of a mental representation containing related and associated knowledge. More specific types of organizational possibilities are also presented. For example, the exemplar notion proposes that the structure contains mostly lists of examples of the category: specific events, episodes, or individuals. No one example defines the category, but there may be some examples that are more typical than others. In contrast, the notion of prototype describes an organizational structure that contains connected sets of attributes that describe a typical category member. It sum-

> **Schema:** A structure or mental representation, stored in memory, that organizes all the knowledge one possesses about a class or category. This can include specific detailed memories of features or behaviors that were learned, as well as abstractions that summarize the class, such as a trait or characteristic.

marizes the set of most probable attributes to be found in a category member, but also represents the less probable features. A theory is an organizational structure that focuses not simply on associated features but the relationships among them that explain why they are associated. It contains propositions that specify the nature of the relationships among the associated concepts. Theorists have argued over which type of structure best captures reality, and why this debate matters.

SCHEMAS, PROTOTYPES, AND EXEMPLARS

The term "schema" was introduced by Bartlett (1932), a cognitive psychologist who proposed that *schemas* were mental representations in which an abstracted set of prior knowledge about a class of people or events was stored. It is a structure in memory that organizes the knowledge one has about a category. Bartlett used the category of "story" in his research, arguing that a schema for a story includes specific elements that everyone in the culture would learn and use when a story was being told. A new story is easy to follow and comprehend because it follows a form familiar to the person. However, what happens when the schema is not being followed and the information one is learning is hard to fit to a schema? For example, stories from other cultures can have content and form that is unusual to the perceiver and that do not fit one's schema about how stories unfold. In this case, Bartlett found that such stories from a culture different from one's own will evolve when the story is told from one person to the next. Each person telling it will alter the story to make it more typical to their culture, to fit their schema for stories, with the story becoming more coherent each time it is retold. This increased coherence came with a loss of original detail and content. Bartlett argued that people learn new stories through a context of the expectations and prior beliefs already held in memory about "stories" as a category, and this served to distort an unusual story to fit the existing "structure," or schema. Schemas alter the way information is encoded and remembered, thus leading, in the case of the Bartlett research, to the production of stories that are unintentionally distorted to be consistent with the schema.

Schemas are not limited to knowledge of stories. We have schemas about any category, including people, even including schemas about the self. Markus (1977) suggested that the self-concept is simply a schema containing all of the information about the self; qualities such as values, traits, goals, and beliefs, as well as concrete behaviors one has previously performed. Thus, schemas can contain features that are in an *abstract form* (see Chapter 1, Figure 1.1A); *concrete behaviors* observed when interacting with specific people, objects, or events (see Figure 1.1B), as well as specific examples drawn from past experience (also called exemplars). A schema describes generalized *types* as well as specific instances. For example, a schema for athletes calls to mind a set of abstracted attributes and concrete behaviors, or it might call to mind specific examples of athletes we know (e.g., Roger Federer, Tiger Woods, Michael Jordan). Since it contains culturally shared knowledge as well as personal beliefs, two individuals can have different schemas for the same construct, as depicted for athletes in Figure 2.2.

In addition, a schema is also defined by having contained within it the *relationships* that exist among the features (Fiske & Linville, 1980; Fiske & Taylor, 1991; Taylor & Crocker, 1981). In this way schemas provide more than a taxonomy of features, but they also provide an understanding of the rules that govern the connections between the features. They contain both associations among individual pieces of information in memory as well as propositional knowledge about the relationship among those items (e.g., De Houwer, 2009, 2014a, 2014b). For example, on the right in Figure 2.2 the person knows more than just to associate persistence with competitiveness, but that the schema for athlete specifies a relationship—competitiveness causes persistence. One final defining feature of a schema is that it will impact the processing of information about a person, event, or place in a way that leads you to see and remember information about the person, event, or place in a manner that is consistent with the schema (e.g., Fiske & Linville, 1980). A purpose of having abstract knowledge about a class of "things" is that it allows one to absorb and assimilate new information into that class, so that the features of the class can be imbued on it, and meaning achieved somewhat easily and effortlessly. New information (such as how to ride a subway in Munich) can be understood through the lens provided by the abstracted representation

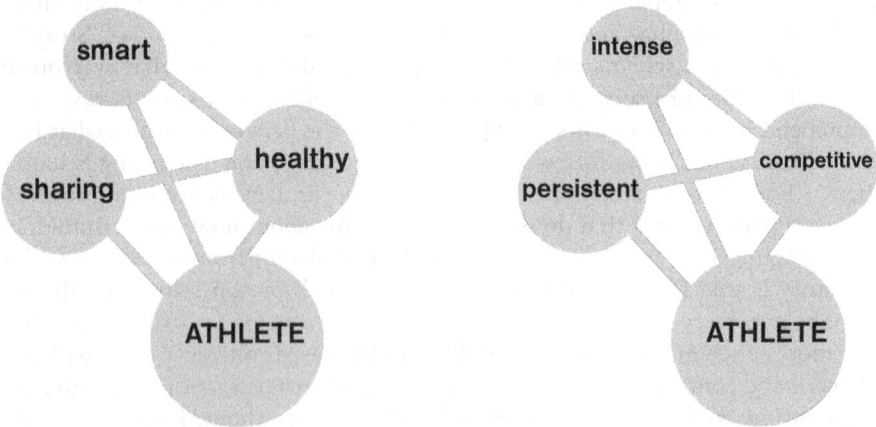

FIGURE 2.2. Schemas of "athletes" for two different persons.

(subways). That which is difficult, alien, and complex is rendered knowable and actionable. In this way we see the principles discussed in Chapter 1 at work—experience in the world leads to associations to develop in a bottom-up way, but once those associations are structured in schemas, they exert a top-down influence on new learning.

The Features and Functions of Our Mental Representations

Regardless of how one conceptualizes the types of information associated in the network, most descriptions of mental representations (prototypes, exemplars, theories, etc.) share some *common features* in describing the structure. The first commonality is that they are mental representations of *socially shared* knowledge about classes of people, events, and things that exist in the world. The second is that the representation *need not be accurate* in representing people, events, or things—they are what the culture associates with the class. Third, representations are *"fuzzy sets" of items* in that they stipulate some central items and some more peripheral items, with items at the edge of the periphery being hard to determine whether they belong in the set. For example, the category "pet" might have central items such as dogs, cats, and birds. However, with more peripheral items—skinks, snakes, pigs, and rats—it becomes hard to determine whether they belong in the category. A fourth shared feature is that the items in the set are part of an associative network, and *activation can spread within a network* from one item to others. The category "pet" will trigger thoughts of dogs, cats, and birds. Finally, they all allow for *making a probabilistic inference* about whether a new person or thing should be categorized as a member of the class.

In addition to these common features that describe the representation, there are also *common functions* that are provided by having such representations. First, *they provide meaning* to any member of the class *through inferences* about membership in the class. Each member is inferred to possess (quickly and easily) the central qualities that are associated with the class, and information is processed faster when it is relevant to a mental representation. For example, regardless of whether one's representation of "Canadian" is a prototype or an exemplar, the inferences associated with the category provide one with a sense (accurate or not) that one knows something about the person by virtue of category membership (such as they celebrate on July 1).

Second, being in possession of such meaning *allows one to make predictions* about what other qualities to expect—what is likely to happen when interacting with a person who fits the representation (such as a role schema) or when entering a situation that fits the representation (such as a place schema). Relatedly, these representations *allow one to fill in the gaps* when information is missing or when information is confusing (such as with stories from a different culture). I may not have been provided with the information, but I can fill in the gaps and believe that by virtue of being Canadian the person celebrates Thanksgiving in October. And I may incorrectly believe that this information was provided for me, rather than filled in by me.

Next, mental representations guide how one will act by *allowing one to generalize* from the category to a specific instance that one has encountered (provide a direction for instrumental activity; a plan for how to act). For example, I might infer that a Canadian colleague working with me in the United States has no plans on the fourth Thursday in November, when Thanksgiving in the United States is celebrated, and invite them over; I might not invite a colleague from the United States because of the probabilistic inference that they have plans. Finally, mental representations provide one with *a sense of control* over the environment through the predictions and meaning that result.

Now that we have reviewed the general concept of a schema, and its functions and features, we turn next to the types of schemas that exist.

Prototypes versus Exemplars

When conceptualizing a mental representation, one could take what is called a **probabilistic view** in which there is not a list of required features that are singly necessary and jointly sufficient. Instead, the attributes that describe any given member of a category are not deemed to be necessary but represent qualities that could be expected to be found in this category of "thing" with some degree of probability. There is a central tendency that contains the most typical features to be found in most category members (that are most probable to be found in a category member), and then other less central features that are likely in some category members but not others. A **prototype** is a mental representation with this type of structure. It comprises the features most typical of the category, yet this set of most common features also contains associations to less probable features (e.g., Kihlstrom & Klein, 1994). An example will help make this distinction clear: "birds tend to fly, sing, and be small, but there are a few large, flightless, songless birds. The category prototype is some instance, real or imagined, that has a large number of these typical features" (p. 160). Ostriches and penguins are not prototypical birds since they lack central features, though they are members of the category "birds" and our schema for birds applies to them. They just have fewer prototypical features. Thus, flight as a feature is not necessary to be a bird. But it is highly likely, or a central feature. Person categories can also be prototypes. As Cantor and Mischel (1979) remarked:

> **Probabilistic view:** When conceptualizing a mental representation, a view in which there are not required features that are singly necessary and jointly sufficient. Instead, attributes that describe any given member of the category are qualities that could be expected to be found in this category of "thing" with some degree of probability.

> **Prototype:** Mental representation that captures the probabilities of the specified features being present for a category member, rather than listing sets of required features that must be present. It specifies most typical features, but allows for less probable features to also be characteristic of category members, such as flightless birds.

> Clearly it would be difficult to find a set of necessary and sufficient features shared by all members of any particular person category that one would want to use as the definitive test of category membership. For example . . . some extraverts seem primarily dominating and active rather than warm and sociable. (p. 11)

Because prototypes are abstractions of sets of likely features derived from personal experience, two individuals can have different prototypes for the same category (different mental images of what the typical category member looks like, or what the central tendency of the category looks like). Despite the fact that prototypes can differ in content from person to person, they do not differ in function. The role of prototypes in how we think is to help us make inferences about what categories people and things belong to, and with category membership comes knowledge of expected features, behaviors, and attitudes.

Cantor and Mischel (1977) proposed that a "prototype seems to function as a standard around which a body of input is compared and in relation to which new input is assimilated into the set of items to be remembered about a given experience or list of stimuli" (p. 39). They argued that if a trait category or group type is used as a label for a person (e.g., geek, jock, princess, misfit, delinquent), then we think they have the other central features that make up the prototype for that group or trait. If so, they will use the prototypes to generate missing information (fill in the gaps in their knowledge) and to generate additional information (inferences) about the person. Thus, information not explicitly observed will be confused with information actually presented because of their association in a mental structure. Their research (reviewed in Chapter 4) shows exactly these types of errors. When people form impressions of others, they use the features detected to help them "type" the person. The features of the prototype that match the person are then activated and used to additionally describe the person, thus biasing one's memory of the person.

The prototype view of mental representation can be contrasted with a description of cognitive structures that consist of **exemplars**. Medin (1989) suggests that categories do not consist of summaries of highly probable features of the typical member, but of specific examples of actual members. Thus, rather than there being an abstracted sense of the sorts of features a typical athlete might possess, the category "athlete" would instead be conceived of as a set of actual athletes one has encountered in one's experience: *exemplars*. When an exemplar exists for a single person, the representation contains examples of features and behaviors of that individual

Exemplars: A mental representation that specifies examples of the category as opposed to probable features. From the examples that exist, one can create an image of the shared features and traits, rather than storing those abstractions directly.

that can range from being a fairly complete list of that specific person's features to one marked by only a few key features descriptive of the person (e.g., Smith & Zarate, 1992). One's concept of one's mother is likely a fairly detailed and complete exemplar, and one's exemplar for Elon Musk is likely inhabited by only a few central attributes. Each exemplar, however, is stored in your mind, as merely reading "mother" and "Elon Musk" likely brought specific images to mind.

Smith and Zarate (1992) suggest that exemplars are stored representations of specific events and people (representing certain types or attributes) that are accessed, typically without one's conscious awareness, and that influence judgment. This view is best summarized with the assumption that "the perceiver has many cognitive representations of persons (exemplars). Each representation includes not only encoded perceptual attributes of the person but also the perceiver's inferences, attributions, and reactions. When the perceiver encounters a new target person, information from stored representations that are similar to the target will be used to make judgments." Which exemplars are retrieved and used is determined by many contextual factors, and the way in which a person is judged and treated, therefore, will be dependent on the exemplar to which that person is being compared. For example, an Israeli professor is an example of someone who could be categorized according to relevant exemplars of Israelis or professors. The context can help to determine which category is most likely to be triggered and what types of exemplars will impact on processing. If the person is encountered at a statistics lecture in front of the class, perhaps the "professor" exemplar will be most salient and determine how this person is categorized and ultimately evaluated/judged.

Thus, when categorizing, if the current person matches or fits the exemplars from a given category, that category is used to describe the new person. According to Lingle, Altom, and Medin (1984), "a new item will be identified as a category member if it cues the retrieval of a critical number of exemplar representations from the category and does so before cuing the retrieval of a criterial number of exemplar representations from some contrasting category" (p. 91). The process is one of comparison between specific instances or examples. Medin, Altom, and Murphy (1984) argue that the exemplar view better represents category structure because it can go beyond the prototype view in explaining how categories function. They argue that variability within a category is not captured well by prototypes. For example, restaurants differ in terms of how the bill is paid, with sometimes the money going to the server and other times being brought directly to the cashier. People know that when a restaurant has a counter with stools (such as a diner) it is likely to be one where the cashier is paid, but when a restaurant has candles on the table (such as a five-star restaurant) it is likely one where the server will collect the money. This variability is easily captured by a representation that stores examples of restaurants one has encountered. It is not as easily captured by a representation that has an abstracted list of typical restaurant features (of course, one merely needs to conceive of adding propositional statements that describe the relationship among features to a prototype to give it the same flexibility as an exemplar).

As elaborated upon in Chapters 9 and 10, these distinctions between mental representations that are organized as prototypes versus exemplars are not mere theoretical points. If a specific example is retrieved from memory to serve as the organizing structure for new information, it creates a very specific standard against which that information is compared. Exemplars as standards have different effects on the evaluation of the person than when a more abstract set of traits is used as the organizing structure for making sense of new information. For instance, exemplars (such as Michael Jordan) impact how we interpret the behavior of another person differently from a prototype representing the same construct (such as professional athlete) does. Exemplars like Michael Jordan are likely to make our new person seem to pale in terms of their athleticism. The same behavior from the same person is seen as less athletic when compared against Michael Jordan than if the prototype "athlete" had been used when judging it. The behavior being judged will likely be seen as having exaggerated differences when compared to an exemplar, since the exemplar is an extreme instantiation of the category. Prototypes, being more ambiguous by nature, are less likely to trigger this reaction. One seems far more dissimilar to Michael Jordan than to an abstract athlete. Heider (1944) noted this type of perceptual contrast effect using the language of Gestalt psychology: The exemplar serves as the context, or ground, against which the figural behavior is evaluated. Like the outer circles in the Ebbinghaus illusion that creates a contrast with the inner circle, the exemplar creates a standard against which the new behavior is judged, and the evaluation is biased to seem unlike the standard. Michael Jordan is like the outer circles setting an extreme standard, and the target person being evaluated is like the inner circle, the perception of which seems unlike the standard by comparison. Exemplars serve as a standard against which a comparison is made. Prototypes can also serve as standards against which a comparison is made, but the contrast is less sharp. This is because the standard being used is vague and abstract, such as the prototype for "athlete," as compared to the narrow and specific standard of an exemplar. Comparison to something narrow and specific often creates a sense of contrast between the two, whereas comparison to something vague and abstract allows for seeing similarity between the two. Thus, the same behavior of a person we are evaluating might be deemed less athletic if compared against Jordan, and more athletic if compared against the more vague concept of professional athlete. The narrower, more exclusive, and more distinctive the mental representation being used to help impose meaning on new information, the more likely the judgment will seem different from that representation. An exemplar possesses features. Prototypes do not; they are abstract concepts (e.g., Moskowitz & Skurnik, 1999).

This logic holds for negative qualities as well. Consider the schema for the quality "racist" or "prejudiced person." When we hold out an exemplar such as the Ku Klux Klan (KKK), it sets an extremely narrow (and extreme) definition. When we compare our own behavior against this standard we pale by comparison and we reassure ourselves we are not racist, not even close. When we hold out a more abstract prototype—such as a list of traits or behaviors describing a person who can act in a way that favors one group and negatively discriminates against another—we can now see some similarities to the self that would never be possible with the exemplar. Most of us can recognize that we favor some groups over others, and that we at times avoid a person because we think the interaction might be uncomfortable because of differences we perceive. This is not to say we label ourselves racist but we allow for more similarity among self and "prejudiced" than we would for self and "KKK member." In this way, using an exemplar to define the schema "racist" reduces one's own sense of being responsible in any way for racism in society. Pointing out racist and sexist examples is important, but it must be done in a way that does not reduce individual responsibility for the problem; that shifts accountability entirely to extremely negative exemplars, or "bad people." Bad people as exemplars can create contrast when assessing the self.

It is beyond the scope of this book to review more complex models, but it is possible that mental representations of people contain a blend of prototypes and exemplars, shifting between them (e.g., Cantor & Kihlstrom, 1987; Lingle et al., 1984). There exist specific models that suggest when each will form the basis of category knowledge, and the interested reader is directed to those sources for a thorough treatment of mixed models of exemplar/abstraction use. Examples include the work by Klein and colleagues on impression formation (Klein, Loftus, Trafton, & Fuhrman, 1992; Sherman & Klein, 1994), as well as Sherman and colleagues' work in the domain of stereotype representation (Sherman, 1996; Sherman, Lee, Bessenoff, & Frost, 1998). As a quick summary, these researchers find that when familiarity with a target is low, exemplars are used. As one's familiarity with a target grows, abstractions are created and are used instead of exemplars. In this way, exemplars serve as the basis for prototype formation, and until a well-developed prototype emerges, some mixture of the two can be seen in mental representation.

Place and Event Schemas

Specific sets of action patterns, beliefs, and attitudes are associated with different types of environments. For specific situations we have schemas that dictate ways of thinking about and behaving. This is a **place schema**. For example, the way in which one would purchase ice cream from an ice cream truck is very different from how one would buy ice cream at a grocery store, and different yet from how one would buy it at an ice cream shop. Merely mentioning these three types of events or places has likely conjured in your mind an image of each of them, along with knowledge about how those contexts each are structured and function, and action plans for what you would do to purchase ice cream from each. This is made possible by the fact that a mental representation, a schema, exists that specifies how to think about and understand an ice cream truck, the dentist, a classroom, a fast-food restaurant (how you act and get food in McDonald's is different from Red Lobster, which in turn is different from fine dining), and so on.

> **Place schema:** A mental representation that specifies the action patterns, beliefs, and attitudes associated with a specific environment or event.

Another example of a place schema is the set of beliefs that a person has about a type of neighborhood. For example, Bonam, Taylor, and Yantis (2017) show that White people in the United States have a set of preexisting beliefs about African American neighborhoods, including such thoughts as having homes with lower property values, having dirtier physical spaces, having unsafe and lower-quality schools, and being crime ridden. These are to be contrasted with the schema they hold for White neighborhoods, which are associated with wealth, safety, cleanliness, and excellent schools (e.g., Bonam, Yantis, & Taylor, 2020; Yantis & Bonam, 2021). These map onto the stereotypes held in the United States about White versus Black people, but the schema for White versus Black places and spaces is even more pronounced (e.g., Bonam et al., 2020). Yantis and Bonam show that this schema is in some ways immune to class distinctions, as middle-class African American spaces are seen to substantially overlap with lower-class African American neighborhoods in the representations of White perceivers. These schemas matter for how people evaluate and make sense of those spaces. Yantis and Bonam show that as the schema for middle-class Black neighborhoods merges with that of poorer neighborhoods, they evaluate homes in the neighborhood as being of lesser value (by $36,000) than in a similar middle-class White neighborhood. Even when told the property value, White participants rate a home in a middle-class Black neighborhood as being less desirable.

A schema for an event or place can lead one to enter into types of behaviors that are uniquely associated with that context if specific preconditions are met. Some schemas are furnished with an action rule that specifies when and where certain actions can be initiated by the presence of features in those environments that signal that specific actions are appropriate. In this way, not only the event/place schema is triggered by the situation but experience in such situations has allowed one to develop an action rule that dictates appropriate behavior in that situation (e.g., Abelson, 1981). Such knowledge is known as a **script**, defined

> **Script:** A mental representation that specifies an action rule to be initiated by the presence of features in an environment. In this way, not only is the event/place schema triggered by the situation, but an action rule that dictates appropriate behavior in that situation—a predetermined sequence of actions—develops.

by Schank and Abelson (1977) as a "predetermined, stereotyped sequence of actions that defines a well-known situation" (p. 41). By nature, scripts specify both procedures (how to act) as well as semantic knowledge that defines the situation and the elements within it. Thus, it contains information that specifies more than expectations about what events will occur, but also contains information about the order of events as well. Scripts are conceived of as a series of IF–THEN clauses that dictate responses in the presence of certain conditions (e.g., *IF* there is a row of cash registers at the front of the restaurant, *THEN* go up and order food there rather than sitting down and waiting for a server). When do we act in scripted ways? After all, not every situation triggers a predetermined manner of responding, nor would we assume that any time a situation is classified as a "type" of event or place, that a script has been invoked. A precondition for scripted behavior is the attachment of an action rule to a schema that ties specific behaviors to specific cues in the context.

The script concept bears resemblance to work on "frames" in cognitive psychology, a term introduced by Minsky (1975). A **frame** was defined as a mental representation that

> **Frame:** Hierarchically structured representation containing information about typical settings/situations, with top levels of the structure specifying broad truths about the situation as well as a default set of specifics, and the lower levels being flexible so that different versions of the situation can be slotted in if the default is unwarranted.

contains information about stereotyped settings or situations, such as attending the opera, taking an exam, or going to work in the morning. Frames were proposed to be hierarchically structured, with the top levels specifying unwavering truths about the situation, such as the fact that one's office will be there when one arrives. The lower levels of the frame have what are referred to as *slots*. The slots detail the specifics of this particular instantiation of the frame. Thus, if one arrives at work to find that one's boss is away on a business trip for the week, a different set of specific behaviors would be entered into the slot than if one arrived to find that one's boss wanted one to lead a group meeting in an hour. The slots are able to be replaced with specific information that the current instantiation of the script invokes, but there is also a default value for the slot that specifies how one typically behaves in the event that nothing unusual is happening within the situation that day. In our office example, the default value might be to first get coffee from the office lounge as one's computer boots up. The frame, therefore, not only tells you how to act in this situation but has flexibility to tell you how to act in different versions of this situation, including how to act if one's typical expectations are disconfirmed (such as when one arrives to learn that one is leading a meeting in an hour). In this regard, it must be noted that even the unwavering truths at the top of the hierarchy may occasionally yield unexpected findings (such as when fire or terrorism has destroyed one's place of work over-night), and the frame still specifies appropriate ways to act in this version of the context.

Self-Schemas

Schemas are proposed to exist for all types of knowledge we possess, not just places and events. This includes the knowledge we have about ourselves! Markus (1977) put forward the idea that our self-concept is in effect a schema. The **self-schema** is all the information we have about the self, with this knowledge organized in memory through associations. It consists of traits, goals, values, beliefs, attitudes, and behaviors with which one has real experience, and with which one has acquired a meaningful attachment to as part of one's self-definition. This includes abstract conceptions of the self that represent one's most cherished values, aspirations, and beliefs, as well as specific examples of behavior from one's past that are central to these attributes. To identify the attributes comprising one's self-schema, a person could respond to a test that asks them to complete the following thought: "I am _____." The attributes that immediately come to mind (e.g., smart, hardworking, a good friend, athletic, attractive, honest) would then be linked to more specific features and behaviors associated with each attribute. The self-schema is also hypothesized to be resistant to change, making the discovery of infor-mation about the self that is contrary to that suggested by a schema unlikely. It allows people to make judgments about schema-relevant behavior or attributes easily and quickly, and predictions about future behavior become easier to make. According to Markus, self-schemas are generated because they

> **Self-schema:** Mental representation containing all self-relevant informa-tion, to which one has acquired a meaningful attachment as part of one's self-definition, such as traits and behaviors. This includes abstract conceptions of self that represent cherished values, aspirations, and beliefs, as well as specific examples of behavior from one's past.

> are useful in understanding intentions and feelings and in identifying likely or appropriate pat-terns of behavior. While a self-schema is an organization of the representations of past behavior, it is more than a "depository." It serves an important processing function and allows an individ-ual to go beyond the information currently available. The concept of self-schema implies that information about the self in some area has been categorized or organized and that the result of this organization is a discernible pattern which may be used as a basis for future judgments, decisions, inferences, or predictions about the self. (p. 64)

In her dissertation research, Markus (1977) performed what is considered the first examination of how schemas impact the processing of self-relevant information, altering how one sees and remembers the world. Research participants were students who rated themselves as having either (1) self-schemas concerning traits relating to independence, or (2) self-schemas for dependence, or (3) no self-schemas relating to the trait domain of independence–dependence (called *aschematics* to signify that this dimension of behavior was not relevant to their self-definition). These ratings were done at the start of the semes-ter and were far removed from the time period in which the actual experiment occurred (so schematics did not know the experiment had anything to do with their self-schemas).

Participants at the experimental session were exposed to a set of traits (one at a time) on a screen and were asked to determine whether the words were self-descriptive (by pressing a button marked "me" or "not me"). The speed to make the responses were recorded. The traits that were being presented on the screen were selected so that 15 were related to independence, 15 were related to dependence, and 30 related to creativity (included as control words to compare schema-relevant responses against). Next, a subset of words of each type were presented, and participants were asked to indicate which words were self-descriptive, and then describe why they were self-descriptive by providing evidence from their past behavior.

Markus (1977) found that people who are schematic for a trait were more likely to say that a word relating to that trait is self-defining than a person who is not schematic for that trait. More interesting (since we would really hope that if a person is schematic for independence, that they choose words related to independence as self-relevant) is the result concerning the speed of responding. Schematics were *faster* to make decisions about whether a word was descriptive of "me" or "not me" if those words were relevant to their self-schema (as opposed to the opposite trait or to control words). Aschematics did not differ in responses to any of the types of words. There is not only the ability to accurately choose words that are self-descriptive but one is faster at detecting and reacting to those words. Additionally, schematics were better at providing behavioral evidence to support the assertion that a trait was self-descriptive. People schematic for independence, for example, wrote more descriptions of independence-related words than did aschematics or people schematic for dependence. They not only claimed to be independent, they remembered having lived a life full of behavioral evidence to support that.

In a second experiment, Markus (1977) illustrated that people with self-schemas are *resistant to receiving information that is counterschematic*. Participants were asked to take a test (actually bogus) said to assess levels of suggestibility. Someone schematic for independence would not include notions of being suggestible as part of their self-definition, and they should be more likely to reject feedback that suggests they scored highly on this test. The results revealed that those who were aschematic found the test to be more accurate and to provide a better description of them than those who were schematic. A person who was schematic was more likely to question the validity of the test; their schema made them defensive, dismissive, and resistant to information that challenged their sense of self.

Rogers, Kuiper, and Kirker (1977) provided further evidence that schemas help one process self-relevant information: "the central aspect of self-reference is that the self acts as a background or setting against which incoming data are interpreted or coded. This process involves an interaction between the previous experiences of the individual (in the form of the abstract structure of self) and the incoming materials" (p. 678). One's vast reservoir of self-knowledge can help one to embellish material that is self-relevant by filling in the blanks and providing extra descriptive richness. Their experiment illustrated how linking information to the self makes the encoding of that information richer and more complex. Their participants were asked to judge words. In some cases, the judgment invoked the self, in others it did not. For example, some of the time participants made semantic ratings of the words by deciding whether a word was similar in meaning to a target word. Other times they made structural ratings relating to the words by deciding whether a word was larger (font size) than a target word. Some of the time the participants made self-reference judgments by deciding whether a word described the self. The participants were then given a surprise memory test. Better memory on a surprise memory test is presumed to indicate a deeper, more complex, memory structure. Thus, if self-reference has benefits for the processing of words, words should be better remembered if presented as part of a self-referencing task as opposed to making a semantic or font comparison task. This is precisely what was found. The self is used as an organizing structure for interpreting new words, altering the way in which that information is processed, giving it a deeper, more thorough, memory trace.

Schemas for People and Classes of People

We have schemas for both specific people (other than the self) and for classes of people. A schema of an individual is most likely to be held for relationships of personal significance. For example, I not only have a schema about mentors (an abstract category or class of people) but I have a specific schema about *my mentor*. Baldwin (1992) proposes that relationships are internally represented, such that one's interpersonal experiences can exert an impact on how information relevant to one's relationships is perceived, interpreted, and remembered. Baldwin defined a **relational schema** as "cognitive structures representing regularities in patterns of interpersonal relatedness . . . the focus, then, is on cognition about relationships, rather than about the self or the other person in isolation" (p. 461). These cognitive structures include action sequences and behavior patterns that define the relationship between two (or more) social entities (such as self and mentor). The relational schema includes not only summaries of typical action patterns but thoughts, feelings, and motivations that define the relationship. Triggering a schema will, through spreading activation, also trigger the elements that define the relationship, making them more likely to impact one's information processing. Thus, if the current environment triggers the relational schema for one's mentor, then thoughts, feelings, and motivations that define the mentor relationship might impact how one thinks about a new person. For example, if someone resembles one's mentor, then seeing that person could trigger the schema for that mentor and impact how one interprets the new person, without one realizing any influence exists.

> **Relational schema:** A cognitive structure that includes action sequences and behavior patterns that define the relationship between two (or more) social entities (such as self and mother). The relational schema includes both summaries of typical action patterns as well as thoughts, feelings, and motivations that define the relationship.

Baldwin et al. (1990) provided an illustration of a relational schema being triggered outside of awareness and then influencing one's evaluations of relevant information, without one realizing an influence existed. In one experiment they investigated the schema of the relationship between a young professional and their mentor. In a second experiment they examined the schema of the relationship between a Catholic individual and the Catholic church (represented by an image of the Pope). For example, participants in the second experiment were Catholic women. They were shown disapproving images of either the Pope or a stranger, outside of conscious awareness (subliminal presentation), and then had to evaluate their own performance on a task. Did the subliminally triggered relationship impact on this self-evaluation? They found that selfratings were reliably lower following a disapproving face of the Pope as compared to a stranger, despite the face never being consciously detected. The result cannot be explained simply by disapproval having been triggered, because all of the participants saw (subliminally) disapproving faces. The best explanation is that specific relationship patterns were being triggered, and disapproval as it relates to one's relationship with the Pope is quite different from disapproval generally. Thus, this relational schema, and the meaning of disapproval within the context of the schema, is what impacts responses. The schema is unconsciously triggered and alters information processing.

Chen (2001) illustrated this effect using significant others. In one experiment, participants were asked to list features that describe a significant other, such as "dad is an extravert." Then, later in the year, participants performed an ostensibly different experiment. They were asked to "meet" several fictional target persons by being presented with a series of descriptions. However, some of the fictional targets were described as having features that matched what the person had earlier said about a significant other (thus, materials were prepared specifically for each person in the experiment). These are believed to trigger the relational schema of the significant other. Participants next completed a memory test about each fictional person. They were presented with a series of descriptive sentences and rated how confident they were that the description is one they had earlier learned about the fictional person. Some statements were presented earlier, others were not, but were statements the participant had listed as being descriptive of their significant other. Participants felt confident about statements describing a fictional person that were never actually presented, but only if both of the following conditions were met: (1) those statements were true of the significant other, and (2) the fictional person was similar to the significant other. A schema of the significant other was triggered and applied to the fictional person.

Schemas relating to specific types of people (the self, mother, mentors, etc.) are not the only types of representations relevant to people. We also possess mental representations for the various roles people play. These are **role schemas**. According to Fiske and Taylor (1984)

> **Role schemas:** Mental structures that specify the rules, norms, and behaviors associated with a social position, or a role.

"a social role is the set of norms and behaviors attached to a social position, so a role schema is the cognitive structure that organizes one's knowledge about those appropriate norms and behaviors" (p. 159). Role schemas provide for us our knowledge of the rules, norms, and expected behaviors associated with broad social categories such as gender, age, and race, as well as the norms and behaviors associated with more specific types of categories relating to social positions, such as occupations (doctor, journalist, trash collector, teacher, etc.). For example, the role "friend" requires one to listen to others when they complain and are dejected, to be supportive and helpful, to generate enjoyable experiences and fun, to stimulate and engage, and to not be harboring feelings of lust (in which case one has exited the friend zone and is now a secret admirer or unrequited lover). Some stereotypes are essentially role schemas, if they are stereotypes about the social roles that people play, such as occupations they choose or organizations and groups they elect to belong to (e.g., police officers, nurses, "snowbirds," professors, conservatives, skinheads, bowlers).

Cohen (1961) illustrated how role schemas guide impression formation. Research participants were asked to watch a videotape that depicted a woman engaged in a variety of behaviors (e.g., having dinner with her husband). The interest was in what sorts of detail participants would recall about the video and how memory for those details would differ as a function of role schemas. Some of the participants watched the video with the understanding that the wife was employed as a waitress, others believed she held the occupational role "librarian." The details recalled were found to differ between the two groups in a schema-consistent fashion. A librarian was more likely to be recalled as having glasses and liking classical music relative to a waitress, who was more likely to be recalled as being a beer drinker. Additionally, such schema-consistent information was more likely to be recalled than schema-inconsistent information (such as a librarian who owns a bowling ball). More recently, evidence for role schemas was shown in the types of inferences people draw from observing behaviors. Chen et al. (2014) found that people are more likely to infer traits about a person based on a single behavior if they have a role schema to guide the interpretation of that behavior. For example, people are more likely to infer that a person they have read about has the trait "helpful" if they also learn that the person is a nurse.

THEORY-BASED MENTAL REPRESENTATIONS

The discussion of mental representation that we have provided thus far has suggested that they contain associations with features, and which of our many mental representations is used at any moment is dependent on the number of matching features between some stimulus and a schema. The more features that are matched between a stimulus and a schema, and the fewer the mismatches, the greater the chance the stimulus will be seen as an instance of that schema. However, several theorists have offered alternatives to these feature-based approaches to schemas (e.g., Medin, 1989; Murphy & Medin, 1985; Rips & Collins, 1993; Wittenbrink, Gist, & Hilton, 1997). They argue that there are an infinite number of features that could potentially be used to determine whether two (or more) stimuli are similar enough to class together as instances of the same "type." Something more than a list of features is needed to constrain these infinite comparisons and to help determine similarity for the sake of organizing items into an existing mental representation. As Chen (2001) noted: "the clearest examples of this shortcoming are categories that group together instances that share little or even no obvious featural similarity, such as the category for 'things to take out of one's house in case of a fire,' which might include pets, money, jewelry, and photo albums as members" (p. 130).

In addition to associations that link information, researchers also speak of **propositional reasoning** that allow a person to understand the relationships among associated items in a schema. As an example, when an association specifies good grades in a class are linked to a specific professor, the proposition explains why. The explanation or reason may be that the professor is easy. Or it may be that the professor inspires harder work. These two propositions change the nature of the processing from what a mere association would suggest. Propositions add the relationship that exists between two constructs to the association among them. A proposition can also define the nature of the relationship when one of the items associated is an emotion or feeling—for example, "I feel disgusted and angry because of the ideological positions of group *X*" (e.g., Gast & Rothermund, 2011). As De Houwer (2018) described it:

> **Propositional reasoning:** A mental representation that contains information about the nature of the relation between stimuli, not only that stimuli are associated, but the relationship that defines the association (such as one causing the other, or one predicting the other).

> A proposition about a stimulus relation is an informational unit that is defined in terms of its informational content: it is a mental representation that contains information about the nature of the relation between stimuli (e.g., A *predicts* B, A *causes* B, A *co-occurs with* B). Because there are many different ways in which stimuli can be related, different propositions can be formed about the same stimulus pair. For instance, the same pairing of stimulus A with stimulus B can lead to the proposition that A *co-occurs with* B, that A *predicts* B, or that A *causes* B. (p. 3) [italics added]

A **theory** is an alternative to a purely feature-based mental representation. By theory it is meant that the mental representation contains information that describes the causal relationship among items and explanations about how items go together. Why did they act that way? Why did they say that? The answer one arrives at may involve a theory the perceiver has about those particular types of people, or the types of situations in which those people find themselves, or the relationship known to exist among certain types of people

> **Theory:** Mental representation containing information about causal relationships among items and explanations about how/why they go together. Theories need not be explicitly applied or reflect conscious reasoning. People often hold implicit theories about the nature of what qualities belong together and why, and the reasons types of people act as they do.

or objects. In this view, schemas are not simply lists of features or examples but theories that make these features coherent and have relationships with one another that can be used for explanation (e.g., Murphy & Medin, 1985). When scientists try to make sense of some phenomenon that they are studying they develop theories about the phenomenon. These theories play a facilitating role in generating explanations for the phenomenon. What the theory notion suggests for social cognition is that people operate in a similar fashion to scientists—the phenomenon in question is the behavior of other people, and perceivers develop theories about behavior to explain it.

Developmental psychologists have called this position—that lay people have knowledge much like scientific theories that they apply to explain behavior—the theory theory (because it is a theory that people rely on theories). More specifically, in developmental psychology, the child's use of theories to explain behavior is referred to as the child having a *theory of mind* (e.g., Wellman, 1990), and there are a variety of types of theories of mind that emerge through the course of development. As an example, Gopnik and Meltzoff (1997) propose some very general theories used by even extremely young children. First, newborns seem to possess a theory about what it means to be human versus nonhuman, displaying an ability to distinguish between people and objects. A newborn knows to imitate people but not machines. Second, newborns look to their immediate environment (what is physically contiguous) to see if there is an effect of their actions, a behavior that is seen as reflecting the existence of the child's theory about mechanical causation. As the child grows, theories evolve about the nature of personal causation—what causes people to act as they do. The theory of "persons as distinct and independent entities" evolves and acquires the notion that people have distinct wants and desires relating to the external world. Wellman referred to this as a child developing a **desire theory**, and the explanations the child generates to account for the behavior of others is usually seen in light of this theory. The child ponders, "Why did he act that way?" The answer returned is "Because he wants to." Even at 16 months old infants can distinguish an intended action from unintended action (e.g., Brandone & Wellman, 2009; Carpenter, Akhtar, & Tomasello, 1998; Hamlin, Newman, & Wynn, 2009; Hamlin, Wynn, & Bloom, 2007; Over & Carpenter, 2009). Cognitive development research suggests that theories modify and become more complex with development. The desire theory is modified to a "belief and desire" theory, where explanations for behavior can now include beliefs as well as wants. The theory acquires the notion that people are not only objects of impulse that act according to wants and desires but creatures of cognition who have beliefs about the world and who can internally represent the external world. The theory then adapts again to include the notion that other people have their own sets of beliefs about the world that are different from one's own and that lead people to see and explain things differently than one might from one's own perspective (what is usually referred to as *perspective taking*). By adulthood, the theory has grown to link the behavior of others to stable traits that provide strong and simple explanations for behavior.

> **Desire theory:** The theory that emerges with development that other people are distinct and independent entities from oneself who are operating under their own unique wants, desires, and intentions.

Theories do not need to be explicitly applied or need to reflect conscious reasoning. People often hold *implicit theories* about the nature of what qualities belong together and why, and the reasons a type of person can be expected to act the way they do, or cause one to feel as they do (e.g., Bruner & Tagiuri, 1954; Clore, Schwarz, & Conway, 1994; Dweck & Legget, 1988; Kelly, 1972a; Nisbett & Ross, 1980; Wegener & Petty, 1995b; Wegner & Vallacher, 1977; Wilson & Brekke, 1994). We do not provide an exhaustive review of all the theories that people use in making sense of one another. Instead, we review a few examples here, and point out that other examples of "theory use" are highlighted throughout this book.

Implicit Personality Theory

We have already discussed how a schema allows for not merely the retrieval of a single item of information from memory but the retrieval of associated constructs. One factor that links one's various mental representations together are **implicit personality theories**. Grant and Holmes (1981) state, "an implicit personality theory can be viewed as sets of clusters of traits that form cognitive schemas representing clear-cut exemplars or prototypes of different personality types" (p. 108). They are theories people have that describe certain types of people or sets of traits that usually co-occur in others (e.g., Cantor & Mischel, 1979; Leyens & Fiske, 1994; Rosenberg & Sedlak, 1972; Schneider, 1973). When one trait is considered to be true of a person, the theory allows for the related qualities in the associative network to be triggered as well, without the individual consciously thinking about person "types" or relationships between traits. One might use an implicit personality theory (IPT) to assume a personality "type" from a simple behavior, or from knowing one quality about a person. From that one quality one might instantly also infer that the person is courteous, kind, and forgiving; or behaves in a way that is gentle, peaceful, honest, and neighborly, with only good things to say. It is a set of beliefs about the relationships between traits, their co-occurrence, and their association. IPT is related to cognitive structures such as stereotypes. Eagly, Ashmore, Makhijani, and Longo (1991) describe stereotypes as a type of IPT where group membership is one trait thought to covary with other traits (such as the stereotype for athletes depicted in Figure 2.1). IPTs are also closely related to prototypes, as we discuss next.

> **Implicit personality theories:** Theories that describe types of people with personality traits that cluster together (sets of co-occurring traits in others of a particular type). When one trait is considered true of a person, related qualities in the network are also triggered, without one consciously thinking about person "types" or relationships among traits.

Some views of the ways traits relate to one another in the mind posit a strictly associationistic view in which people think about others in terms of correlations among traits. IPTs, however, should not simply reflect a correlation among semantically similar adjectives (such as courteous, kind, and forgiving). There must be a unique person-specific component of the inferred *relations* among traits (De Soto, Hamilton, & Taylor, 1985). An IPT specifies propositions, as well as associations. People think of others in terms of "types," such as prototypes (e.g., Ashmore & Del Boca, 1981; Hamilton & Trolier, 1986; Taylor & Crocker, 1981), that are united by more than features, but explanations about the relationships among the features and the causes for the set of features being related (e.g., their religiosity causes them to be courteous, kind, and forgiving). The qualities are connected by a theory that specifies why they are associated (e.g., Anderson & Sedikides, 1991; Cantor & Mischel, 1977; Schneider & Blankmeyer, 1983; Sedikides & Anderson, 1994). Thus, an IPT is an organizational structure that contains the attributes associated with a person type and relationships (causal interconnectedness) between them. Triggering one can trigger them all through their association and spreading activation.

Theories about Significant Others

As we saw when discussing relational schemas, one group of people for whom we have mental representations stored in memory are significant others. Whereas IPTs address theories we have about generalized types of people (e.g., religious people, egalitarians, women, extraverts, nerds), we also have cognitive structures for specific people, most notably those who are central to our everyday life and those who occupy a favored status in our hierarchy of people: friends, parents, spouses, siblings, grandparents, lovers, mentors, and so on. Thus, these are exemplars. So, we may ask, what is so special about exemplars that denote significant others? Andersen and Cole (1990) propose that mental representations of significant others have rich associations. Significant-other representations have feelings, motivations, and roles related to them; they contain more knowledge about internal states than representations of nonsignificant others (e.g., Andersen, Glassman, & Gold, 1998; Prentice, 1990). Additionally, perceivers spontaneously list a greater number of distinctive features to characterize a significant other. These features are distinctive in that they are less likely to be associated with stereotypes and traits, but characterize something unique about the person. Finally, given how relevant such individuals are to one's own emotional and motivational outcomes, one is likely to try hard to make sense of and understand one's significant others (e.g., Read & Miller, 1989). This richness and distinctiveness in the category suggests that there is greater structural complexity relative to other types of mental representation (e.g., Andersen & Klatzky, 1987).

Chen (2003) examined whether mental representations of significant others are best thought of as lists of features about a person (e.g., Dad is outgoing and extraverted) or as theories about why a person has certain features (e.g., Dad is outgoing and extraverted because he likes to have fun). The existence of theories as part of one's mental representation was measured by examining the extent to which IF–THEN relations are present in the cognitive structure. By IF–THEN relations Chen refers to the notion that a causal relationship exists between some state (IF) and a response (THEN). For example, the mental representation would not simply contain the knowledge that "Dad likes to have fun" or "Dad is extraverted." It would contain a relational clause that says, "If Dad is at a party, then Dad likes to have fun." IFs are the situations people encounter ("IF at a party," "IF at work . . ."), and THENs are responses observed in those situations (" . . . THEN he is extraverted," " . . . THEN he is focused and serious"). What is important is that not all IF–THEN relationships are considered theories. Simply noting an association between two events does not a theory make. It requires the inference of a psychological state as a mediator and cause of the relationship. A theory specifies when and why a trait or behavior can be expected to be elicited. When an IF–THEN relationship is mediated by psychological states that serve as the causal link between them, a theory is said to exist. "If Dad is at a party, then he is extraverted" is turned into a theory when feelings, goals, and expectancies about "Dad" serve as the causal link that connects the IF and THEN.

Chen (2003) asked research participants to read a list of "IF" statements about specific situations, such as "If at a party . . ." and asked participants to complete the sentence with a response ("THEN . . ."). They were asked to do this with a significant other as the person whose behavior was being described, with a member of a stereotyped group as the person whose behavior was being described, and with a nonsignificant other as the person being described. Next, participants were asked to read each IF–THEN observation they had listed, and to provide a reason for the behavior they described. They were asked to provide a BECAUSE phrase for every behavior (e.g., "If at a party, then Dad talks to everyone BECAUSE . . ."). These statements served as causal explanations that could then be evaluated to determine the extent to which people implicated psychological states, such as feelings and goals. If people have theories, the logic is that psychological states will be listed as the reasons (the BECAUSE) for the link between the IF and THEN. As an example, a BECAUSE that reflects a mediating psychological state (and hence a theory about the person) is "If at a party, Dad talks to everyone BECAUSE he is worried that others do not like him." The psychological state of insecurity is the theoretical link between the situation and the behavior observed. The results revealed that participants generated more BECAUSE statements (explanations) for significant others. More importantly, the reasons offered in the explanations for significant others mentioned psychological states a greater proportion of the time than responses made for stereotyped and nonsignificant others.

Research on romantic relationships shows a similar use of theories, focusing here on theories about the meaning of conflict (e.g., Holmes & Cameron, 2005; Murray, Holmes, & Collins, 2006). When a conflict arises with a relationship partner, it also raises issues of trust in that each partner now has to pit their own self-interest against the other person's interests, and against those of the relationship. A theory about the nature of such conflicts dramatically changes how the outcome resolves. Does one have a theory that conflict will involve self-protection or relationship promotion? If one has a theory that conflict invokes self-protection, then processing rules will follow in which one is doubting one's partner's motives and is sensitive to signals of rejection. Signs of rejection will be interpreted as an infliction of pain and a lack of trust, with such feelings of rejection increasing avoidance. If, however, one has a theory that conflict will promote relationship-enhancing goals, it will increase trust and lead one to seek signals that one should take risks and see an opportunity for growth. For example, Murray et al. showed that married couples with different theories about marital conflict reacted differently to similar types of everyday conflicts (feeling connected vs. angry, drawing closer vs. distant).

Implicit Causal Theories

Dweck (1995, 2017) posits that people hold theories about the performance and ability of others that they use for making sense of others' behavior. One set of people are described as theorizing about ability as a fixed entity, a stable quality about the person they are observing. They use what is known as an **entity theory**, which construes behavior as attributable to fixed factors (such as traits) that are unlikely to change over time or with development. For example, an entity theory would be applied by perceiving that "people are either good at math or not," or "people are either athletic with good instincts for a sport, or not." The implication of attributing a stable quality to the person is that ability will not change; practice may make one better, but not alter the basic fact of having skill or not. In contrast to this type of theory is one used by a separate set of people who believe that ability can change and grow in a particular domain. They use what is known as an **incremental theory**, which is a theory that construes ability as malleable and dynamic, and suggests ability grows over time and with practice as one learns and develops new skills. People with different implicit theories believe either that people can change, or that you are "who you are and that's that," which alters how they make sense of other people.

> **Entity theory:** A theory that construes behavior as attributable to fixed factors (such as traits) that are unlikely to change over time or with development. Practice may make one better, but not alter the basic fact of either having skill or being inefficacious.
>
> **Incremental theory:** A theory that construes ability as something malleable and dynamic, and suggests ability grows over time as a person learns and develops new skills with practice. A belief that all people can change due to ability being unfixed.

For example, Chiu, Hong, and Dweck (1997) showed that a person's implicit theory shapes the type of attributions they make. Participants read about a target person who exhibited a trait in one situation. They were next asked to predict whether that person would exhibit the same trait in a new situation. Entity theorists make predictions about the target's behavior in a new situation based on their traits to a greater extent than incremental theorists. Indeed, incremental theorists did not believe that a trait seen in one situation would be exhibited in another, and could even reverse (if Henry was friendlier than William now, it could be William who was friendlier later). In another experiment participants read a series of behaviors that ranged from very positive to very negative. They then indicated the extent to which each behavior revealed something about the person's inherent goodness or badness (their moral character). Entity theorists were shown to rate *behaviors* as indicative of moral character to a greater extent than incremental theorists, and also were more likely to believe that a person's character could be inferred from a single behavior. This is even seen in judgments about the self. When given feedback about a failure in an intellectual pursuit, Dweck and Legget (1988) showed that entity theorists saw this as evidence of a fixed quality they lacked, ascribing global and negative ability to themselves based on limited failure experiences. In contrast, incremental theorists attribute their performance to lack of practice and believe their ability will improve in the future.

In addition to impacting the types of predictions people make about future behavior, different implicit theories are also associated with different types of goals people set for their own performance (e.g., Elliott & Dweck, 1988; Grant & Dweck, 2003; Robins & Pals, 2002). People with entity theories are more likely to set what are known as **performance goals**. Performance goals focus the individual on the specific outcomes that are achieved

Performance goals: Goals that focus the individual on the specific outcomes that are achieved during goal pursuit, using those outcomes as a measure of competence or relative ability in relation to outperforming others.

during goal pursuit, using those outcomes as a measure of one's ability. If one performs in a superior way in relation to others, one feels competent and capable. As Robins and Pals show, when negative feedback is received about one's performance in relation to others, then adopting a performance goal can lead to experiences of debilitation, helplessness, and vulnerability. Rather than being motivated by being told one has not done well, instead entity theorists with performance goals interpret such negative feedback as an unmovable lack of ability. Thus, one sets a goal of performance and achievement, but failure is doomed to be interpreted through the lens of a theory that says that strong performance is unlikely, ever, given the feedback that one lacks the ability. In contrast, people with incremental theories are more likely to set what are known as **learning goals**. Learning goals focus the individual on the new knowledge or

Learning goals: Goals that focus individuals on new knowledge/skills that can be acquired during goal pursuit rather than the outcomes that might be achieved. These goals set ability-determining situations as opportunities to assess and then increase competence (opportunities for growth), rather than decrees about what one can or cannot do.

skills that can be acquired during goal pursuit rather than the outcomes that might be achieved (e.g., Dweck & Elliott, 1983; Dweck & Leggett, 1988). These goals lead one to see ability-determining situations not as decrees about what one can or cannot do, but as opportunities to assess and then increase competence. They are goals that lead to framing tasks as opportunities for growth, and as such lead people to interpret negative feedback in a way that is motivating, increases striving, and triggering a mastery-oriented pattern of behavior, not helplessness. Robins and Pals illustrate this in the intelligence domain. They followed students throughout their college career. Learning goals led incremental theorists to seek mastery in a challenging task, increasing effort if feedback suggested they had not done well. The performance goals of entity theorists produced attempts to avoid further feedback that one is stupid or lacking in intelligence—disengagement from the task.

Grant and Dweck (2003) used a challenging environment at an elite institution to examine how such goals matter for performance. Many universities have courses perceived to be opportunities to "weed out" students from an inappropriate path of study, courses where more than half the class gets a grade of C or worse. For elite students accustomed to being the best in their high school, such courses are a shock to the system. Who perseveres and succeeds under such difficult and challenging conditions, when facing failure in a cherished domain for the first time? Grant and Dweck asked students at Columbia University who were enrolled in a first year chemistry class to list their goals with respect to the class. Of course, all students want an A—however, they also differ in terms of whether their focus is simply this performance outcome. Whereas some students saw performance alone as important and an indicator of their intelligence, others saw the class as an opportunity to learn and develop their skills in chemistry. Tracking the grades over the semester, they found that students with learning goals not only received better grades in the course but improved with each exam through a pattern of behavior that responded to a lower-than-expected grade with increased effort and seeking out resources to improve (study groups, teaching assistant [TA] meetings, etc.). Research reveals a variety of real-world (e.g., school, business, sports) performance differences as a function of such goal differences (e.g., Duda & Nicholls, 1992; Dweck & Sorich, 1999; Elliot, McGregor, & Gable, 1999).

There is a large literature on implicit theories, which is summarized well by Plaks, Levy, and Dweck (2009). One last point to be made here about these theories is that they are not only chronic orientations held by specific types of people. Theories can be manipulated in situations to create different types of learning environments with different goals made salient; learning environments can be constructed to establish the goals that are deemed best for that environment—that is, when experimental manipulations are used to create either an incremental theory or an entity theory in that moment, we see that people then adopt either learning goals or performance goals to pursue in that situation. As a result, we see the respective mastery-oriented response of increased effort and remedial action versus a helpless response (e.g., Bempechat, London, & Dweck, 1991; Elliott & Dweck, 1988; Hong, Chiu, Dweck, Lin, & Wan, 1999).

EMBODIED COGNITION

Theorists such as Herb Simon, Gene Mandler, and George Lakoff propose that, starting early in life, and in the absence of mental representations to make sense of them, there are a set of physical qualities that infants are able to perceive and understand: gravity, warmth, pain, color, coldness, and so on. Mental representations of these concepts then begin to build by associating, for example, physical warmth with a caregiver who literally—through close contact—eliminates the aversive state of being uncomfortable via warming hugs and wrapping us in blankets. The more metaphorical use of the term "warm" to mean close, kind, supportive, and so on arises from these bodily sensations (e.g., Williams & Bargh, 2008). Thus, warm not only means one has achieved a physical state but also means (1) closeness of a relationship, or (2) a type of person said to have qualities such as trust, help, and nurturance—that ultimately have nothing to do with actually feeling warm. These new qualities become associated with the bodily state of physical warmth.

Embodied cognition as discussed by Lakoff and Johnson (1999) is the theory that all of human cognition is rooted in bodily experience, with our metaphorical and conceptual thought being extensions of how the body reacts to and functions in response to stimulation. Philosophical issues such as whether the concept of dualism of mind and body is accurate, or whether all experience is reducible to sensorimotor activity and sensation is beyond the scope of this book. The concern here is merely with the idea that bodily states and the experience of the senses can be foundational to mental representations, and, as Williams and Bargh (2008)

> **Embodied cognition:** Theory that cognition is rooted in bodily experience, with metaphorical and conceptual thought being extensions of how the body reacts to and functions in response to stimulation. It posits that bodily states are integral to mental representations, with conceptual understanding built like a scaffold atop lower-level early learning about physical states.

propose, that more complex conceptual understanding is built like a scaffold onto lower-level early learning about physical and bodily states. The knowledge stored in a mental representation necessarily includes information about bodily states (e.g., Barsalou, 2008, 2010) since such states are the starting point for these concepts (our experience with being made to feel physically warm is now associated with an abstract type of person—a warm person). Psychological traits such as cold, stable, warm, and calm are linked to the corresponding physical state due to associations forged from early experience with the physical state (e.g., Landau, Meier, & Keefer, 2010).

It is not only traits such as cold and warm that are associated with bodily sensation. Many bodily states develop associations with abstract concepts. For example, being intimate involves leaning in, happiness involves smiling, and feeling powerful involves an expansive body posture. When you encounter a mountain lion on a hiking trail the advice is to make yourself big to display your power. However, a physical display of power, easily perceived by an animal, is also likely to trigger a metaphorical sense of power in a human perceiver. The lion may see you as physically strong, a human will see you as influential and important. If the mental representation for a psychological state/trait/goal (such as power) contains associations like these to a physical state (such as an expansive body posture), then any one element can trigger the other. Happiness will not only cause smiling but smiling should trigger happiness. Power in the boardroom has nothing to do with physical power (the way a lion understands it), yet feeling metaphorically powerful will adjust your body posture to the "power pose." And adjusting body posture to be more expansive can trigger a metaphorical sense of power to others (e.g., Cuddy, Schultz, & Fosse, 2018).

An example was provided by Strack, Martin, and Stepper (1988). They argued that physiological feedback provided by the movement of facial muscles will trigger (without one's awareness) the cognitive experiences with which that physical alignment of muscles is associated in a mental representation. For example, frowning should trigger sorrow, and smiling happiness. They induced research participants to frown or to smile without needing to consciously ask them to frown or smile. They induced a frowning expression by asking participants to hold a pen with their lips only, which contracted their orbicularis oris muscle (the muscle used when we frown). They induced smiling by having participants hold a pen with their teeth only—they argued this would result in the contracting of the zygomaticus major or the risorius muscles that are used in smiling. A control group held a pen in their hand, which would have no impact on bodily feedback. Fritz Strack and his colleagues posited that facial posing, when done without one realizing it, triggers the psychological state associated with the alignment of facial muscles created by the pose. Their results supported this prediction. Implicitly frowning or smiling provided bodily feedback that triggered the associated states of sadness or happiness. To illustrate this, the participants were asked to evaluate a set of cartoons on a scale from 0 (*not at all funny*) to 9 (*very funny*). People who held a pen in their lips saw them as the least funny, those with the pen in their teeth rated the cartoons funniest, and those with pen in hand fell in the middle. Triggering the precise facial muscles, though undetected, triggered the corresponding metaphorical state, evidenced by the difference in how participants rated cartoons.

Williams and Bargh (2008) showed a similar effect in the domain of interpersonal warmth. They argued that many classic works in psychology show the centrality of the "warmth" dimension. From Harry Harlow on the physical importance of warmth (where baby monkeys preferred to spend their time with an inanimate surrogate mother that had warmth as compared to one that had food but provided no warmth) to Solomon Asch on the conceptual importance of warmth as a central trait, we see that warmth as a conceptual quality (a psychological trait) is tied to the association with physical warmth. Williams and Bargh argue that physical warmth should trigger the associated trait of warmth, much like a pen in one's teeth triggers happiness, even if people do not realize this link exists. To illustrate this, they replicated the work of Asch (1946) by having people make judgments of a person who is described by a set of qualities. Asch manipulated whether the quality warm or cold was included among the set. Williams and Bargh eliminated the concepts of warm or cold from the set, but manipulated the bodily feedback of warmth or coldness by having participants hold either a hot cup of coffee or an iced coffee just prior to the judgment task. In a next experiment they replaced the task of judging traits with a behavioral measure, looking to see whether warmth or coldness as a bodily state impacted whether a participant acted selfishly or prosocially with a friend. Across both studies they showed that physical warmth was associated with social warmth (higher ratings, prosocial acts), even though participants were unaware of the connection.

Ijzerman and Semin (2009) similarly explored the connection between physical warmth and warmth as a psychological quality. They found that when people are asked to hold a warm cup of coffee it triggers (through spreading activation) associated types of warmth. They used various measures of how close to others the participants felt as the measure of psychological warmth. For example, when asked about how much they overlap with others, participants construed the self as more part of the other, seeing a greater amount of self–other overlap. Using a separate measure of warmth, they found that when holding a hot cup of coffee people start to use more verbs as part of their speech pattern. Verbs were described as indicative of being close to others when used in describing social situations, so that physical warmth once again triggered closeness. As one last example, physical coldness is associated with social exclusion (we metaphorically give someone the cold shoulder, or leave them out in the cold). Thus, it could be the case that physical coldness could trigger exclusion and ostracism (the related metaphorical concepts). If true, feelings of bodily coldness could motivate people to seek out affiliation with others. This would eliminate the feelings of social isolation that had been (implicitly) triggered by the physical sensation. This is what they found: When cold, people sought to restore a feeling of belonging to the group.

Interestingly, some researchers posit the reverse pathway for the association as well, so that not only does coldness trigger feelings of isolation but isolation and ostracism could trigger increased judgments of physical coldness. This is perhaps why snuggling in a warm bed or a hot bath or building a cozy fire can make one feel better after feeling ostracized or neglected. Physical warmth perhaps eases the effects of social coldness. To illustrate this connection, Zhong and Leonardelli (2008) found that when people are socially excluded they estimate the temperature as lower (see also Ijzerman & Semin, 2010, who triggered notions of psychological distance and showed that people estimate the ambient temperature as lower). In fact, they not only judge the temperature as colder, their own physical state seems to be rendered colder by social isolation. Cacioppo et al. (2002) showed that loneliness leads to vasoconstriction where blood moves away from the periphery of the body, leading to colder skin and goosebumps. Ijzerman and colleagues (2012) also suggested that when faced with loneliness or ostracism, these psychological changes would actually cause physical coldness (lowered skin temperature). In their research they manipulated whether participants were excluded or included in a social task, and then measured the temperature of their skin using a device used to measure temperature in industrial coolers that is accurate to .0005 degrees Celsius. The participants who were excluded had significantly lowered skin temperature relative to the included participants. Finally, in one experiment, Bargh and Shalev (2012) had people experience a social rejection and then measured whether they seek affiliation. People who were rejected while also physically cold sought affiliation with others to compensate for their social exclusion. However, people who were rejected while also physically warm did not seek out affiliation. Physical warmth eliminated the impact of the social rejection, whereas physical coldness seemed to exacerbate it.

The Implicit Nature of Embodied Cognition

The literature seems to strongly suggest that the relationships among bodily states and how one uses the metaphorically linked psychological constructs hinges on a *lack of awareness* of the connection or influence. A physically unstable chair and table make one translate those feelings of physical instability into relationship instability, causing the research participants to overestimate the likelihood of divorce (judging relationships as more unstable). These feelings of metaphorical instability, once triggered by physical instability, can even lead one to seek out or prefer more stable qualities in a potential mate to compensate for the feelings of relationships as being unstable (e.g., Kille, Forest, & Wood, 2013). However, if one knew that the feeling of instability in a relationship was correctly attributed to a chair being unstable, it is unlikely it would have any impact. As we later see in Chapters 8 and 10, when one comes to consciously recognize that one's judgment is being influenced, people typically seek to remove the influence, not embrace it. If one learns that the word "warm" in a list causes a judgment to skew positively, they attempt to counteract this influence rather than rate someone as warm.

Using another example, power poses and facial feedback can trigger associated psychological states, but if one deliberately faked a smile or strategically adopted a power pose, the effects would seemingly disappear. Research on power posing shows that when people are tricked into assuming a body posture that is associated with power, they feel more powerful (Carney, Cuddy, & Yap, 2010). However, if they were to intentionally use such a pose, it is unlikely they would feel more powerful (e.g., Cesario, Jonas, & Carney, 2017). It is true that in one of the most watched TED Talks of all time, Amy Cuddy (a coauthor on power-posing work) advocated for a strategic use of power posing to boost self-esteem. I would argue that evidence suggests doing so strategically in that way is unlikely to work to boost one's sense of power (unless after deliberately striking the pose frequently enough, the behavior ultimately became habitual so that one no longer consciously struck the pose, but did so without awareness). Power posing should work to make other people (and mountain lions) see you as more powerful. But it would be hard to consciously strike a pose and then personally feel the associated power, unless the pose was accompanied by a set of other motivational tactics meant to "pump oneself up" (in which case it is not one's bodily state that increases the sense of power). Much of the work on embodied cognition hinges on the assumption that people are not aware of the association between their bodily state and the associated concept for an impact to occur from one's bodily state. When one decides to take a hot bath or sit by a roaring fire when feeling lonely or rejected, one is usually not explicitly thinking it is because the physical warmth will address one's social isolation. We know it feels good, but if we thought too much about why it feels good, then the physical warmth might lose its power to soothe. We jump in the tub out of habit, not specifically to reduce feelings of social isolation by increasing physical warmth. Not knowing the mechanism is what makes it work to soothe us.

Mimicry

If physical states are connected to psychological and emotional experience, one way to have greater empathy for people is to reproduce their embodied state. Mimicry of another person's actions and facial expressions should enhance the similarity of psychological experience through one's own embodied cognitive processes now mirroring the other person. If they are sad, mimicking their sad expression will help you experience sadness. Our ability to understand social and emotional information that we receive from others is dependent on our ability to simulate the state of the other person (e.g., Niedenthal, Barsalou, Winkielman, Krauth-Gruber, & Ric, 2005). **Mimicry** is the enacting of the behaviors and facial expressions we see in others. Chartrand and Bargh (1999) propose that mimicry serves this empathy function. They provided an illustration of this by showing that the brain areas activated when one is experiencing disgust are the same areas activated when one is observing another person experiencing disgust. This heightened empathy produced by mimicking the embodied states of others also allows for social interaction to flow more smoothly, since one has a more accurate "reading" of the needs of the other person. In facilitating interpersonal bonding in this way, mimicry promotes liking and trust (e.g., Chartrand & van Baaren, 2009; Maddox, Rapp, Brion, & Taylor, 2008). As the motivation for interdependence in social interaction grows greater, so too does mimicry (e.g., van Baaren, Maddux, Chartrand, de Bouter, & van Knippenberg, 2003).

> **Mimicry:** Our ability to simulate the state of another person through enacting the behaviors and facial expressions we see in others.

Chartrand and Bargh (1999) proposed that mimicry of others is passive and nonconscious: "One may notice using the idiosyncratic verbal expressions or speech inflections of a friend. Or one may notice crossing one's arms while talking with someone else who has their arms crossed. Common to all such cases is that one typically does not notice doing these things—if at all—until after the fact" (p. 893). We often mock people as insincere when their accent slightly changes to match people in their immediate surrounding, or if they do what others are doing. But this can be a functional response that we do without realizing it and without the conscious intent to mimic and experience greater connection (and signal our trustworthiness). However, mimicry can undermine liking and trust if misapplied. Another person mimicking me may be a signal of empathy and trust if my behavior is reflected back appropriately. Yet if the behaviors are not exact or misapplied by the other person, it can reduce feelings of trust by signaling to me that something is "off" (e.g., Dalton, Chartrand, & Finkel, 2010; Finkel et al., 2006; Leander, Chartrand, & Bargh, 2012).

Ideomotor Action

During my first year as a member of the faculty at Princeton, the psychology department hosted a conference to honor its beloved former member, Ned Jones, a storied mentor of many of the researchers whose work is reviewed in this book. From among them, Dan Gilbert used the opening of his talk at the conference to relay a story. A young Gilbert, we were told, had found himself in the passenger seat speeding at 90 miles per hour along the New Jersey Turnpike with his advisor, Ned, when a common occurrence was observed: A police car had someone pulled over on the side of the road. Gilbert observed how all the drivers on the road acted in the exact same way—they slowed down. Except for Ned, who sped up. When young Gilbert asked about this, Ned said he saw getting away with speeding as a game, a matter of guessing where the police are, and to play the game well meant to adjust speed accordingly at the right moments. Slowing down at the sight of the engaged police officer, Ned explained, was irrational. Police cars, he explained, need to be spread out over many miles of turnpike. Slowing down just before you reach one is rational, but you don't know where they will be, and they are not evenly spaced out. That is what makes the game challenging. However, there is one instance where it is not challenging. When one sees an officer busy on the side of the road, it is rational to assume that another won't be seen in the immediate future. This is the time to adjust speed up, not down. In his talk, Gilbert relayed Ned's words: "Speeding by the cop is the best move you can make. . . . But most people don't. They react in ways that are totally illogical. . . . It never ceases to amaze me."

What might have amazed Ned more, had he lived just another few years to see it, was research that tells us that perhaps people were not being so irrational. Rather than using the wrong rules in construing their environment, it is possible that the people driving their cars were acting using a more basic rule: to let their mental representation trigger associated behavior. It is possible that people are slowing down not because they are incorrectly playing a game or misconstruing their context. Perhaps they are instead *behaving without the influence of any thought* (rational or not). The suggestion is that behavior is triggered by a mental representation that has the behavior stored within it; when the representation is triggered, the associated action is triggered (e.g., Bargh, Chen, & Burrows, 1996). To return to Gilbert's story, it could be that our schema for "police" includes the fact we should be cautious around them. If the schema is triggered upon seeing an officer, then behavior linked to it, such as being cautious and driving slowly, is as well. Rather than slowing down at the wrong moment because of bad decision making, people act without thinking at all. They slow down without knowing why or deciding to do it. The embodied state of slowing down is associated with the concept of caution, and it is engaged when the concept is.

What is being suggested is that we act without even knowing we are acting or being involved consciously at any stage of the decision to act; the mere presence of a cue in one's environment that is relevant to a construct is followed immediately and unhesitatingly by the act, without the intervention of construal processes or consciousness (Dijksterhuis & Bargh, 2001). The logic behind this assumption is derived from James (1890/1950), as evidenced by the following quote:

> It is a general principle in Psychology that consciousness deserts all processes when it can no longer be of use . . . if we analyze the nervous mechanism of voluntary action, we shall see that by virtue of this principle of parsimony in consciousness the motor discharge *ought* to be devoid of sentience. If we call the immediate psychic antecedent of a movement the latter's *mental cue*, all that is needed for invariability of sequence on the movement's part is a *fixed connection* between each several mental cue, and one particular movement. For a movement to be produced with perfect precision, it suffices that it obey instantly its own mental cue and nothing else. (pp. 496–497) [italics added]

Ideomotor action: The idea that we behave because the mere presence of a cue in one's environment that is relevant to some construct is followed immediately and unhesitatingly by behavior associated with that construct, without the intervention of construal processes or consciousness. It is action without consciousness of the decision to act.

In his chapter on the will, James posed the question of whether the representation of a behavior can be directly triggered by a cue in the environment: "must there be an additional mental antecedent, in the shape of a fiat, decision, consent, volitional mandate, or other synonymous phenomenon of consciousness, before the movement can follow?" James answered his own question by turning to the notion of **ideomotor action**, or the "sequence of movement upon the mere thought of it. Wherever movement follows *unhesitatingly and immediately* [italics added] the notion of it in the mind, we have ideo-motor action" (p. 522).

One excellent way to illustrate that the will is not involved in the production of behavior is to show that people act in the exact opposite way than they intend! If one's conscious will dictates not to do something, only to find oneself engaging in the undesired act, then it cannot be a behavior one intended or consciously chose to enact. Elegant and easy-to-grasp examples are offered by James (1890/1950). First is the example of a woman who, in the early morning, finds herself getting dressed despite her last conscious thought having occurred while in bed and dreading the cold awaiting outside the covers. Her will had her desiring to stay in bed, yet thoughts of work and the chores of the day ahead impel her to get dressed before she has even realized she is no longer in her desired place snugly under the blanket. A second example is of the "stuffed" man who, after finishing a big dinner, further stuffs nuts and chocolates into his mouth on perceiving them on the table. People eat without thinking. James also gives the example of a host retiring to his bedroom to dress for a dinner party only to find himself moments later in his pajamas, in bed, instead of in his tie and walking down the stairs to welcome his guests. The cues in each of these situations trigger an associated behavior, not the behavior the individual willed.

Bargh et al. (1996) were the first to examine whether triggering a schema leads individuals to behave in a manner consistent with behavioral representations that are part of that schema. In one of their experiments, participants were subtly exposed to words linked to the stereotype of old people ("Florida," "old," "wrinkle," "ancient," "wise"). None of these words implied the concept of "slowness," which is also part of the stereotype. The idea was that this task would make people, without realizing it, contemplate the stereotype of older adults, and as such would also trigger the concept of physical slowness, since it is also stereotypically associated with older adults. People should come to act in a way consistent with the mental representation. They should start to move more slowly! The measure of interest was how fast/slow the participants walked from the experimental room, down the hallway, toward the elevator. The experimenter, unbeknown to the research participants, timed their trek down the hallway. They found evidence for ideomotor action—people led to implicitly contemplate the older adult walked more slowly than people who had not contemplated this stereotype. The mental act (thinking about slowness) seems to have become the physical act. In subsequent experiments, Bargh et al. replicated the finding by doing the exact same experiment again in the exact same manner. It was also conceptually replicated by triggering a different schema (stereotypes of African Americans) and a different behavior (aggression). People acted what they were thinking, without realizing they were thinking it.[1]

MINDSETS

To this point, the chapter has focused on how the *content* of what people think is organized in a mental representation. Next, we discuss structures that tell us how to manipulate information—that is, we explore mental representations that specify *procedures* for thinking. Külpe (1904) noted that asking people to solve a specific task created a related cognitive orientation (i.e., a set) that facilitated that task (and related tasks), while hampering unrelated tasks. For example, when asked to serve on a jury one is asked to not make a judgment until all the facts are heard and to put any biases aside. This requires a "set" such as being open-minded about the type of information considered. This approach to meaning making will not last forever, but will govern the cognitive procedures used while in that context. The concept of a collection of processing strategies that are relevant at a given moment for producing a particular type of outcome (such as being open-minded) is now known as a **mindset**. A mindset is perhaps most easily thought of as like a script, but one that specifies cognitive processing steps instead of action. Examples of such steps include being open and flexible in the variety of information considered versus rushing to use the quickest and easiest explanation, inhibiting associations among

Mindset: Processing strategies relevant at a given moment or type of task that produce styles of thinking about the stimuli. Rather than processing aimed at producing specific conclusions (like "he is athletic"), they are cognitive procedures utilizing particular forms of meaning making (such as being defensive, open-minded, narrow-minded, open to growth, etc.).

constructs versus activating them, activating remote associations to a construct versus the most immediate associations. Mindsets select, from various alternatives, the style of processing that is used. One can be instructed to adopt such a set explicitly (as with the case of a juror), or a mindset and its related cognitive procedures can become triggered when working on a task. Once triggered a mindset will initiate processing that facilitates the task and that is functional to task completion.

The Growth Mindset and the Fixed Mindset

The term "mindset" did not truly gain notice in the popular culture until about 100 years after Külpe introduced the term in 1904. This was sparked by the publication of Carol Dweck's best-selling book from 2006 for a lay audience called *Mindset: The New Psychology of Success*. Earlier in this chapter we reviewed research from Dweck and her colleagues focused on two types of implicit theories (entity theories and incremental theories). These theories that people hold about ability help them to set two distinct types of goals (performance goals and learning goals). Dweck described each of these two theories, and the two distinct goals they trigger, as associated with two specific types of mindsets. An entity theorist pursues their learning goals by analyzing information through what Dweck described as a **fixed mindset**. In contrast, a **growth mindset** is triggered when people have incremental theories and are pursuing learning goals.

Fixed mindset: When analyzing information, people use an attributional style that emphasizes traits and immutable aspects of the situation.

Growth mindset: When analyzing information, people use an attributional style that emphasizes goals of the person (which can be altered with commitment and changes in opportunity) and changing aspects of the situation as the explanation for what happens to people.

In the fixed mindset people use a style of thinking in which they attempt to find something stable and long-standing about a person or situation that will remain a consistent explanation over time. People use an attributional style that emphasizes traits and immutable aspects of the situation. Thus, when observing a person who does poorly on a test, the perceiver with a fixed mindset will search for explanations that invoke the person's personality and stable capabilities. With a growth mindset people use a style of thinking in which they attempt to find changing aspects of the situation as the explanation for what happens to people. They see situational influences and factors that determine effort and opportunity as central to meaning making. They use an attributional style that emphasizes the person's goals (which can be altered with commitment and changes in opportunity). When observing a person who has done poorly on a test the person with a growth mindset searches for explanations that are malleable and that invoke a person's effort in that moment, distraction by other goals, and pressures that exist in the situation.

Deliberative Mindsets

Gollwitzer, Heckhausen, and Steller (1990) found that there are unique mindsets associated with *how* people go about pursuing goals, and that these mindsets can be triggered at different phases of goal pursuit. For example, consider the goals of applying for your first job, studying for an exam, working out at the gym, and posting content on social media. These are difficult to pursue simultaneously, and in any moment one may need to choose which to pursue (goal setting). In another moment one may have selected which to pursue, but need to develop a plan as to how to do it (implementation of the goal). There are different mindsets for each of these phases of goal pursuit. A **deliberative mindset** is a cognitive orientation used when people are evaluating and selecting a goal from among many alternative goals that could possibly be pursued at a given point in time. The choice as to which goal to pursue involves deliberating over the *feasibility* of attaining a goal (i.e., thoughts about whether and how the goal can be realized), the *desirability* of attaining a goal (i.e., the value of the goal), and the ability of the current situation to afford an opportunity to pursue a goal (see Atkinson, 1964; Gollwitzer, 1990, 1993). Rather than avoiding certain types of information to protect a particular goal or way of thinking, one is open in one's assessment of all sides in deliberating about what is best. A deliberative mindset leaves one open to analyze the value associated with each of the possible goal pursuits.

Deliberative mindset: Style of processing aimed at evaluating and selecting from among alternatives, leaving one open-minded when considering/analyzing information rather than protecting particular conclusions. This requires assessing *feasibility* of successfully attaining each alternative (including whether the situation affords opportunities to succeed) and determining the *desirability* of attaining each alternative.

To illustrate these features of this mindset, Gollwitzer et al. (1990) first had research participants enter a deliberative mindset. They did this by asking the participants to deliberate about an unresolved personal problem and to weigh the pros and cons of different plans of action they could take to resolve the problem. Participants next performed a "second experiment"—they were presented half-finished fairy tales, and were asked to complete the stories. The impact of the mindset from the "first experiment" was gauged by how the person described the actions of the characters in the fairy tale of the "second experiment." Were they described as being deliberate and lost in thought like Hamlet, or quick to act like Laertes? The results revealed that a participant's mindset led them to ascribe deliberative qualities (contemplative and advice seeking) to the main character (as compared to a control group without this mindset).

Savary, Kleiman, Hassin, and Dhar (2015) showed that goal conflicts (where one must select from among conflicting goals) also lead to a deliberative mindset. Resolving conflict requires either restructuring the situation to attain each goal or selecting among goals, and thus evaluating them openly and evenly. Either way, one needs to consider information in a broader and more balanced way, extending rather than quickly ending information search. The deliberative mindset is a type of open-mindedness where conflicting points of views are examined, different perspectives are taken, and one extends thinking rather than rushing to a particular path of action. The impact of this mindset can also be illustrated by using a hypothesis-testing task. Goal conflict (which triggers the mindset) then leads to the consideration of information that would both confirm and disconfirm a hypothesis (e.g., Kleiman & Hassin, 2013; Kleiman, Stern, & Trope, 2016).

Implemental Mindsets

In contrast to being deliberative, a separate cognitive orientation is associated with *pursuing* a goal once one has selected a goal. This is the **implemental mindset** where one is concerned with specific *planning* on how to best implement a course of action to achieve the selected goal. A plan for a particular goaldirected action requires focus, warding off distracting thoughts, and searching for specific cues that will support the plan of action. This narrow and decidedly unopen style of thinking promotes achieving a goal. In the study described above by Gollwitzer et al. (1990), a control condition was mentioned. In that alternative condition the participants were given an implemental mindset by asking them to plan how to achieve a chosen personal project. Once again,

Implemental mindset: Style of information processing focused on warding off distracting thoughts, and searching for cues that support a specific plan of action. This narrow and un-open style of thinking promotes action by associating action with specific cues—when, where, and how to act is proactively planned and cues trigger the plan.

participants were next asked to finish a fairy tale. Now the participants described the main character as plunging into action. Rather than questioning alternatives and being open-minded, they were laser focused on what to do. Instead of extending thinking, they reached conclusions quickly. In complex cases, where goal achievement may be hard to initiate or maintain, the implementation of goaldirected action needs to be prepared through the individual reflecting on when, where, how, and how long to act, thus creating a concrete plan for implementing action when appropriate cues are detected (e.g., Gollwitzer & Moskowitz, 1996).

Flexibility Mindsets

In research on creativity (e.g., De Dreu, Nijstad, Bechtoldt, & Baas, 2011; Finke, 1996; Newell & Simon, 1972) a **flexibility mindset** is described where people engage in divergent thinking, active switching among possible categories, consideration of alternatives, and an openness to conflict that makes people less stuck on traditional solutions or approaches to problems. While it is perhaps best demonstrated through creative performance, a mindset that allows people to "think outside the box" can be used in any type of cognitive pursuit. Sassenberg et al. (2022) argued that any task that requires abandoning traditional approaches, or breaking from habit, can benefit from a flexibility mindset since it leads to considering alternatives beyond a "gut reaction" or dominant approach that is typically taken. Once this mindset is triggered it can be applied to subsequent judgments (e.g., Kleiman et al., 2016). Sassenberg et al. review research on conflict, creativity, ambivalence, decision making, and stereotyping that all benefit from this mindset.

> **Flexibility mindset:** Style of information processing focused on divergent thinking and switching among possible categories and an openness to conflict that makes people less stuck on traditional approaches to problems. It is not just openness, but breaking from habitual ways of responding and recruiting alternatives beyond the dominant approach typically taken.

For example, **attitudinal ambivalence** (having positive and negative attitudes at the same time) is often characterized as negative, and as leading to an experience of an undesirable state of uncertainty, or lack of resolve. People are often motivated to remove this uncertainty, to have confidence in their attitudes. However, attitude ambivalence is not always undesirable, and the flexibility engendered by entertaining both positive and negative beliefs is of value. There are specific situations where a person will benefit from embracing attitude ambivalence and the flexibility mindset it triggers. Such instances include when certainty or commitment needs to be delayed in favor of continued elaboration (e.g., Reich & Wheeler, 2016), or when an issue or person that one is encountering is controversial (e.g., Maio, Greenland, Bernard, & Esses, 2001; Maio & Haddock, 2004). Research on a different type of ambivalence, **emotional ambivalence**, reveals a similar flexibility mindset that accompanies the ambivalent state. Emotional ambivalence is when a person experiences both positive and negative emotions at the same time. Unlike attitude ambivalence where the mixed reactions are directed toward a specific target, emotional ambivalence can be a more diffuse state where the affect is not specific to anyone or anything. Also unlike attitude ambivalence, it is not usually a threatening state, but experienced as promoting openness and divergence in how one thinks (e.g., Rothman & Melwani, 2017; Rothman,

> **Attitudinal ambivalence:** Having both positive and negative attitudes toward a particular attitude object simultaneously. This can be aversive or arousing, unless this opposition poses no threat. Such mixed feedback can even be sought out, rather than eliminated, when uncertainty is desirable to an individual.

> **Emotional ambivalence:** When one experiences both positive and negative emotions simultaneously. Unlike attitude ambivalence where the mixed reactions are directed toward a specific target, it is a more diffuse state where the affect is not specific to anyone or anything. Rather than being threatening, it is experienced as promoting cognitive complexity.

Vitriol, & Moskowitz, 2022; van Harreveld, van der Pligt, & de Liver, 2009). For example, Rees, Rothman, Lehavy, and Sanchez-Burks (2013) found that emotionally ambivalent people considered positive and negative feedback about a job candidate, whereas those with just one emotion (happy) sought out mostly positive feedback. The ambivalent person was more flexible in what was considered. Another line of research shows that people high in ambivalence are more open to persuasion than people low in ambivalence (Zemborian & Johar, 2007).

While conflicting attitudes or emotions cause ambivalence, so too does experiencing internal conflict more generally, which in turn triggers the flexibility mindset—people have broadened attention spans and are open to a balanced consideration of information from a variety of perspectives. For example, Vasiljevic and Crips (2013) found that cognitive conflict, where inconsistent beliefs are introduced, initiates a flexible processing strategy to try and resolve the inconsistency. Participants see two category descriptions that intuitively and stereotypically do not go together well. They read about a female mechanic, or a priest who is entering a mosque. This task increases cognitive flexibility in that participants mentally restructure the situation in an attempt to make sense of the conflict—for example describing the priest as seeking to improve intergroup relations and reduce religious bias.

The mere act of thinking about alternatives can also create the flexibility mindset. Thinking of alternative functions for an object can make one open to thinking of alternatives more generally. Higgins and Chaires (1980) had research participants think about "interrelational constructs," which is the type of relationship between objects/people that exists when we use prepositions such as *of* versus conjunctions such as *and*. They posited that conjunctions make us think of two things as belonging together, which creates a mindset where one will now see future things more broadly and flexibly, grouping things together in novel ways, and encouraging divergent thinking. Connecting the same two things with a preposition leads one to focus on one specific function. To test this, they presented participants with a list of objects and their containers as part of a memory task (e.g., bag, vegetables; jar, cherries). The object and its container were described with either the conjunction "and" or the preposition "of"—for example, "jar *of* cherries" versus "jar *and* cherries." They next worked on a creativity task, a problem whose solution required divergent thinking. They found that the different mindsets created by the manipulation of the use of prepositions and conjunctions impacted performance on the task. Conjunctions led to more divergent thinking, with greater creativity following "jar *and* cherries" versus "jar *of* cherries."

A similar finding is seen when people are prompted to think about alternative outcomes to an event that could have made the outcome better (e.g., Galinsky & Moskowitz, 2000a; Markman, Lindberg, Kray, & Galinsky, 2007; Roese & Epstude, 2017). When participants are asked to think about a negative event, and then about how that bad event may have gone differently if only a small change had been made, their mindset shifts. It is not just how they think about that event, but the task leads people to a more flexible mindset that allows them to think more creatively on a subsequent task. This happens through relational processing where one thinks about relationships that exist among a set of stimuli, or through "thinking outside the box" via expansive processing where one switches back and forth in considering all items in the set.

LEVEL OF ABSTRACTION

Any given behavior we observe or any goal that we adopt can be identified or interpreted at various levels. For example, we can focus on the mechanics of an action (that explain how the act was completed) with a detailed description of behavior. Alternatively, we can focus on more abstract explanations of why a behavior was conducted, and with what effect (that explain the consequences of the action). As an illustration of this range of abstractness, "putting a stamp on an envelope" is a lower level of abstraction than "sending a message," yet each is equally valid in explaining the exact same action. The same act can mean very different things to two different people who see it at different levels of abstraction. The same act can even mean two different things to the same person at two points in time if the level of abstraction shifts. One may start with the categorization of one's behavior as "sending a message" only to have that turn to "putting on a stamp" as one searches in vain for the stamp that one needs to send the letter.

Goal pursuits also can vary in abstraction (e.g., Grant & Dweck, 1999). The highest level of abstraction is conceiving of a goal in terms of the need or value of the organism that it will fulfill. This high level of abstraction (such as to increase self-esteem) makes setting specific approaches to goal pursuit difficult. It is hard to determine how an abstract goal such as self-esteem promotion should be pursued. The lowest level of abstraction is conceiving of a goal in terms of solving a very specific problem. This low level of abstraction also makes setting specific approaches to goal pursuit difficult since it is too concrete to set a general pattern of behaving. Consider a new year's resolution to lose weight. A goal set this abstractly might be hard to achieve because it does not specify detailed approaches to doing so. However, the same goal expressed at too low a level, such as a resolution to go to the gym every day at 6 A.M., may also fail because life events will continually disrupt the ability to stick to this pattern. More moderate levels of abstraction for framing a goal are more adaptive and allow one to pursue appropriate strategies. For example, the goal of improving self-esteem might be better framed as gaining competence through learning new things. The goal of losing weight might be better framed as making healthier food choices and exercising during one of several possible points in one's day. In this way, the goal can be triggered by cues—a piece of cake becomes a cue to seek a fruit, one's morning meeting being delayed might be a cue to hit the gym. Such moderate levels of abstraction enable one to set adaptable action plans that promote goal commitment.

Action Identification

Vallacher and Wegner (1985) referred to this process of categorizing an action at a certain level of specificity in some hierarchy (from concrete to abstract identities) as **action identification**. Essential to this categorization is the notion that only one identification for an action is made at any moment. People adopt a single, prepotent identity for an action. The level at which behavior is categorized, and the meaning attached to the behavior as a result of that categorization, is dependent on one's naïve theories about what the appropriate level of analysis/identification is. They adopt a strategy for identifying information at a certain level of abstraction. Is it best to focus on the most mechanistic level, the most abstract, or somewhere in between? One's theory of the appropriate level of action identification is said to be linked to the difficulty of the action (Vallacher & Wegner, 1987). Effortful and difficult actions are typically identified in low-level terms, whereas practiced and effortless actions are typically identified in high-level terms.

> **Action identification:** Categorizing action at one level of specificity in a hierarchy ranging from concrete to abstract identities. Concrete identifications include detailed descriptions focusing on the mechanics of the action; abstract identities explain why a behavior was conducted and with what effect (explaining the action's consequences). Only one identification exists at any moment.

People intuitively know this to be true, with most of us having naïve theories specifying that it is advantageous to use a lower-level identification for action when learning a new task. Thinking about the mechanics of one's action on an unfamiliar and difficult task will make it easier to perform the action. When learning to dance a waltz, one must focus on the exact movement of each foot at each point in time. Identifying the behavior at this mechanistic level is necessary to perform the behavior successfully, even if the behavior is not enacted smoothly. However, using an inappropriate theory of action identification can result in a debilitated performance. For example, self-focused attention on the details of one's own behavior, while advantageous when a novice, can be devastating when an individual is already skilled in a domain (e.g., Vallacher, Wegner, & Samoza, 1989). Experts need not focus on mechanics. A tennis star should not be thinking about how high to throw the ball before serving. In fact, if we start to focus on the things we typically do fluidly and without thought, performance suffers. Baumeister and Steinhilber (1984) propose that this is what causes athletes to commit unusual errors and to at times **"choke" under pressure**, or to see routine actions suddenly become clumsy and lose their fluidity when in stressful situations (such as being watched by many or in a big game). The pressure is said to cause one to focus attention on the self, which in turn leads to unnatural (for skilled behavior) attention to the mechanics of behavior; the normally routine becomes strained and disrupted. An experienced tennis player is better off concentrating on beating the opponent (a higher-level action identification) rather than hitting the ball (Vallacher & Wegner, 1985).

> **"Choke" under pressure:** When pressure causes one to focus attention on the self, which in turn leads one to an unnatural (for skilled behavior) attention to the mechanics and details of one's behavior. This shift in action identification causes behavior that is normally routine to become strained and disrupted.

People prefer to think about behavior at a level that provides comprehensive meaning, and low-level identification does not provide a very satisfying way of thinking about one's own behavior or as providing sufficient meaning (Vallacher & Wegner, 1987). Indeed, when experimenters force people to think about behavior in low-level terms, people seem to seek out cues of higher meaning in the environment. Higher-level action identities can define the actor as well as the action, and essentially tell us about the superordinate goals of the actor. For this reason, naïve theories of action identification point the person toward a somewhat more abstract level of identification. Theories that point to lower-level identities can be prompted in certain contexts and with certain behaviors, but naïve theories more generally point away from a focus on the lowest levels of abstraction (Vallacher & Wegner, 1987). Rather than "moving our lips" or "making utterances," we are "being supportive" and "providing words of comfort." But, as described above, using too high a level of abstraction can also be faulty. If we describe our behavior not as being supportive but as connecting with my ingroup, it may be too vague to be meaningful. Once again, finding a moderate level of abstraction (that leans more toward the high end) is what people use. Of course, if the level of abstraction being used is manipulated in one or the other direction, then it will change the nature of thought.

Construal Level

Yaacov Trope and his colleagues have pursued an interesting line of research on this theme. They discuss the importance and consequences of what they referred to as **construal level**, a mindset in which behavior is construed of as either concrete or abstract. Construal level focuses a perceiver on different aspects of a behavior. Abstract construal focuses the person on high-level goals, whereas a concrete construal focuses the

> **Construal level:** A mindset that determines whether behavior is construed of as either concrete or abstract, focusing the perceiver on high-level goals or concrete actions. Although people have default styles for construal, it can be manipulated within a situation.

person on specific actions. This will then impact how well that behavior seems to fit to one's goals. If the level of abstraction of the behavior aligns with the level of abstraction of one's goals (such as a concrete behavior and a concrete goal), then it helps us to achieve our goals. If they are misaligned (an abstract construal of a behavior and a concrete goal), then the theory says we should miss opportunities to act because we fail to see the behavior as goal relevant. For example, Trope and Liberman (2003) performed an experiment in which some of the research participants had an abstract construal of their behavior and others had a concrete construal of their behavior. They predicted that this difference in construal would affect goal pursuit by determining one's ability to see the relevance of information to a given goal; opportunities to initiate goal pursuit are detected differently based on how the behavior is construed. Important to keep in mind is that what is changing across the groups of participants is the way in which the behavior is construed, not the level of abstraction with which the goal is held. They found that concrete construal of behavior reduced the ability to see the connection of that behavior with a goal, if the goal was abstractly construed. As construal of the behavior also becomes abstract, and aligns with the abstraction of the goal, the behavior is more readily seen as relevant to the goal, and this allows the behavior to be used in goal pursuit. If one has an abstract goal, then high-level construal of behavior (vs. low level) will help to match the behavior to that goal (e.g., Fujita, Trope, Liberman, & Levin-Sagi, 2006; Liberman, Sagristano, & Trope, 2002).

With another example, Fishbach, Dhar, and Zhang (2006) describe an increased level of abstraction when construing a behavior focuses the individual on the purpose of the action and why it occurs (its more abstract functions). Focusing a person on why they wish to do something has the consequence of highlighting their commitment to the action. In contrast, when there is a low level of construal it focuses the person on how the goal will be achieved and on issues relating to progress toward the outcome being reached. Abstraction should make people more committed and more likely to approach complementary forms of action. Concreteness should operate like an implemental mindset, narrowing people to focus on how to accomplish the low-level actions elected. This is what they find, with increased abstraction of the behavior leading to greater interest in complementary actions also being pursued, and a greater focus on commitment versus progress.

Although people have default styles for construal, it can be manipulated within a situation. Trope and his colleagues propose that construal level can be easily manipulated. In their research they illustrate how subtle changes in what they call psychological distance can alter construal level. **Psychological distance** refers to thinking about people, things, or events in terms of nearness to the self, with "nearness" being able to be conceptualized both in terms of physical distance (literal nearness) and in terms of time (e.g., Fishbach et al., 2006; Trope & Liberman, 2000). Research shows that increases in psychological distance promote higher construal levels, with abstract framing of information. Reducing psychological distance creates low-level construals, resulting in concrete framing of information. Using time as an example of distance, a goal is "near" if it is proximal and relating to what one will do in the here and now. However, a goal framed in terms of outcomes in the future—a distal goal—is psychologically "distant." If an action is scheduled in the distant future, the rewards it may produce are delayed. The value of that reward can change if psychological distance changes. Consider research on a phenomenon in decision making known as **delay discounting**. This is characterized by people seeing less value in the exact same action or outcome if the rewards associated with it are delayed into

> **Psychological distance:** Thinking about people/things/events in terms of nearness to self, with "nearness" conceptualized both as physical/emotional distance and in terms of time. Goals framed in terms of outcomes far in the future—distal goals—are more psychologically distant than goals relating to what one will do here and now.

the future. Its value is minimized if the payoff is far in the future. A person given the choice of receiving $20 now or $100 in 6 months will more often choose the lesser value in the here and now. The value of the more distal option is discounted (for a variety of reasons, one of which being that the immediate offer feels more concrete and thus aligns with one's concrete goals of finishing the experiment and a certainty of being compensated). As another example, a goal to do well in a class can be framed as one that is psychologically distant in time (to prepare me for getting a good job) or as one that is near in time (to prepare me for making the dean's list, or to impress my mom when I see her next week). Nearness in framing makes a goal concrete, which makes one better able to detect concrete actions that will help one get the desired good grade. Distance makes the goal abstract, and focuses one on abstract construals of behavior that will promote getting the desired good grade.

> **Delay discounting:** When the perceived value of a reward is reduced when the delivery of that reward is simply delayed in time. For example, $100 feels less valuable if promised to you in 1 month versus tomorrow. When given a choice between immediate versus delayed rewards, the delayed reward must be far greater to be selected.

This shift in framing from abstract to concrete has an important influence on the nature of cognition. Consider the example of how people manage their money. The goals of saving for retirement and being secure in older age are extremely abstract concepts to people under the age of 40. The future seems far off, and one's focus is typically on concrete things in the here and now: how to pay the rent or mortgage, the nice new shoes one could have, the vacation that feels needed and deserved, and so on—that is, one's construal of money is more concrete, and this aligns with one's concrete goals of doing well today. So, less money gets saved, as more of it is spent on the concrete goals. A shift in either the goal (to focus more on the needs one will have in the distant future) or in the construal of money (to see it more abstractly as a way to build security) will change the behavior. Less may be spent in the here and now and more saved for the future. In such an example, one's salary has not changed, and one's immediate or future needs have not changed. But the abstraction with which they are construed changes. A focus on what is near in time makes concrete acts, such as using money to buy a great dinner, seem more valuable. The same dinner seems less valuable if one's focus is on retirement. Construal can shift one's mindset from buying what is right in front of me, to saving and detecting opportunities to save.

CONCLUSIONS

As noted in Chapter 1, meaning is made when stimulation from the external world meets not only the perceptual apparatus of the perceiver but the existing mental representations used by the perceiver to shape and absorb that stimulation. These representations serve as filters that can vary in level of abstraction and in strength of association to related representations. Meaning is "made" by its distortion through these filters, and thus the nature of the filter will alter the nature of the meaning. A person may seem not at all racist when the concept of racism is filtered through an exemplar—comparing that person against a skinhead, Klansman, or Nazi makes them seem decidedly not racist. The same person may seem racist if the concept of racism is defined with a prototype, where the person in the abstract can be seen to share some of the features that make up the category. Thus, I could perceive the same person dramatically differently if that person is viewed through one type of representation (a prototype) versus another (an exemplar). Indeed, even a simple shift in the level of abstraction with which information is categorized can dramatically change how one interprets it and to what goals it is relevant.

This chapter has illustrated the variety in types of mental representations, and revealed how these differences in types of organizational structure of information can change what we think, and how we think. Embodied cognition research highlights the importance of physical experience in forming our structures and most basic associations. These physical experiences then get tied to more metaphorical meanings that associate psychological qualities with those physical states. Heaviness as a physical state comes to mean burdensome, difficult, or ponderous. Coldness as a physical state becomes associated with aloofness, ostracism, and lacking in emotion. Pressure as a physical state is associated with stress, anxiety, and severity of conditions. Warmth comes to mean kindness, support, and caring. These more complex representations continue to build, being linked together in complex nets of associated meaning. The associative networks contain not merely links among related concepts but theories and propositions that can specify why and how the concepts are related. These representations can then serve as a filter for absorbing new information. They provide the function of making new stimuli knowable, and hence actionable.

NOTE

1. This finding has not been replicated by several other labs. The same is true of the facial feedback study of Strack and colleagues (1988) described above. Replication failures like these were central in triggering a debate about methodology that has helped to revolutionize transparency and data sharing in psychological research. An impassioned description of why this is important is provided at *www.cos.io/blog/why-are-we-working-so-hard-open-science-personal-story*, and in the open science handbook (Bezjak et al., 2018).

CHAPTER 3

Self-Report Is Unreliable Because Cognition Is Often *Automatic*

Like other sciences, psychological science faces daunting methodological challenges. How can you study the very thing you wish to study if it is invisible? Over the centuries, other sciences have developed tools that we know and trust—microscopes, telescopes, calculus (and more complicated forms of mathematical reasoning), centrifuges, and so on—that allow scientists to study even the things that cannot be seen by the naked eye and that once existed only in theory. Psychology has two disadvantages relating to its tools relative to other sciences: (1) it is a young discipline, having only used scientific methods for about 100 years, with tools that are less developed and trusted relative to older sciences; and (2) the object of study is ourselves.

There is an old adage that when humans know their behavior is being studied, it changes the way that humans behave, so that "natural" responding is altered (the **Hawthorne effect**). This is complicated even further when studying social cognition as opposed to behavior. Methods for studying social cognition are not only complicated by people becoming unnatural when aware they are being studied but by people being *unable* to accurately report how they are thinking even if they wanted to. How can you tell what someone is thinking, what they intend, and how they produce the responses of which they are consciously aware if we rely on an unreliable conscious response

> **Hawthorne effect:** How people naturally behave is obscured by the knowledge that one's behavior is being studied, leading people to alter their behavior so that it does not reflect what is natural.

as the method by which we learn these things? Psychological science is often disparaged with the quip "it's not rocket science." But, at least rocket scientists have the tools they need to do the job. Allport (1954) stated that "Civilized men have gained notable mastery over energy, matter, and inanimate nature generally, and are rapidly learning to control physical suffering and premature death. But by contrast we appear to be living in the Stone Age so far as our handling of human relationships is concerned. Our deficit in social knowledge seems to void at every step our progress in physical knowledge" (p. xiii). It is both a difficulty and an allure of social cognition that the tools that can penetrate the true nature of thinking needed to be developed.

In the earliest days of psychological science, Wilhelm Wundt's lab (with students such as James McKeen Cattell, Oswald Külpe, and Edward B. Titchener) used **introspection** as a method for examining psychological processes. Unlike how it is used in everyday language, introspection as a tool for psychological discovery did not refer to casual processes of reflection. Instead it referred to extensive training in attending to elemental sensations and images experienced in the mind (Wundt, 1862). Through practice, over thousands of introspections, one could develop skill at self-reporting on low-level cognition: "perception, apperception, discrimination, judgment, and choice" (Boring, 1953, p. 172). Yet, within Wundt's own lab, Oswald Külpe came to conclude that this technique was ineffective for examining thought processes. He argued that one did not have access through introspection to examine the processes that direct thinking. Thus, one category of reasons to distrust self-report is a lack of ability for one to access the information with which we investigators are concerned. [1]

> **Introspection:** A methodological tool that relies on self-report about one's own psychological experience, but a specific type of self-report that requires intense training in how to observe one's own perception, discriminations among stimulus features, judgment, and choice.

Another, entirely different reason that trust in self-report as a tool can erode is a lack of desire on the part of the individual to report to investigators the true nature of their experience, even if able to access it. Perhaps self-report is reliable if the task is to decide which of two lights shine more brightly; is it equally reliable when the task is to distinguish which of two people is more skilled? As the targets of our inquiry acquire social value, that value can deter us from wanting to share the truth. People can be motivated to lie when reporting on their social cognition. In some cases, the perceiver may make a conscious choice to lie during self-report—in other cases they may not even know they "lie." We turn next to more fully examining reasons to distrust self-report: decisions to deceive others, deceiving the self, and lacking the ability to access what to report.

STRATEGIC DECISIONS TO DECEIVE: STEREOTYPING AND LIES OF SOCIAL DESIRABILITY

Self-report is often fallible as a measurement tool because of **social desirability bias** (e.g., Paulhus, 1991; Schlenker & Leary, 1982). People have a desire for others to view them in a way that will contribute positively to self-esteem. This creates concerns about being seen negatively by others, an apprehension, or social anxiety, about being evaluated negatively that threatens to lower self-esteem (e.g., Stephan & Stephan, 1985). Such anxiety about looking bad, or a desire to look good, motivates people to make a positive impression when they have doubts that natural responding would do so. A strategic intention to deceive others with one's self-presentation can occur when people feel they are being observed or are the focus of attention. It also occurs when concerns are raised about how one's natural response corresponds with what others expect, such as expressing beliefs that do not conform with the norms and standards for what ought to be done that are held by a valued social group (e.g., saying something inappropriate or harassing that would lead others to think those statements stem from a biased person). When one worries about interpersonal failure, especially those that people find threatening to self-esteem because they imply one is an immoral person, social desirability can lead to deception.

> **Social desirability bias:** Concerns about being viewed negatively by others and apprehension (social anxiety) about being evaluated negatively that threatens to lower self-esteem. It is a desire for others to see the self in a way that contributes positively to self-esteem, including strategic concerns about presenting the self to avoid being seen negatively.

Not Stereotyping as a Lie: The Case of Normative Pressure to Be Unbiased

To avoid public disapproval, people can be unwilling to express publicly a stereotype that they privately believe (e.g., Lambert, Cronen, Chasteen, & Lickel, 1996). They allow the lie to conceal an unflattering personal fact that they are unwilling to admit to others. This type of lie not only happens among friends but people lie to strangers. For example, people lie to pollsters and on self-report measures by reporting they support a normatively popular person or thing they actually dislike. Stereotypes often operate in this way. A specific version of this type of lie relates to political candidates from disenfranchised or minority groups that have popularity in the culture. To oppose such a person, even if for reasons that have nothing to do with being prejudiced, could appear to be due to prejudice. Thus, social desirability suggests saying you support the minority candidate, even if you do not. This has been called **the Bradley effect**, named after an African American mayor from Los Angeles who lost the race for governor of California in 1982 after polls over-estimated his support. The accepted belief about why this happened is that White voters attempted to appear unbiased in what they told pollsters and news organizations. Succumbing to social desirability concerns, they claimed to support this African American candidate. What they reported was a lie in that they did not truly intend to vote for the minority candidate. In the privacy of a voting booth many did not.

> **The Bradley effect:** When people lie on self-report measures by reporting that they support/approve of a normatively popular person or thing they actually dislike. Stereotypes often operate in this way. To avoid public disapproval, people can be unwilling to express publicly a stereotype that they privately believe.

In cases of stereotyping such as this, there is the potential to cause harm by one privately acting in ways that are the opposite of what one says. If many people do so, it creates an appearance that a problem does not exist, but private actions promote stereotype-guided behavior and disparities. Moving beyond elections, consider important jobs in which the public places trust: doctors, teachers, nurses, police officers, and so on. If such people publicly assert they have no bias against women, against Black men, or against transgender individuals, then it creates an illusion in the society at large that no disparities exist. However, if they privately endorse such stereotypes, it can lead to treating those individuals differently and perpetuating or extending disparities, with the cultural impact never being detected due to their explicit denouncement of bias.

Consider the example of sentencing decisions made by jurors (Glaser, Martin, & Kahn, 2015). Jurors claim to believe in an unbiased judicial system and to agree with the principle of "statutory (and ethical) irrelevance of race in the determination of suspicion, guilt, or punishment" (p. 2). However, past research has shown that race plays a role in how jurors actually mete out punishment for identical crimes. White defendants are treated more leniently for the same crime, and this effect is even found for the death penalty, where Black defendants are more likely to be sentenced to death, especially if the victim is White (e.g., Eberhardt, Davies, Purdie-Vaughns, & Johnson, 2006). Glaser et al. performed an experiment to examine this matter. Do jurors find a person guilty and susceptible to the death penalty differentially as a function of race, despite stating they would never use race as a factor in determining the decision to convict? Research participants were asked to decide whether to acquit or convict a suspect in a murder trial and were provided with a case summary that suggested guilt. The summary left it ambiguous as to whether the victim was Black or White, but manipulated whether the defendant was Black or White. When the jurors thought the maximum sentence was imprisonment, they did not treat a Black defendant any differently than a White defendant. The private decision about sentencing a person to prison made in the experiment matched what they publicly endorsed. However, when the maximum sentence was *death*, a bias appeared. They were reluctant to provide a death sentence to a White defendant relative to a Black one—that is, they were more likely to convict a Black defendant who faced the possibility of the death penalty. They publicly say that justice, to them, is blind. But when a life is on the line, what they privately do is not matched to what they publicly say.

A similar break between what people publicly say and privately do is seen with research with police officers. White police officers make the claim that their training and experience makes them relatively immune to anti-Black biases that are displayed by laypeople who are White. On one stereotyping task, where a research participant is asked to simulate firing a weapon if they encounter a person holding a gun (as opposed to holding a wallet or a phone), participants fire more quickly if the person holding the gun is Black, and they make the decision to not fire more quickly if the person holding a wallet is White (e.g., Correll et al., 2007). Police officers show this exact same bias. And the bias is greatest in officers who work in areas with the highest concentrations of Black and minority citizens. In fact, officers trained to work on street violence and gang activity show the bias as much as laypeople (Sim, Correll, & Sadler, 2013). Where the experience they publicly tout as immunizing them from bias is greatest, private bias is greatest.

One final example comes from the medical community, where strong normative pressures create a need to provide the best possible care and to do so without prejudice, yet racist and sexist responding still prevails in private. Even when doctors explicitly proclaim to adhere to their Hippocratic oath, they treat patients from different social groups differently. Green et al. (2007) showed that when medical doctors reported feelings for Black patients that were equally positive to those of White patients, many nonetheless held private negative feelings toward Black patients (private feelings of bias were assessed using a tool we review in Chapter 4: the IAT). Do these hidden negative prejudices contribute to a bias in their treatment recommendations? The doctors of medicine (MDs) in this experiment were provided with a description of a 50-year-old man with chest pain, accompanied by an electrocardiogram implying he had anterior myocardial infarction. A picture of the patient was included as well, with half the MDs seeing a picture of a White man, the other half received a picture of a Black man. All other information was identical from doctor to doctor. Their findings showed that Black patients were diagnosed more often with coronary artery disease (CAD). However, the preferred treatment for CAD—thrombolytic drugs—was not recommended more often to Black patients. The more that the test of their private attitudes revealed prejudice in the MDs, the less likely they were to recommend thrombolysis for the Black patients. Public attitudes did not impact treatment recommendations. A preferred medical treatment was being systematically denied, but the doctors did not report having any bias at all in how they would treat patients. But differences exist.

One might argue that this is not the doctor yielding to a norm and hiding their "true" negative feelings but a case of the doctors simply not recognizing their negativity and truly believing they are unbiased (as is explored next in the section on aversive racism). This is possible. However, it is also possible that doctors are merely saying what is normative in public and are aware of their private prejudice. They lie. Evidence in support of this would be provided by doctors being more likely to show bias when they have greater social desirability concerns. For example, Wolsiefer et al. (2023) found that physicians with higher levels of social desirability concerns had higher levels of private anti-Hispanic bias.

Stereotyping as a Lie: The Case of Normative Pressure to Be Biased

We just reviewed cases where the normative pressure is to like someone (such as pressure to not stereotype a member of a different group), or to label someone as qualified and good, while privately one feels otherwise. The inverse of this happens as well. In such instances stereotyping and bias emerge because people feel pressured to publicly express bias when privately they do not feel any. Imagine a person who is low in prejudice yet is living or working or studying among people who they believe to be high in prejudice. An unbiased person could express bias in these situations because they fear not fitting in. The pressure to acquiesce to bias is great. Many of us have felt this pressure when hearing a sexist or racist joke that we seemingly supported, allowing our fake approval to give legitimacy to the bias. To this day I am haunted by a shameful smile from my childhood to a terribly offensive joke told by a friend's father while giving me a ride home from nearby Manhattan as a favor to my family. I wanted to condemn him or jump out of the car and walk home. But we were 20 miles from home, and I was 15, in a car pool full of adults. All I could muster was a fake smile—a lie—as he and the other adults in the car laughed at a racist joke.

There is an entire literature on racist humor that explores this way that stereotyping can be a deceit exacted to gain social approval from people who, unfortunately, may be doing reprehensible things. Ford and Ferguson (2004) proposed a **prejudiced norm theory of humor**. In this theory, jokes are said to be used to communicate group norms and can be used as a way to signal agreement with the group (and as Ungson, 2019, suggested, they can also signal dissent from the group if jokes are used to challenge a norm). For example, when male research participants heard sexist jokes they then believed that a norm of anti-sexism was less strongly in place, and that being sexist was more acceptable (e.g., Ford, Boxer, Armstrong, & Edel, 2008). Some of the men then acted in a more sexist manner as a result, and for those who did not, a pressure to not dissent was felt. A joke is more than a joke, but an expression of a norm, and many men may find themselves

> **Prejudiced norm theory of humor:** Theory that jokes are used to communicate group norms and can be used to signal agreement with the group (even if one privately disagrees). For example, when male participants heard sexist jokes they believed that the norms of anti-sexism were less strongly in place, and that being sexist was more acceptable.

in locker rooms and boardrooms where sexist norms are communicated through humor. Nonsexist men may decide to lie and not voice their opposition to sexism because of such social pressure. In keeping quiet they do more than give the false impression that everyone shares the sexist norm. Jokes are only humorous when we all agree they are benign, or done without malicious intent (e.g., Warren & McGraw, 2016). Thus, laughing at sexist jokes also communicates that sexism is more than just normative, but it is benign or harmless.

It is not just in humor where people "lie" by stereotyping. Social pressure within one's circle (family, friends, carpoolers, work colleagues, teachers, fraternity brothers, teammates, etc.) can exist to pressure one to denounce certain groups that are disliked within that circle. Socially shared sets of beliefs are transmitted, and a good group member is supposed to share those negative beliefs. People may privately not agree with a stereotype but may publicly agree with it so they are seen as agreeing with their group (Katz & Braly, 1933). An example from politics would be if a valued social circle had a shared dislike of a candidate because of their race. In the opposite of the Bradley effect, one would now fail to publicly endorse a candidate who one privately supports out of concerns about social disapproval. In this case, polls underestimate the vote, leading a figure that polling suggests is trailing (or with a narrow lead) to win (or win by a landslide). Some believe this is why polls underpredicted the victory of Barack Obama in 2008.

Let us look at one last example of how we lie with a public statement that is misaligned with private beliefs. People will publicly say they disagree with a minority, when private measures show far more agreement than they self-report. People are reluctant to express public agreement with a negative group. At times this is a true reaction (there is actual power in numbers and we feel those in the minority are less correct). Yet at times this is a lie, and we say we disagree with the minority even though the minority has convinced us to agree with their view—there is **minority influence**. Moscovici, Lage, and Naffrechoux (1969) conducted studies in which four research participants and two confederates (people who actually work for the research team pretending to be fellow participants) were asked to report the color of a series of slides. All were blue slides that varied in their light intensity. The two confederates (a numerical minority) were asked by the experimenter to give an incorrect response and report seeing the color green. The participants still reported seeing the color blue on 92% of their responses, thus mostly disagreeing with the minority that consistently reported seeing the color green. This was a lie because more subtle measures showed that the participants actually agreed with the minority far more often than 8% of the time and were just reluctant to say so publicly. When later brought into a private room and exposed to blue-green disks, over 35% of them reported seeing green.

> **Minority influence:** The power of minorities (often defined numerically) to persuade people. Often, influence is initially private, with people reluctant to publicly express agreement with minorities (due to normative pressures to agree with the consensus). With time, the stereotype of minorities as wrong can fade within individuals and public opinions may shift.

Moscovici and Personnaz (1980) made this same point in an experiment that utilized chromatic afterimage. If an individual fixates on a white screen after focusing on a color, they will see the complementary color on the screen. Thus, if a participant actually perceives the slides to be green, they will be more likely to report seeing red (the complement of green) than others who actually perceive the slides as blue, who should report seeing yellow (the complement of blue) during the test of their chromatic afterimage. They found that when a minority reported seeing green, the participant's public report was that they saw blue. However, they saw red during the chromatic afterimage test with a greater frequency than research participants who were confronted with a majority who reported seeing blue on the initial task. While minorities have a small influence publicly, the influence is much larger in private, indicating that the public response was a deception (see also Nemeth, Swedlund, & Kanki, 1973).

Lying to Say What Is Socially Desirable Can Be Detected from Nonverbal Behavior

As just reviewed, when we have social desirability concerns, we may say and do things that will align us with what is "appropriate" even if we privately disagree. However, as shown above, researchers can detect such misalignments with cleverly designed experiments. One set of clever procedures takes advantage of the fact that when our true beliefs and feelings are misaligned with overtly expressed beliefs and feelings, we betray our hidden views with our *nonverbal behavior*. As we review in more detail later in this chapter, nonverbal behavior is more difficult to control than the things we consciously say. We may say we are not mad but our anger screams out in other ways. We may lie and say we have not broken the law but in doing so we may be nonverbally admitting to the crime. Researchers can use measures of nonverbal behavior to reveal true attitudes and beliefs despite what is being publicly said.

Dovidio, Kawakami, and Gaertner (2002) used this fact to explore how racism might be expressed through one's nonverbal behavior, even when one overtly reports having nonracist views and feelings. They argued that while consciously intended behavior is typically predicted quite well by publicly expressed beliefs, it is not predicted by private beliefs and attitudes. These more implicitly held beliefs and attitudes instead predict more subtle types of behaviors, such as nonverbal displays of bias. The fact that overt and explicit bias is predicted by what people explicitly say is nicely illustrated in an experiment by Fazio, Jackson, Dunton, and Williams (1995). They looked at biased responding to a case of police brutality that had great publicity in the early 1990s (the beating of a Black man named Rodney King). Responses to this incident, including reactions to the subsequent trial of the officers and support for the Black community, were predicted by measures of the participant's publicly expressed racial prejudice (see also Dovidio, Kawakami, Johnson, Johnson, & Howard, 1997). However, privately measured attitudes did not predict these conscious responses. What is predicted by privately measured attitudes? Nonverbal behavior. McConnell and Leibold (2001) showed that the degree of private prejudice toward Black people held by a White participant predicted less smiling, less speaking, and more speech errors with a Black versus White interaction partner. This pattern of findings tells us that people will often be saying one thing, but sending signals that betray that their true feelings are the exact opposite. How does this impact the interaction, when one's interaction partner picks up on these signals and essentially knows you are untrustworthy?

Dovidio et al. (2002) explored such interactions of people whose overt actions and subtle actions were misaligned in this way. Is this noticed? Which behaviors (the overt or the subtle) have greater weight in one's judgment of the interaction partner? How do people feel in such interactions? To explore this, Dovidio et al. placed two research participants in an interaction where a noncontroversial topic (unrelated to race) was discussed. Of special interest were the dyads that contained one White person and one Black person. They found that for the White people in these interactions, their focus was mostly on their own overt behavior. If they said friendly things, they judged the interaction as having gone well. However, what happens when despite their overtly positive behavior, they have implicitly negative feelings being expressed by their nonverbal behavior? They do not see these reactions. As Dovidio et al. put it:

> Whites have full access to their explicit attitudes and are able to monitor and control their more overt and deliberative behaviors. They do not have such full access to their implicit attitudes. . . . We expect that as a consequence, Whites' beliefs about how they are behaving . . . are based primarily on their explicit attitudes and their more overt behaviors, such as the verbal content of their interaction. (p. 63)

Although the White people do not think they are sending negative nonverbal signals, their Black interaction partners detect them. The interaction partners see both communication channels—what is being overtly said and what is being communicated nonverbally. The results showed that measures of the White person's "hidden prejudice" (and once again, in Chapter 4 we discuss in detail how to measure this) predicted greater amounts of negative nonverbal behavior. And more importantly, the negative behavior that went undetected by the White person displaying it, was easily detected by their interaction partner. The more implicit prejudice held by the White person, the greater the amount of negative nonverbal behavior detected by their Black partner.

When such a misalignment in the verbal and nonverbal behaviors of one's interaction partner is detected, what consequence does this have? Research has shown that a misalignment of one's verbal and nonverbal communication can create feelings of communication awkwardness and general distrust in one's interaction partner. If members of minority groups detect a majority group member saying nonprejudiced things, but have this mismatched to negative nonverbal acts, this creates a sense of distrust, a feeling that a deception is being perpetrated. This reduction in trust from the misalignment makes the minority group member less satisfied with the interaction than the majority group member, who fails to detect this discrepancy (e.g., Shelton, 2000). Consider the repercussions in an important domain such as medicine. Dovidio and Fiske (2012) argue, "a mismatch between a physician's positive verbal behavior (as a function of conscious egalitarian values) and negative nonverbal behavior . . . is likely to make a physician seem especially untrustworthy and duplicitous to those who are vigilant for cues of bias" (p. 949).

Other research shows that such negative nonverbal behaviors are exaggerated when White participants are also faced with social desirability concerns and are explicitly worried about appearing racist (e.g., Amodio, Harmon-Jones, & Devine, 2003; Goff, Steele, & Davies, 2008). Ironically, one's concerns about appearing biased make one send nonverbal cues suggesting just that, and make one seem less trustworthy, as if one is suppressing true feelings and lying. Evidence for this is provided by Blair and colleagues (2013), who report that Black patients saw White physicians as being less trustworthy and less skilled as a function of the physician's social desirability concerns. The greater the physician's need to hide feelings of discomfort, the more the physician's body communicated that discomfort, and the less satisfied the Black patients were with the medical experience (see also Penner et al., 2010).

Finally, if detecting a mismatch between a person's feelings of discomfort held at the private level and the positive things the person is saying causes feelings of distrust and dissatisfaction, it would make sense if such feelings are then reciprocated. Being the recipient of repeated negative treatment, even if it is nonverbal, can cause ethnic minorities to compensate for this treatment by sending their own signals that they detect the discomfort and feel awkward in such a situation. They may start to signal that they wish to escape this situation in which they are being rejected by their partner (e.g., Shelton, Richeson, & Salvatore, 2005). With one person signaling dislike and the other signaling a desire to escape, such interactions can be anxiety provoking and tense, and can spiral into a negativity that leads both sides wishing to exit. This in turn can strengthen beliefs that members of other groups are less interested in legitimate and equal contact and make people more avoidant of it in the future (e.g., Shelton & Richeson, 2006). In essence, negative treatment by one partner in the interaction will draw out more cautious, uncomfortable, and awkward reciprocal responses from their partner. In one classic experiment, Word, Zanna, and Cooper (1974) found that White research participants displayed a set of negative nonverbal behaviors that communicated discomfort and dislike when interviewing a Black job candidate: an increased rate of blinking, more speech errors, decreased eye contact, and body posture such as leaning away from the person. While they did not detect their own prejudice, it led to disparate treatment and microaggressions. **Microaggressions** are subtle acts, poten-

> **Microaggressions:** Subtle acts, potentially not consciously initiated, that are perceived as hostile and derogatory by the person toward whom those acts are directed.

tially not consciously initiated, that are perceived as hostile and derogatory by the person toward whom those acts are directed (e.g., Sue, 2010). Importantly, Word et al. further showed that being treated in this way produces negative reciprocal behavior. In a second experiment they examined what happens when a person in an interview is treated in this manner and is the recipient of the type of nonverbal behavior these Black interviewees experienced. They found that when you treat people differently with nonverbal cues, they react in kind. Participants who were the targets of microaggressions were then seen as reciprocating and were judged more negatively than people not treated this way. Negative views led to treating people with negative nonverbal acts (e.g., Dovidio et al., 2002) and elicited negative behavior that confirmed the initial negative view.

The Motivation to Control Prejudice

Any discussion about stereotyping and prejudice is a personal matter, and we can imagine that an individual might not wish to self-disclose this information, and might lie if asked about it. Thus, separate from how any of us think, feel, and value are our social desirability concerns. These are matters of impression management and projecting an acceptable image to others. Will other people perceive us to be biased? Are we going to be rejected for being immoral or "canceled" for failing to meet a cultural ideal about bias? We can imagine that an individual might lie about these matters when asked about it directly. When a person declares "I am the least racist person you will ever meet," there are two distinct reasons they might espouse this concern for prejudice control and a goal of being egalitarian. First, they may be reporting a true belief. Second, the declaration may be strategically false, a deception reflecting simply their concern with *how they look*. A person might be concerned with both of these reasons, or one but not the other.

Plant and Devine (1998) introduced this distinction as two reasons people might be motivated to control prejudice. One is an **internal motivation to control prejudice** (IMCP), which reflects privately held goals to be fair and unbiased, as well as personal beliefs relating to concerns for equality, social justice, and nurturing diversity in one's social life. Members of *other* groups afford one an opportunity to pursue these goals and support those beliefs and are not a threat to one's IMCP, but an affordance. A second is an **external motivation to control prejudice** (EMCP), which reflects a concern with social desirability: concern with doing the socially incorrect thing, worry about the opinions of others, and not wanting to seem biased. Members of *other* groups afford an opportunity for one's social incompetency and bias to be revealed, and create heightened arousal; heightened self-consciousness; and a desire to report beliefs, attitudes, and behaviors that highlight how one is not biased (e.g., Amodio et al., 2003; Bean et al., 2012; Blascovich, Mendes, Hunter, Lickel, & Kowai-Bell, 2001; Mendes, Blascovich, Hunter, Lickel, & Jost, 2007; Moskowitz, Olcaysoy Okten, & Gooch, 2017; Plant & Devine, 2003; Richeson & Trawalter, 2008). Both motives capture so-called principled opposition to bias, but the differences emerge in application of those principles, as seen in work on "laissez-faire racism" and ideological principles (e.g., Bobo, Kluegel, & Smith, 1997; Feldman & Huddy, 2018; Reyna, Henry, Korfmacher, & Tucker, 2006; Sears & Henry, 2003).

Internal motivation to control prejudice: A personally held goal to be egalitarian and fair, with the desire to be nonprejudiced stemming from one's value system and individual needs.

External motivation to control prejudice: A goal to appear egalitarian and fair in the eyes of others and not be seen as doing anything socially incorrect. A desire to report to others that one holds beliefs, attitudes, and behaviors that highlight that one is not prejudiced in order to avoid the anxiety of being labeled biased.

Despite IMCP and EMCP each being motives aimed at controlling prejudice, they do not always produce the same response. IMCP may lead one to say they are an ally, support minority causes, and wish to work toward social justice. The same person whose IMCP leads them to say such things can also have an EMCP that sends the opposite signal. They can appear nervous, anxious, and uncomfortable around a person from a minority group. Even low-prejudiced people with a very high IMCP can have concern with *appearing* prejudiced. In fact, the anxiety associated with EMCP is especially acute for a person who is also high in IMCP. Being nonprejudiced is central to their identity, and having core elements of that identity challenged is especially threatening (e.g., Vitriol & Moskowitz, 2021). Thus, a person high in both IMCP and EMCP will have beliefs and attitudes that denounce bias, but will be exceptionally nervous and anxious about appearing biased and having others questioning their moral credentials. Despite truly believing they despise bias, the signals sent nonverbally communicate anxiety and bias.

Cross-race interactions can be stressful and arousing for this very reason (e.g., Richeson & Shelton, 2007). Both the majority and minority group representatives in the interaction may have no personal bias toward the other group. However, for the minority representative in this interaction there can be a concern with being stereotyped and treated in an unfair way, and this causes anxiety. Their anxiety may lead them to monitor their behavior to make sure they are not sending any signals that might affirm the stereotypes others hold (stereotype threat concerns; e.g., Steele, 1997) and to monitor their partner's behavior for signs that they are biased. They proactively attempt to make sure the interaction goes smoothly, creating a need to monitor and regulate behavior that does not exist in same-race interactions (e.g., Richeson & Shelton, 2003; Shelton et al., 2005; Shelton & Richeson, 2006; Taylor, Garcia, Shelton, & Yantis, 2018; Trawalter & Richeson, 2006; Vorauer, Main, & O'Connell, 1998). This is hard work. For the majority-group representatives there is social anxiety introduced by the interaction associated with potentially being seen as prejudiced, an anxiety that does not exist in same-race interactions. Their anxiety may lead them to engage in impression management to make sure they say only things that can lead to a positive impression and give off no whiff of racism. This is hard work. And may mismatch what they are communicating nonverbally. Such interactions are complex.

Richeson and Shelton (2007) show that all this hard work is draining and actually makes people less effective at performing other tasks that require self-regulation. In one experiment it was illustrated how a cross-race interaction led to decreased performance on a subsequent task that required cognitive control (the Stroop task, reviewed later in this chapter), thus indicating a reduced capacity to self-regulate among people who needed to regulate their stereotypes during the interaction. The devotion of cognitive resources to monitoring the expression of stereotypes and disproving that one may be biased during the interaction worsened performance on a task assessing executive functioning. As Richeson and Shelton stated:

> Engagement in one task that requires self-regulation (e.g., inhibiting behaviors, thoughts) impairs later tasks tapping the same resource. Self-control draws on a central executive attentional resource that can be depleted. Based on the model, therefore, interracial contact impairs performance on tasks that require executive control because individuals engage in self-control during the interaction, which depletes their executive attentional capacity. (p. 317)

They also show that such interactions are distracting, with attention diverted to monitoring these secondary matters of impression management (see also Vorauer & Kumhyr, 2001). Concerns with social desirability from both interaction partners—not affirming a negative stereotype, not seeming to endorse a negative stereotype—lead the interaction to be fraught. Interestingly, Richeson and Shelton report that Black research participants actually preferred a more openly (as compared to less openly) biased White person as an interaction partner because they knew where the person stood. There was no misalignment of verbal and nonverbal behavior, and no feeling of distrust and deception. No need to regulate. At least they knew why the interaction was negative.

Avoidance

The anxiety that social desirability concerns create in cross-race interactions has so far been said to have consequences such as deception, creating distrust, triggering arousal, draining people, and distracting them. As a result of these unpleasant consequences an individual will, often unintentionally, avoid people who are not from their own group. Research in a wide variety of domains (e.g., avoiding eye contact, sitting farther away, ending conversations sooner, exiting an interaction more quickly, avoiding an encounter altogether, speaking less) shows people engaging in such avoidance. At times the avoidance is explicit, as in a classic study of attitudes from the 1930s where hotel owners expressed a desire to avoid contact with minorities by denying them a room at the hotel. This type of denial and avoidance can occur even when the person running the hotel is not overtly prejudiced (e.g., Howerton, Meltzer, & Olson, 2012). At other times people can be subtly avoidant. For example, one way a person can be avoidant is by exiting a situation where social anxiety is present. Peck and Denney (2012) provided evidence of such avoidant behaviors in the health care professions. They studied doctor–patient interactions to see whether doctors exited cross-race interactions more quickly than same-race encounters. To assess this Peck and Denney looked at the medical interviews conducted within the doctor's office. This is not arbitrary chitchat but follows a structure and format in which the doctor has been trained. It should *not* vary based on race, yet it does. Looking at 221 doctor–patient encounters, they found that the amount of patient input solicited and the amount of control exerted by doctors in the interaction fluctuated as a function of race. This resulted in non-White patients having shorter medical visits than White patients (23.9 vs. 28.5 minutes). The 4.5-minute difference represents a 20% shorter visit for patients who are not White (two-thirds of whom were Black).

A similar type of subtle avoidance can emerge in job interviews that invoke social desirability concerns. Hebl, Foster, Mannix, and Dovidio (2002) showed bias in a job interview toward gay and lesbian job applicants, despite participants not realizing they had bias. The bias did not manifest in the form of overt hostility and dislike, but in the form of discomfort and avoidance. Less interest was shown in gay applicants; interactions ended sooner. Specifically, they found that fewer words were spoken by a heterosexual interviewer to gay than straight applicants. Also, the length of the interview was shorter with gay versus straight applicants (M = 245 seconds vs. 383 seconds). The interviewer exits the interview sooner when they are with a member of a social group that is not their own. Avoidant strategies are also indicated by measures showing that the potential employer exhibits less eye contact, and acts more standoffish, with a gay applicant. While clearly prejudice behavior such as lying about the availability of the job, or not being allowed to fill out an application when asked, is not seen, subtle negative behaviors are.

Avoidance is also seen in an experiment by Kawakami, Dunn, Karmali, and Dovidio (2009). Their participants met two confederates posing as other participants . One confederate was Black, the other White. The situation was scripted so that the Black "participant" needed to leave the room momentarily and on the way out gently bumped the White confederate accidentally. Some participants saw only this accidental bump and then were asked to choose who they would want to be their partner on the next task. Half chose the Black confederate and half chose the White confederate. Other participants saw the same accidental bump but also saw the White confederate *utter a racist comment about the bump while the Black confederate was out of the room*. Some heard a moderate racial slur ("I hate it when Black people do that") and some heard an extreme racial slur (the use of a word widely regarded as extremely offensive in the English language). Who does the research participant pick to be their partner? Rather than rejecting them, participants embrace the person who made the racist remark. In both slur conditions they avoid the Black person and choose the racist White person (63% of the time). Observing a racist act makes racism salient, and highlights the racial nature of the interactions that can follow. That anxiety and threat makes people avoidant. So much so that they choose to partner with the racist and avoid the target of the racism. Of course, when asked to predict how they would act in such a situation, people say they would summarily reject the racist. Similar avoidant behavior is seen in an experiment by Plant and Devine (2003) where research participants were asked to return to the lab at a later date for an interaction. They found that as participant anxiety about an upcoming interracial interaction increased, they were less likely to return for the interaction.

Finally, avoidance can also be seen in very low-level responses. In one experiment, Bean et al. (2012) found that White participants who were high in EMCP had a bias in visual attention to faces of Black men that was indicative of threat. Using eye tracking they revealed that, without realizing it, participants would shift their gaze toward faces of Black men and away from faces of White men within the first three-quarters of a second from when the faces appeared. However, at about 1 second (as conscious control began to set in) their gaze quickly shifted so that they became avoidant of the faces of Black men. The immediate response was as if a threat was present (focus attention on the threat), and the more controlled response was avoidance (to divert one's gaze).

Cross-race interactions become an arousing chance for bias and social incompetency to be discovered (e.g., Plant & Devine, 2003; Vorauer & Kumhyr, 2001). Research has established that although external motivation to avoid prejudice is not a general form of arousal that cuts across domains, it is predictive of arousal in intergroup responses, even when White participants are simply briefly shown faces of Black men (e.g., Amodio et al., 2003; Bean et al., 2012; Plant & Devine, 2003). This type of arousal makes individuals motivated to avoid experiencing the anxiety—they avoid cross-race interactions. In this way, people who report themselves to be high in EMCP can be quite poor at controlling the bias they so desperately want to control. Ironically, the very social desirability concerns that they report as making them legitimately not want to be biased will make them anxious and threatened. These feelings can make them avoidant, which is a type of bias. Even when not avoidant, it can make them signal unease and discomfort to an interaction partner, another form of bias. Thus, their self-report is unreliable and inaccurate; it is called into question by their nonverbal behaviors. This is a type of deception. People say they are not biased, they intend to be not biased, but they act in a biased way anyway. However, it is not a deliberate deception. They did not intend to lie.

AVERSIVE RACISM AND SELF-DECEPTION

In the previous section people were shown to lie to others due to social desirability concerns. At times the lies are deliberate (as with the Bradley effect, or minority influence, or conforming to offensive jokes or politically correct attitudes). At times the lies (e.g., saying all is good while displaying nonverbal signaling of dislike, avoiding others) are an outgrowth of unintended processes, such as when private feelings misalign with public norms and cause anxiety. In all of those examples the lie was that a person's true feelings were being concealed from others. Here we turn to lies to the self: where people deny their true feelings in both what they self-report to others and in what they consciously admit in their private thoughts.

Self-Deception and the Desire to Look Good

People at times cannot handle the truth. They deny and suppress inconvenient truths. *People often lie to themselves*, which means they do not recognize their act of self-deception. The lie is engaged to protect self-esteem from damage. Above you were asked to imagine a person without bias, but who had anxiety about appearing biased. Here, we ask you to imagine a more complicated person. Imagine a person who legitimately does not want to be biased and has anxiety about being biased, but who nonetheless has bias that they do not recognize. This is a person who wants to be fair and unbiased and without prejudice, yet deep down they have such biases and prejudices that they do not consciously see. These unwanted thoughts are hidden from the self because they violate important self-standards and values.

Self-deception can shield one from unwanted and non-normative beliefs and feelings. People who desire to be low in prejudice often do not wish to face the reality that they have biases and can at times respond in biased ways. To protect themselves from this negative view of the self, they self-deceive by believing wholeheartedly in their nonbiased sense of self. When you do not want to face your own biases and so you repress and deny them, you have engaged in what is called **aversive racism** (Dovidio & Gaertner, 1986; Gaertner & Dovidio, 1986). One is not only unable to see one's biases, but what one does see is that one is not prejudiced and a need to reject prejudice. To do this people will often (1) exaggerate their own sense of self as unprejudiced, and (2) believe that bias in the culture is extreme by pointing to terrible exemplars (so one's own views are positive in comparison). When engaged in this type of self-deception, the suggestion that one is prejudiced will be experienced as highly aversive, yet at the same time one does in fact possess unconscious thoughts and feelings that label another group as aversive. Despite one not consciously seeing it, one holds negative outgroup beliefs and feelings and consciously has strong egalitarian beliefs.

> **Aversive racism:** Implicit prejudice that emerges among people for whom the suggestion that they are prejudiced is aversive, who simultaneously have unconscious thoughts/feelings that another group is negative or to be avoided. It is a dissociation from the reality that biases exist in the self and reflects a legitimate desire to lack biased tendencies.

As just described, overtly the aversive racist is convinced of their lack of bias and has no overt antipathy. Instead they experience discomfort and anxiety. As discussed earlier, when people have anxiety due to consciously worrying about being seen as prejudiced, they can be avoidant, and they can feel threatened and anxious. Aversive racists experience these same subtle avoidant responses, but for different reasons. Rather than the anxiety arising from a bias they know they have and do not want others to discover, the anxiety arises from a conflict they cannot see. Aversive racism describes a "new" type of bias that complements old-fashioned racism. This is not to argue that the more prototypical forms of explicit and overt prejudice no longer exist. Certainly, prejudice can be expressed openly, and the willingness to do so waxes and wanes with the times (and we are unfortunately in a time where it seems to be waxing).

Aversive racists are continuously providing evidence to support their self-deception that they reject prejudice. When they find themselves in situations where discrimination would be obvious and the social norms to reject bias are strong, aversive racists will act in clearly nonracist ways. They are motivated to illustrate their egalitarian intent. They can point to nonracist beliefs, actions, and attitudes in these situations as a way to avoid facing the bias lingering below the surface. Pearson, Dovidio, and Gaertner (2009) argue that what the aversive racist does not see are the subtle ways in which bias can often leak out through how one acts. In situations that are clearly ones where bias can manifest, they act in an unbiased way that can be contrasted with the bias seen in others. However, there are other situations, that are less clearly about race, where the aversive racist does not think they have acted in a biased way, but an experimenter can easily observe it. Pearson et al. reviewed four types of situations in which aversive racists produce discriminatory responses without realizing their bias. Three situations in which bias can leak out without one realizing it are "situations in which normative structure is weak, when the guidelines for appropriate behavior are unclear, [and] when the basis for social judgment is vague" (p. 318). A final way bias leaks out is in a situation in which one's actions can be justified or rationalized on the basis of some factor other than race. We begin our review of how to detect aversive racism there.

Bias Can Leak Out When It Is Unclear That the Situation Is about Race

When a situation is clearly about race, an aversive racist knows to control how they act. When the situation is not seemingly about race, they are less controlled. What is meant when we say "the situation is not seemingly about race"? It is when race is confounded with other possible reasons to disagree with or dislike a person. When people are **using legitimate issues that are ambiguous to mask bias**, pointing to their principled stance as the

> **Using legitimate issues that are ambiguous to mask bias:** Pointing to existing facts as justification for a response, when in reality that fact is used as a mask to hide a bias that is the true basis for the response. For example, saying existing policies are the reason one dislikes a candidate when it really is gender bias.

reason for the dislike. For example, it is unclear the situation is about race when there are reasons other than race present for disparaging a person—their political views, their inexperience, their having been accused of a crime, their acting badly at an awards show. These are all legitimate reasons to dislike a person that do not need to invoke race. With "cover" being provided by such legitimate reasons, race can be allowed to drive how one responds without fear of being labeled racist. However, such responses are indeed racist if one responds differently when a Black person performs the behavior in comparison to a White person. If your response to a Black politician seeking office, or a Black academic receiving an award, is "they lack experience, I cannot support it," you would be exhibiting aversive racism if your response to a White politician or academic with the same inexperience was "what a young superstar." In such examples the response of the White person to the Black person's situation seems to that White person to not be about race, allowing them to not see that the response is a biased one. Such situations where race is a possible reason for dislike, but another cause is also seemingly legitimate, allow us to diagnose aversive racism since the aversive racist will not see (or control) their bias. They will just lean on the seemingly legitimate explanation.

It is not that one dislikes Black political candidates but this candidate's set of policy positions. It is not that one dislikes Black men but one sees the data as showing that Black men commit more crime. It is not that one disfavors Black applicants for college but the qualifications show the White applicants to be superior. It is not that one does not want more Black people hired at work but that one has a principled opposition to the policy of affirmative action since it is not based on merit. Or to make things very real as I write on a Sunday morning in March of 2022, it is not that one prefers White Ukranian refugees over Syrian or Sudanese refugees but the conditions of the Ukranians warrant special treatment. Of course, it is possible that any of the above expressed beliefs are not race based and are formulated based on the data and good evidence. One could truly oppose affirmative action because of a principled feeling about meritocracy that has nothing to do with race. Not all people espousing such beliefs above are racist. However, aversive racism research is able to show *when* it is race, since the evidence used to justify the choice is shown to shift to whichever available information is negative about the stigmatized group. For example, if a White person opposes affirmative action because it is not meritocratic, yet supports other types of deviations from meritocracy when they benefit White people, then it is race not meritocracy that is the real issue, and meritocracy is used as diversion. One might oppose a mayoral candidate who is Black using their positions on issues as a justification for one's opposition to them, yet if a White candidate with very similar positions on the same issues receives one's support and is deemed acceptable, then it is race not policy that is really directing one's response. The seemingly legitimate cause is shown to be a crutch. McConahay and Hough (1976) stated:

> Behaviorally, it is a set of acts (voting against black candidates, opposing affirmative action programs, opposing desegregation in housing and education) that are justified (or rationalized) on a nonracial basis but that operate to maintain the racial status quo with its attendant discrimination against the welfare, status, and symbolic needs of blacks. (p. 24)

To illustrate this phenomenon, McConahay (1982) performed an experiment that asked White research participants about the policy of using buses to more equally distribute children across schools. In 1970s Louisville, Kentucky, where the study was being conducted, this meant the percentage of Black children in predominantly White schools was increasing due to busing. There are many issues relating to one's own self-interest that one could say is a reason to oppose such busing that are not racially motivated. McConahay examined issues such as having school-age children, being the parent of a child who would be bused, having an interest in maintaining the social stability of the neighborhood, owning a home in the neighborhood, and so on. However, White participants who claimed their opposition was about the policy and not about race were shown to have it truly be about race. McConahay stated:

> Various measures of high and low self-interest among whites were virtually useless in discriminating degrees of support or opposition. On the other hand, measures of racial attitudes were correlated strongly and consistently with the anti-busing position: the more racist, the more opposed. In short, it is not the buses, but the blacks that arouse the ire. (p. 714)

In this instance the White participants truly believed they opposed the practice of school busing, and that objections to this policy had nothing to do with race or the increase of the percentage of Black children in their own child's school. However, opposition to a legitimate issue—busing—was used to mask an illegitimate bias against a group of minority children from entering one's circle. The participants rationalized their preferences on the basis of political beliefs rather than race. A White person will allow racist feelings to seep out if they think they are expressing beliefs regarding issues they do not see as about race. A similar illustration using the more modern example of opposition to Obamacare was provided by Knowles, Lowery, and Schaumberg (2010).

In a second example, Hodson, Dovidio, and Gaertner (2002; see also Dovidio & Gaertner, 2000) showed how people will justify a biased college admission decision by pointing to the credentials of the candidate as the reason for the applicant's rejection. From an aversive racism framework, we would predict that when the qualifications of the prospective applicants *were clear, an unbiased* decision would be made—that is, if an applicant had excellent credentials on every dimension (e.g., both grade point avaerage [GPA] and SAT scores were excellent), there would be no bias. It would only be when a résumé was *questionable* that decisions might reflect bias due to the ability to point toward the insufficient qualifications as the justification for the rejection. Such studies allow us to see bias in action because the White participants show a tendency to reject the Black applicants in favor of White applicants regardless of why the Black applicants lack strength. If a Black applicant has stronger SAT scores but a weaker GPA than a White applicant, White participants say GPA matters and choose the White applicant. Yet, if a White applicant has the exact same qualifications of stronger SAT scores and a weaker GPA than a Black applicant, the White participants now say SAT scores matter and again prefer the White applicant. A pro-White choice is made no matter the data but justified as purely data driven.

In a third example, this has also been shown in hiring decisions. Son Hing, Chung-Yan, Hamilton, and Zanna (2008) investigated discrimination against Asian job applicants in Canada and found that when assessing candidates with identical qualifications, evaluators recommended White candidates more strongly for the position than Asian candidates with identical credentials. Yet they claimed it was credentials that were the basis for the decision. Even though the reality was that whenever the credentials on which the job applicant was best shifted, the participants shifted what credentials they chose to highlight as the basis for the decision. If a White person was superior to the Asian candidate on quality "*x*" but not "*y*," people justified the choice of the White candidate by saying it is clearly quality "*x*" that matters most and is therefore why I selected the White candidate. However, when the White candidate was superior on quality "*y*" then the importance of quality "*y*" was now seen as self-evident and the correct basis for the choice. The same credentials disparaged when held by an Asian applicant were seen as strong when held by a White applicant. The decision always seemed to the participant to be based on evidence, but they could not see how their assessment of the evidence was biased by prejudice. This bias was greatest among participants who scored highest on measures of implicit prejudice.

Self-Deception Can Leak Out When Norms of How to Act Are Unclear

Another time aversive racism can leak out is when there is a **weak normative structure**. Situations vary in regard to how clearly there are rules for how to act, with some situations constraining us entirely, and others where there are no rules (and all points in between). The normative structure is said to be weak when the rules for how to act are poorly defined or nonexistent. For example, if you are alone and come across a person in dire need of help, the norms tell us it is incumbent on us to call for help (at a minimum). If you are one of thousands of people at a festival and see the same person in dire need, then norms of how to act are far less clear. Aversive racism can be diagnosed in such situations, where there is uncertainty about how to act. Helping situations provide a nice way to illustrate the point: Does racism leak out by failing to help a Black victim when one would help a White victim?

> **Weak normative structure:** Situations vary in regards to how clearly rules specify how to act. Some situations' rules constrain us entirely, others situations have no rules. The normative structure is said to be weak when such rules are poorly defined or nonexistent (such as emergency situations with many other bystanders also present).

For example, when a person is in a situation where norms of helping are clear, it would be inappropriate to deny help, and failure to do so when the person "in need" is a member of a minority group would clearly suggest the inaction was a form of bias. However, if your role as a bystander less clearly dictated intervention was required (e.g., Darley & Latane, 1970; Latane & Darley, 1970), then failure to act based on race can be masked by the weakness of the situational norms. Gaertner and Dovidio (1977) provided one of the first experimental illustrations of aversive racism using such a situation. Research participants were White female undergraduates who overheard a supposed emergency in which several chairs seemed to fall on either a White or a Black female confederate. The participants were either alone or in the presence of two other bystanders. No differences in helping behavior were found when alone: The norms were clear. This is a helping situation, and when alone you must be the one to help. When others are present the norms about helping are weaker, and a helping situation that was not seemingly about race can now be seen to be clearly about race. A Black person in need of help in such a situation was provided that help about half as often as a White person.

Gaertner (1973) provided another example. Research participants were U.S. citizens who were called on the telephone at their home with a wrong number that presented a crisis situation to the call recipient. The person calling (long before the days of cellular phones) claimed to have a car broken down on the side of the road and had walked to a phone booth and used their last coins to make this call to what they thought was a service station. Having dialed the wrong number, and now out of coins, they had a simple request: The participant was asked to call the service station for them and report the incident so that help could be sent. The phone number for the "service station" was actually the research lab, where it could be recorded how many people called. Here are two additional keys to the research: (1) half of the participants heard callers with voices that indicated they were likely Black men and half of them heard voices that indicated the person was likely a White man, (2) half of the people called were White and registered as political liberals and half were White and registered as political conservatives. Gaertner found two distinct types of racism evidenced by these unsuspecting research participants. One type was to simply hang up on the Black caller before the emergency situation could be explained. Another type was to listen to the complaint, but then to not take action if the caller was believed to be Black. Conservatives did not differ in hang-up rates, but were far less likely to help a Black caller who explained they needed help (65%) than a White caller (92%). This is an example of more overt bias. They heard that help was needed yet did not offer it at the same rate for Black versus White people. Liberals, in contrast, were just as likely to help each group if they waited to hear the problem—however, they were far more likely to avoid hearing the problem if the caller was Black—they hung up early on a Black caller (20%) more often than a White one (3%). They may believe the inaction was caused by the call being a scam, not because the person was Black. But in this normatively weak condition, the pattern of behavior to these callers suggests a subtle bias is present.

Aversive Racism Leaks Out When the Basis for Social Judgment Is Vague

Aversive racism also manifests when the stimulus being observed is ambiguous. For example, Dovidio and Gaertner (2000) showed research participants the profiles of the personnel at a peer counseling center that were supposedly culled from their job interview. In the key conditions of this experiment the qualifications of the person revealed in their interview showed them to be ambiguous in regard to how well-suited they were for the job. Some of these were White and others Black job candidates. The results were clear—though participants reported having no bias, there was in fact a pro-White bias. Ambiguously qualified Black candidates were evaluated more poorly and were less likely to be recommended for the job than White candidates with the same qualifications. When the records were not ambiguous, and the applicants were clearly strong, there was no bias.

AUTOMATIC PROCESSES AND THE NOTION OF "BELOW-THE-SURFACE" THINKING

The cognition that we experience consciously (such as experiencing the sky as blue) is the end product of a series of processing steps that deliver that experience. A focus on the end result, the conscious experience, can obscure the fact that the experience arises from cognition that we (1) do not see, or (2) cannot see. As described in Chapter 1, there is a *phenomenal immediacy* that makes the conscious experience seem to just appear suddenly, as if delivered by the properties of the stimulus and not produced by the processes of the mind. This does not mean people do not ever recognize the role of their own perception and attention and learning processes in producing what they consciously experience. However, when they do, their assumptions about how they arrived at their conscious experience are often incorrect. It is difficult to introspect upon such inaccessible processes, so people lack the ability to see and to know what to report about how those processes unfold. Yet they still *feel confident* that they know. Humans have a lifetime of experience convincing themselves that they know how they think and what they think. This "feeling of knowing" about their cognitive process gives people high levels of confidence in their conscious experience. The beliefs people hold about their cognitive processes are often wrong, despite the confidence with which they are held.

Nisbett and Wilson (1977; see also Wilson & Brekke, 1994) provided an important illustration of just how much people lack awareness of the processes contributing to their perception of one another. In one clever experiment, Nisbett and Wilson asked participants to memorize a series of word pairs. For some of the people the pairs of words included the pair "ocean–moon." Shortly after finishing this task the participants were asked to answer some mundane questions, and this included among them a question that asked them to name a laundry detergent. The number of people who responded with the brand "Tide" was double for people who had previously seen the word pair "ocean–moon." Are people aware that the word association task influenced their responses about laundry detergent? No. They have a wholly different explanation for the cognitive process that brought that brand to mind. Nisbett and Wilson found that people not only lack awareness of an influence on them (such as thoughts of the ocean or moon unknowingly influencing production of the brand "Tide") but they are also unable to accurately report on the nature of the influence when they correctly suspect one exists. In one experiment students watched a video of a teacher who spoke with an accent. Some people saw the teacher respond in a "warm" way, others saw the teacher respond in a "cold" fashion. The warm/cold behavior determined how much they liked the teacher, and the degree to which they liked the teacher influenced other ratings, even ratings of the teacher on dimensions that should not have been influenced—his attractiveness, how much they liked his accent. The important point is not the fact that such *halo effects* exist, where ratings on one dimension spread to other dimensions. It is that participants cannot accurately guess the direction of the influence! They know their ratings of the teacher are biased, but they believe it is the teacher's attractiveness that influences liking, when it is actually the other way around. When asked to reflect about what we do when forming impressions, we do not have good access to what it is we are doing, and cannot reproduce it accurately when asked.

In the above examples people lack access to accurate knowledge about their cognition because they do not comprehend the actual mechanisms involved. However, a separate reason people lack access to accurately describing their cognitive processes is because they are unable to recognize that any mental activity is taking place. We turn now to a focused discussion of cases of cognition being inaccessible due to its invisibility—to cognition that is automatic. An *automatic process* is not simply a cognitive process for which one lacks conscious awareness. Since most cognitive processes contain some components that occur outside of awareness, practically all processes would be called automatic if automaticity was defined by a lack of conscious awareness at any point in the process. For example, even complex behaviors such as driving lack awareness of one's responding at times. If such actions were to be called "automatic," it would render the term so vague as to be useless. A cognitive process must have all four of the features described below to be defined as automatic (Bargh, 1984, 1989, 1994, 1997). First, an automatic process is one that lacks conscious intent in that it is triggered immediately and directly from stimuli in the environment rather than initiated by a conscious choice. Second, automaticity is marked by a lack of control—once triggered the process will run to completion without disruption (even if one wanted to control it). Third, automatic processes are efficient in that they cannot be disrupted by other ongoing mental activity and usurp very little processing effort. Finally, they occur without awareness; consciousness is not involved at any stage of processing. Driving is not an automatic process because, despite at times lacking conscious monitoring or attention, it is consciously willed (the mere presence of a car does not cause one to jump in and begin driving) and consciously terminated.

The root of the concept of an automatic process can be traced to Charles Darwin's (1872/1998) description of the nonverbal emotional signals humans send to communicate with important others. When describing how complex behavior such as this is routinized, Darwin stated, "some actions, which were at first performed consciously, have become through habit and association converted into reflex actions, and are now so firmly fixed and inherited, that they are performed, even when not of the least use" (p. 45). Similar language is used by James (1890/1950) to define habit: "a strictly voluntary act has to be guided by idea, perception, and volition, throughout its whole course. In habitual action, mere sensation is a sufficient guide, and the upper regions of the brain and mind are set comparatively free" (pp. 115–116). Wegner and Bargh (1998) defined an automatic process as a *mental habit*, "patterns [that] become the deep grooves into which behavior falls when not consciously attended" (p. 459). How does a process become automatic? Through practice, repetition, and habit. Bargh (1990) proposed that a response that is routinely paired with a specific set of environmental features can, over time and practice, lead to the activation of the response given the presence of those environmental features. Let us next turn to examining in detail each of the four elements described above as necessary for identifying an automatic process: lack of conscious intent, efficiency, lack of control, and lack of awareness.

Lack of Conscious Intent

An automatic process is not consciously initiated, but triggered by the stimuli to which one is exposed. When one looks up at the sky one does not consciously intend to perceive its color. In our perception of the people we encounter there is also a good deal of processing that proceeds without our conscious intent: assessing race, gender, facial expressions, and so on. What about complex inferences such as beliefs about a person or attitudes toward a social group? Can these form without intent? How can we illustrate that a process is initiated without intent?

Let us start with the process of detecting a person's facial features. One way that researchers illustrate that facial features can be detected without conscious intent is to present an image of a face subliminally—below the person's threshold for conscious recognition. This is called **subliminal presentation**. If one never consciously detects the presence of a stimulus, yet that stimulus is able to trigger responses associated with it, then the processes associated with detecting it and responding to it must not have been consciously intended. For example, Murphy and Zajonc (1993) subliminally showed faces to research participants, manipulating whether the facial expressions depicted positive or negative emotions. Since the faces were not consciously seen, the participants could not intend to detect the expression and could not intend to have a mood triggered in them by virtue of the expression. Nor could they intend to be influenced by their mood in their judgments of some new and unrelated picture. Nonetheless, the valence

> **Subliminal presentation:** When stimuli appear and disappear so quickly that they are never able to be consciously detected, yet they are detected outside of conscious awareness by the perceptual apparatus.

associated with the faces was shown to influence the judgment of an ambiguous (neutral) stimulus. The stimulus was liked more when preceded by an "unseen" face with positive (as opposed to negative) valence.

Subliminal exposure to stimuli is a useful way to show lack of intent, but not very typical in everyday life. But the lack of conscious intent is easily demonstrated in other ways, most powerfully when people engage in thoughts and actions relating to other people that are the exact opposite of what had been consciously intended—that is, a good way to prove a response is unintended is when people explicitly intend to do something else. Wegner (2002) explains a host of "mystical" phenomena observed through the ages as cases of a person having a conscious intent, and then unconsciously acting against it. The person then misattributes the unexpected behavior to the supernatural rather than to the powers of the automatic processing system. Divining rods, Ouija boards, automatic writing, séance tables lifting or spinning, pendulum divining, water dowsing, and alien hand syndrome all share a common cause. One does not intend to move the object, yet it moves. How can this happen? People imbue the objects with "spiritual" power to explain it. But spirits and magic are not needed. Just because one does not consciously intend to move an object (such as with pendulum swings being used to decide a baby's gender) does not mean that the movement reflects something magical. Instead, people may consciously intend to keep their hand still and let the pendulum "speak," all the while allowing their behavior to be unconsciously guided by their own expectations and desires. One may have an expectation of the result (such as I expect the baby will be a boy) that is never consciously recognized, and such an expectation can cause shifts in muscular movement that produce the expected result (the pendulum swings in the direction that indicates the baby will be a boy). There is no feeling of personal agency or willing. In fact, the agency is to do the exact opposite. People feel as if they know they are not causing the motion (e.g., Ansfield & Wegner, 1996). And because of this **feeling of knowing**, the response feels magical. But it is not. It simply lacks conscious intent.

Feeling of knowing: When one has a conscious intent/belief that one knows why one acts, even when the cause is an automatic process one does not see, and this sense of knowing is wrong. This produces the sense that some outcomes are magical, mystical, or spiritual because one "knows" they were not intended.

There are many examples of people responding in ways that are the exact opposite of what they consciously intend to do. As another interesting example, people often wish to conceal how they truly feel about someone or something. Rather than "wear the heart on the sleeve," a person may want to keep their feelings personal, or even communicate the opposite (acting pleasant when encountering a person who is despised). Concealing emotions when we engage in deception may be what we intend, but we unintentionally continue to send signals that reveal the emotion we wish to conceal. Ekman and Friesen (1969) proposed that while it may be possible to verbally suppress certain ideas or emotions, the body is not always a willing accomplice to our attempts at deceit. Nonverbal signals communicate our true feelings and beliefs with others even when we intend to hide those beliefs through what we say (e.g., DePaulo, Kashy, Kirkendol, Wyer, & Epstein, 1996; DePaulo, Lanier, & Davis, 1983). Despite our intentions, it is difficult to monitor our nonverbal behavior, and the information we intended to keep hidden leaks out. We saw this above when reviewing cross-race interactions. Although we do not intend to send signals, perceivers detect the unintended messages coming from different channels, such as body posture and facial expression (e.g., Ekman & Friesen, 1974; O'Sullivan, Ekman, Friesen, & Scherer, 1985).

It is likely not surprising to learn that we conduct communication with others through a nonverbal language—our personal sign language. Our bodies, faces, social distance, and tone of voice communicate information that interaction partners are constantly sending to and receiving from each other. A wave, a wink, leaning in, a furrowed brow, the middle finger, a shameful smile, pushing away, pulling toward, an outstretched thumb, and a look of disgust are all part of a silent exchange in social interaction. What may be surprising is *how* silent these exchanges are. One illustration was the nonverbal anxiety communicated during cross-race interaction (e.g., Dovidio et al., 2002; Richeson & Shelton, 2007). Chawla and Krauss (1994) provided an experimental illustration of how people unintentionally send and detect nonverbal cues in a domain not involving race. Research participants were to determine whether a person was delivering a rehearsed speech or speaking spontaneously. Two tapes were created of the same speech, one delivered spontaneously, the other a re-creation of the same speech by an actor. Each research participant rated how spontaneous the speech was, and the experimenters then correlated these ratings with the use of nonverbal cues by the speaker. Participants were not intending to use nonverbal cues to help them make this decision, nor were they intending to focus on a specific type of nonverbal cue to help them make this decision, but they did so. Spontaneity ratings made by the perceivers were significantly correlated with certain types of gestures and pauses. These were hand gestures and pauses in speech known to be related to problems with lexical access (trouble pulling words and thoughts from memory). Without intending to, perceivers scanned the behaviors for these cues, and used these cues to help them decide whether the behavior was spontaneous. The types of cues used were nonverbal acts such as observing someone tilting their head when trying to think of just the right word, or someone pausing as if trying to "off-the-cuff" think of a good example.

Efficiency

Efficient processes are able to operate even in the face of limits to one's processing capacity (like being rushed, working on many tasks simultaneously, having divided attention, etc.). An efficient process requires little mental energy and effort and is not constrained by ongoing mental activity; it runs to completion without being disturbed regardless of processing constraints that disable other forms of cognition. Color detection is an efficient process. You can detect that the color of a passing car is red while simultaneously straining memory for the year Martin Luther King was murdered (it was 1968). In person perception research, many of the processes used to characterize other people (and the self) proceed with such efficiency. Being lost in deliberation, or straining to retrieve information from memory, or trying to remember the grocery list does not incapacitate the ability to form impressions of other people (e.g., Uleman, Hon, Roman, & Moskowitz, 1996).

> **Efficient processes:** A process that operates even in the face of limits to one's processing capacity (like being rushed, multitasking, or having divided attention) because it requires relatively little mental energy and effort and is not constrained by ongoing mental activity. It runs without being disturbed regardless of processing constraints or cognitive load.

For example, Bargh and Thein (1985) provided evidence that the processing of highly relevant information is efficient. For some of their research participants' traits related to honesty were highly relevant; other participants had no particular affinity for the trait of being honest. Participants then read a set of behavioral descriptions about other people. A given set had 24 behaviors, 12 of them implying a relevant trait (such as honest), 6 implying an inconsistent trait (dishonest), and 6 were neutral. Descriptions were presented one at a time on the computer. Some people were asked to read the sentences in only 1.5 seconds, making the task highly demanding of their mental energy. Such people were described as being under time pressure to respond, having to make a rapid response. Although rapid response is not exactly the same thing as making responses when inundated with large amounts of information, for the sake of convenience we group all such types of responses that place a person under highly limiting conditions as a response made under *cognitive load*. For other participants the task was performed while they were not under cognitive load. In summary, there were people who either did or did not value honesty who received informa-tion about another person that was either relevant to honesty or not, and they received this information while either under or not under cognitive load.

If forming an inference is an efficient process, it should occur regardless of whether one is under cognitive load. If not efficient, the time pressure (load) should create limita-tions that disrupt one's ability to process the behaviors and form an impression. The data show that people who do not value honesty have no trouble processing the information when there is no load (so they come to see the person as honest), but when doing the same task under cognitive load they no longer come to form an impression of the person as hon-est. Their ability to form a coherent impression is interfered with by the limit placed on their processing. However, people for whom honesty was a relevant trait do not have such an impairment. For these people the proportion of honest traits that were presented was able to be detected and used to guide their impressions. This was true both when cognitive load was absent and when it was present. This suggests that processing information that one deems as highly relevant is efficient. It happens even when responding occurs too rapidly to stop and think deeply.

The **cocktail party effect** is another illustration of the efficiency of self-relevant infor-mation. You have likely experienced your own ability to detect your name being spoken in a loud and crowded room when you were engaged in a conversa-tion with someone and not paying attention to what people engaged in other conversations were saying. Yet somehow when they speak your name, it turns out that you were, at some level, attending to what others were saying in the din. How is this possible? Much of perceptual experience takes place prior to your conscious awareness getting involved. The mind efficiently perceives many more things than get reported to consciousness. This ability is linked to a differen-tiation between short term and iconic memory. Due to the huge amount of information that bombards our senses at any given moment we have developed the ability to store large amounts of information, for very brief periods, without con-sciousness getting involved. The vast sensory storage house of visual information is known as **iconic memory** (called *echoic memory* for auditory stimuli). Once information enters this storehouse, people are able to "decide" what information, from this bombardment, enters consciousness, capturing our focus of attention, and is represented in short-term memory.

> **Cocktail party effect:** Phenomenon whereby one detects one's name spoken in a loud and crowded room when otherwise fully engaged and not paying attention to what people in other conversations were saying. Yet one's name jumps out from the din. It indicates the vast attentional capacity humans have beyond what they con-sciously recognize.
>
> **Iconic (echoic) memory:** A vast sensory storage house of informa-tion where perceived stimuli are held before consciously detected. Once in storage people can "decide" what information enters consciousness, capturing our focus of attention, and this is represented in short-term mem-ory. This vast amount of information is in storage only very briefly.

These "decisions" about what information to keep and what to filter out occur prior to conscious reflection and are done efficiently, without being constrained by conscious men-tal activity. Thus, although you may not have been consciously attending to another conver-sation in the room, the contents of other conversations were being scanned and placed in the iconic storehouse. When that content is self-relevant, perception and attention shift to alter what enters consciousness.

Lack of Control

Lack of control refers to one's inability to stop a cognitive process from happening. Once the stimulus that triggers the process is present, one cannot stop the process from starting. Once started one cannot stop it. Even if one consciously decides to not perform the process prior to seeing the triggering stimulus, knowing full well that the stimulus is about to be presented, one still cannot stop its occurrence in the face of this preparation. If I asked you to look at the sky and not perceive its color, you could not do it. The mere presence of the stimulus (sky) triggers the response (color perception) regardless of any goals you might have to prevent the response.

As another example, if I ask you to ignore the meaning of the words written in this sentence and focus only on whether the shapes of the particular letters are curved versus angled, you would still likely extract the meaning of the words. Extracting word meaning occurs even when we consciously try to control it. Stroop (1935) provided a classic experimental illustration of this fact. Research participants were shown either words that named a specific color ("red," "blue," green," etc.) or patches of the color. The words were always printed in colored ink, but the color of the ink did not always match the word. For example, the word "red" might be written in blue ink, while the word "blue" might be yellow colored. The task was extremely simple: Name the ink color. This is facilitated by not reading the words. Naming the ink color is difficult when it is in a word as opposed to a rectangular patch. When the word "red" is written in blue ink, people instead start to name the printed word ("red") rather than the ink in which it is printed (blue). The processing of word meaning occurs immediately upon perceiving the word. They then need to stop and correct themselves, which interferes with the ability to do the task asked of them (naming the color) relative to just seeing a patch of color. Why? Indicating you have seen the color blue when encountering the word "red" in blue ink is in conflict with an uncontrolled response of reading the word (what we usually do with words). The inability to control one response (reading) slows the designated response (naming colors). This **Stroop effect** illustrates interference due to lack of control over an automatic process.

One can use a similar methodology to illustrate that processes in person perception are beyond control. For example, Geller and Shaver (1976) presented words to people and asked them to name the color of the ink. This time, however, instead of the words being color names, the words were either self-relevant to the people who were reading them or neutral words that were not relevant to the research participants. The logic was that stimuli that are relevant to us will be detected and processed without being able to control it. We cannot help reading words that are presented to us, and when those words are relevant to us we find ourselves distracted by them and wanting to linger on them. This increased attention to the word meaning is in conflict with the task. Rather than saying the color of the ink as fast as possible, we are sidetracked by the processing of self-relevant information in our environment. A similar finding was produced by Bargh and Pratto (1986). Words pretested to be part of a participant's self-concept were shown in colored inks, along with words that were not self-relevant. Participants were to name the color of the ink. The reaction times to naming ink colors were reliably slower when the word content (which should be ignored to efficiently do the task) was consistent with the participant's self-concept. Attention was uncontrollably drawn by word content that was self-relevant. As Shiffrin (1988) stated: "If a process produces interference with attentive processes despite the subject's attempts to eliminate the interference, then the process in question is surely automatic" (p. 765).

> **Stroop effect:** When automatically detecting a word's semantic meaning is illustrated by interference with another task. For example, if "red" is written in blue ink and the task is to name the ink's color, we can discern that the semantic meaning "red" is automatically triggered if interference with saying "blue" occurs when naming the ink color.

Lack of Awareness

Lack of awareness of a cognitive process is perhaps the easiest from among the features of automaticity to grasp intuitively. Many of the cognitive tasks we engage in occur without our awareness; the feeling of gears churning is absent. We can drive while lost in thought, without any awareness of what we did during the last 4 miles. We earlier reported an experiment by Murphy and Zajonc (1993) in which people were influenced by facial expressions in photos that were presented subliminally. If the facial expressions were never consciously seen, the person would obviously not be aware of its influence. Yet an influence was evidenced all the same. In the Murphy and Zajonc research, perceivers are not aware of the processes through which a subliminally presented picture of a face impacts on their evaluation of an object. Indeed, they are not even aware of the existence of the influencing force (the facial expressions).

Varieties of Automaticity

Most information processing contains some subset of these four criteria for automaticity, but not all of them. A running example has been that of driving a car. It does not meet all these features, yet driving does not always occur with full consciousness and one's awareness focused on the task. To call this activity fully under control would seem to misrepresent the process. But so too would calling it automatic. To capture the full complexity of most processes, especially those involved in perceiving other people, Bargh (1989) proposed that there are varieties of automaticity. This allowed for the possibility that the four features of automaticity could appear in various combinations. If a process possessed all four features, such as when one perceives color, it was said to be a particular variety of automatic processing: **preconscious automaticity**.

If one does not intend to initiate a response and even lacks awareness that the response has occurred, but its occurrence requires some type of conscious processing, then a second variety of automaticity is said to exist: **postconscious automaticity**. For example, you may unintentionally and unknowingly find yourself sending nonverbal cues to someone you are interacting with, yet are conscious of the interaction and of the fact that nonverbal signals of some type are being sent. These cues could unintentionally signal to that person that you are uncomfortable around them (e.g., you lean away from them, fail to make eye contact). The perceiver might not realize they are seeking out facial cues and the person whose face it is might not intend to have anything but a neutral facial expression. Yet information about broad personal qualities, such as dominance, power, and trustworthiness, are sent through facial features and are detected by perceivers (Todorov, Said, Engell, & Oosterhof, 2008). Micro-expressions one does not intend to send can reveal when one is lying (Ekman & Rosenberg, 2005). However, such unintended responses would not have occurred had you not consciously decided to interact with the person who is detecting these unintended facial expressions.

Finally, some processes occur without conscious awareness and with great efficiency, but require that one has a conscious goal in place for the response to be initiated. This variety of automatic processing was labeled **goal-dependent automaticity**. A perfect example has already been discussed at length: driving. Driving is efficient (you can go miles without

Preconscious automaticity: A cognitive process that has all four features of an automatic process—it is not consciously intended, it is efficient, it happens outside conscious awareness, and it is unable to be controlled.

Postconscious automaticity: A cognitive process that is efficient and occurs without awareness but that can be controlled when conscious processing demands it. For example, you may unintentionally and unknowingly send nonverbal cues during an interaction, but can control it when desiring to control it. Consciousness allows for control over the process.

Goal-dependent automaticity: A cognitive process that requires one to have a conscious goal for the response to be initiated, but runs outside awareness and without conscious monitoring. For example, you may intend to mentor another person but unintentionally trigger microaggressions when doing so that would have been absent without a mentoring goal.

it being disrupted by simultaneous tasks such as making a call, being lost in thought, and singing quite loudly). But it requires having the goal to drive, and starting and stopping can be controlled by willing it.

EFFICIENCY AND IRRATIONALITY

Identifying the various features of automaticity and incorporating them into the definition is important if one hopes to distinguish an automatic process from other responses people make that are similarly efficient. Why is it essential to make this distinction? Because equating the term "automaticity" with low effort can give rise to the false conclusion that unconscious processing is irrational processing. Automatic processing is often "rational" and accurate, while conscious processing is at times low in effort and irrational. It is important to distinguish automatic processing from processes that simply reflect irrationality and mindlessness.

Mindlessness

Automatic processing is not simply a shortcut people use to avoid thinking deeply. Rather than laziness, it is a routine set of responses that are associated with a stimulus that allow one to develop increased efficiency at a task. It allows one to trigger associations (which may or may not be accurate) once detecting a cue that is diagnostic of the category. For example, one may detect a person wearing a turban, and this might trigger one's associated knowledge of the various cultures in which people wear headwear with cloth winding in this fashion. If one's schema matches that specified by Wikipedia, then one would have knowledge that a variety of cultures have people who wear turbans and this includes communities located in "the Indian subcontinent, Southeast Asia, the Arabian Peninsula, the Middle East, the Balkans, the Caucasus, Central Asia, North Africa, West Africa, East Africa, and among some Turkic people in Russia, as well as Ashkenazi Jews." It need not be an automatic process that causes a person with such a schema to incorrectly categorize a person wearing a turban as Middle Eastern. The automatic process associates turbans with this group, but with many other groups as well. If a person with such a schema were to misidentify another person wearing a turban as Middle Eastern solely on the basis of them wearing a turban, this would be an incorrect use of conscious processing, not a flawed automatic process.

In this example there is an automatic process that triggered many possible groups that are all associated with the category. Yet the error occurs not in associating these groups with the category but in the irrational narrowing of focus on one of these groups to the exclusion of the others when there is no other reasonable evidence to do so, and perhaps good evidence to suggest a different group is more relevant (such as Balkan). The easy triggering of information should not be confused with the low effort use of conscious reasoning to limit what we think. Bargh (1984) makes this point by contrasting automatic processing with **mindlessness**: a type of thinking about other people in which mental energy and effort seems to have been eliminated in how we consciously attend to their behavior and features. Langer, Blank, and Chanowitz (1978) introduced the term, and defined it as responding initiated in a situation when "attention is not

> **Mindlessness:** A type of thinking where mental effort is apparently eliminated and we instead operate using existing knowledge about situations/people. For example, scripts, frames, and schemas specify appropriate ways to act that can merely be triggered by cues in the environment, allowing one to respond without the need for mental elaboration.

paid precisely to those substantive elements that are relevant for the successful resolution of the situation . . . new information is actually not being processed . . . what is meant by mindlessness here is this specific ignorance of relevant substance" (p. 636). Like an automatic process we operate on the basis of existing knowledge about situations and people, but unlike an automatic process that knowledge is triggered because of a faulty and incomplete conscious assessment of the features of the stimulus. Whereas automatic processing reflects unconscious processing, mindlessness involves an incorrect use of conscious processes in an effort to not think deeply. The difference is subtle. Automaticity is when a cue that has, through habit and conditioning, been associated with a representation triggers that representation without one knowing (and perhaps without even knowing the cue is present). Mindlessness is when the same responses are triggered by the same cue, but because one consciously chooses to focus on that cue to the exclusion of other information in the situation that would render the responses inappropriate. A selective ignoring of some information, the choice not to process relevant stimuli in the situation in favor of the simplicity offered by the script, is its hallmark. While automatic processing may make it easier to detect some stimuli over others, this is not the same as choosing to ignore some stimuli because it would be effortful or undesirable to do so. One is about the efficiency of thought, and one is about a conscious choice to not exert necessary effort.

Langer et al. (1978) assumed that mindlessness resulted in behavior produced without the benefit of conscious consideration of the cues in the situation; behavior initiated because a superficial assessment of a situation triggers a script or schema. It is mindless not because the response is automatically associated with a schema but because the schema is triggered by a superficial assessment. Situations we enter into, such as getting a beverage at the coffee shop, have features and cues that tell us how to act. Conscious processing is focused on verifying the script as appropriate for this situation. The script may tell you that first you wait on line, then you order, then you pay, then you walk to the other end of the counter, then you retrieve your beverage. But if you wait behind a group of people only to learn they have already ordered, this is not a problem with automatic processing being irrational. You have simply failed to dedicate enough conscious processing to detect that there is no line, so the script is not relevant in this situation. According to Bargh (1984), with mindlessness "the result is that certain pieces of information are selected by the script over others that may actually be more relevant and useful in the current situation" (p. 35). People scan the environment in a way that fails to detect germane information and avoid using information they should use (if operating rationally).

A well-known experiment by Langer et al. (1978) makes this point using the category of "a favor." If a favor is requested, then the triggering of an associated response would be a type (or variety) of automaticity. There are scripts that specify how to act if a favor is requested. However, if another person does not make a legitimate favor request, it is not an automatic process if you respond with the scripted response. This is simply you, the perceiver, getting the category wrong because not enough attention was paid to realize that the script for "favor" is not appropriate in this instance. This is superficial processing of the features and assigning the wrong label, but then using the right associations to that wrong label. The association would not be irrational had the schema for "favor" actually been invoked. But one's low effort at attending to the situation caused the wrong category to be invoked, and hence the response is irrational. Langer et al. had an experimenter approach unsuspecting people who were using the copy machine at the library. These people were asked if they would step aside and allow the experimenter to use the copy machine immediately. They reasoned that this request could trigger a script in the mind of the person using the copy machine that a favor was being requested, and that favors reflect either an urgent need, or an emergency. The triggering of the script for "a favor," they reasoned, would depend on whether or not *a reason* was provided by the person making the request. If the person merely said, "please stop what you are doing and allow me to cut in and make copies immediately," without providing any reason, they would likely be seen as rude and the request denied. However, if the person offered a reason, then the script for a favor would be triggered. Langer et al. argued that because of mindlessness, all that was needed to trigger the script was for the person making the request to *seemingly* offer a reason. It should not matter if the reason offered was legitimate or ridiculous. If the person being asked is mindlessly processing the request, they would relinquish the copy machine.

Langer et al. (1978) argued that if any reason offered—even a ridiculous one—resulted in the person acquiescing, then we would have evidence of mindlessness. The person at the copy machine would simply follow the rule of "if a favor is requested and is accompanied by a reason and I am not being burdened in any way, then comply." They would stop assessing whether the reason was legitimate. To show this, some of the people using the copy machine were approached and asked, "excuse me, I have five copies to make, can I use the machine instead of you *because I am in a rush*." Other people using the copy machine were approached and asked, "excuse me, I have five copies to make, can I use the machine instead of you *because I have to make copies*." Each of these requests seem to follow the script for a favor by the person offering a reason for the request. Yet one of these requests offered no reason at all, but just followed the format of providing a reason—can I make copies because I have to make copies. Evidence for mindlessness was found because each "reason" was equally effective at having the request granted; both requests led the person to relinquish their use of the copy machine more than when the person was approached at the copy machine and asked without a reason being provided—"excuse me, I have five copies to make, can I use the machine instead of you." Adding "because I have to make copies" offers no additional information, and is thus not a real reason. But it is effective. Why? Because it triggers mindlessness where people stop paying attention to relevant details and then surrender their action to the scripted response. Even though the script for a favor does not really apply. They irrationally treat a person with a nonsensical and vapid "reason" better than a person with no reason. It is not the script and the process of triggering responses associated with it that is irrational, but the mindlessness on the part of the perceiver consciously invoking the wrong category and hence the wrong script. Mindlessness is a poor deployment of conscious processing, not irrationality of the automatic processes. It exists when people act and think with a low level of conscious involvement and end up not making use of (or paying attention to) all the relevant details in their environment. To quote Langer et al. (1978): "only a minimal amount of structural information may be attended to and that this information may not be the most useful part of the information available" (p. 641).

Are Conscious Processes More Irrational Than Automatic Processes?

Research on mindlessness points out that consciousness does not guarantee that people will think rationally, and research on automaticity highlights that not all processes that lack conscious awareness are irrational. Automatic processing is not to be equated with irrational outcomes. When an automatic process leads us to retreat into the unconscious it can service our ability to detect relevant information in the environment, just as conscious processing can lead us to ignore relevant information. Huang and Bargh (2014) argued that in many areas, such as self-regulation, automatic processes were an evolutionary earlier development relative to conscious processes; during self-regulation people often operate better without the burden of consciousness. Conscious processing can yield undesired results, and an implicit form of regulation might avoid these errors and biases. Typically, a process becomes automated through practice, and that practice is engaged in because the process is making responding easier and more efficient. Irrationality is not a feature of automaticity, but efficiency is.

For example, a conscious goal to control the use of stereotypes can have unintended consequences that promote stereotyping (e.g., Macrae, Bodenhausen, Milne, & Jetten, 1994). Asking people to explicitly try and be colorblind leads to them using race more rather than less (Norton, Vandello, Biga, & Darley, 2008). These acts of consciousness result in the opposite outcome. As another example, telling people to be creative, and giving them direct instructions about what not to do (e.g., do not plagiarize, do not copy the names of existing products when generating new brand names), leads to a lack of creativity. People in such experiments plagiarize more and copy brand names to a greater degree (e.g., Marsh, Bink, & Hicks, 1999; Marsh, Ward, & Landau, 1999; Smith, Ward, & Schumacher, 1993). Wegner and Erskine (2003) describe an entire class of unintended effects that result from people trying to exert control over their own unwanted acts. Conscious thought is not always better than automatic processing.

There are many lines of work that illustrate that at times the elimination of consciousness creates better efficiency, a reduction in bias, and better outcomes (e.g., Dijksterhuis, Bos, Nordgren, and van Baaren, 2006; Dijksterhuis & Nordgren, 2006; Sassenberg & Moskowitz, 2005). Let us return again to the example of being creative, which by definition requires that one avoid conventional ways of thinking and typical associations. Research has shown, as noted above, that asking people to try and be creative has the opposite effect. However, when creativity is triggered outside of conscious awareness and the pursuit is turned implicit, the desired outcomes of heightened creativity are achieved (Sassenberg et al., 2021; Sassenberg & Moskowitz, 2005). Similar benefits of unconscious cognition can be seen in decision making. Dijksterhuis et al. (2006) gave some participants a conscious task of choosing between several products (e.g., from among four apartments to rent). They were given time to consciously evaluate the qualities of each option and then make a choice. Other participants were not given time to consciously evaluate the qualities that differentiated among the options. They found that the people who were not able to consciously deliberate made objectively "better" choices than people with conscious effort exerted. The logic of this research is that when denied the chance to consciously evaluate, people still had the goal of making a choice and continued to deliberate and assess the options outside consciousness. The processes used to regulate this goal were happening outside awareness and were less prone to bias than the conscious ones.

In another illustration of the benefits of automatic processing, Shah (2003) showed that when people had a goal of performing an analytical reasoning task that required conscious effort, performance on that task was facilitated if a second goal had been unconsciously triggered in the same participants. This was only true if the two goals were compatible with each other (such as an unconscious goal to be creative). Thus, whereas trying to meet two conscious goals would be effortful and overloading, trying to meet an implicit goal is not an overload to the conscious goal. It can actually make a conscious goal easier to reach. People are more efficient when a single behavior can serve multiple goals that can each help toward performance (e.g., Chun, Kruglanski, Friedman, & Sleeth-Keppler; 2011). Fishbach, Friedman, and Kruglanski (2003) showed that when an unconscious goal was incompatible with a conscious goal it could still produce more efficient responding by inhibiting the conscious goal (especially if the unconscious goal was the more important). For example, people with an unconscious goal of eating healthy were able to inhibit their conscious goals relating to pleasure eating that were harmful to them in the long term.

Macrae, Milne, and Bodenhausen (1994) argued that if automatic processes are to be thought of as promoting efficiency and better responding, there should be demonstrable benefits; information processing should be easier, more efficient, and cognitive resources preserved when automatic processing accompanies a conscious task. For example, even though we think of stereotypes as negative, if they evolved to make us more efficient, then they could serve as a useful means for economizing cognition. People who use stereotypes on a task should be able to think less and arrive at decisions about people more quickly than people who do not (e.g., Gilbert & Hixon, 1991). This "savings" afforded by the use of the stereotype should be reflected elsewhere with increased efficiency; they should be better at another task they perform at the same time. Macrae et al. found that people who unconsciously used a stereotype in an impression-formation task had attentional resources liberated that were then used to assist in executing a reading comprehension task that required intense focus. People without a stereotype to use on task 1 performed worse on task 2.

Throughout this book we see many examples of automatic processing producing unwanted outcomes and biases. Indeed, this is how many people think of unconscious processes: either through the Freudian lens of trauma or this more modern lens of bias. When bias is produced by automatic processing, conscious processing can help to overcome those errors and mitigate the bias. Our point here is that this view is unbalanced. Both automatic processing and conscious processing can produce better cognitive outcomes, and both are capable of leading to bias. The argument put forth here is that automatic processing is the child of desires for efficiency and ease, and not of trauma and error. Even some of the errors produced by automatic processing are beneficial to the organism. Balcetis and Dunning (2010) showed that people perceive things that they are motivated to acquire as closer to them than objects they do not desire. Thirsty people perceived a bottle of water as 1.1 times closer. Less wealthy college students saw a $100 bill they could win as 1.2 times closer than a $100 bill they could not win. People who felt strong disgust for insects perceived a spider to be 1.5 times farther away than people with no such aversion (Cole et al., 2013). Women who saw a man urinating in public perceived him to be 1.4 times farther away than an angry man (Cole et al., 2013). When people need to act to acquire a desired reward or avoid danger, their automatic processes bias their perception of distance. But this bias is helpful to them and serves their well-being.

AUTOMATIC ATTITUDES AND BELIEFS: THE IMPLICIT NATURE OF IMPRESSIONS OF GROUPS

The capacity to evaluate other people is essential for navigating the social world. Humans must be able to assess the actions and intentions of the people around them, and make accurate decisions about who is friend and who is foe, who is an appropriate social partner and who is not. Indeed, all social animals benefit from the capacity to identify individual conspecifics that may help them, and to distinguish these individuals from others that may harm them. Human adults evaluate people rapidly and automatically on the basis of both behavior and physical features.
—HAMLIN, WYNN, AND BLOOM (2007, p. 557)

What Is an Attitude?

An **attitude** is an evaluation of a person or an object encountered in the social world—an assessment of the target as positive or negative. Attitudes specify how we feel, dictate our positive and negative reactions, and this naturally guides our behavior (though the links between attitude and behavior are a complex topic that is best reviewed by a more specialized book or chapter; e.g., Albarracin, Johnson, & Zanna, 2005; Fazio, 1986, 1990b). As such, evaluations orient the person for interacting with the social world, so that the person approaches or engages the stimuli they view favorably and avoids or disengages with the stimuli they view negatively (e.g., Eaton, Majka, & Visser, 2008). Due to their functionality, attitude activation is seen in the psychological literature as among the most primary and important mental activities in which humans engage. Even infants show a preference for a character who helps others and an avoidance of a character who hinders others. If shown animated characters who help another character up a hill, versus characters who prevent another from trying to get up that hill, a 10-month-old will like those characters who help and dislike those who hinder. When presented with both characters, infants choose to play with the one they had seen help (e.g., Hamlin et al., 2007). From infancy we are *evaluating others based on their actions and intentions*. It is not just people but any object, place, or thing is also evaluated. The target of these evaluations is known as an **attitude object**. Fazio, Sanbonmatsu, Powell, and Kardes (1986) argued that people spontaneously retrieve stored attitudes from memory when an attitude object is seen, and that they use this initial attitude as the basis to evaluate, judge, and make decisions about the current attitude object—that is, the attitude is associated with the attitude object, so that when the object is encountered the attitude now has heightened **attitude accessibility**. Once accessible, the association of attitude and attitude object is reinforced.

Many theories of attitudes specify that an attitude is more than just the "affect" experienced toward a stimulus. The attitude is thought of as a structure represented in memory that contains this evaluative or affective response, but also specifies behavior relevant to how one might appropriately respond to the attitude object, as well as related cognition—knowledge and beliefs—about the attitude object. For example, Greenwald (1968) showed that when an evaluation of an attitude object occurs there is an accompanying **cognitive response**. People actively engage their existing beliefs when evaluating, and the content of this internal dialogue regarding what they know about the attitude object is their cognitive response. This can include thoughts that affirm the existing attitude, but also counterarguments that create doubt about the existing evaluation. And as reviewed in Chapter 2, attitudes can contain associative learning that connects it to affect, but also to propositional learning (e.g., De Houwer, 2014a, 2014b; Gawronski & Bodenhausen, 2018; Kurdi & Banaji, 2023) that dictates the relationship among attitude objects.

Attitudes differ from one another not only in the affective response they trigger but in how strongly those reactions are held (e.g., Fazio, 2007). **Attitude strength** is determined by factors such as (1) how important the attitude object is to the person (its association to goals to which one is highly committed and to the vested interests of close friends, family, and social in-groups), (2) its embeddedness among one's value and belief system (its association in an interconnected network of one's philosophical, political, moral, and religious

Attitude: An evaluation of an object as positive or negative. Many theories specify it is more than "affect," it is a structure in memory that also specifies how to appropriately respond to an attitude object (behavior), as well as related knowledge and beliefs (cognition) about the person/thing being evaluated.

Attitude object: A stimulus (person, place, or thing) that is the target of a person's evaluation; the thing to which they have an attitude.

Attitude accessibility: The attitude object serves as a prime that makes the existing attitude have heightened accessibility. Once accessible, an attitude can reinforce its association to the attitude object by being applied yet again to the evaluation of the attitude object that triggered it.

Cognitive response: When attitudes are formed or changed by actively engaging existing beliefs and an internal dialogue regarding what one knows about the attitude object is triggered. This can include thoughts that affirm the existing attitude, but also counterarguments that create doubt about the existing evaluation.

Attitude strength: The degree to which an attitude is important to a person and richly embedded in a network that ties it to one's knowledge, committed goals, social identity, moral beliefs, and vested interests.

values), (3) how well-informed the person is when developing the attitude (more knowledge when forming an initial attitude will lead to it being more strongly held), and (4) its association to social identity concerns. Fazio et al. (1986) illustrate that the more strongly held the attitude is, the faster and easier it is activated from memory when the attitude object is encountered, making stronger attitudes more likely to be reinforced through repeated use. Thus, stronger attitudes can be detected by their ease of accessibility. For example, attitude objects associated with morality should be linked to strongly held attitudes and trigger affect and inferences about whether a person is honest and trustworthy (e.g., Brambilla & Leach, 2014). This is supported by functional magnetic resonance imaging (fMRI) research that shows that the association of trustworthiness with a face (as an attitude object) shows corresponding activity in the amygdala (Winston, Strange, O'Doherty, & Dolan, 2002), which is active when detecting dangerous and threatening stimuli (e.g., Todorov, Dotsch, Porter, Oosterhof, & Falvello, 2013; Todorov, Dotsch, Wigboldus, & Said, 2011).

Are Attitudes Automatic?

Bargh, Chaiken, Govender, and Pratto (1992) argued that attitudes are more than easily made accessible, but that there are **automatic attitudes** (e.g., Bargh, 2017; Fazio, 2007)— activation occurs whenever the attitude object is encountered without the conscious intention to retrieve the attitude. The process of evaluating the stimuli (especially people) we encounter, due to its frequency and repetition, comes to be *automated*. Bargh et al. proposed that people have attitudes relating to *everything* they encounter, and those attitudes are triggered within *milliseconds* of having encountered whatever the thing may be. As described in the quote from Hamlin and colleagues (2007) that starts this section, this triggering of affect is described by researchers as having a functional and adaptive value, and it is this functionality that is believed to be the cause of its habitual use and ultimate automation. And this automatic attitude activation is not dependent on attitude strength. Even weakly held attitudes are activated automatically. Attitude strength might impact whether an attitude guides judgment and behavior, but accessibility of the attitude—its associated evaluation being triggered and made ready to use—depends only on the presence of an attitude object.

> **Automatic attitudes:** Positive or negative affective evaluations that are immediately triggered by stimuli; the mere presence of the stimulus leads to activation of an evaluative response associated with the stimulus. Such implicit affective responses allow us to know if the stimulus is a threat or an opportunity; whether to approach or avoid.

Chen and Bargh (1999) provide an illustration that nicely shows the automatic triggering of attitudes, and the adaptive nature of attitudes via their link to approach and avoidance goals. They argued that if an attitude is activated automatically, then people should be faster to respond in a manner consistent with the attitude, such as approaching a positive attitude object and avoiding a negative one. They reasoned that approach motivations and liking are associated with pulling something toward you, such as with a response that involves an arm flexion. Avoidance and dislike are associated with pushing something away, such as with a response that involves an arm extension. Therefore, if a positive attitude is implicitly triggered, it should make one faster to flex. If a negative attitude is triggered, one should be faster to extend. They asked research participants to simply move a lever when a word appeared. Half of them were told to move the lever toward them (a flex) and the other half were told to push the lever away from them (an extend). They then manipulated whether the words that appeared were positive or negative. Although this task was not ostensibly about attitudes, responses were faster to the positive words (vs. negative words) when participants had to move the lever toward them when the word appeared. The opposite was true when the arm movement was extension, people responded faster to negative words. The words automatically triggered an attitude, and this activation is reflected in the way approach and avoidance behaviors were facilitated.

Automatic attitude activation even occurs if we do not consciously know we have even seen anything. As Bob Zajonc (1980b) said, "preferences need no inferences" (p. 151). When images of, say, the Pope are flashed at people so fast they cannot report having even seen an image, let alone the Pope, the positive (or negative) attitudes associated with the Pope will be triggered in one's mind (e.g., Baldwin et al., 1990). We evaluate everything, and we evaluate everything immediately, even without knowing we are doing it, and even without knowing we have even seen anything to evaluate. However, the automatic triggering of an attitude should not be confused with a lack of awareness that an attitude exists—that is, one can have explicit awareness of the attitude (e.g., that one dislikes cauliflower) without awareness of how it was formed or how it is activated, or that it was activated in any given moment. Fazio and Olson (2003) point out that a perceiver may not have separate structures for implicit attitudes and explicit attitudes. One might have awareness of the experience of the evaluation itself, but could still lack awareness of the associations that exist in that structure that produce that conscious experience. This means one can have an attitude triggered without realizing how or why, but still consciously experience the negative or positive affect (e.g., Hahn, Judd, Hirsh, & Blair, 2014; Phillips & Olson, 2014). It is also possible for one to *not* experience the affective response, so that the entire process of evaluating is automatic.

Where do automatic attitudes with such easily triggered associations come from? As with learning more generally, attitudes can be learned through conditioning. An object that is novel or evaluatively neutral can develop a positive or negative evaluative association if it is repeatedly paired with an attitude object that has valence (e.g., Crano & Prislin, 2006; Eagly & Chaiken, 1993; Hofmann, De Houwer, Perugini, Baeyens, & Crombez, 2010; Olson & Fazio, 2001, 2003, 2006). The neutral stimulus is known as the conditioned stimulus (CS), and the positive or negative object with which it is repeatedly paired is known as the unconditioned stimulus (US). The CS comes to take on the valence of the US and an attitude has been formed through a process known as **evaluative conditioning**. This process may also involve the encoding of propositional information that describes relationships among the stimuli (e.g., De Houwer, 2018; De Houwer & Hughes, 2016).

> **Evaluative conditioning:** A stimulus-driven process in which an attitude is formed through repeated pairing of an object with an unconditioned stimulus (US) that has either positive or negative affect. Through this pairing the conditioned stimulus forms an association to the US in long-term memory, and is linked to its affect.

Is Prejudice toward a Group of People Automatic?

The automaticity of attitudes extends to all people and objects for which we have mental representations. This means we have attitudes toward groups of people as well. **Prejudice** is such an attitude. It is a prejudgment of a group of people, usually a negative one, where *evaluations* of a group are held in our mental representation for that group, and typically applied to individual members of the group. Just like any attitude, the attitudes toward a group can develop through conditioning, and these associations can be triggered automatically. For example, prejudice toward a group of people could be conditioned by a person forming associations in memory among the group (that might start out as neutral

> **Prejudice:** A shared prejudgment of a group, usually negative. It is an association between *evaluations* of a group—positive or negative attitudes—with a mental representation for that group. If triggered, these attitudes are typically applied to individual group members, with little awareness of the attitude accessibility or its influence.

or unknown) and negative behaviors or traits (such as violent, criminal, unintelligent, or generally bad) with which the group is associated via repeated exposure. This can happen unintentionally, or intentionally, through selective media exposure. Weisbuch, Pauker, and Ambady (2009) found that when participants were exposed to television programs portraying White characters expressing negative nonverbal behavior to Black characters, the participants subsequently had increased prejudiced to the group "Black people." Similarly, Lamer and Weisbuch (2019) found that participants who saw images of men consistently placed in a higher position on the page than images of women associated men with dominance. Prejudiced attitudes were conditioned.

Once such associations among negative evaluation/affect and a specific social group develops, it remains possible that such associations become triggered outside conscious awareness. A wide variety of measures now exist that allow us to illustrate the "automatic" activation of prejudice. Though people would deny it explicitly, these measures reveal that research participants associate positive reactions with groups to which they belong and negative reactions to groups that are stereotyped in their culture. For example, Fazio, Jackson, Dunton, and Williams (1995) presented an attitude object followed by a positive or negative adjective. The participant was to respond whether the adjective was "good" or "bad," with the speed of this response facilitated if affect had previously been triggered by the attitude object. In this case the attitude object was a photograph of either a White or a Black man's face. The adjectives were positive (e.g., attractive, likable, wonderful) and negative (e.g., annoying, disgusting, offensive) words that are irrelevant to the stereotypes of these groups. This allows a test of whether positive or negative affect is immediately triggered upon seeing the face. The findings revealed that White participants were faster at making the evaluations when positive adjectives were preceded by faces of White men and negative adjectives were preceded by faces of Black men.

Wittenbrink, Judd, and Park (1997) used a similar procedure, except White participants saw the *subliminal* presentation of a group label ("Black" vs. "White") rather than a face. Also, instead of judging whether an adjective was "good" or "bad," participants simply were asked to indicate whether a string of letters was a word (a lexical decision task). When the string was in fact a word, it could be either positive or negative. The results revealed that participants responded faster to positive words when they followed the label "White," yet they responded faster to negative words when they followed the label "Black"—despite the labels being presented outside of conscious awareness. And the effect was strongest when the words were stereotypical of the group. An affective response was triggered by the mere presence of the group label, with participants remaining unaware of either the label's presence or their affective reaction to it.

In the next chapter, we focus on a variety of measures that have been developed to assess implicit cognition, including many that have been used to reveal prejudiced attitudes. We end this discussion of prejudice by noting that we have not really answered the question posed by the heading to this section. Is prejudice automatic? What we have seen is that people often do not realize they have prejudice, and if they are not aware of it, this makes control over it less likely. You do not have to be an explicit racist to be biased and make racist assumptions and choices. That is what preconscious influences do to you—it seems like the person *is* this way but it is really just an assumption; it is information added in by attitude activation. As a perceiver we feel as if the information came in from outside, via our senses, because it is fast and efficient. But does this efficiency and invisibility make our prejudice automatic? The answer to this is complicated, since we have defined a variety of types of automaticity. To fit the definition of preconscious automaticity these processes would need to be uncontrollable. In Chapters 11 and 12 we review evidence that argues these affective reactions—though outside awareness and efficient, and perhaps triggered silently by cues—are controllable. While more difficult to control than an explicit reaction, even a process that is fast, efficient, and implicit can be controlled. In this way prejudice is not fully automatic but goal dependent.

CONCLUSIONS

In psychological science, there is an emphasis on individual reporting as a primary method of discovery about the nature of cognition. There are modern tools such as fMRI and event-related potential (ERP) that allow insight about what is happening in the brain, but since we are studying human cognition, our most common course of action is to ask those humans to report about their own cognitive experience. This is not problematic for some areas of investigation. If our interest is in the perception of two very similar stimuli, we can trust the individual to report whether they notice a difference between them. For example, which stimulus is faster or is brighter? If we are interested in the selective nature of attention, we could flash an array of stimuli at a perceiver and ask them to report what they can recall having seen from among the set. In each of these examples, the report might be inaccurate, but there is little reason to suspect the person is not reporting what they believe to be true of the stimulus. Self-report can be a trusted tool if our concern is with what people consciously see and recall (and they are motivated to be honest). However, that trust starts to erode if our concern shifts from what people see and recall to how people know what they see and recall. Can people accurately report on *how* they think? Can people accurately report on the mechanisms of cognition?

As you know from personal experience, people lie to others during self-report for a variety of reasons that allow them to look good and be accepted: ingratiation, conformity, manipulation, flattery, kindness, rhetoric, and so on. When people self-report they are often not reporting what they actually think but creating a socially desirable impression in that moment. The most generous interpretation is that they do not know what they truly think and are simply reporting what is most salient to them at that moment. Their processing is automatic and they cannot see it, so they report as best as they can. But it is inaccurate. A less generous interpretation is that people lie to others so they can look good. Being seen as biased is especially threatening to people who believe they are not, and the fear of being mislabeled as a biased person causes anxiety and arousal in such people.

Of course, people also lie to themselves, seeing themselves as more unbiased than perhaps reality dictates. This can be seen in the disjunction between self-reports about their own bias and more subtle measures, as well as in the different types of behaviors predicted by each of these measures of bias. For example, direct and overt ratings of prejudice can reveal low amounts of bias when in the same person more subtle measures of bias (which we review in the next chapter) can reveal high levels of bias. The explicit and implicit attitudes diverge. Additionally, the overt measure is correlated with explicit and deliberative behavior, such as what a White person says when interacting with a Black person (such as promoting the legitimacy of anger in the Black community). But the indirect and implicit measures of the same attitude are correlated with spontaneous acts and nonverbal behavior that signals avoidance and aversion (e.g., Dovidio et al., 2002; Fazio et al., 1995). Because people are less able to monitor their nonverbal (and other forms of spontaneous) behavior, such behaviors are often seen as more honest, and relied upon more heavily than what people say and do with more deliberation. When the two do not align, the deliberate behavior is seen as untrustworthy.

An automatic process is not only one that people have difficulty seeing and monitoring but is also one that they cannot control, and never intended to initiate. For example, categorizing another person's facial expressions as happy or sad will happen upon mere exposure to that expression. One does not need to want to infer their state, nor can one stop oneself from knowing what emotion is being communicated. Similarly, having an attitude does not require a request to form an opinion. The mere detection of an attitude object triggers the corresponding affective response. When people process automatically this is not the same as saying they are lazy, or irrational, or thoughtless, or thinking poorly, or lacking a desire to get it right. Automatic processes can be efficient, and can avoid errors that conscious thinking would produce (e.g., Hasher & Zacks, 1979; Shiffrin & Schneider, 1977).

Importantly, automatic processing and control are not opposites. Lack of control is an element of automatic processing, but not the only defining feature of automaticity. So, a process over which one has control is not correctly called the opposite of automatic thought. People too readily see these two constructs as endpoints of a continuum of processing: automatic and controlled. They actually address different things. Control relates to one's ability to self-regulate. People typically use it to mean to exert conscious effort to regulate. However, as discussed above, self-regulation is at times better when it lacks consciousness. The idea of unconscious control is counterintuitive to most people, but you should be able to call upon examples of it from your own life. Many people report that when driving home they need to go to the restroom as soon as they hit the street where they live. This is no coincidence. They had been controlling this urge unconsciously, and cues that signal "home" signal an opportunity to act on it. Examples of such invisible control are around us all the time. We will suddenly see the mailboxes on a street we walk every day when we have the rare need to mail a physical letter. The mailboxes were not invisible. You just have current goals that lead you to seek them out even though you are not consciously seeking them out. Just as with the cocktail party effect, our goals control how we scan the environment and what reaches consciousness. To control is to self-regulate or for a process to be modifiable by intentions. But those intentions and goals do not need to be consciously initiated, the control exerted does not need to be aware to you, and control need not be characterized as lacking efficiency or being effortful. It can be either effortful or effortless. It can be exerted with or without awareness. It is not the opposite of an automatic process. It is a feature of an automatic process. This gets confused when people incorrectly define an automatic process as a lack of awareness and effort, and control as the effortful attempt to reach some goal of which one is fully aware.

The unconscious is not a warehouse for trauma (though it can be) but a tool to produce functioning cognitive responding in a complex social world. Abelson (1981) provided an iconic illustration of how common situations are processed mindlessly, with people following a standard script for how to act in that situation without needing to engage conscious thought. Scripts and schemas were said to be helpful in guiding our behavior in positive and useful ways, allowing people to rely on past experience to guide appropriate action in the moment. Miller, Galanter, and Pribram (1960) stressed that if we had to do everything consciously and deliberately we would never be able to get out of bed in the morning, rendered immobile by having to control each and every muscle with our limited processing capacity. This brings us back to William James's axiom that consciousness drops out of any process where it is no longer needed. Adults forget how difficult many of our hard-earned skills are—we take them for granted. As John Bargh recently told me,

> "I just taught my daughter how to drive a car and was reminded again that what seems so easy for us is really difficult when you are learning—there is enormous savings and

reduction of strain on conscious resources from experience and practice and so much of the activity is done 'for us' by these automatic processes."

Social cognition has allowed us to figure out how to study such important but invisible phenomena that are so central to social life. We delve into some of the methodological accomplishments for studying invisible processes in the next chapter.

NOTE

1. Wundt himself did not rely solely on introspection and was instrumental in ushering in an age of methods used to explore unconscious thought, methods we introduce in this chapter's section on "Automatic Attitudes and Beliefs" and review in detail in Chapter 4. For example, Feldman Barrett (2009) stated that Wundt "invented the reaction time experiment to measure the speed of perception by presenting participants with a tone or light of a particular color and measuring their latency to press or release a button in response. With these first experiments in psychology, Wundt's goal was to identify and measure the atoms of the mind—the most elemental processes that are the basic ingredients of mental life" (p. 314).

CHAPTER 4

We Can Know What People Think Even When They Don't Know

For much of history there had been a focus on higher-level thinking as conscious and deliberate. Decisions were thought to be driven by systematic analyses of facts; persuasion was assumed to be governed by the quality of the rhetoric presented; emotions and motivations were certainly seen to be capable of guiding judgment, but by altering which facts we cherry-pick, from the multitude that are available, on which to place our conscious attention. We may not be accurate and rational in our approach to information processing, but even when we are nonrational and driven by motives other than accuracy (such as self-esteem promotion, ego defense, bonding with a group, etc.) we are still effortfully striving to serve that motive. Posner and Snyder (1975) called this **controlled processing**, and today it is typically referred to as explicit processing.

A shift in how we define cognition began with the cognitive revolution in psychology in the 1950s and 1960s. At first this shift meant a focus on less effortful processing and the use of heuristics and shortcuts in how people think (e.g., Chase & Simon, 1973; Tversky & Kahneman, 1974). Yet this processing was still fully aware to the individual—they were simply using rules instead of thinking deeply. What was novel was the *amount of effort* exerted was less than once conceived.

> **Controlled processing:** Conscious or deliberate processing of information that is executed with an intended purpose that requires effort. Because it requires intent and effort, such thought is limited by what people are capable of doing in terms of their processing resources and efficacy.

Previously we asked that if a person was not being rational (seeking accuracy), what motives were they instead effortfully pursuing. Now we also were asking what shortcuts do people use (e.g., Markus & Zajonc, 1985). Conscious effort, however, was still paramount to higher-level cognition—it was just a matter of how much. This is depicted in Figure 4.1.

However, along with a focus on less effort, a focus soon emerged on no effort. Chapter 3 introduced an important theoretical distinction that human thought could be characterized as automatic. The notion of automatic processing was so important because it introduced a new way of conceptualizing human thought as efficient, outside awareness, unintended, and unable to be consciously controlled. Not all of these features are always present, and today researchers use the term **implicit process** to refer to thinking that has

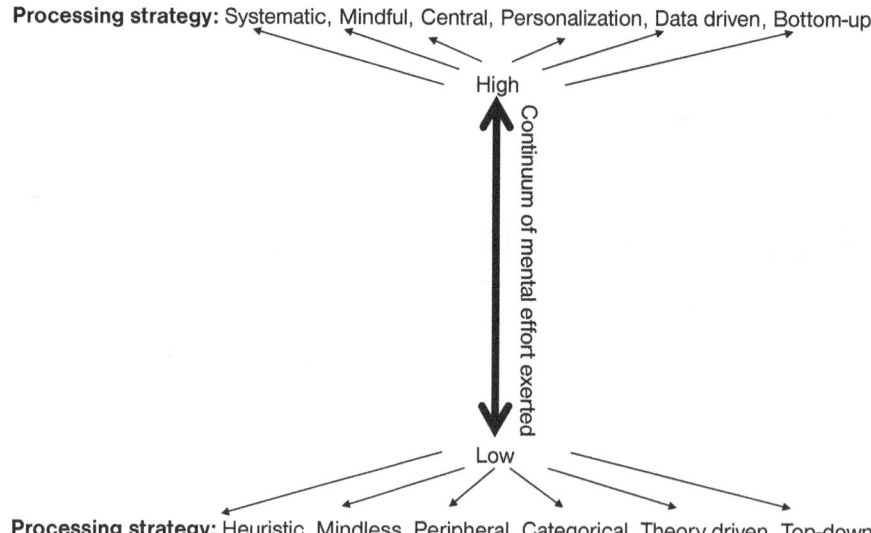

Processing strategy: Systematic, Mindful, Central, Personalization, Data driven, Bottom-up

High

Continuum of mental effort exerted

Low

Processing strategy: Heuristic, Mindless, Peripheral, Categorical, Theory driven, Top-down

FIGURE 4.1. A continuum of processing effort.

Implicit process: A cognitive operation that one is unaware of and that proceeds without conscious intent. Unlike an automatic process, which also specifies notions of uncontrollability and efficiency, an implicit process is one that merely happens outside consciousness, leaving open the possibility for it to be controllable or disrupted.

Implicit measure: A tool for measuring psychological processes where one is not aware of the true nature of what is being measured. The inability to know one is having a process examined allows for the assessment of reactions in a way that the person cannot manipulate so that the response is genuine.

some of the features of automaticity, notably being a cognitive process that one is unaware of and that proceeds without conscious intent. Any given process can at times be implicit and other times be explicit, and often has a mixture of both. Our current concern is that whether we are speaking of low effort in explicit processing or implicit processing, the person is often not aware of how their thinking is produced. If they do not know, how can we as researchers examine that cognition? Self-report is unreliable. Before we address the matter of investigating and assessing implicit processes, it is important to start by making a *distinction between an implicit process and an implicit measure*. An **implicit measure** is one that reports on an attitude, attribution, belief, inference, emotion, judgment, or decision in a manner that conceals what is being measured from the person being tested. For example, if a researcher wished to assess your attitude without you realizing it, then asking you how you feel would not work. However, in Chapter 3 we saw that we can instead measure the speed with which one pushes a lever away from the self when a word appears, and recording differences in the reaction time with which this response is made when the word is positive versus negative. The person does not know what process is being examined. Implicit measures reveal what is being thought without asking, with people unaware that a reaction is being measured. An implicit measure can be used to assess an implicit process. The example just offered is such a case. The attitude is not only being measured without the person knowing it, the process of generating an attitude is an implicit process, with a stimulus merely triggering an evaluation without one's conscious intent or awareness.

However, this does not mean that an implicit measure cannot also measure explicit cognition. Just because one is using an implicit measure, we do not know that one is assessing an implicit process. In the example above, where the measure is the speed of a lever push, the person does not know an attitude is being assessed. However, if they were to see a string of extremely negative words (such as "dead," "war," "cancer") and extremely positive words (such as "joy," "love," "happy"), they may very well be aware that they have an attitude for each word. Repeatedly being exposed to such words could make it hard not to notice that one is having an affective reaction. The reaction can be explicit even if one lacks awareness that this attitude is being measured by the task. In such an instance an implicit measure is being used to measure an explicit attitude (and because it is not subjected to the social desirability concerns reviewed in Chapter 3, it is likely a more accurate assessment of the explicit attitude than an explicit measure could provide). The fact that implicit measures can reveal both types of processes means we need to be careful to know which one is being measured when using such tools. Too often journal articles report that an implicit process has been studied simply because an implicit measure has been used.

PROJECTIVE TESTS AS IMPLICIT MEASURES

During and following World War II, many psychologists immigrated to the United States and became concerned with understanding why hate, demagogy, and fascism could thrive in modern times. They believed that open and obvious forms of hate could not explain how many of their former neighbors in Germany became Nazis, or how so many of their new American neighbors expressed their feelings about race. One explanation was that personality factors other than overt hate might support and promote prejudice. They sought to study elements of discrimination and prejudice that, despite being part of one's personality, were hidden from one and not hate based. Sigmund Freud had famously argued that people hide essential truths from themselves. At an unconscious level the person *wants* such information to remain hidden. It is suppressed. Unconscious thought for Freud was the domain of repressed and undesired events; his interest was in the perils such thoughts would have if they were to reach consciousness, and how people therefore shield trauma and harsh negative experience from consciousness. The Freudian approach is mentioned here merely as a well-known notion of the unconscious to which a social-cognitive approach can be contrasted. Unlike Freud, who saw dark and foreboding motives as the reasons why thoughts are driven from consciousness, social cognition researchers see a variety of motives that could lead one to hidden prejudices that are banished from consciousness. Freud focused on fear and anxiety to parents and sexual shame; early prejudice researchers believed that many types of antisocial feelings, that might lower self-esteem if faced, could be repressed. The logic was that if an individual could not integrate their unwanted impulses with their conscious sense of self, the unwanted impulse would be repressed. In addition, it would be masked publicly as a dislike for an easily targeted group (such as dislike for immigrants).

This introduced a methodological problem. If a person could not face their own unwanted impulse (such as loathing for one's ingroup), how could it be studied? Researchers turned to using projective tests as a measure of implicit bias. A **projective test** is a type of measure that allows people to unwittingly express their hidden motives and beliefs by discussing a target that seemingly has nothing to do with oneself. The target serves as clay to be molded by one's hidden impulses, or, using a more apt metaphor, serves as a blank screen onto which one's impulses can be projected. Although we repress unbearable thoughts in dealing with our own lives, those thoughts seek an outlet of expression, and seep out in how we interpret other people

Projective test: A test that assumes repressed thoughts cannot be assessed through self-report, but because they seek an outlet of expression, they come crawling out in the manner in which we interpret others and situations. The individual projects these thoughts onto external targets who become scapegoats and bear responsibility for the repressed thought.

and situations. What we are unable to face in the self, we can project onto other people, so these others become the scapegoats that can bear these negative responses that we will not face. Projective tests allow one to describe other people as having motives and qualities one cannot face in the self, thus providing insight into the self for the trained eye to see.

We cannot project our feelings of inadequacy onto others who are themselves clearly defined. We need people or objects that serve as a blank screen, for which there is not much information about. One example of a projective measure is the **Rorschach test**, which uses inkblots as stimuli. These ambiguous shapes allow the individual to provide a stream-of-consciousness description of what they believe they see, with the stream then analyzable for themes that the individual would not consciously put forward to describe themselves. Yet these themes that sit waiting to be expressed when describing an ambiguous target (an inkblot) can be assumed to be prevalent in the person's mind. Allport (1954) refers to minorities as "living inkblots" since they are used as ambiguous targets onto which a person unknowingly projects their own emotional failures. Just as hidden agendas can be revealed in the pictures we say we see in the inkblots, motives we fear in ourselves can be seen by looking at the way we describe ambiguous, foreign, and unfamiliar others. Another projective measure useful for revealing implicitly held beliefs and feelings is the **Thematic Apperception Test** (TAT). In the TAT, respondents are shown pictures (typically 10 of them) and asked to describe what is happening, what dialogue might be carried on between characters, and how the story might continue. The TAT is designed to be ambiguous as to what is depicted, and to therefore elicit interpretations of the depicted social situations. Although the pictures used must be interesting enough to encourage discussion, they should be vague enough to be open to interpretation and to not reveal what is actually being studied.

Rorschach test: A projective measure that uses inkblots as stimuli. These ambiguous shapes allow the individual to provide a stream of consciousness description of what they believe they see, with the stream analyzable for themes that the individual would not consciously put forward to describe themselves, yet are accessible in one's mind.

Thematic Apperception Test (TAT): A projective test where respondents see pictures (typically ten) and describe what is happening, what dialogue might be carried on between characters, and/or how the "story" might continue. It is designed to be ambiguous/vague as to what is depicted and to therefore elicit interpretations of the depicted social situations.

Frenkel-Brunswik and Sanford (1945) identified a group of girls as being high in prejudice, and they then gave these girls the TAT to explore what personal qualities, to which they did not consciously admit, might be the true source of their prejudice. Rather than self-disclose any personal problems, these girls instead put forward a surface image of being composed and untroubled, with a high interest in social standing and emphasizing proper appearance. The TAT revealed a hidden personality structure that seemed to characterize these individuals. First, the stories they told on the TAT expressed ambivalence toward parents, and even an underlying aggression that was masked in their self-reports. Their TAT stories reflect hatred, meanness, jealousy, and suspicion toward parental figures—even death of parents. They also reflect aggression more generally, with stories depicting murder, dismemberment, punishment, burning to death, electrocution, concentration camps, and so on. The aggressive acts that occurred in their stories never involved the heroine, but an external force imposed on somebody else. Allport (1954) called this an extrapunitiveness—blaming others, blaming everyone but yourself as a cover up for your own inadequacies. Additionally, their stories reflect a rigidly moralistic view marked by expressions of a strict insistence on good manners, cleanliness, orderliness, and sticking to convention. While there is no organized social–political outlook, there is strong support for the status quo. The characters who are seen to be breaking these conventions in the TAT stories of these prejudiced girls are, for example, criminals and the poor. To these girls, moral transgression is what keeps such people in prisons and slums, deserving of aggression and their diminished fate. There is blame and separation rather than seeking a solution. Their stories also reflect (at least superficially) a devotion to institutions such as religion and country, with religiosity being more utilitarian as opposed to being tied to a system of ethics. Such work suggests that there are personality types that are prone to prejudice that have factors other than disdain for the group as the root cause. Instead, disdain for the group is a manifestation of the things they have disdain for in themselves—their own unseen anxiety and immorality.

Throughout the history of psychology there has been an exploration of such personality types that are prone to prejudice that is not rooted in hatred for the other. Block and Block (1951) defined **ethnocentrism** as having a pervasive and rigid tendency to distinguish ingroups from outgroups, with negative beliefs and attitudes regarding outgroups, and a "hierarchical, authoritarian view of group interaction, in which ingroups are rightly dominant and outgroups subordinate" (p. 304). Yet it is not hate they see as defining these ethnocentric individuals. Block and Block suggested that one way to identify such people is through what Frenkel-Brunswik (1949) called an intolerance of ambiguity—a need to structure the world around them. They argued that such intolerance leads people to excessive blaming of minorities to make sense of ambiguities, such as the ills in the world. Block and Block measured intolerance of ambiguity with a projective test. Block and Block had participants observe a light that was seemingly moving in a dark room. They measured the need to quickly arrive at a stable amount of movement that was perceived in the light (this was ambiguous because the light did not actually move, it was an illusion). A need to impose structure on such ambiguous stimuli was shown to be highly correlated with ethnocentrism.

> **Ethnocentrism:** Having a pervasive and rigid tendency to distinguish ingroups from outgroups, with negative beliefs and attitudes regarding outgroups, and a hierarchical view of intergroup relations. In this somewhat authoritarian approach, one's ingroup is seen as dominant over a subordinate outgroup.

Adorno, Frenkel-Brunswik, Levinson, and Sanford (1950) described another personality structure called the **authoritarian personality** in which fears, dangerous impulses, and insecurities that people cannot face in themselves are repressed out of a concern for harsh and punishing consequences.[1] In defining an authoritarian Allport (1954) stated,

> He seems fearful of himself, of his own instincts, of his own consciousness, of change, and of his social environment. Since he can live in comfort neither with himself nor with others, he is forced to organize his whole style of living, including his social attitudes, to fit his crippled condition. (p. 396)

> **Authoritarian personality:** A personality type where the world is seen as dangerous/threatening due to humanity's selfishness and stupidity. To protect the self from such threats, a strong leader who will guarantee survival with their power to dominate others is embraced. Others are seen as rivals to be controlled in a cruel/sadistic way.

This creates a division between their conscious and unconscious views of the self, a division that is resolved through projecting their deficiencies onto others through scapegoating and prejudice. This often leads to identifying scapegoats, or convenient groups of others on whom dominance can be asserted, seeing these others in simplistic or black and white terms (Maslow, 1943). Their own unwanted impulses leak out in the stories they tell that are expressed as prejudice.

IMPLICIT MEASURES THAT USE MEMORY

In Chapter 1 we reviewed Asch's (1946) seminal research on impression formation, where he presented lists of traits to people and asked them to form an impression. In doing so, people did more than just average or summarize the qualities listed, but used some of them—*central traits*—as the heart of the impression around which the other qualities were organized. A coherent narrative was built that (1) stressed some qualities consistent with the emerging narrative, (2) turned others into modifiers that help extend the impression in nuanced ways, and (3) took qualities that were inconsistent with the narrative and either ignored them or had their meaning distorted so as to not seem inconsistent. Perceivers created impressions of the people described by going beyond the traits provided and told a story that was consistent with the overall impression. Reversing the order in which the traits were learned changed the impression despite the information being equivalent. A change in a single word in a set of words, if it is a central trait, changed the entire impression. However, there is a problem with this methodology—it *asks* people to form impressions. In psychology, and cognitive science more generally, the tasks and goals provided to research participants have the power to determine the types of responses they produce, as opposed to revealing what they do in reality. The finding that people form coherent and well-integrated impressions may be an artifact of this methodology. We need methods that provide a window to the subtle operations of the cognitive apparatus; we need implicit measures.

In the early days of social cognition research on implicit measures centered on a particular cognitive operation: memory. The idea was a simple one—due to developments in memory research one could access implicitly held attitudes, impressions, and beliefs about the social world without needing to directly ask about them. Instead, the researcher could explore the *memory* perceivers had for social objects (people, behaviors, etc.) learned about during the experiment. Why would a memory measure provide a more realistic window into how people think? The logic was that (1) information that is more memorable exerts an unusually strong impact on how we judge people (what comes to mind easily is used when judging people), and (2) when we have formed an impression of a person we organize that information in memory so that associative links form around the related pieces of the impression (the behavior, the person who performed the behavior, the traits we infer about the person, the feelings we develop based on those actions, etc.). Thus, rather than asking a person what they think about someone, and have them engage in what might be a somewhat unnatural way of tapping their impression, we could examine their memory. Memory would reveal what inferences came to mind when learning the information and how those inferences were being weighted and organized. This exploration of **person memory** could be done through a variety of methods by examining patterns of accuracy and systematic biases in different memory paradigms (free recall, cued recall, probe recognition, etc.). Examples of these "mind-reading" techniques are provided below. The point being that probing memory is an unobtrusive way to explore true attitudes and beliefs without requiring self-reflection on these matters on the part of the perceiver, and keeping the perceiver unaware that their perceptions of a person are even being explored (e.g., Srull & Wyer, 1989). Such perceiver naïveté allows for the responses to be free of impression management and attempts to say what is normative or socially desirable. The groundbreaking book that helped to establish social cognition as a field of inquiry had the title *Person Memory* (Hastie et al., 1980) to reflect this methodological foundation. Over the years, methods evolved to incorporate tools to tease apart different stages of memory (encoding, storage, and retrieval). We explore these next.

Person memory: Measures assessing memory to reveal what inferences came to mind in a perceiver when they were learning information about a person. Further, it can reveal how information was weighted and organized. Perceivers are never asked to form an impression or report one, so it evades reporting biases that plague self-report.

Measures of Clustering in Memory

One way to tell what a person had been thinking without directly asking is to have them engage in **free recall** of the information. Free recall is a type of memory measure in which people receive no hints, but need to remember information they read about or saw earlier. A researcher can then examine that free recall to see how the information is **clustered in recall**. The logic is that how we pull information out of memory is a reflection of what we were thinking when we put the information into memory. Memory researchers had shown that information is organized similarly in retrieval as it is at encoding (e.g., Bousfield, 1953; Shuell, 1977). Thus, the way it is clustered at recall (retrieval) will tell us how people were thinking about and organizing the information as they learned it (at encoding). To study whether Asch (1946) was right about how people spontaneously form impressions, we do not need to ask them to form impressions. To explore the spontaneous process, we could examine recall for the information to see if it is clustered according to individual people, personality types, and central traits. When using clustering as a measure of impression formation it is essential to initially present the information in a scrambled order. If the person forms an impression by unscrambling the information and putting it together into a meaningful cluster, then this will be reflected by the patterns in which the information is recalled. Are items recalled in a way that organizes them to describe a "shy" person?

Free recall: A type of memory measure in which people receive no hints, but need to remember information they read about or saw earlier. It is a listing of everything one can recall about an episode or person without any further prompting other than to report what they recall.

Clustered in recall: When information is grouped together during free recall in a systematic or thematic way. Such groupings provide a measure of how information is stored in memory and the types of associations the perceiver formed. The logic is that items recalled together in clusters were inferred together and stored together.

For example, if memory was clustered with all the information about Emily recalled first and all the information about Erik next, followed by all the information about Sue, then we would know the perceiver was thinking in terms of individuals and structuring the information around those individuals. If, instead, the perceiver was stereotyping by group membership, they will cluster all the behaviors of people from the same group together. "Physical information such as age, race, height, and sex are all readily apparent when meeting a number of new people. . . . In such circumstances, one might remember that all the women were outspoken, but not remember which woman said what" (Ostrom, Pryor, & Simpson, 1981, p. 26). Thus, clustering all the information along a dimension such as gender, as opposed to individual people, would reveal gender stereotyping had been happening in the mind, even if the person did not know it.[2]

Ostrom et al. (1981) review several alternate ways of organizing information that we receive about people that could be revealed by a clustering measure. One possibility is around people, as just reviewed (e.g., traits of Roger, and traits of Erik). Another is organization around personality type, such as behaviors that imply shyness, behaviors that imply aggression, and so on. Another is temporal organization, where information is stored in the order it occurred. Imagine you learned that "Roger acted rudely on Monday," "Roger acted sarcastically on Tuesday," "Erik acted selfishly on Monday," "Erik acted egotistically on Tuesday," and so on. Temporal organization would not have all the Roger qualities clustered, but all the Monday qualities clustered. Alternatively, information could be clustered around descriptors. Ostrom et al. (1981) described an experiment in which participants learn information about three different people—Dave, Tom, and John. They are told: Dave is a part-time usher, Dave is from Wichita (Kansas), Tom is from Richmond (Virginia), Tom collects beer cans, John collects coins, Tom is a part-time dishwasher, John is from Denver (Colorado), Dave tinkers with cars, John works part-time on a farm. Descriptor clustering could emerge where people made sense of the information using categories such as hobbies, jobs, and hometowns. The results reveal that unlike what Asch (1946) showed when asking for impressions, a clustering analysis revealed no evidence that participants were using persons or traits as organizing principles for this information (see also Hamilton et al., 1980a, 1980b). Instead they found that descriptor categories were being used. This is not to say we do not frequently use traits for making sense of people. We do. It is simply to say that if we want to know *when* we use traits versus some other way of sense making, implicit measures are a better approach since they capture processing in a more pure and unadulterated form.

Asch (1946) predicted that perceivers try to make information about a person "fit" and seem coherent. Clustering is a procedure that allows for a way to more naturally detect how people make such coherence. The answer may be different from the one you get when you ask people what they think, which perhaps forces them to use traits more than they naturally would. Asking people to use traits not only can alter what people would naturally do but it provides a richer way of thinking than just learning the material. The instruction to form impressions engages people in more complex thinking, with richer associations being made; this makes the information more memorable as a side effect (e.g., Hamilton et al., 1980a; Srull, 1983; Srull & Brand, 1983; Wyer & Gordon, 1984). Ironically, people asked to remember information have poorer memory than people asked to form an impression. The two groups were structuring and organizing their impressions differently, and inferring traits had the benefit of helping memory.

Encoding Specificity

Asch (1946, p. 258) not only claimed people form impressions in a way that merges qualities together to form a coherent narrative, he claimed this is among the most natural things we do. We look at a person and immediately a certain impression of their character forms itself in us. A glance, a few spoken words are sufficient to tell us a story about a highly complex matter. We know that such impressions form with remarkable rapidity and great ease.

Once again, how can we tell whether a person naturally and immediately accounts for an observed behavior by inferring a trait as its cause if asking a person to form impressions is neither natural nor immediate? Forming impressions in response to a directive is artificial, and it is something that directly calls for conscious reflection (and is not immediate). A solution to this conundrum once again comes from memory research and procedures borrowed from cognitive psychology.

With memory measures we can ask and answer the important question: Do people form impressions of others in a somewhat automatic way (e.g., Uleman, Newman, & Moskowitz, 1996)? When we observe another person's behavior, do we produce an inference about the trait that explains that behavior *without being aware* an inference has been formed and in the *absence of an intention* to do so? Moskowitz and Uleman (1987) coined the term **spontaneous trait inference** (STI) to describe such a process. For example, if you observed a woman at the coffee shop inform the cashier she got too much change, an inference of "honest" could be spontaneously made, without you even knowing it. If you were at a wedding and in the corner of your eye saw a man tripping over his date's feet while dancing you might infer he was "clumsy" even if you do not recall ever watching him, let alone having formed an impression about his attributes. A variety of memory measures have been used to study this question, and many rely on a type of memory measure called **cued recall**. Unlike free recall where memory is unprompted and is reported in a stream-of-consciousness fashion, cued recall provides people with hints or memory aids, called cues. These

Spontaneous trait inference: An inference made outside of awareness and without conscious intent about an observed trait of a person. Such rapid first impressions are among the most common acts of social cognition humans engage in, instantly providing meaning about a highly complex matter—another person.

are typically single words that are associated with the to-be-recalled information and thus provide access to that information. Even when one has difficulty freely recalling something, a cue can serve as a hint that triggers the information with which it is associated, and renders what had previously been unrecollected easily recalled.

Winter and Uleman (1984) devised a clever procedure for discovering such implicit inferences that relied on what is known as the **principle of encoding specificity** (Tulving & Thomson, 1973). This principle states that if two items of information are encoded in memory together, then this link among them makes them useful cues for each other. If two unrelated words—"chair" and "elephant"—are presented together when asking people to memorize pairs of words, then they will be stored together. When memory is later tested one may feel as if they have no recall for either of those words. But as soon as I prompt you (provide a cue) with "elephant," you can suddenly recall "chair." If memory is better when retrieval cues are presented than when they are not, this can only be

> **Cued recall:** Unlike free recall, where memory is unprompted and reported in a stream of consciousness, in cued recall people are provided with hints or memory aids called cues. These are single words associated with the to-be-recalled information and thus provide access to that information. Memory reported in response to such hints is cued recall.
>
> **Principle of encoding specificity:** If two items are encoded in memory together, this link between them makes them useful cues for one another. When memory is later tested, being cued with one word might improve recall for the other. This would indicate the word being recalled was stored (encoded) together with the cue.

because the words were stored (encoded) together initially and they are now associated in memory. How can we use this to know what someone was thinking, even if they do not know they were thinking it? Winter and Uleman devised an ingenious procedure.

Winter and Uleman (1984) reasoned that if a trait inference was made when a behavior was observed, then both the trait inference and the behavior should be encoded into memory and stored in memory together. This should be true even if the person was unaware they made an inference. A person can swear they made no judgment of another person, be accurate in saying they have no awareness of having done so, but encoding specificity allows us to tell whether they actually did so. If they did form an STI, then even though they never consciously thought of the trait "honest" it would nonetheless have been inferred and stored in memory with the behavior "returned the extra change to the cashier." This association in memory would make "honest" an effective cue for the remembering the behavior. Rather than asking people if they formed an inference or asking them to form an impression, we can simply test their memory for the behavior by providing them with a *cue*. If they inferred a trait, then the trait would improve memory for the behavior. An unrelated word serving as a cue, such as "elevator," would not improve memory. "Honest" would only work as a cue if it had been inferred. And it would only help memory for one specific behavior—returning the excess change.

Savings in Relearning

Carlston and Skowronski (1994) devised another ingenious way to read people's minds and discover the inferences they themselves do not even know they made. Once again borrowing from memory research in cognitive psychology, they used the principle that information that has already been learned, that is already stored in memory, is easier to learn again. This is true even for implicit memory, or memories one does not consciously recall having made. In the simplest way to say it, it takes less time to learn something if you already know it at some level. This is why learning material in a class is easier to learn if it was covered in an earlier class, even if you have no explicit memory of the earlier learning. Carlston and Skowronski created an implicit measure that capitalizes on this fact, one that examines relearning. In a typical experiment, a participant reads about a series of behaviors performed by different people (one behavior per person). The behaviors are also paired with a picture of the person being described in the sentence. Some of these sentences imply traits, and others do not. Their goal is to memorize the behaviors performed by each person. They have no explicit instruction to form an impression or infer a trait, and they do not report having done so when questioned about it after the experiment is over. However, for half of the sentences they should have inferred a trait spontaneously since half of the sentences implied traits. The logic of the implicit measure is a simple one. If someone spontaneously inferred a trait, that trait would have been paired with the picture of the person provided (and with the behavior provided). These things should be stored together in memory—that is, even though they are not aware of it, the participant has learned that person A has trait X. If person A and trait X had already been paired due to having formed an STI, then it should now be easier for participants to attempt to learn that person A possesses trait X if they are now explicitly paired together and the participant is asked to learn this "new" information. It is easier to learn something if one already knows it, even without explicit memory that one knows it (e.g., Carlston & Skowronski, 1995).

There are two phases in this procedure. In Phase 1 the participants memorize a set of behaviors that were paired with photographs of the person who performed the behavior. In Phase 2 the participants are given the task of memorizing entirely new pairs of items. This time they once again see photographs of faces (some of which were seen earlier in Phase 1), but this time they are paired with single words—trait words, such as "honest." Some of the traits were implied earlier by the behaviors in Phase 1. These traits were now paired with the same person who had earlier performed the behavior that implied the trait. In these instances, the participant is essentially relearning a pairing they already learned, even though they have no memory of having learned it. Other traits were not implied earlier. These traits were paired with the face of a person whose earlier behavior did not imply a trait. In these instances, the participant is being asked to learn something entirely new (see Figure 4.2). If traits had been inferred spontaneously, then it should be easier to learn the pairs that represent a relearning than the pairs that represent new learning. There is a **savings in relearning**. Research consistently reveals this to be the case.

> **Savings in relearning:** The principle that information already learned, that is already stored in memory, is easier to learn again. This is true even for implicit memory, or memories one does not consciously recall making. That is, it takes less time to learn something if you already know it at some level.

Gap Filling

To continue this brief summary of implicit measures that use memory, let us recall that Asch (1946) also claimed we go beyond the qualities provided to see new, related qualities. Do people go out of their way to provide such more elaborate impressions only because they were asked? Or do they naturally extend the impression by **filling in the gaps** in their knowledge? Important phenomena such as stereotyping assume people make inferences that are not warranted from the data because they fill in the gaps of their knowledge using a stereotype. An implicit measure can address this question of whether perceivers do naturally go beyond the information given.

Cantor and Mischel (1977) proposed that traits have this function of filling in the gaps and adding information

> **Filling in the gaps:** Perceivers use prior knowledge—stereotypes, schemas, scripts, implicit personality theories—to make inferences not specified in the existing data. They round out knowledge of the person by combining prior knowledge with existing data to form a more complete impression/memory of the person than warranted by the data alone. They go beyond the information given.

Step 1: Learn sentences (some implying a trait, some not) that are paired with images.

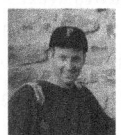   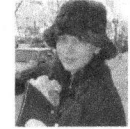   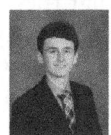

Gordon took the orphans to the circus.   Cindy went for a walk to the store.   Ben thought he did not deserve the praise.

Step 2: Learn traits (some inferred in Step 1, some not) that are paired with images.

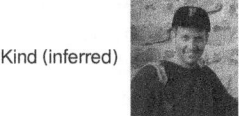   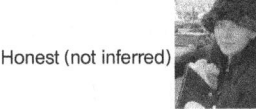   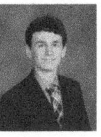

Kind (inferred)   Honest (not inferred)   Forgetful (not inferred)

Step 3: Have memory tested for the pairings learned at Step 2.

Kind 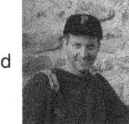 Memory for the relearned items (such as this pair) should be best.

FIGURE 4.2. Relearning as a measure of spontaneous inference.

to the emerging impression of the person that was not actually presented. Personality traits and group stereotypes—such as labeling someone as being of a certain type (e.g., geek, jock, princess, misfit, delinquent)—define a set of prototypical features for that trait or stereotype. People may not realize they use such traits or stereotypes if explicitly asked, but we can examine whether they do by using a memory measure. Participants first learn behaviors that describe a person who is labeled by a quality (such as introvert) that has prototypic behaviors associated with it (such as does not like loud parties). They next learn new behaviors about the person, some of which are unrelated to the label, some of which are related to the label. People are then asked to rate how confident they are that each new behavior was not in the original set of behaviors learned. When the new behaviors are unrelated to the label (introvert), this should be easy. However, when the new behaviors are related to the label—they are prototypic of an introvert—this task now becomes harder. These behaviors feel familiar, and they might be likely to mistake a new behavior for one seen before. They might generate a belief that something they had not seen previously was actually seen, because it fits what they expect. This is what is meant by "filling in the gaps"—items associated in memory by a prototype, schema, or stereotype are triggered when the label is encountered, making one likely to think those items had been seen when they had not. Information not explicitly seen (such as being quiet) is confused with information actually seen (not liking loud parties) because of their association in memory.

Cantor and Mischel (1977) tested this by asking people to rate how confident they felt about whether a new item was in the original list of behaviors learned about a person. That person was first labeled with a trait (such as introvert). The prediction was that when the new behavior is unrelated to the label, one should feel quite confident it was not in the original list. However, when the new behavior is related to the label, people should start to lose confidence that they had not seen the behavior before. They might even convince themselves that they had seen it. Their results confirmed that participants were less confident in thinking a quality was new (and had never been seen before) if that quality was related to a label provided. If the person was labeled an introvert, then a new introverted behavior was not as confidently identified as new as an unrelated behavior. Having a prior label for a person makes us feel uncertain about whether new behaviors that are consistent with that label were previously seen. A label causes us to think of related behaviors, creating a confusion about what was actually seen versus merely triggered by association. This can cause us to believe that we see things we did not, filling in the gaps in our knowledge. At a minimum, as shown by Cantor and Mischel, it leads to uncertainty over what was seen versus what was not. The memory measure reveals a process where, without realizing it, participants form impressions influenced not only by what was seen but by inferences they add. The inferences come from associations among a label and related, prototypical behaviors. They are less confident that something they never saw was actually never seen.

Reverse Correlation

One final memory measure we review takes advantage of the fact that people have stored in memory a typical set of facial features that are associated with a particular trait or group. When the word "criminal" is read, a particular image comes to mind; the same is true for the social group "women," where an exemplar of the group that includes their most typical facial features comes to mind. We can uncover these mental images—that people may not realize they have—by asking people to judge a face repeatedly, each time partly hidden behind patterns of random noise (e.g., Brinkman, Todorov, & Dotsch, 2017). The participant observes two images of the face side by side. Each is obstructed by a pattern of random noise that makes categorizing it difficult, to different degrees depending on what features of the face are being blocked by the noise. Their task is to pick the image that looks most like their mental representation of the group. In Figure 4.3 we use the example of undocumented immigrants. This task is repeated over hundreds of trials, with different patterns of noise obstructing the faces on each trial. On each trial of the task the participant selects one of the two obstructed images (as seen on the left in Figure 4.3) as the one that best approximates what the group looks like them.

Then, from the image selected on each of the hundreds of trials, the researcher calculates the average noise pattern and superimposes this noise pattern on the face. The resulting face (as seen on the right in Figure 4.3) is a picture of what the person's memory for what a typical member of the group looks like. This procedure is known as **reverse correlation**.

> **Reverse correlation:** An implicit measure of what a category member looks like. A group member's face is shown twice, each obscured with random noise patterns, and participants judge which looks more like a typical group member. An enormous number of such judgments are combined to reproduce the mental image for the category.

Dotsch, Wigboldus, Langner, and van Knippenberg (2008) showed that we can use this procedure to reveal biases people have. Their Dutch research participants performed the task by identifying which image was the most "Moroccan" (a group that Dutch society associates with a stereotype of criminality). Not only could the procedure identify the typical face of a "Moroccan" among the Dutch participants (and show that the facial features align with threat and danger) but they also showed that the more prejudiced the participants were, the more "criminal" the mental representation of the typical Moroccan face. This despite the fact that criminality (or any trait) was never mentioned as part of the task. Just a judgment of which face was more Moroccan (see also Ratner, Dotsch, Wigboldus, van Knippenberg, & Amodio, 2014).

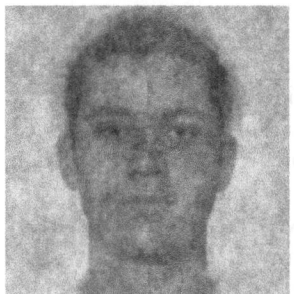 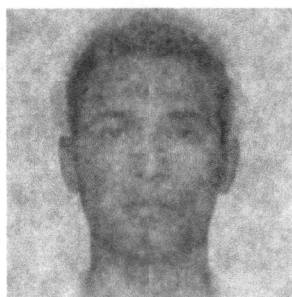 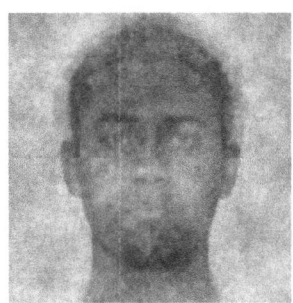

FIGURE 4.3. Reverse correlation: Which of the two images on the left looks most like an undocumented immigrant? For each participant, hundreds of such choices produce a composite image, such as that depicted on the right.

IMPLICIT MEASURES THAT USE REACTION TIME

One way to measure a cognitive process without one realizing what is being measured is to use a task where speed of responding, or **reaction time**, can be recorded. If the response is asked for at a speed that is too fast for conscious control to be exerted, then the person is unlikely to know what the response is measuring. This gives the additional benefit of the response being genuine. Because a controlled process is marked by conscious effort, the ability to be consciously controlled, and is initiated by conscious intent, it does allow for a person to have the time and ability to mask their genuine response should they want to. One way to ensure a genuine response is to not allow the time for such social desirability biases to be implemented—to force people to respond at speeds where only an implicit response could occur because the time and effort needed for control simply does not exist. When using a reaction time measure, the task should not overtly reveal what the process of interest is, but ask one to do something that seems unrelated. We saw an example earlier when an attitude was being measured, but the response asked for was simply to push (or pull) on a lever whenever a word appeared.

> **Reaction time (RT):** A measure of speed of responding on a task where responses are asked for too quickly for conscious control to occur. Any RT itself is often less important than a reliable difference in RTs among conditions in the experiment. Are reactions in condition X faster than condition Z, and why?

What other types of responses can be measured that quickly tell us something about cognitive processing? In Chapter 2 it was reviewed that knowledge is connected in memory through associative links, with associations among shared pieces of knowledge forming an *associative network*. Each item in the network can (in milliseconds) trigger other items in the network, pulling that item from memory (even if the person is not aware of this) so that there is *spreading activation* across the network. The more strongly linked or closely associated two concepts are, the faster the activation spreads, and thus the faster one can respond to related knowledge once the initial piece of knowledge is triggered (e.g., Logan, 1989). We are faster to respond that a moral person is helpful as compared to literate because "helpful" and "moral" are more closely linked. Closely linked items (such as "bread" and "butter") require less time to trigger each other than less closely linked, or less strongly associated, items (such as "bread" and "soup"). In a sense, this association creates a preparedness to respond so that when one sees "bread" one is prepared to see closely associated information. Flipping this logic on its head, one can use reaction time and preparedness as a measure of how closely two pieces of information are associated. If I can respond more quickly to simply reading the word "butter" than "soup" after seeing the word "bread," it suggests that bread and butter are more closely associated. In this way, reaction time tells us if two concepts are associated and how strongly they are associated.

A classic experiment from Rosch (1975) illustrated this point. Participants were asked to judge whether a stimulus (such as a penguin) was a member of a particular category (such as a bird). The task was to indicate as quickly as possible if a statement—such as "A penguin is a bird" or "A pigeon is a bird"—was true. Reaction times were recorded. The critical manipulation in the experiment was the strength of association among the category (bird) and the category member (penguin vs. pigeon) being judged. Types of birds that were more strongly associated with the category due to being more typical, such as a pigeon, were responded to faster. Collins and Quillian (1969) illustrated the usefulness of reaction time as a measure in an experiment where participants read sentences with information that was either true or false, such as "A doctor is a college graduate," "A doctor has eyes," and "A doctor is a suitcase." The task was to indicate as quickly as possible whether the statement was true. What differentiated the true statements from one another was the directness of the connection among the concept "doctor" and the concept paired with it. "Doctor" and "college graduate" are each members of the larger category "people." However, they are also directly linked because all doctors are college graduates. Body parts, such as eyes, are also features of people. As such, they are features of doctors, despite the fact that there is not likely a direct link between doctors and eyes. People have eyes, doctors are people, so doctors have eyes. The path from "doctor" to "eyes" is traveled by first associating doctors with a higher-level category ("people") and then traveling along a path back down to the features people possess. This is more indirect than the links that allow one to know that doctors have college degrees. We can easily respond that doctors have eyes, but it is easier yet to respond they have college degrees *if memory is organized through a series of hierarchical connections*. Given this structure, it would ironically require that it is somewhat harder to retrieve the fact that doctors have eyes, something true of all people, than to determine that doctors went to college, something true of only a minority of people in the world. Figure 4.4 uses knowledge about the musician John Lennon to illustrate the variety of ways that associations could be structured. The dark arrows in Figure 4.4C represent more strongly held associations. Thus, we could diagnose what a person thinks about Lennon by their reaction time to various qualities about him, with response speed being faster, in this example, to the fact that he was a musician and guitarist.

Reaction time measures not only help to tell us interesting information about how we structure information in memory (whether there is a hierarchical arrangement, whether we store specific behaviors to the person or only more abstract traits). That information might be interesting to only a small set of people who are concerned about how the mind is structured and functions. Perhaps of greater interest to more people is the fact that reaction times can help us "read minds" so that we can diagnose, for example, whether a person is stereotyping or not. Reaction time can tell us if people associate things, and the strength of that association, even when they might not be able to consciously report it. If you think I am a jerk rather than helpful, then you would respond faster to the word "jerk" than "helpful" after seeing my name. This is especially useful for diagnosing negative thoughts that people might be reluctant to self-report, such as stereotypes about a group. A man might be unwilling to say he has stereotypes of women, but a reaction time test could assess whether he is faster to say "emotional" versus "strong" after seeing a woman. This would tell us that he associates the stereotypic term "emotional" with women, even if he was unwilling to say it, and even if he truly believed he did not associate those things. Aversive racists will consciously report they have no dislike for a particular minority group. However, if they strongly

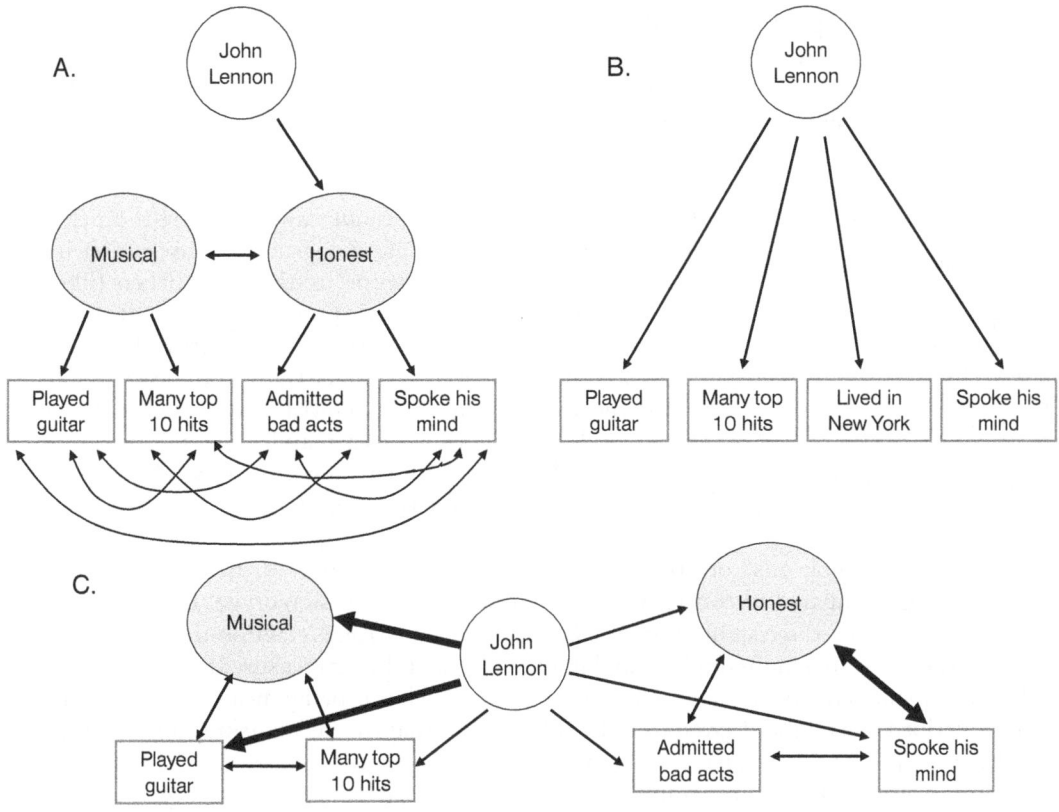

FIGURE 4.4. Types of associations in memory; darker lines indicate stronger associations.

associate that group with feelings of dislike, then this association suggests the conscious response is the less valid one. The purer response is the one they cannot control that reveals a link between the group and negative feelings. Gaertner and McLaughlin (1983) were the first to use reaction time measures to diagnose stereotypes in this way. They had research participants respond to either stereotypic words or to control words after being exposed to a category label for a group ("Black"). They showed that stereotypic words (compared to control words) were responded to more quickly when they followed the category.

Attitude and Stereotype Automaticity Measures

One type of implicit measure uses reaction times to positive and negative words to assess prejudice, or the positive versus negative attitudes associated with a social group. As discussed in Chapter 3, stimuli, such as members of a stereotyped group, are associated with positive or negative responses. The association of the affect with the group, experienced immediately and without awareness, can be assessed using reaction time even if one is unaware that this affect exists. In real life there often is not enough time to react in a controlled fashion, making reaction time measures not only useful as a way to parse what is genuine versus not but as a measure that might more accurately predict how people will respond to the pressures of daily life. A classic example is the research of Fazio et al. (1995). Participants saw a face of either a Black man or a White man followed by an adjective. The logic was that the speed of responding to whether an adjective (e.g., wonderful versus disgusting) is a "good" word or a "bad" word will be facilitated if the attitude was previously triggered by the face. They found that White research participants were faster to identify a positive adjective as good when preceded by White faces and faster to identify a negative adjective as bad when preceded by Black faces. This can only be explained by people associating "good" with White and "bad" with Black. This technique is sometimes called the **bona fide pipeline**, which is a reference to an older technique called the bogus pipeline where participants believe physiological responses are being recorded that provide a "pipeline" to their true beliefs (like a lie detector test). Here, automatic processes of attitude activation provide an unobtrusive measure of true attitudes.

> **Bona fide pipeline:** Feelings about a group are measured where participants simply believe they are categorizing words as "good" or "bad" while observing faces. Associations of good with one category of faces, bad with another, is assessed by speed-up in RTs for these good/bad judgments when simultaneously accompanied by some types of faces.

Reaction times are not only useful to show associations to negative feelings but can also reveal associations between groups and stereotypes. Gaertner and McLaughlin (1983), as mentioned above, had participants respond to either stereotype-relevant or control words after being exposed to words that represent a social group (such as, for stereotypic words, "White–ambitious" or "Black–athletic"). People were faster to respond to stereotypical words compared to control words, revealing an implicit stereotype that is not consciously expressed—the responses are too fast to reflect control. A reaction time measure is perhaps best able to remain implicit (and not reveal what is being measured) if set up so that the participant is unable to see, even if given the time, what is being measured. In the task just described one might, if given time, be able to learn that the task is asking about groups and stereotypes. The task can be set up so that the cognitive process at hand is harder to see. A lexical decision task is an example of a measure where people are never asked to directly associate the qualities being studied.

Lexical Decision Task

Rather than asking people to evaluate a word as good or bad, or to categorize a word as a certain type (e.g., is "ambitious" a quality of the group "White"), Meyer and Schvaneveldt (1971) used a task where people simply decide whether a string of letters on the screen was a word or just gibberish. Pairs of letter strings appeared together and the research participant had to decide whether both of the items were in fact words. If this was the case they hit a button marked "yes," and they hit "no" if they were not both real words. This is known as a lexical decision task. Research participants perform many of these decisions, and sometimes the strings contain two words (e.g., "nurse" and "doctor," "nurse" and "butter") and other times they contain nonsense strings (e.g., "nurse" and "grispe"). The concern is with reaction times. If people associate the two items, then they should be faster to make the lexical decision. I can know if you think doctors are associated with nurses if you respond faster to identifying those items as words than when asked to do the equally easy task of identifying "nurse" and "butter" as words. It is not the actual amount of the speed up in the responding that matters (is it 20 milliseconds or 100 milliseconds) but that any statistically reliable facilitation in reaction time can only be explained by an association between the two. Having first seen the word "nurse" should trigger associated items in memory and make one faster to respond to those items. Even if the response is simply identifying it as a word.

Lexical decision tasks became a popular way to test whether people stereotype others. Do people store information about social groups (e.g., Jews as a category), and does that category contain certain attributes (e.g., stereotypes)? We could address this question by showing a person the word "Jew" (or a picture associated with Jewishness) and then measuring how quickly they identify letter strings as words. If they identify stereotypic attributes faster, then the person is known to be thinking about the stereotype when they see the word "Jew." Even if they consciously detest such thinking. As mentioned above, implicit measures should allow us to naturally tap how people think, without giving them goals that could alter how they respond and to make socially desirable responses. Stereotyping and prejudice are particularly prone to such social desirability biases in how

> **Lexical decision tasks:** Tasks where people decide if a letter string is a word or gibberish. Pairs of letter strings appear together and the task is to decide if both are words or not. When both are words, an association among them is detected by faster reaction times than for unassociated word pairs (doctor–nurse vs. doctor–soup).

people respond because being labeled as biased in this way is particularly aversive. A lexical decision task is quite good at avoiding such social desirability effects since the link between what one is doing and what is being measured is hard to detect. While the task might not look like something we do naturally, what it measures is something we do naturally.

Galinsky and Moskowitz (2000b) used a lexical decision task to illustrate an ironic point: that people who are asked to *not stereotype* will stereotype even more than people to whom nothing about stereotyping is explicitly mentioned. This helps to illustrate the implicit nature of the response. Even though conscious responding provides no evidence of stereotyping, stereotyping is revealed by a lexical decision task. The explicit measure of stereotyping was an essay about a person that participants were asked to write (coded for how stereotypic it was); the implicit measure was a lexical decision task. Participants were first shown a photograph of an old man sitting on a bench and were asked to write a short essay about his day. Some were asked to not stereotype when doing so. Afterward they performed a lexical decision task that the participants did not know measured stereotyping. In addition to a set of nonwords, participants saw a set of words pretested to be known as related to the stereotype of older adults (traditional, stubborn, lonely, forgetful, dependent), and a set of words unrelated to the stereotype (jumpy, envious, scheming, cowardly, deceptive). We can tell whether people stereotype older adults if they respond more quickly to identifying the stereotypic items as words as compared to the unrelated items. They do, and they are especially fast if asked to try and not stereotype when writing the initial essay.

The Weapon–Tool Task

This same reaction time logic can not only be used to determine whether people associate traits with a group (such as forgetful and older), or feelings (such as "bad" and "Black"). It can also show specific types of objects and situations that we associate with people or groups. For example, recent research shows that White people in the United States associate impoverished and crime-ridden neighborhoods with Black people (e.g., Bonam et al., 2020). Payne (2006) used a reaction time procedure he developed to illustrate an association held by White people between violence/criminality and Black people. In this **weapon–tool task** participants have a face flashed at them extremely quickly—for one-fifth of a second. The face is either of a Black man or a White man. Immediately after it disappears an object is flashed extremely quickly (also one-fifth of a second) and is then replaced by the screen getting all "snowy." The participant has no time to lie, and has very little conscious sense of what they saw. The "snowy" screen dominates consciousness. The trick to this task is that the object that gets flashed is either a gun or a hand tool (such as a

> **Weapon–tool task:** An implicit test revealing if weapons are stereotypically associated with Black men. Participants see either a Black or a White man's face flashed extremely quickly. Next, a weapon or tool is quickly flashed. Reaction times for judging whether a weapon or tool was flashed following each face type reveal if stereotypic associations exist.

wrench). The response is a simple one: Press one button to indicate if the object was a weapon and another to indicate if it was a tool. Participants responded to guns faster in the presence of a Black man as compared to a White man, and no such difference appears for tools. This procedure reveals that there is a stereotypic association in the mind of some White Americans that has thoughts of African Americans immediately and unconsciously triggering thoughts of violence and guns. The task allows this impulse to be revealed, even if it is not consciously recognized by the person who holds these associations.

The Shooter Task

In this task, as part of playing a video game, one is asked to determine whether a person is holding a gun or a harmless object, and they are asked to shoot the person (press a button marked "shoot") if they are holding a gun, and to not shoot (press a button marked "don't shoot") if they are holding a harmless object (like a cell phone). This type of an approach allows us to extend the idea that reaction times tell us what people think and feel, to allowing us to also see what people are likely to do (shoot or not) and whether they make errors (e.g., Correll, Park, Judd, & Wittenbrink, 2002; Correll, Wittenbrink, Park, Judd, & Goyle, 2011).

Does a person's race affect a participant's (or a police officer's) decision to shoot? The logic is that an association exists in American culture between Black men and threat or violence, and this association leads one to have notions of threat ready when perceiving a group member. This association can be revealed by looking at the reaction times with which people respond to White versus Black men who hold guns (and those who do not hold guns) in the **shooter task**. Results of these types of experiments (of which there are many) show that White participants fire at an armed Black man *more quickly* than an armed White man. They were also faster to hit the button indicating they would not fire at an unarmed White man as compared to responding to an unarmed Black man. Even police officers, who are trained to use guns in such situations, show this reaction time bias (e.g., Correll, Hudson, Guillermo, & Ma, 2014). Importantly, the implicit stereotyping evidenced by such results was not related to a participant's explicit beliefs about race. Even people who do not personally endorse stereotypes or prejudice show the bias. Even Black people show the bias. The self-report and the implicit measure diverge, because the implicit measure taps an association. Later in this chapter we return to discuss the errors made by participants in this task, since it is the errors (such as shooting an unarmed person) with which most people are concerned. However, the reaction time measure helps us to understand that a stereotype is associated with the group and that such associations facilitate seeing a weapon that is clearly present. This bias to readily see a weapon not only allows one to more quickly make the decision to shoot when a gun is present but it could lead one to incorrectly see a gun when one is not present. In ambiguous situations, where it is not clear whether a weapon is present, this bias could lead one to erroneously see a threat that does not exist.

> **Shooter task:** Participants in a "video game" are to shoot if a person has a gun and not shoot if holding something harmless. That person's race varies across trials. Reaction times and error rates for this choice are used to determine if there is an association between threat and Black men.

The Implicit Association Test

A popular measure of the implicit association between affect and a group is the **Implicit Association Test (IAT)** (Greenwald, McGhee, & Schwartz, 1998). How does the IAT work? It maps two tasks (e.g., categorizing a face as Black or White and categorizing a word as positive or negative) onto a single pair of responses. In other words, people make two different decisions (judge faces and judge word affect) by doing the exact same thing: choosing between two keys on a keyboard to press. For example, to indicate that a face was White you would press the "*S*" key when a White person's face was presented. To indicate that a face was Black you would press the "*L*" key when a Black person's face was presented. Additionally, there is a second task that requires pressing the same keys. To indicate that a word was "good" you would press *S* when a good word (such as "peace") was presented. To indicate that a word was bad (such as "war") you would press *L* when a bad word was presented. In this example the Black person's face is responded to with the same action required to respond to negative words (pressing *L*).

> **Implicit Association Test (IAT):** A tool that measures feelings about a group without participants knowing attitudes are being assessed. Instead, they simply believe they are categorizing one set of stimuli as good/bad while categorizing other stimuli as group X/Y (such as Black/White). Reaction times on what are called compatible and incompatible trials reveal bias.

The IAT can be used to detect an association without one realizing this task is assessing race. If the responses are set up in the way described above, then pressing *L* when a negative word appears will be facilitated only for people who associate "Black" and "bad" in the mind since the responses will be compatible (they require making the same response). If, however, the response to categorize a face as Black (press "*L*") is paired with a different response used to indicate a word is "bad" (press "*S*"), then the responses are incompatible for people who associate Black and bad. Despite never being asked to say whether one likes or dislikes specific types of people, an association can be revealed by the speed of making the choices on compatible and incompatible trials.

To perform an IAT requires multiple judgments done in blocks. First one needs to practice pressing *S* and *L* to make judgments about what race a person is (or whatever category one is interested in). Then one needs to practice pressing *S* and *L* to make judgments about whether a word is good or bad. Then the two tasks are combined so that people do one or the other across many trials—they might see a face or they might see a word, and they need to respond appropriately to whichever one they see on that trial. Finally, people are trained again to flip the mappings. If they had been pressing *L* to indicate they had seen a bad word, they now practice pressing *L* to indicate a good word. Once they have reprogrammed their responses, they again put the tasks together and juxtapose making decisions about group membership alternated with decisions about word affect. Pairings that had once been compatible (such as *S* for White and good, and *L* for Black and bad) are now incompatible (they press *S* for White and bad, and *L* for Black and good). Juxtaposing the tasks allows for an implicit association to be detected. If the category "Black" is associated with bad feelings, people will more easily press the appropriate key if the same key is used to indicate a word is bad. There will be a facilitation in response times on compatible trials of the task in comparison to the incompatible trials of the task. It must be pointed out that the experiments that use this technique always train some people on the incompatible pairings first and some people on the compatible pairings first, so it cannot be argued that what they learn first is what they respond most quickly to.

Greenwald et al. (1998) introduced the procedure in a now classic set of experiments. They used a variety of groups to illustrate that the effect measures associations quite generally, not just race bias. For example, one experiment used groups of flowers and insects—the participants' overt dislike for insects is also uncovered by the IAT. More importantly, their dislike for groups one would not report consciously is also revealed. One experiment showed negative associations between Japanese American students judging Korean American students (and vice versa). The IAT results showed that implicit negative feelings felt by Japanese people toward Korean people (and vice versa) led to faster responses to negative words when doing so required pressing the same button as identifying a name as Korean (and Korean participants were faster when "bad" was paired with the same response for indicating a Japanese surname). The same pattern was found in another experiment using White research participants making judgments about whether a name is that of a Black person or a White person. When the response to indicate a name is "Black" is the same one used to indicate a negative word, White participants are faster than if the response to indicate that a name is that of a Black person is the same as to detect a positive word. This reveals an association between the category "Black" and negative attitudes in White people. This is an association they do not intend to reveal and do not know they have expressed. Despite the IAT being a popular methodology (e.g., Charlesworth & Banaji, 2021, 2022), as with almost any psychological test, critics have raised methodological reasons to suggest it is a flawed measure of attitudes (e.g., Dasgupta, Greenwald, & Banaji, 2003; Kurdi et al., 2019; Rudman, Greenwald, Mellot, & Schwartz, 1999). This is an important debate (see Jost, 2019b, for a review). However, our concern in a book such as this cannot be to dive into the details regarding the efficacy of any one measure. If it were the *only* measure of implicit attitudes, then such a deep dive might be necessary. But there are many ways to measure implicit evaluation (see also Fazio & Olson, 2003; Olson & Fazio, 2003), as seen above with attitude automaticity and as reviewed next.

MISATTRIBUTION MEASURES

When earlier discussing aversive racism, it was mentioned that one way to detect such a bias was to place people either in a situation that was not seemingly about race, where there were no clear norms about what type of behavior is appropriate. In such ambiguous situations, the true source of one's behavior is a bias that the participants do not see. The participants believe their reaction to be caused by the situation they are in—the person did not need their help; a candidate had weak qualifications; the policy being asked about was inappropriate. The ambiguity allows them to misattributed the response from their own bias to a stimulus they are judging. **Misattribution** refers to such a shifting of responsibility for one's reac-

> **Misattribution:** When what one is privately thinking is incorrectly attributed to being aroused by something other than the true source. For example, feelings recently experienced toward one person are attributed to a new person, with the incorrect belief that the new person's behavior is responsible for the reaction one is having.

tion; it shifts from the true source, which is not detected, to some other cause that is not actually responsible. It is a case of mistaking an effect that is caused by one source (such as an implicit process) as caused by another source. Misattribution is a specific type of error where there is an outcome one is trying to explain (why I liked my dinner, why I hired that person, why I invited that person on a date, etc.), and there is one true explanation. However, other explanations are grabbed hold of instead, even though they are not actually responsible for the outcome. One may believe the reason dinner was liked was because the restaurant has a superior chef, but it may actually be that you attribute the enjoyment to the chef, when it was actually your dinner companion that made the meal feel more enjoyable. It is more than an error. Confusing one fact for another, or forgetting and needing to guess, is not a misattribution. Remembering that your father cooked you a birthday dinner when it actually was your mother is likely not a misattribution, but an error of recollection accompanied by a guess.

Writing for *The New York Times* (September 3, 2021), Amia Srinivasan provides a good example of misattribution by describing the situation where a client develops feelings for a therapist, or students develop romantic feelings for teachers:

The teacher–student relationship arouses in the student a strong desire, a sense of thrilled if inchoate infatuation. That desire is the lifeblood of the classroom, and it is the teacher's duty to nurture and direct it toward its proper object: learning. The teacher who allows his student's desire to settle on him as an object, or the teacher who actively *makes* himself the object of her desire, has failed in his role as a teacher. (section SR, p. 4)

Passion for the material and the excitement of new discovery can be misattributed to the teacher. The arousal felt in therapy can be misattributed to the therapist. (This is similar to the clinical notion of **transference**.) There are many examples of misattribution in social psychology.

Dutton and Aron (1974) famously illustrated the sort of misdirected feelings of passion just described. They placed some participants on a dangerously high and shaky bridge. When physiologically aroused by the bridge, participants misattributed that arousal to another person. Arousal caused by the precarious situation was misattributed to the next person they met, finding that person more attractive than a person who was met after a participant had crossed a safe bridge. Another well-known example of the misattribution of one's own arousal was provided by Schachter and Singer (1962). They showed that when they injected participants with the drug epinephrine, participants experienced the natural result of the drug, which is physiological arousal. The participants were either told that the injection would cause arousal, or they were told it would have no effect. Participants were then placed in a room with a confederate who exhibited a strong emotion (such as anger). When participants believed the injection would have no effects, they now were experiencing arousal that required an explanation. They misattributed their arousal from its true source (the injection) to the person with whom they shared the room. The arousal was assumed to be caused by sharing the emotional experience (anger) of the highly emotive person in the room. However, when participants were told the injection would make them aroused, this misattribution of arousal failed to occur. In another experiment, people were experiencing arousal that was actually caused by an inconsistency in their beliefs or attitudes (as reviewed in Chapter 9, such inconsistency causes an arousing state of inner turmoil). When they correctly assessed that their inconsistent attitudes were the source of their arousal, they changed their attitude to remove the inconsistency and eliminate the arousal. However, if participants were asked to take a pill that they were told would make them physiologically aroused, the arousal that was actually caused by the inconsistent attitudes was misattributed to the pill. This is seen by the fact that they no longer change their attitudes (Zanna & Cooper, 1974). A variety of measures use misattribution as a diagnostic tool to tap implicit cognition. We review some next.

> **Transference:** A case of misattribution occurring in therapy when a patient has feelings they experience toward a significant other that they do not consciously detect or face and instead misattribute those feelings as due to the behavior of their therapist, who becomes the target for the emotional reaction instead.

Misattribution in Social Judgment

Higgins, Rholes, and Jones (1977) developed what has become a classic implicit measure that relies on principles of misattribution to reveal how people are biased when judging others. A perceiver will think their judgment is caused by the behavior of a person they have met (or read about), when in fact the judgment is reflecting an implicit thought the perceiver previously had about a totally different person. The true source is unseen and the reaction is misattributed.

A typical study of misattribution in social judgment is divided into two parts: (1) triggering a source of influence, and (2) a judgment task. In the first task, people are incidentally exposed to information—such as a stereotype, attitude, trait, a negative facial expression—in order to trigger that concept in memory (make it accessible). For example, seeing "reckless" as part of a list of words to be memorized in a "memory task" increases the accessibility of associated concepts (such as notions of riskiness, danger, and constructs related to reckless). As another example, flashing a face subliminally will make accessible the emotions communicated in the face nonverbally. The goal in this first task is simply to trigger a response (a trait, a stereotype, an emotion, a belief, etc.) without the person thinking it will have any impact on them now or later (see also Bargh & Pietromonaco, 1982; Srull & Wyer, 1979). Next, an ostensibly separate "judgment task" is performed, where participants learn behaviors describing a person and form impressions of the person. In this example, they judge the person as more reckless than people not exposed to "reckless" in Task 1. Accessible concepts from a first task impact on a second task without one realizing it. One thinks it is the person's behavior that determines how one responds, when in reality this judgment is misattributed *from* its true source, which is not in actuality the person.

Stereotypes of women at work unfortunately suffer from these types of misattribution in judgment. An existing social problem facing many women is men's use of stereotypes in how they judge women at work (e.g., Carli & Eagly, 2007; Fiske, 1993b; Heilman & Okimoto, 2007; Rudman & Glick, 2001). Rather than a man seeing a negative assessment of a woman with whom he works as attributable to its true source (the man's stereotypes), it is instead attributed incorrectly to be due to the woman's behavior. The triggering of a gender stereotype will bias us by leading us to believe we see evidence for that stereotypic belief that does not exist, and to make judgments about the person accordingly. Banaji, Hardin, and Rothman (1993) performed an experiment to illustrate how stereotypes can be misattributed to a woman's behavior. They followed the standard procedure of asking participants to perform two "unrelated" tasks. Male research participants first performed a task that triggered their stereotypes of women. They next were asked to perform what they believed was an unrelated second experiment where they read about a person's behavior and made judgments about what type of person this was and what caused their behavior. The story they read described a person who was acting in a manner that was mostly irrelevant to gender stereotypes, but that contained a small subset of behaviors that were weakly related to the trait of dependence (a quality that is part of the stereotype of women). Thus, the behavior was ambiguous and open to interpretation, as opposed to clearly an example of dependence. After reading about the behavior, the participants were asked to make judgments about the person and rate the degree to which the person could be described as "dependent."

The judgments that participants reported provide a clear illustration of stereotypes guiding judgment in that the male participants saw the woman's behavior as providing the evidence of the quality "dependent," rather than attributing that judgment correctly to their own stereotypic expectations. How do we know the stereotype is the true source of the judgment, and that a misattribution has occurred? Because (1) the behavior was not a clear example of dependence, and (2) perhaps more importantly, Banaji et al. (1993) had also manipulated whether the target in the story was a man or a woman. When it was a man named Donald the male participants correctly saw a behavior that was not particularly dependent. However, when it was a woman named Donna they believed they saw behavioral evidence that was clearly dependent. When Donna performed the same ambiguous behavior—that was at best weakly related to dependence—she was interpreted in a stereotype-confirming manner. It is not that women are simply rated inferior to men but that they are seen as having qualities, supposedly based on behavioral evidence, that confirm specific stereotypic expectations. They are judged to be dependent even though the evidence is weak. The evidence comes from the already existing stereotype and is misattributed to the woman's behavior. A false belief that a perceiver has actually observed clear evidence of a woman's heightened dependence and lack of dominance creates a barrier to women hoping to be promoted. Unfortunately, for many women, the precise conditions that allow for misattribution are often met in the workplace. Women may be in smaller numbers and thus likely to be categorized according to gender. If not in smaller numbers, the job may be sex typed, making gender roles likely to be triggered. Work environments are typically a constant source of cognitive load, with people racing to get many tasks done, and thus providing them with incentive to stereotype. These conditions can lead men to misattribute their own implicitly held stereotypic bias to the woman's actions.

Another example of gender stereotypes leading to misattribution is seen when such stereotypes prescribe what we consider to be acceptable behavior, such as how assertive or aggressive a person can be. Gender stereotypes allow for less assertiveness in women. Therefore, if a man and woman at work are shown to exhibit objectively the same amount of assertiveness, the judgment could still be that the woman has acted inappropriately assertive. This has been called a **backlash effect:** a process where a person (in this example, a woman) is judged negatively for the same behavior performed by another person (in this example, a man) because stereotypes have prescribed different expectations of what is allowable for people who come from each of their two groups. It is not an instance of one person actually being more extreme (in which case the judgment might be accurate) but of the perceiver using their expectations as a standard for what is acceptable and basing the judgment on the deployment of those standards without realizing it. They misattribute judgment to the person's unwanted actions, not to the true source,

> **Backlash effect:** When a person is judged negatively for the same behavior performed by another person because stereotypes prescribe different expectations of what is allowable for people from each group. Thus, the person is stereotyped (faces backlash) when performing in ways that, for others, are seen as acceptable and perhaps necessary.

which is their own stereotypes. A person faces backlash for performing in ways that, for others, are seen as necessary to get ahead at work. An excellent example was provided by Fiske, Bersoff, Borgida, Deaux, and Heilman (1991).

Fiske et al. (1991) were researchers called upon by the U.S. Supreme Court to testify about how implicit stereotyping and prejudice toward women operates and could impact an employer's evaluations of men versus women employees, without the employer realizing it or consciously intending it. Can misattribution in social judgment inform Court rulings on sexual harassment and hostile workplaces? Fiske et al. argued before the Supreme Court, in the case of *Price Waterhouse v. Hopkins*, that an agentic woman (such as the accountant at Price Waterhouse named Anne Hopkins) could be seen as abrasive and unlikable due to the backlash from having violated prescriptions that dictate agentic behaviors are inappropriate for women. Yet, the same behavior from a man would be seen as valued and necessary. The lawsuit alleged that backlash in the form of negative attributions led Hopkins to be seen as less suitable for promotion than her male peers (who had objectively less success with clients). Backlash further led to alleged insulting and sexist commentary to Hopkins about needing to be more "feminine." If a woman is told that she should be weak, emotional, and dependent, and is instead demeaned for having the qualities that enhance the probability of promotion, then hiring and promotion decisions that exclude women will seem justified. To overcome the stereotype, she may need to act in a way that clearly disconfirms that stereotype, yet that behavior will be misattributed to the women's inappropriateness and not to the true source of the problem: the prescription held by the man that only men should act that way. Thus, by being appropriately assertive, a woman may risk backlash effects. In Chapter 9 we discuss how this places women on a *tightrope*, with the double bind of needing to maintain enough of the stereotype to be seen as normative (warm), but violating the stereotype sufficiently to be seen as efficacious (e.g., Williams, 2014).

Affect Misattribution Procedures

Misattribution of affect: The error of transferring a reaction from its true source to an incorrect target is not limited to semantic assessment such as "confident" or "reckless." General affective reactions, such as liking a person, can be misattributed as well. Transferring good/bad reactions arising from one source to another.

Affect misattribution procedure (AMP): Task for assessing true attitudes where a positive or negative image is seen at Step 1. Attitudes are assessed implicitly at Step 2 by pleasantness ratings of a Chinese pictograph. Bias in these ratings provides a window to the true attitudes toward step one stimuli being misattributed to the pictograph.

We already saw a case of **misattribution of affect** when we reviewed the work of Murphy and Zajonc (1993) in Chapter 3. A subliminally presented face displaying a negative emotion led people to see another object as more negative (relative to when exposed to a positive face). The emotional reaction to the face gets misattributed on to something else. Participants believe the object being judged is negative and dislikable, not that a facial expression caused them to experience negative affect. Misattribution when judging something or someone does not require that the influencing agent is subliminal. If one does not detect the source of the influence (as with the Higgins et al., 1977, study reviewed above), the person will believe they are not influenced. Payne, Cheng, Govurum, and Stewart (2005) used these ideas to develop a way to test a person's true attitude to a stimulus. In their **affect misattribution procedure (AMP)** people are never asked to self-report their attitudes, and further, are explicitly asked (in some cases) not to evaluate or develop attitudes toward the target of their judgment. This measure follows what should now be a familiar two-step process. In a first step an image of either a positive (a cute baby, a puppy, etc.) or a negative (snakes, spiders, etc.) stimulus is presented. This triggers an attitude (without one realizing it, since one has been explicitly asked not to evaluate the images). If the attitude has been triggered, it can be detected through misattribution. This is measured in a second step where participants judge the pleasantness of a Chinese character. The task is to rate a Chinese pictograph by pressing one of two keys labeled "unpleasant" and "pleasant." The bias seen in ratings of the pictograph provide a window to the true attitudes held toward the people and objects from the first step of the task. Participants misattribute those attitudes as having been caused by the pictograph (the two phases of the procedure are depicted in the top half of Figure 4.5).

Affect misattribution procedure (AMP)

Phase One: Exposure to Attitude Object   Phase Two: Evaluate a Chinese Pictograph

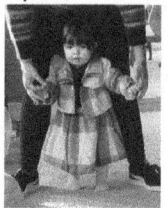

"Good" or "Bad" 我

Misattribution to a subliminal word (MSW) task

Phase One: Learn a Set of   Phase Two: Supposed   Phase Three: Was It
Behaviors Paired with Pictures   Flash of Subliminal Word   a Good or Bad Word?

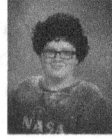 Isaac stopped to help an older woman carry her groceries across the street.

********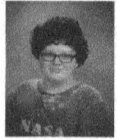

Press "S" if   Press "L" if
"Good."   "Bad."

FIGURE 4.5. Two examples of misattribution procedures.

A similar logic for assessing attitudes toward people was used in our own lab with the **misattribution to a subliminal word (MSW)** task. Olcaysoy Okten, Schneid, and Moskowitz (2019) had participants read positive and negative behaviors about people paired with their picture. Did our participants immediately form positive and negative attitudes about each person based on their behavior? Rather than ask them, we used misattribution to find out. Participants first read a set of behaviors, each paired with a picture of the person (Task 1). Next, they saw the same pictures again, but were told a subliminal word was going to be presented immediately before seeing the picture, and that the task was to guess whether the subliminal word that preceded the person's picture was a good word or a bad word (by pressing one of two keys labeled "Good" and "Bad"). The trick is that there actually was no subliminal word. Thus, when participants select a key to push they are actually revealing their attitude toward the person. They misattribute their attitude toward the person to a (supposed) subliminal word (the three phases of the procedure are depicted in the bottom half of Figure 4.5).

> **Misattribution to a subliminal word (MSW):** Participants read behaviors paired with faces. To assess if the behaviors impact impressions of the person, participants see the faces again, now paired with a word flashed subliminally. Participants choose what the word was—for example, good/bad. There actually was no word; the task taps affect associated with each face.

Feeling That Someone or Something Is Familiar

One reason misattribution is important is because it allows us to detect the ways in which people are biased. Just as people at times do not know their true beliefs, stereotypes, or attitudes, they often do not see the ways their judgments and decisions are biased, perhaps even denying bias. The examples reviewed so far have illustrated how our emotions, liking of objects and people, and the experience of arousal are misattributed due to an inability to detect our cognitive processes. One of the most troubling types of misattributions is one that helps to explain why misinformation is easy to spread and why people believe false things to be true. Misattribution has been used to shed a light on a bias known as the **availability heuristic**. This is a cognitive process where people assign an explanation to why some information is readily available in the mind. If it comes to mind easily, people generate a reason as to why. The reasons we use to explain why information comes to mind easily can be faulty, misattributing the cause from the actual reason to an incorrect reason. One common misattribution for why information comes to mind quickly and easily is that it signifies that it is encountered frequently, happens often, and is likely to be true. Something may come to mind easily because it was recently seen on social media, yet we might misattribute the feeling of coming to mind easily to the fact that it must be true.

> **Availability heuristic:** A bias leading one to associate the ease of retrieval of information from memory with a theory about what such ease of retrieval means, such as assuming that it indicates the frequency with which that information is encountered or the probability that this information is true.

This is not always a misattribution. Typical and common things can come to mind easily. When you think of a "bird" the image that comes to mind most easily probably is a bird that is commonly seen (such as a robin, or pigeon). You are less likely to have imagined a more atypical bird (such as an owl, or penguin). It is a "misattribution" when we assign a reason for something coming to mind easily as being due to its commonness or factual nature, when in fact it is neither common nor factual. Feelings of information as easily retrieved do not always arise because these feelings represent things that are common or true. At times they are "perceptually ready" for reasons that have nothing to do with truth, such as how frequently or recently one had been exposed to it. If we hear something frequently, it starts to feel familiar. Especially when we cannot remember where we heard it, but it feels like we know it (it is easily recalled), our tendency is to misattribute such feelings of familiarity to truth. Experience in life teaches us that things we easily remember, that feel familiar, are things that are either true or frequently seen.

This is precisely how advertisers and agents of misinformation try to persuade people. If something is presented often enough it will feel familiar, and the person hearing it may misattribute the familiarity to truth. We believe that because a product is easily brought to mind it must be best. Its quality is the reason it comes to mind, not its repetition in a commercial. If we see a piece of information shared on social media by many people, it may feel more familiar to us than an alternative piece of information. The alternative may be what is true, but the one that feels familiar is the one we believe to be factual. This is a misattribution of the feeling of familiarity; it is an incorrect assignment of what the ease of retrieval signifies. A quote from Tversky and Kahneman (1973) explains the rationale behind the availability heuristic: "That associative bonds are strengthened by repetition is perhaps the oldest law of memory known to man. The availability heuristic exploits the inverse form of this law, that is, it uses strength of association as a basis for the judgment of frequency" (pp. 208–209).

Let us review two examples of this error. In one experiment, research participants severely overestimated the probability that a Black student on their college campus was also an athlete. Popular athletic teams, such as football and basketball teams, have high percentages of Black men. The popularity of the sport makes these men highly salient. They stand out in memory. When thinking about Black men on campus, this identity—athlete— comes easily to mind. The students believe that the reason "athlete" comes to mind easily is because it is a frequent and true thing of Black men. In reality, only a small percentage of Black men on these campuses are athletes. The salience of Black athletes on popular teams makes thoughts about athletics come to mind easily when thinking about the group. Participants' true source for thinking about athletics is this salience, but they misattribute the ease with which they think about Black athletes to the (incorrect) fact that most Black students are athletes (Higginbotham, Shropshire, & Johnson, 2021). Salient things (as a source for availability) are often misattributed to frequent or true things. This is why the typical U.S. citizen believes Americans are more likely to be killed in plane crashes or terrorist incidents than bathroom accidents. They have no data to inform which is more frequent, just the fact that plane crashes and terrorist events are vivid, salient, and newsworthy. They are easier to call to mind than bathroom accidents (which lead to far more deaths annually). Ease of retrieval due to salience is misattributed as due to frequency.

The very first empirical illustration of the availability heuristic was provided by Tversky and Kahneman (1973). Research participants memorized a list of names that contained an equal mix of "celebrity" men and women. In some of the cases the men were more famous (e.g., Richard Nixon vs. Lana Turner), and in other cases the women were more famous (e.g., Elizabeth Taylor vs. William Fulbright). Participants were asked to judge the frequency of men and women in each list. Participants judged the gender with the better-known celebrities to be the more frequent one, even though the numbers were equal. Fame made names salient, increased salience made those names easier to recall, and this made people overestimate the frequency of that group in the list. Jacoby, Woloshyn, and Kelley (1989) provided another illustration of how fame is misattributed by flipping this effect. Where Kahneman and Tversky showed that fame leads people to make incorrect attributions about frequency, Jacoby et al. showed that frequency leads people to make incorrect estimates about fame— that is, if one does not explicitly recall having ever seen a particular name before, or met a person with that name before, the reason it feels familiar must be due to one knowing the name for another reason. One explanation is that the person is famous. In their experiment, participants first saw a list of names. When later tested about a new list of names that included some from the first list, the participants now felt as if some of these names were familiar, but did not recall that this was because they were on the first list. Participants did not recall having seen them before. To attribute this feeling of familiarity, this availability of the name, to something, they assumed the names felt familiar because the person was famous (having, incorrectly, ruled out the true source—the names were seen earlier in the experiment). They called this the **false-fame effect** (see also Banaji & Greenwald, 1995).

Any time something feels familiar, but you have no memory of having seen it before, the opportunity exists for misattribution. The misattribution allows us, as the experimenter, to see the cognitive process that is influencing the person—one they themselves cannot see. Jacoby and White-house (1989, Study 2) performed an extremely clever study to show this. They made a word feel familiar by flashing it at people subliminally. They had participants study a list of words for a memory test (Task 1). The memory test (Task 2)

> **False-fame effect:** A misattribution of the feeling of familiarity from having been exposed to name earlier (but not being able to recall having seen it before) to the name being that of a famous person. Although the true source is the earlier exposure, the familiarity is misattributed to the fame of the individual.

presented them with a mix of new words and old words and simply asked people to identify the old ones. There was one trick. Participants sometimes had a new word flashed at them subliminally just before they were asked to decide whether it was "new" or "old." In this way, the "new" word felt familiar to participants, but not because it was on the earlier list. Participants were more likely to label a new word as an old word when it was preceded by such a subliminal presentation. They misattributed familiarity due to the subliminal presentation as due to prior learning. (As a control condition, participants also sometimes had a new word flashed at them so that it was consciously seen. When it next appeared as part of the new versus old task the reason for its familiarity was clear. It was because the participants just had it flashed at them. With an obvious explanation for the feeling of familiarity, they no longer call these "new" words "old.")

INTERFERENCE TASKS

Some tasks allow us to know what someone is thinking outside of consciousness by examining how a conscious task you have asked them to do is interfered with. One example has already been reviewed. In Chapter 3 we discussed the Stroop effect. We could tell people automatically extracted word meanings because they were explicitly asked to ignore word meanings and just name the color of the font. However, when a word meaning was incompatible with the conscious task of naming the font color (e.g., the word "blue" in red font), it interfered with it. Responses were slowed. Participants could still appropriately say the font was red when that red font was used in the word "blue." But the response was interfered with—disrupted (see Figure 4.6). A variety of procedures use interference as a way to diagnose what people are truly thinking.

Probe Recognition Task

We have already discussed the idea that people often infer traits outside of awareness. The encoding specificity principle and relearning procedures were reviewed above as implicit measures to diagnose such invisible trait inference. Uleman, Hon, et al. (1996) created another way such inferences could be revealed that relied on interference. The idea is straightforward. If you read about a person (*Gordon returned back to the cashier the extra money he accidentally received*) and inferred a trait (honest) about that person without realizing it, that trait would attain a state of heightened availability or perceptual readiness. Even if you do not recall having made any inference, the quality would still feel as if it was something familiar about that person. If you were then asked the question "Did the sentence you read about Gordon explicitly mention that he was honest?" or "Was the word 'honest' in the sentence you just read about Gordon?," the correct response is "no." However, your ability to respond "no" would be interfered with if (and only if) honesty had been inferred. This interference could be reflected in two ways. You could make an error and respond "yes." Or you could correctly respond "no," but be delayed in doing so. You start to say "yes" and then stop yourself. The interference would slow your reaction time. The **probe recognition procedure** of Uleman, Hon, et al. asked participants to read sentences—some implied traits, and some did not. They then were asked to indicate whether a given trait (such as "honest") was in the sentence. Reaction times to correctly respond "no" (the trait was not in the sentence) were shown to be slower on sentences that implied the trait relative to sentences that did not. This interference indicates that an inference had been made.

> **Probe recognition procedure:** Task where participants respond if a probe word is familiar. When it is not, but it feels familiar, "no" responses to the probe are slowed. Assessment if a person had recently been thinking about something is revealed by reaction times to saying "no, I didn't just see this" now being slower.

False-Recognition Task

Todorov and Uleman (2002) introduced another method for revealing the unconscious inferences we make, the **false-recognition task**. In a first phase, participants read sentences that each imply a trait, and each is paired with a face. The task is to memorize the sentences and faces. In a second phase, participants are shown a face, this time paired with a trait. Some of the time that trait is paired with the face of the person who acted in the manner that implied that trait during Phase 1 (this is called a critical trial). At other times the trait is paired with a face that originally accompanied a sentence that did not imply the trait (this is a control trial). The task is to decide whether the trait was actually included in the sentence originally paired with the face. On the critical and control trials the answer to this question is always "no." The traits were never in the sentence, they were only implied by the sentences some of the time.[3] The logic of this method is that if people inferred the trait upon reading the sentence, then this trait would have been encoded in memory along with the face of the person. Thus, when the face later appears, it serves as a cue that triggers recall of other events stored in memory at encoding (see Figure 4.6), including the inferred trait. If that is what is happening, an error will result. Participants will assume the reason they remember seeing the trait is because it was in the sentence about that person. They will have a false recognition of an inferred trait as one that had been presented. They are more likely to incorrectly reply "yes." To calculate this, one should take the number of false recognitions on the control trials and subtract it from the number of false recognitions on the critical trials of the experiment. If there was an inference made on the critical trials, the difference score would be greater than zero. If the participants correctly respond "no," then we should also see an **interference effect**. They will be slower to make this correct response if the trait had earlier been implied (and inferred) relative to how quickly they make this correct response when the trait had not been implied.

> **False recognition task:** An interference task similar to probe recognition except instead of speed of responding indicating interference, memory errors are used to indicate interference. People mistakenly recall having seen a word because it feels familiar due to their having thought about it, even if they do not realize such thoughts occurred.

> **Interference effect:** When one response disrupts or slows the performance of a related task. For example, implicitly inferring a trait that was never actually seen would slow responding to a separate task where one must respond if that word had been presented earlier. Or when information one is asked to ignore disrupts attention to another piece of information on which one is asked to focus attention.

Learning Phase   **Testing Phase**

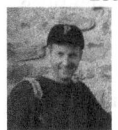

He walked up and
introduced himself
to the strangers at
the office party.

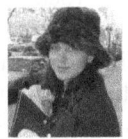

She left only a 5%
tip for the quick,
cheerful waitress.

*Do you remember having seen the word
in this actor's behavior?
Press "Y" if yes and "N" if no.*

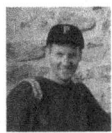 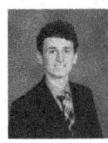 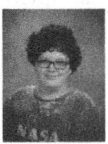

Social   Cheap   Selfish

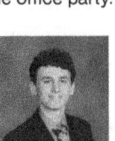

He refused
listening to his
doctor's advice on
health practices.

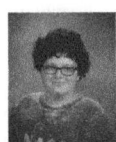

He was very selfish so
he would not loan his
extra blanket to the
other campers.

critical   *control*   *filler*

FIGURE 4.6. The false recognition task (Todorov & Uleman, 2002).

Capture of Attention Tasks

Finally, interference can occur when one is explicitly asked to ignore a stimulus, or to focus on one particular stimulus, but attention is drawn away from this focal task to be displaced on a different stimulus. These types of tasks allow us to see what people are focusing on, even if they consciously say they are focused on something else. Is the ambivalent racist focused on a person's race? Is the person with an important goal dedicating attention to that goal even when they are asked to focus attention elsewhere? In Chapter 3 we reviewed several examples of how the capture of attention could reveal an automatic process from the cocktail party effect to research by Bargh and Pratto (1986). For example, Bargh and Pratto showed that when words are relevant to us we find ourselves distracted by them and wanting to linger on them. Even if our attention is meant to be focused elsewhere, our increased attention to the self-relevant words is in conflict with that task and interferes with performance. Words relevant to each participant were presented in colored inks, along with words that were not self-relevant. The task for participants was to name the color of the ink. The reaction times to naming ink colors were reliably slower when the word content (which should be ignored to efficiently do the task) was consistent with the participant's self-concept. Attention was captured by the self-relevant word. We review several other tasks that rely on interference with a conscious task to reveal implicit processing.

Gollwitzer (1996) used an attention task called a **dichotic listening task**. People wearing headphones have separate information presented in each ear. They are told to ignore the information in one ear and attend to the other (by repeating out loud words presented to that ear). If the information one is asked to ignore actually grabs attention instead, this would interfere with the focal task (saying words aloud). Speed and accuracy on the focal task will be interfered with (impaired) if attention is directed to information in the ear that is supposed to be ignored. Many types of information

Dichotic listening task: People wearing headphones have separate information presented in each ear. They are told to ignore the information in one ear and attend to the other. If the information one is asked to ignore automatically grabs attention, this would interfere with the focal task, slowing reaction times and reducing accuracy.

have the power to grab attention, despite explicit attempts to focus attention elsewhere. Gollwitzer focused on information related to one's current goals. The experiment required creating a goal for each participant by having them name an important project they wanted to complete, and to write out a plan as to how they would attain this goal. Using these descriptions, words related to their goal were selected. These words were then used in the dichotic listening task by presenting them to participants in the ear they were supposed to be ignoring. The results showed that despite being asked to focus on one task, participants, without realizing, were implicitly pursuing their goal. This was evidenced by interference—when goal-relevant words (vs. words unrelated to their goal) were presented in the ear they were asked to ignore, performance on the focal task deteriorated (slower reading speeds, increased errors).

Research in cognitive psychology has shown that threatening information has this same ability to initially capture attention. However, despite attention being initially drawn to threat, as conscious control begins to be exerted people turn away from threat and seek to avoid it. This is known as a **vigilance–avoidance pattern in attention** (Mogg & Bradley, 2002; Mogg, Matthews, & Weinman, 1987; Pflugshaupt et al., 2007; Williams, Watts, MacLeod, & Matthews, 1988). This is a response in which people respond to anxiety-inducing cues (such as angry faces, guns, and spiders) with initial (more involuntary) visual attention directed toward the threatening cues, but then turn away from the cues as consciousness gains control over directed attention. This pattern of attention capture, followed by avoidance, can be used to diagnose whether a person finds a stimulus to be threatening, even if

> **Vigilance–avoidance pattern in attention:** A response in which people respond to anxiety-inducing cues (such as angry faces and spiders) with initial (more involuntary) visual attention directed toward the threatening cues, but then turn away from the cues as consciousness gains control over directed attention.

their explicit report is that they do not. An illustration of this was provided in Chapter 3 in an experiment conducted by Bean et al. (2012). They used a camera to track the eye movement of White research participants as they observed displays that contained both a picture of a Black man's face and a White man's face. The White participants, who did not recognize their own anxiety concerning interactions with Black people, exhibited looking behavior that followed the vigilance–avoidance pattern. Gaze was initially directed toward a Black man's face, but within 500 milliseconds it shifted away from that face to the face of a White man.

Richeson and Trawalter (2008) showed that racism in White research participants could be diagnosed in this way using attentional capture as an implicit measure. If faces of Black men are held to be threatening by White research participants, then if those faces are presented at speeds too fast for conscious control (such as 35 milliseconds), visual attention should be drawn to them. Yet the same participants should exhibit avoidance of these faces when presented for a longer duration (450 milliseconds). This is precisely the pattern seen in their White research participants, and it suggests that they were experiencing arousal and threat when seeing faces of Black men. This vigilance–avoidance pattern (initial capture of visual attention, turning to avoidance with conscious control) was especially likely among White participants concerned with social desirability and appearing nonprejudiced (with high scores on EMCP). Trawalter, Todd, Baird, and Richeson (2008) show a similar attentional capture from "threatening" faces using a dot-probe task. Pairs of faces of Black men and White men appeared on the screen for a brief interval (35 milliseconds). A dot appeared on the screen after the faces disappeared, and the dot was located in the place where one of the faces had previously been. The task is to locate the dot as fast as possible. If participants are having attention drawn to the faces of Black men, then this will interfere with the ability to quickly locate the dot when it appears in the place where the face of a White man had been. They find this capturing of attention and resulting interference. The logic of this measure is that if threatening stimuli uncontrollably grab our attention, then faces of Black men presented in an experiment to White participants should cause such a capture of attention and interfere with performance on a task that needs their attention focused elsewhere (see also Hugenberg & Bodenhausen, 2003). In fact, March, Gaertner, and Olson (2021) suggest that threat may be the modal affective response that White individuals have to Black individuals in priming tasks.

TASKS THAT ASSESS A SHIFTING STANDARD OF COMPARISON

Most people would agree that the words we use to describe people and things are relative in nature and depend on the context in which the word is used. A "large" melon will be smaller than a small chair. The comedian George Carlin had a classic bit about "jumbo shrimp." Even within the same category, the same word can shift in its information value—a small American Bulldog and a large Japanese Terrier teach us that descriptive terms (such as "large") have a subjective value that can shift based on who or what is being described. The dog called small in this example is substantially larger than the dog called large. This is implicitly understood by people who know dogs and how the standard for large and small shifts as one moves from using an American Bulldog as the standard to a Terrier as the standard. When the Japanese Terrier is called large, what is really meant is "large for a Terrier." Stereotypes of people work the same way. What is meant when a White person calls a Black man articulate? Does it mean a different thing than when that person calls a White man articulate? Earlier we saw how an assertive woman at work can mean a different thing than an assertive man in the same company. Stereotyping occurs when implicit in statements such as "she is assertive" is the fact that a different standard is used for different groups. What may seem like a compliment is actually a way of saying that expectations were set lower by a stereotype that led one to presuppose a woman would not be assertive. Or that a Black man would be less articulate. The person might be unaware that they thought such things. Being able to assess their shifting standards in this way help us to see the hidden stereotype that the person would not otherwise know. Their use of seemingly innocuous descriptors can reveal bias due to shifting standards. How? To prove a person is using a word differently for two different groups requires more than simply showing they use the word. The word "articulate" is not an insult. What needs to be shown is that the standard applied for using the word shifts when you move from talking about one category to another. A Japanese Terrier might accurately be called "large," but the same-sized American Bulldog would not. The different standard reveals that the person understands the accurate stereotype about the sizes of these two categories of dogs and applies them. The expectations are not always accurate but are drawn from stereotypes one may not recognize in oneself. Consider a student who writes an essay to be graded by a White teacher. If we find that the exact same essay is seen as "better" and assigned a higher grade when it is written by a Black student versus a White student, what have we learned? One possibility is that the teacher has a pro-Black bias. However, somewhat counterintuitively, another possibility is that the teacher is biased against Black students. The teacher's expectations for Black students are low, and the standard that the teacher uses for evaluating the paper is lower. Ultimately, in this scenario, the negative stereotype helps the Black student's grade by lowering the bar. The boosted grade is not favoritism but the result of an assumption of incompetence, of a lower standard being used. Against that lower standard the work is subjectively labeled as "excellent."

A line of research from Biernat, Manis, and Nelson (1991) show that when using adjectives to describe people, the standard used for defining the adjective will shift as the category shifts (e.g., Manis, Nelson, & Shedler, 1988). A personal trait might take on new dimensions when discussing a Black person versus a White person or a woman versus a man. Thus, when we describe a White man as "athletic" this might convey different information, because of a **shifted standard of comparison**, than when we say a Black man is "athletic."

> **Shifted standard of comparison:**
> A bias where a construct's meaning changes as the standard it is measured against changes. For example, the meaning of "tall" changes when the standard is a man versus a woman because what one thinks is typical for each group is used as the standard against which "tall" is compared.

A person who calls a woman analytical might be using that adjective very differently than when it refers to a man. Rather than using the same standard, such as the *average person*, when judging how analytical (or assertive, or independent) a man versus a woman is, one might use the average woman when judging women and the average man when judging men. If the trait being judged is relevant to the stereotypes of these groups, then the average person would look very different in a woman than in a man, and a different standard for evaluating the person would be used. Thus, our description might suggest that we are unbiased (we describe to an equal degree a woman as very analytical and a man as very analytical), but the description does not reflect what we mean or how we experience those traits in one group versus the other. We might think of a given man whom we have called analytical as much more analytical than a woman described identically, even though we have seemingly judged them the same. What the prejudiced person might mean is "she's very analytical, for a girl," for whom they have low expectations on this dimension.

How can such low expectations be revealed if the person holding such biases is convinced they do not evaluate people differently based on race or gender (or any category)? Biernat et al. (1991) had research participants make judgments of women and men. Participants saw a picture of a man or a woman and needed to make a judgment—how tall is this person? This judgment could be made using either an objective scale or a subjective scale. For example, an objective scale would be estimating height using feet and inches. A subjective scale would be judging whether the person is short or tall. The prediction was that when using a subjective scale a perceiver might describe a woman as tall and a man as tall, to equal degrees. The same word would be used to describe each ("tall"), and we would perhaps think that this person perceives no difference between the groups on this dimension. However, the objective scale would tell us whether people really do perceive a difference. The women might be rated as smaller than the men when estimates are made using feet and inches, despite the fact they are called "tall" just as often as the men in subjective ratings. Such a finding would suggest people use different standards when making the subjective judgment. The data show that when making judgments in feet and inches, the participants saw men as significantly taller than women. However, when they were instructed to make judgments by evaluating height relative to a typical person, the difference noted on the objective measure was reduced by 80%. A "typical" person was a "typical woman," if judging women, and a "typical man," if judging men. Since stereotypes suggest a typical woman is shorter than a typical man, the standard used for judging women is shorter than that used for judging men. The objectively short woman would now be called tall using a subjectively shorter standard.

Biernat and Manis (1994) illustrated this shifting standard effect in judgments made about category members using a wide variety of social groups and stereotypic qualities. Stereotypes that men are more competent than women, that women have better verbal skills than men, that Whites have better verbal skills than Blacks, and that Blacks are more athletic than Whites do not seem to exist when subjective measures are used. Whites are judged as just as "athletic" as Blacks on a subjective rating of athleticism, and women are judged to be just as competent as men. This suggests an apparent lack of stereotyping. However, despite describing both groups using the same language and apparently making no distinction among the groups, objective measures show there is a distinction being made. It requires greater levels of athleticism for a Black man to achieve the same rating that a White person gets. A woman need not be nearly as competent as a man on an objective scale to be subjectively called "very competent" as often as a man is. What it means to be athletic or competent shifts when a Black person or woman is used as a standard of evaluation (because the perceiver has stereotypes about their low ability in these domains). When subjective measures are used, each group is judged relative to the standards created within their group, not by the same standard. In this way people may seem to not have stereotypes when they really do (see also Biernat & Kobrynowicz, 1997).

The Shooter Task and Shifting Standards

Think back to the shooter task described above. This task was described only in terms of the reaction times to make a response (shoot, or do not shoot). However, one can also look at the pattern of errors one could make relating to these decisions. One could fail to shoot an armed person (what is called a "miss" in the language of signal detection theory). A wholly different (and perhaps more dire) error is that one could shoot an unarmed person (what is called a "false alarm" in the language of signal detection theory). A "hit," or correct decision to shoot, and a false alarm both result in the participant deciding to shoot. Together, these two responses (correct and incorrect choices to shoot) reflect an overall propensity to shoot. Since the decision to shoot is predicated on the presence of a threat (a gun), one's propensity to shoot reflects one's experience of a sufficient level of threat to warrant making the decision to shoot. The **criterion** is the cutoff used for decision making and represents when this sufficient level of threat is experienced. It is the point at which the experience of threat exceeds this level, and one will shoot. If the criterion is set low, then that decision to shoot will be arrived at sooner and more often. If the criterion is set high, then greater amounts of threat need to be experienced before that decision is reached and it will be made less often. A person performing this task might say that a White person without a gun and a Black person without a gun pose an equal level of threat. However, if their standard for "threat" shifts when judging the Black man versus the White man, then behavior will differ. The same behavior from a White person might not feel as threatening; the *criterion* used for defining threat is different. Despite calling them threatening to an equal degree, the behavior that leads to that label is more extreme from a White person and less extreme from a Black person. The participant would end up deciding to "shoot" the Black man more often than the White man because of this lowered criterion.

> **Criterion:** Threshold for deciding when sufficient confidence exists to initiate a specified response. If the decision is to shoot when, and only when, sufficient threat is experienced, the criterion is the point where that level of threat is set (which can vary across groups). A lower criterion means one shoots sooner.

Correll et al. (2014) review many experiments utilizing this task, and are able to show that the race of the person who appears on the screen during the task shifts the criterion that is used. The standard used to define a sufficient level of threat is altered. Using signal detection theory as a guide, they use a formula that allows them to calculate the criterion being used when making the decision to shoot. They show that research participants have a more lenient criterion when they respond to Black men as compared to when responding to White men. This different criterion leads to a greater sense of a sufficient cause to open fire. Hence, they shoot more at Black men. When he is holding a gun, this is a correct decision for this task. But they also shoot more at men not holding a gun, which is a fatal error in real life. Interestingly, another possible cause for the disparities in the shooting of unarmed men in this task could be what is called a problem of **sensitivity**. A stereotype might not only make people have a lower criterion for experiencing threat but it could make one more ready or prepared to seeing threats. In an ambiguous situation—such as when it is dark or a person is far away—one might incorrectly see an object (such as a wallet or cell phone) as a gun. Correll et al. concluded that this is not the cause of differential shooting rates in the shooter task experiments. In these experiments it is apparently clear enough what the person is holding, and participants are not shooting because they think they see a gun when there is none. It is not a sensitivity issue in this instance but a matter of a shifting criterion.

Sensitivity: The ability to detect a cue's presence and to discriminate among stimuli presented during different task conditions. In ambiguous situations, such as in darkness or a person being far away, cue detection will be harder and sensitivity will be lower. An expectation or stereotype that a cue is present might make one more sensitive to detecting it (or falsely detecting it). Using the shooter task as an example, accurately detecting whether a person is holding a gun or another object (under different conditions, such as when White versus Black men are holding an object) would demonstrate sensitivity.

For those who think better visually, Figure 4.7 illustrates this point using distributions. In this figure we see that a participant who sees a person without a gun should have low levels of threat. However, given this fact, their perception of threat should still vary to some degree and be normally distributed. Similarly, a participant who sees a person with a gun should have higher levels of threat. However, given this fact, their perception of threat should still vary to some degree and be normally distributed. These two distributions should not overlap much because people can easily discriminate the threatening targets (gun) from the unthreatening target (no gun). *Sensitivity* is high. Where race matters is in the *criterion* used. On the left-hand side of the figure we see the two distributions for when a Black man appears on screen and the participant has set a lower criterion to decide to shoot (they experience threat more easily). On the right-hand side of the figure we see the two distributions for when a White man appears on screen and the participant has set a higher criterion to decide to shoot. The area under the curve that falls beyond the criterion reflects the percentage of people who get shot. What we see is that when the low criterion is set for the Black man more people get shot accurately (fewer misses) but more false alarms get made, with an unarmed Black man shot more often than an unarmed White man.

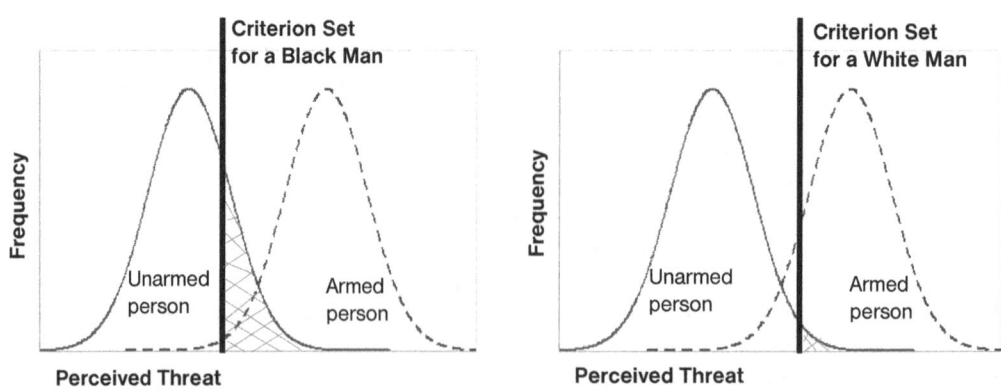

FIGURE 4.7. A shifted criterion and the increased rate of false alarms.

CONCLUSIONS

People are easy to read if one knows the language. Despite the distraction of what they say and do, what people truly think and feel is open to discovery using implicit measures. In the early days of psychology this meant using projective tests that allowed true feelings to leak out in stories and narratives that the people being investigated did not realize were a window to their inner self. In more modern times this has meant reverse engineering what we know about cognition to create measures that can accurately capture what is being thought below the surface. In the best cases these tools can help to reveal unwanted influences on cognition and create awareness of biases that lead people away from their goals. They can inform interventions to help prevent such misdirected goal pursuits.

To end this chapter, let us address the question of why there are so many different types of processes of which a person is not aware (and so many different implicit tests to tap them). The discussion of automatic processing in Chapter 3 focused on the fact that, in general, people lack awareness of how they process information, and thus self-report would be inadequate. Miller et al. (1960) had already asserted that all thinking occurs outside of awareness, and we really only are aware of the outcomes of these implicit processes. We are not aware of how we think, only of the final product of processes that are invisible to us. More recently, Reber (2013) argued that a distinction between explicit and implicit processes (such as implicit and explicit memory) is simplistic: "implicit learning does not depend on a single circumscribed neural system but instead occurs in changes within processing systems across the brain. These ubiquitous changes result from plasticity within all the neural circuitry of the brain" (p. 2039). It is, from this view, useless to dissociate explicit memory systems from implicit memory systems, because there is no general "implicit memory system" or "implicit learning system." Reber further states:

> The core idea is that implicit memory reflects a general principle of plasticity within neural processing circuits that leads to adaptive reshaping of function to match experience. This approach provides a way of grouping the variety of phenomena described as implicit learning and identifying similarities across domains in the way that this type of learning proceeds. (p. 2027)

Rather than a few measures to tap a finite set of systems, there are many different implicit processes or circuits that do not necessarily correlate with one another or substitute for one another. To tap each of these processes requires distinct implicit tests.

NOTES

1. To protect the self from such threats they embrace a strong leader who will guarantee survival with their power to dominate others. They exhibit a tendency to hierarchy, seeing others as rivals who are either superior or inferior, and seeking to have power over them in a cruel/sadistic way.

2. If you are interested, Shuell (1977) and Ostrom et al. (1981) provide details about how a clustering score can be computed so as to determine if a cluster exists.

3. There are also filler trials where the trait did appear with the face at Phase 1 (so that the answer at Phase 2 is not always "no," since for these trials the answer is "yes").

CHAPTER 5

First Impressions Are "Sticky" and Difficult to Update

An impression is our experience of a sense of "knowing" and "feeling" about a target; it is a judgment, evaluation, or emotional reaction. The target of an impression can be an individual person (my impression of a new professor on the first day of the semester), a group (my impression of the types of students who attend my college), a place (my impression of the college I attend), or thing (my impression of the bus that takes me around campus). The impression can be based on an attitude, an emotional reaction, a belief, or some combination of these different types of responses. It can be based on inferences we have formed from an observed behavior, on learning transmitted to us from another source (media, books, friends, strangers, etc.), or on prior beliefs and attitudes we have about the same target or associated targets. An impression can be as simple as a single inference, or as complex as a network of interconnected beliefs and attitudes about the target. It can be formed and held implicitly or explicitly. An impression, when first formed, removes a sense of uncertainty about the target.

Intuitively, we know that first impressions are resistant to change, or "sticky." This topic is of importance because our first impressions often form without us knowing, and even if we know they exist, they can be incorrect. Changing a false first impression, or simply modifying one that needs to be updated, is central to interpersonal interactions. The ability to see how one was wrong about another person shapes psychological reactions such as accountability, apology, behavior change, self-awareness, and emotional reactions (such as guilt, gratitude, anger, blame, and forgiveness). Misinformation (about vaccines, politicians, etc.) arise when others deliberately seek to create a false first impression, and it persists if not modified. Changing a false first impression is also central to important intergroup dynamics. Stereotyping, prejudice, and discrimination can arise from incorrect first impressions about groups. Such impressions are often rooted in historical forces and culturally taught associations that need revision.

To address both the interpersonal and intergroup dysfunction of impression "stickiness" typically involves two important types of psychological understanding. First, we need to understand why a first impression is hard to update. This involves a set of questions concerned with the following topics: why first impressions form so easily, what types of first impressions exist (attitudes, beliefs, stereotypes, traits, etc.), how does existing knowledge shape our first impression and give it a sense of being accurate and useful for action, how are first impressions incorporated into other knowledge through associations, and how and why do we protect and bolster first impressions. Second, we need to use the knowledge gained from the first step to understand how to change an impression or stereotype. This too involves a set of questions concerned with topics such as why we resist information inconsistent with a first impression, what motivates a person to want to change an impression, why people resist being motivated to change, and what does updating an impression do to memory about a person or group (how are mental representations changed).

Over the last 50 years there have been parallel literatures on these two sets of question that address them from either the level of group perceptions (showing why stereotypes are resistant to change and how to ultimately change them) and person perception (showing why first impressions of individuals are resistant to change and examining what factors lead to their revision). Kurdi and Banaji (2023) have argued for a better integration of these two approaches, with one informing the other. However, a handful of scholars (myself included) have always straddled both lines of research and attempted to integrate findings from the two (e.g., Brewer, 1988; Hamilton & Gifford, 1976; Moskowitz & Roman, 1992; Neuberg & Fiske, 1987). This chapter uses findings from each of these parallel lines to address the first question: the reasons why first impressions are sticky and resistant to movement. We return later in the book to the second question of how we use this knowledge about first impressions to change them.

A SUMMARY OF WHY FIRST IMPRESSIONS ARE SO PERSISTENT

A first reason that first impressions persist is the efficiency and simplicity of relying on what is already known. Changing an impression is more difficult and draining than sticking with what is already known, which is easier to do. There can be an aversion to effortful processing unless specifically motivated to do so. This can be described as laziness, or it can be described as efficiency, but there is a propensity to use less processing effort by seeing what one is prepared to see and affirming the attitudes and beliefs we already possess when gathering information and making sense of the behavior we observe. A first impressions is efficient not only because it is relatively effortless. As reviewed in Chapter 1, people need to have a sense of meaning and a feeling of control. This is achieved by being able to prepare appropriate action based on an ability to predict what another person is like, and likely to do. A first impression provides this, and abandoning the impression creates the possibility for uncertainty and suggests abandoning the security of knowing what to expect and how to act. This first reason for the stickiness of a first impression is *not a motivated process* where people try to reach a particular conclusion; instead the stickiness emerges as an outgrowth of natural cognitive processes. People have attitudes, beliefs, schemas, and stereotypes that make sense of the world for them and that are used as a lens through which new information is understood. This tendency to efficiently see information through the lens of existing attitudes, schemas, or beliefs—free of motivations to desire to see the information in a specific way—is known as a **confirmation bias**.

> **Confirmation bias:** A bias to see what one is prepared to see and to affirm attitudes and beliefs already possessed when gathering information and making sense of the behavior of people we meet and situations we enter. This bias is unmotivated and arises from cognitive processes that render some information more available.

Confirmation bias may on the surface feel similar to a **self-fulfilling prophecy** (which is also called behavioral confirmation), so let us briefly review how it is distinct. With a self-fulfilling prophecy (e.g., Rosenthal, 1974; Snyder & Swann, 1978; Snyder, Tanke, & Berscheid, 1977) *a perceiver's own behavior* toward the person for whom they have an impression shapes the interaction and *draws out expectancy-confirming behaviors from the other person*. The perceiver expects the other person to be cheap, for example, so the perceiver initiates the interaction in a way that expects stinginess (e.g., by offering to pay for dinner). This behavior then is more likely to compel a seemingly stingy behavior. If the other person is compelled to respond in kind, they have just fulfilled what had been expected of them (see Figure 5.1).

Self-fulfilling prophecy (behavioral confirmation): When a perceiver has an impression of a person that shapes their own behavior when interacting with that person. These behaviors then draw out expectation-confirming behaviors from the other person, compelling them to act as the perceiver expected. The other person confirms or fulfills the behavior that was expected.

With confirmation bias the perceiver *does not produce the expected behavior in the other person*. Indeed, the expected behavior need not even be exhibited by the interaction partner. A perceiver merely believes they see the expected behavior. A person might act in an ambiguous way that a perceiver twists and distorts to see as confirming their expectation. In the current example, the other person will not actually act cheaply (does not allow someone else to pay for dinner), yet the perceiver still concludes the person is cheap, seeing confirmatory evidence that is not there.

Confirmation bias is unmotivated; a person is merely operating efficiently. A second reason first impressions persist is a motivated one. We have values, identities, goals, and attitudes that lead us to desire to have a particular conclusion reached. We think in a way that will help sustain and promote the impressions that our motives and identities dictate (rather than being motivated to be accurate). Unlike with the ease of confirmation bias, there can be a great deal of effort exerted to preserve a first impression if we are motivated to see that impression persist. The set of cognitive strategies used to *preserve a desired conclusion* is known as **motivated reasoning**. According to Kunda (1987):

> People use cognitive inferential mechanisms and processes to arrive at their desired conclusions, but motivational forces determine which processes will be used in a given instance and which evidence will be considered. The conclusion therefore appears to be rationally supported by evidence, but in fact the evidence itself is tainted by motivation. (p. 637)

Motivated reasoning: A style of thinking in which cognitive processes are directed toward producing specific outcomes that support the individual's goals. If one is motivated to hate a rival institution, data about that institution is distorted in a way that highlights the negative elements, and twists what is positive into a negative.

A third reason first impressions persist is that they can be tied to important social identities and to norms of important social groups. This socially shared nature of the impression is not only resistant to change because of social desirability concerns. More than just worrying about a dissenting view causing ostracism from the group, or worry about being dismissed from the group altogether for being deviant, socially shared impressions are sticky because they are more strongly held. A group provides consensus that the impression is correct. A group helps to polarize the impression or make it more extreme. At the very least, it will seem more extreme to others. As reviewed in Chapter 2, we perceive group beliefs to be more extreme than they actually are (Robinson, Keltner, Ward, & Ross, 1995). Miller and Prentice (1999) posit that this makes impressions tied to a social group seem harder to change, and this perceived extremity and intransigence of the impression make people challenge it less frequently. For these reasons—being challenged less,

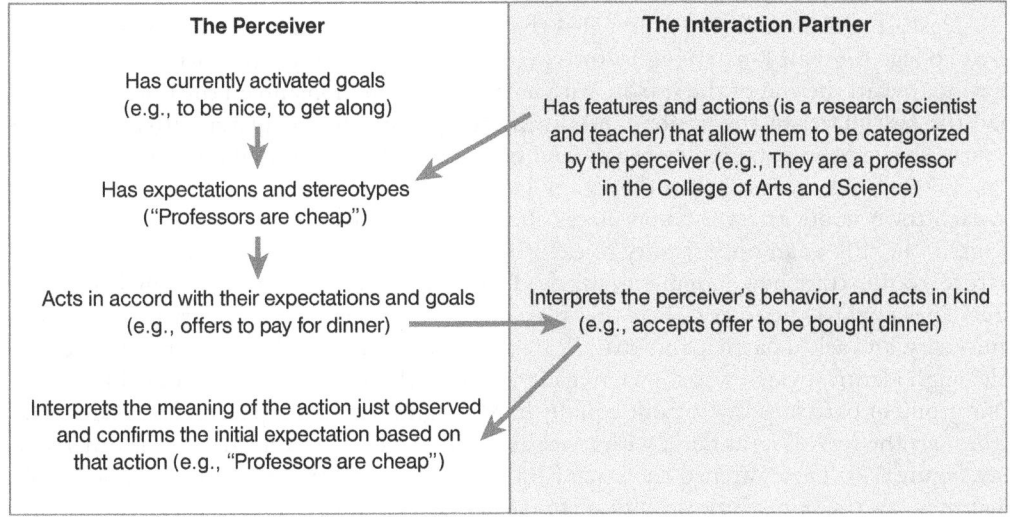

FIGURE 5.1. Self-fulfilling prophecies.

gaining strength from consensus, the comfort of being accepted rather than ostracized—first impressions tied to an important social identity (group membership) resist updating.

A fourth reason first impressions persist is that people have a variety of cognitive biases that reinforce first impressions. For example, Tversky and Kahneman (1981) describe a bias to anchor on a belief that has already been formed, with that anchor preventing subsequent judgment from drifting away. Such biases are discussed more fully in Chapter 7.

CONFIRMATION BIAS

As noted above, confirmation bias occurs when both one's memory for past events and making sense of behavior that one is currently observing are skewed toward seeing information in a way that aligns with what one already knows. The old saying "seeing is believing" has an inverted meaning from how it is typically used. Rather than meaning we will only believe something if we first see it, the confirmation bias reveals that **seeing is believing** can also mean that we will only see things in a way that confirms what our first impressions already tell us to believe—that is, two people can disagree over what it is that they "see," so that the seeing is not the believing, but the believing becomes the seeing. The exact same person doing the exact same behavior who is observed by two different people will be seen in a way that confirms what each person had expected.

> **Seeing is believing:** When perception is distorted so that it aligns with what one already believed to be true, or wished to be true. When what one sees and perceives and knows is what one already believes to be true.

Those expectations come from a first impression. With the first impression serving as a lens through which information is filtered, it is constantly being confirmed. Vehement disagreements—about what an athlete did on the field (in bounds or not, safe or out, goal or not), or what a politician meant in a speech, or if an officer's use of force was justified, or whether the media is biased or fair, or whether an act of protest is patriotic or treasonous—often result from distorted seeing due to confirmation bias.

Hastorf and Cantril (1954) provided the first illustration of confirmation bias. They used college football fans trying to interpret the events of a big game. Rival teams were playing toward the end of the season, with a national championship on the line. One team had the best player in the nation, and during the game this star player suffered a severe injury. The game was marred by rough (and potentially dirty) play and multiple injuries to players. Each side accused the other team as being dirty, tempers flared, and newspapers in each town wrote angry opinion pieces about the other team and its fans. Hastorf and Cantril saw this as an opportunity to examine how person perception is confirmatory in nature, to illustrate how judgment is skewed toward a first impression already held to be true. They ran an experiment where they played video of the actual game to students at each university, and asked participants to indicate the number of plays that could be called dirty. Although identical video was shown to each group, each fan base *saw* the game differently. One group of partisans saw a game equally hard fought, with dirty play on both sides. The other saw their rivals as at fault, with twice as many penalties committed by the other side (see Figure 5.2). They watched the same film, but saw a different game. It was not simply that they saw the same thing, but liking for their team led them to judge their team as better. It was that participants saw different things—in confirming their first impressions they judged what they perceived differently. Hastorf and Cantril stated:

> It seems clear that the "game" actually was many different games and each version of the events that transpired was just as "real" . . . it is inaccurate and misleading to say that different people have different "attitudes" concerning the same "thing." For the "thing" simply is *not* the same for different people. (pp. 132–133)

An even older illustration of this confirmatory strategy in how we "see" the world was provided in the political realm by Lorge and Curtis (1936). American participants were asked to rate how much they liked statements such as "I hold it that a little rebellion, now and then, is a good thing, and as necessary in the political world as storms are in the physical." Some of their participants were told the statement came from Thomas Jefferson, others were told it came from Vladimir Lenin. The number of statements they read was so large that some could be listed twice without the participant noticing. When a statement did appear a second time, its author was changed. This yielded two ratings of one statement,

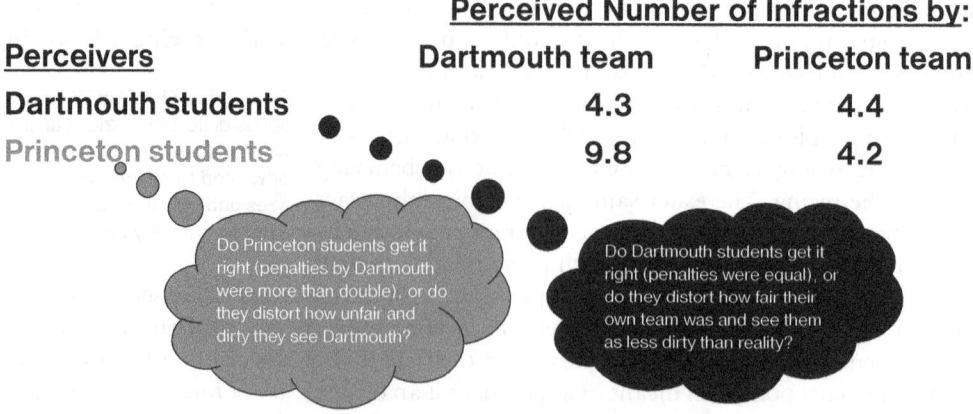

	Perceived Number of Infractions by:	
Perceivers	**Dartmouth team**	**Princeton team**
Dartmouth students	4.3	4.4
Princeton students	9.8	4.2

Do Princeton students get it right (penalties by Dartmouth were more than double), or do they distort how unfair and dirty they see Dartmouth?

Do Dartmouth students get it right (penalties were equal), or do they distort how fair their own team was and see them as less dirty than reality?

FIGURE 5.2. "Seeing" the same event differently.

differing only in who was believed to have stated it. Lorge found that changes in liking for the statements corresponded with the impressions of the people who made the statement. Asch (1948) argued that this is because the quote changes meaning when ascribed to Jefferson versus Lenin (for example). People "see" a different statement as a function of its author. The meaning of "rebellion" when uttered by Jefferson is seen as New England farmers throwing off the yoke of corrupt authoritarian rule. When uttered by Lenin it is seen as streets running red with blood and an authoritarian regime sweeping in to power. Maoz, Ward, Katz, and Ross (2002) showed a similar shift in how a document is judged based on its author. They found that a Mideast peace proposal was viewed quite differently when Israelis believed the plan had been written by a fellow Israeli, as opposed to a Palestinian. The impression that is held in advance leads one to see confirming evidence in the document.

From sports and politics, we turn next to the media. Today's media environment is fragmented, with outlets that cater to specific ideologies. It is easy to see what one expects in such a media culture where information often does have a specific "spin." However, in the time before social media and hundreds of television channels, news was typically perceived to be more fair and objective. There were only three or four television outlets for receiving news prior to 1990, and they were premised on the idea that facts were essential, multiple sources were required for something to be reported, and opinion was for another venue. However, even in such a balanced media environment, confirmation bias still allowed perceivers to see what confirmed their first impressions in what the news reported. To demonstrate this bias, Lord, Ross, and Lepper (1979) had members of opposing ideological camps read an identical newspaper article. The article presented some arguments showing the effectiveness of capital punishment, and an equal number of arguments showing its ineffectiveness. It was balanced in its examination of the pros and cons. Participants had strong beliefs and attitudes about the issue prior to the experiment. Some were advocates for, and others were against, capital punishment. Rather than the inconclusive data bringing the two sides closer together in their judgment, they instead polarized their views. Each side easily saw the evidence that confirmed their existing impression as indisputable fact, but saw evidence from the opposing side as open to alternative explanations and as methodologically flawed. The same information was used to confirm either side of an ideological divide by leading people to see the world in a way that bolstered the impressions already held. **Attitude polarization** occurs where an already held belief or attitude is accentuated after exposure to a complex sets of facts that argue both sides.

Such complexity allows one to cherry-pick the facts that enhance the position that existed prior to receiving the new information, and to devalue and dismiss those that undermine the existing position. Since these early studies, there have been many experimental illustrations to support what every fight on Facebook or Twitter has revealed: that exposing partisans to objective information will fail to persuade them, and the opposing evidence may even make them dig in deeper and strengthen initial attitudes or impressions (see Byrne & Hart, 2009, for a review).

> **Attitude polarization:** When exposure to complex facts allows one to cherry-pick those that enhance the position that existed prior to receiving the new information. Supportive evidence is accepted, while information challenging existing views is dismissed. This leaves the perceiver to see the world in a way that bolsters the impression already held.

Turning to other forms of media, we see a similar finding. Vallone, Ross, and Lepper (1985) had pro-Arab and pro-Israeli perceivers watch the same information from the evening news about the death of refugees in Lebanon. Each group saw the media as *biased against* them. Vallone et al. argued that each group used the news report to confirm their impression that the media was hostile toward them and biased. They called this the **hostile**

media effect, which is a belief that the media has a distorted view that is hostile and oppositional to one's group, even when there is no evidence to suggest this is true. Often this is caused by one's own views being so extreme that even a neutral media presentation seems discrepant and, therefore, adversarial. During his presidency, Donald Trump repeatedly labeled the mainstream media as biased and presenting "fake news." It is possible the media did collude to provide unfair and distorted news. But it remains wholly possible that rather than there being actual hostility in the many media outlets accused, it was simply that their failure to report supportive and Trump-promoting news was *perceived* as a bias when none existed. When a partisan holds a view, especially if extreme, it sits far afield from moderate views and from an objective presentation of the facts. One can attribute one's distance from those facts to those facts being fake (and its purveyors being antagonistic), or to one's own extreme stance. Most partisans prefer to see a conspiracy of these unsupportive others rather than identify their own views as extreme. The media, to them, seems hostile. Long before Trump saw a hostile media, politicians for decades had made similar claims of "fake news" if they were not supported by the media, as did any person whose group was not being supported by the "supposed facts." Vallone et al. illustrated this beautifully in their experiment. Student advocates for either Israelis or Arabs, each with extreme opinions, saw the same moderate and fair news story about refugee deaths in Lebanon as biased against them. The news presentation seemed far afield from their own view and felt biased. For example, to support the position that the two groups came to "see" totally different news reports, they showed that pro-Arab participants felt that 42% of the references to Israel were favorable, but pro-Israel participants thought that only 16% of the references to Israel were favorable.

> **Hostile media effect:** The belief that the media has a distorted view that is oppositional to one's group when no evidence suggests this to be true. These beliefs typically arise from one's own views being so extreme that even a neutral media presentation seems discrepant with one's own position, and, therefore, adversarial.

These findings reported by Vallone et al. (1985) seem on the surface to oppose confirmation bias as reported by Lord et al. (1979). We initially described confirmation bias as when people see evidence to support their views, even in a mixed message. Yet, Vallone et al. showed that partisans do not see supportive evidence in a mixed media message, they see the message as biased against their group and argue that the media is hostile to them. However, this too is an illustration of confirmation bias. What is being confirmed is the expectation that the media must be biased because the view they present regarding one's group is not as positive as one thinks it should be. One rejects the negative information being presented as fake, and confirms one's sense that its purveyors are biased. Confirmation bias is a flexible tool that wards off negative information while embracing the confirming information. The bias can of course vary in its impact. Not all evidence that argues against an existing belief is rejected and discredited. However, the more well-informed one is on a topic, and the more strongly committed one is to a group, the more one will have firm expectations about the issue that will guide what is seen. When others present attitudes and beliefs that do not align with those strong expectations, even if a moderate and balanced view is being communicated, the elements that disconfirm one's expectations will be rejected as ignorant or hostile; the positives will be embraced or confirmed.

Confirmation Bias in Perception

Even extremely low-level processes, such as how we perceive a stimulus, are biased by what we expect to see. For example, Levin and Banaji (2006) asked research participants to observe the face of a person and to try to perceive the lightness–darkness of the image. The task measured the perceived lightness by having the participants match the image's lightness as they were looking at it to the color of squares that were provided that varied in their lightness–darkness. How did they establish an expectation that could potentially be confirmed by the perceptual experience? They provided labels that identified each face as either being that of a Black man or a man of mixed race. They found that the label that assigned the face to one group or another changed the perception of the darkness of the image, even though participants were looking at the image as they were matching it (not relying on memory, but a direct perceptual experience). If the face was identified as a Black man, the color of the square was adjusted to be darker than if the exact same face was labeled as biracial. The perception was distorted to confirm an expectation.

Another example of perceptual confirmation bias was provided by Goff, Jackson, Di Leone, Culotta, and DiTomasso (2014). They illustrated a confirmatory bias in the perception of age. White research participants examined photographs of children and judged how childlike and innocent they looked. They also provided direct ratings of how old the children were. They manipulated the race of the children, so that, for example, one might see images of 14-year-old Black children and 14-year-old White children. Goff et al. found that the Black children were perceived to be less innocent than other children. Additionally, when looking at such pictures along with a description of a crime that the person was said to have been accused of committing, perceptions of guilt not only differed by race, but perceptions of age. White participants overestimated the age of Black children by an average of 4.5 years. Thus, a Black 14-year-old is not only seen as guiltier than a White 14-year-old (despite the exact same description of a crime) but mistakenly perceived to be much older.

Confirmation Bias in Memory

Beyond the tendency to perceive the information in front of us in a way that confirms what we already believe, there is also a tendency to have **stereotype (expectation) confirming memory**. We *remember* evidence that confirms what we believe, even when no such evidence ever existed (e.g., Alba & Hasher, 1983; Snyder & Uranowitz, 1978). First impressions lead one to (1) disproportionately remember evidence that supports that first impression (better memory for confirming information), (2) remember things that were never there by falsely thinking such confirming evidence had existed, (3) not remember (or disproportionately underestimate the prevalence of) the things that undermine the first impression that were once present, and (4) distort the inconsistent information that one does remember so that the memory for this information is less able to alter the first impression (e.g., remembering it to be more ambiguous or less relevant than it actually was). As an example of the first point, Zadny and Gerard (1974) had research participants memorize the exact same information about a college student. There was one difference in what was learned— the student's major (the first impression provided) was manipulated so that some people learned they majored in music and others learned it was chemistry. This shaped how the other information was recalled. Research participants who were told that the student majored in chemistry (vs. music) recalled more information about the student's enrollments in science courses, and had better memory for other details about the student that were consistent with a chemistry major, such as objects and books the student owned. Memory was better for confirming evidence relative to other evidence.

> **Stereotype (expectation) confirming memory:** When people have enhanced memory for events that happened that are consistent with a stereotype (or any prior belief about a person) as compared to memory for behaviors that were also observed that disconfirmed or did not support the stereotype (or prior belief).

Similarly, Rothbart, Evans, and Fulero (1979) showed that people have *better memory for information that confirms a first impression* than information that is irrelevant to a first impression. Their participants were shown a list of 50 behaviors about a group, and in that set there were an equal number of intelligent behaviors and friendly behaviors. Some participants were told in advance of reading the behaviors that the group was more friendly than most. Other participants were told the group was more intelligent than most. After reading the list of behaviors the participants were asked to (1) estimate what percentage of the list was friendly versus intelligent behaviors, and (2) remember as many of the behaviors from the list as they could. The results showed that people had a bias in memory where more confirming items were remembered, and where they believed the list had more confirming items (rather than accurately recalling the split between intelligent and friendly behaviors to be 50–50).

Ross, Lepper, and Hubbard (1975) found that people will scan their memory for evidence that confirms an impression, selectively recalling supporting examples and forgetting the inconsistent evidence. In their experiment they gave research participants a false belief, such as telling them that a personality test reveals the participant to be a socially sensitive person, much more than the average person. The participants generated their own evidence to confirm this impression about themselves by selectively searching their memory for examples from their lives that confirm the test result. Amazingly, they found that even when participants were told the test results were fake and the impression provided was based on bogus feedback, the participants continued to believe this attribute was characteristic of them and were able to find evidence from their memory to support it. People will perceive a positive correlation between the self (or between some other person/group) and categories of behaviors or traits that an impression suggests will exist. And they will perceive a negative correlation between the self (or between some other person/group) and categories of behaviors or traits that an impression suggests will not exist. They do so by distorting their memory for confirming items.

This same distortion can happen with stereotypes. For example, if a stereotype creates a bias that women are more emotional than men, then you might remember evidence that women you work with are more emotional than the men. This can happen even if such evidence did not exist. This can happen if there was some evidence, but no more than evidence for other types of behavior (as in the 50–50 condition above). Hamilton and Rose (1980) asserted that stereotypes associate group membership (e.g., woman) and a set of traits (e.g., emotional; poor at science, technology, engineering, and mathematics [STEM] fields). If one of the associated items is activated, such as group membership, people pay more attention to the associated items—the traits and behaviors that define the stereotype for that group. If a person encounters a member of a stereotyped group at work (e.g., a woman), then stereotypes (e.g., emotional) will be more prevalent, and the person may believe they have seen stereotypic behaviors more than other behaviors, even if they are less frequent than stereotype-irrelevant behaviors. Even if the person acts *inconsistently* with the stereotype just as often as they act in a way irrelevant to it, the inconsistent behaviors will be remembered as being less frequent. Because these relationships are not based on evidence, but are correlations that arise from a first impression specifying a set of associations, they are referred to as **illusory correlations**. An illusory correlation is when people incorrectly assume a high correlation between two things that are not actually related. A spurious association is believed to exist for reasons not tied to facts.

Illusory correlations: When people incorrectly assume a high correlation between two things that are not actually related. For example, two unusual events are seen as going together more than an unusual event and a typical event, even if equally common. A spurious association is believed to exist for reasons not tied to the facts.

Chapman (1967) illustrated that such incorrect associations arise when two unusual or rare events co-occur. When two distinct and unusual events randomly occur at the same time people have a tendency to remember them each better and to see a causal relationship linking them that is not real. For example, Chapman asked research participants to memorize word pairs and found that if each word in the pair was unusual (e.g., exceptionally long), then people remembered that pair as frequently occurring together. The length of the words attracted attention, and attention led to better memory for these words, and the better memory was interpreted to mean they must have been associated frequently. In reality, the unusually long words were not paired more often than any other word pairs. Hamilton and Gifford (1976) argued that negative stereotypes develop from such illusory correlations. On the one hand, minority group members (by definition) are rare and more distinctive than majority group members. On the other hand, negative behavior is rare and more distinctive in relation to positive behavior (e.g., Schaller & Conway, 2001). Therefore, when a minority performs a negative behavior, illusory correlations could develop that tell us these two rare events are associated, even if they are no more linked than negative behavior and a majority group.

In a typical illusory correlation experiment a perceiver might learn a set of behaviors about Group A, and half as many behaviors implying the same traits about Group B. Group B is a minority by virtue of having less information about them. Also, in such studies the behaviors provided have a ratio where one type of behavior (e.g., impolite) is shown twice as often as another (e.g., dishonest). This makes dishonest behaviors rarer than impolite ones. In such an experiment, Group A might be described with 10 dishonest behaviors and 20 impolite behaviors, whereas Group B would have 5 dishonest and 10 impolite behaviors. Despite there being only half the number of dishonest behaviors paired with Group B, and despite the ratio of behaviors being the same in the two groups, it is Group B that is seen as more dishonest and is recalled to have performed a larger percentage of dishonest acts (see Figure 5.3).

Group A: 20 members

John visited a friend in the hospital.
Craig helped a friend move.
Bill is rarely late for work.
Tom shared his lunch with a coworker.
Scott cheated on an exam.
Alan planted seedlings in a park.
Nathan took neighborhood kids swimming.
Chad always talks about himself and his problems.
Josh finished his homework on time.
Davis read a story to his daughter.
Ron made prank phone calls to his teacher.
Ken helped a lost child in a supermarket.
Fred gave blood to the Red Cross.
Alex kicked a dog.
Devin donated his clothes to charity.
Gary earned an A on his research paper.
Ted ran a red light.
Jeff volunteered to tutor needy students.
Eric drove his older neighbor to the grocery store.
Vincent forgot about his job interview.

Group B: 10 members

Allen hit a car and did not leave his name.
Bob helped a child.
John is a very dependable coworker.
Lane is well liked by his colleagues.
Bruce never returns library books on time.
David converses easily with people he does not know well.
Mark learned how to fly an airplane.
Keith organized a birthday party for a friend.
Norman often tailgates when he is driving.
Roger repaired his neighbor's lawnmower.

The ratio of positive to negative events was the same for Group A and Group B: 7:3.

Illusory correlation—we associate the two atypical things (Group B and negative events).

FIGURE 5.3. Illusory correlation from learning behaviors about a majority and minority group.

Even when there is no relationship between group behavior and dishonesty (and an absolute greater number of dishonest behaviors performed by Group A), people associate the two atypical things—Group B and dishonesty. The distortion in memory of the minority group (*B*) is not seen in recall of majority group behavior, where participants' memory is accurate (e.g., Hamilton, Dugan, & Trolier, 1985; Mullen & Johnson, 1990). This is precisely what Hamilton and Gifford (1976) found: Despite majority groups and minority groups engaging in equal proportions of positive and negative behaviors, negative acts were associated with a minority group to a greater degree.[1]

We have just reviewed how an illusory correlation can help to create a stereotype. However, our concern here is with now applying the same logic to help us understand how illusory correlations can confirm stereotypes. Illusory correlations allow stereotypes to persist if perceivers repeatedly misremember a heightened prevalence of the stereotypic qualities they already believe to exist in the members of stereotyped groups. People confirm the stereotype by remembering a correlation that is not there—a correlation that suggests more stereotypic qualities as compared to nonstereotypic qualities were present when a member of a stereotyped group was also present. Hamilton and Rose (1980, experiment 2) illustrate that stereotypes already believed to be true are more likely to be recalled, even though not more likely to be initially presented. In their experiment, information about two people was presented. The people were members of two different stereotyped groups: doctors and salesman. The information was either irrelevant to the stereotype (such as a doctor labeled as humorous) or confirmed the stereotype (such as a doctor labeled as helpful). For some participants the trait "helpful" was presented six times, and in four of those times it was used to describe the doctor (helpful was associated with the doctor more than the salesman). The trait "humorous" was also presented six times, and in four of those times it was used to describe the doctor (it was associated with the doctor more than the salesman). Thus, the stereotypic trait (helpful) was used no more often to describe the doctor than a trait that is irrelevant to stereotypes of doctors (humorous). However, the illusory correlation led people to see the stereotypic information as more prevalent than it really was. Participants remembered the doctor in a way that confirmed the stereotype. He was recalled as more helpful than humorous. While true that the doctor was more helpful than the salesman, he was equally more humorous than the salesman. It is a bias to think the doctor was more helpful than humorous. Memory is distorted to overestimate the prevalence of the qualities that confirm the first impression. This pattern of confirming the stereotype with memory reinforces it, making it harder to overturn.

Illusory correlation provides one explanation for stereotyping that requires only cognitive mechanisms that do not function with a motive to produce bias. However, people who are motivated to promote stereotyping can take advantage of this natural tendency. For example, social media and cable television allow social communication bubbles to exist where, in the absence of facts or true correlations, people can "merely pose questions" that suggest a correlation, and allow the perceiver to naturally infer such correlations to be real. If what a media platform chooses to do when "posing questions" is repeatedly pair a particular group with a particular negative set of behaviors, ultimately illusory correlations will form among the consumers of this information. The communicator has broken no laws of misinformation or libel or defamation, they have merely used what is known about illusory correlation to create the defamatory beliefs nonetheless. The purveyor of such "news" is explicitly trying to create and sustain stereotypes. However, the perceivers who adopt these stereotypes may have no realization that normal processes of illusory correlation are allowing them to implicitly form associations among the group and the stereotype, creating in them a bias they do not recognize.

Confirmation Bias in Judgment

Illusory correlations impact judgment as well as memory. For example, Acorn, Hamilton, and Sherman (1988) found a general influence on judgment so that not only the specific trait implied by the illusory correlation was remembered to be prevalent in the group but related stereotypic traits were judged to be prevalent as well. Research participants read a set of behaviors describing Groups A and B (a majority and minority group). Regardless of the specific negative trait implied about Group B in these sentences, the judgments of Group B were more negative than the judgments of Group A across a variety of other traits. The global evaluation of the group was biased so that group members were judged to have qualities unrelated to the learned behaviors.

The stereotyping literature provides many examples of **stereotyping as confirmation bias**, where people confirm an impression (a stereotype) by seeing support for it in the complex and ambiguous behavior of the people they observe. They use the stereotypic impression already held as part of their schema for the group as a lens through which the behavior that they are currently observing is given meaning (e.g., Hamilton, 1981; Fiske, 1993a; Neuberg & Newsom, 1993; Stroessner & Heuer, 1996; Swim, Borgida, Maruyama, & Myers, 1989; Young & Hugenberg, 2010). Such a distorted pattern of judgment that confirmed a stereotype was illustrated in an experiment by Darley and Gross (1983). They showed how stereotypes about social class impacted judgments of intelligence.

> **Stereotyping as confirmation bias:** People confirm an existing stereotype by seeing support for it in the complex and ambiguous behavior of the people they observe. They use the stereotypic impression already held as part of their schema for the group as a lens through which new behavior from group members is given meaning.

Research participants watched a young girl taking a test measuring her academic ability. Her performance was ambiguous and provided inconclusive evidence about her ability. She correctly answered both difficult questions and simple questions. She also provided incorrect answers to both difficult and simple questions. The trick was that prior to seeing her in this school environment, information about her home environment was manipulated. Some of the participants first saw video of her life in an affluent neighborhood, while others saw her life in an impoverished neighborhood. They also received information about her parent's occupations that, together, set up stereotypic impressions of her as either rich or poor. The results showed that these impressions were confirmed by how her ability was judged. A rich girl was judged to have above-average academic ability. Yet, based on the exact same test performance, a poor girl was seen as having below-average ability. As described above, confirming evidence (a rich girl correctly answering hard questions) is taken as support, whereas disconfirming evidence (a rich girl incorrectly answering easy questions) is ignored.

In many such examples the research participant observes a behavior that is ambiguous, and from that ambiguity they come to confirm the negative beliefs and attitudes they hold about the group. They "see" the evidence to support the impression. As one last example, Gawronski, Geschke, and Banse (2003) identified White research participants who varied in the degree to which they held negative attitudes toward Black Americans. Participants were shown to react quite differently, as a function of their prejudice, to a Black person they then observed. Despite the fact that all participants observed the same behavior, and that the behavior was ambiguous regarding its positivity–negativity, the participants with more negative associations to the group "African Americans" (with negative first impressions) interpreted the ambiguous behaviors of a Black person more negatively than same behavior observed in a White person. Negative attitudes to one group were confirmed, yet no negativity was seen in the exact same behavior of another group. These studies show a confirmation bias in how *ambiguous behavior* is judged. However, the behavior does not need to be ambiguous for a confirmation bias to emerge in one's judgment.

Even if the information we learn is quite clear and unambiguous, we can process it in a biased way that promotes the confirmation of an already existing belief. One way this occurs is if the information learned provides modest support for an existing belief, but we instead interpret it as providing strong support. Another way this can happen is if the information learned does not provide support for an existing belief, and even disconfirms or invalidates the existing belief. Later in this chapter we discuss how people confirm an attitude, expectation, or belief by dismissing clear evidence that is inconsistent with it. Rather than just dismissing disconfirming evidence, Maass, Milesi, Zabbini, and Stahlberg (1995) describe an even more subtle form of confirmation bias that emerges when people encounter information that is clear with regard to how it confirms, or disconfirms, a stereotype. The bias they describe is one where different styles of language are used; people use more abstract versus concrete language when describing a behavior as a way to uphold stereotypes—what they called **linguistic intergroup bias**. They found that when behavior confirms a stereotype it is described in a more abstract way when compared against behavior that does not confirm the stereotype, which is described more concretely. Keeping with an earlier example, if a rich girl answers a difficult question correctly, we might say "she is smart," but if a rich girl answers an easy question incorrectly, we might say "she got question 5 wrong." How does this help a stereotype persist? An impression built on a set of abstract descriptions is harder to challenge with specific facts than one based on concrete descriptions. Abstractions are more difficult to poke holes in. By seeing behavior that confirms a stereotype in more abstract ways, one is showing a form of confirmation bias that helps the first impression stay resilient and better able to persist in the face of challenging new facts. And by seeing the disconfirming information concretely, it can more easily be dismissed. The bias here is not to see mixed evidence as confirming. The bias here is to see behavior that clearly confirms a first impression in a way that is more abstract, and disconfirming behavior as more concrete.

> **Linguistic intergroup bias:** When behavior confirms a stereotype it is described more abstractly than behavior that does not confirm the stereotype. This helps the stereotypic impression to persist because abstractions are more difficult to poke holes in (compared to impressions built on concrete descriptions that can be countered with specific facts).

Imagine you read about a person for whom you have a negative impression engaging in what you consider to be a very negative behavior: driving on a dark, wet road while under the influence of alcohol. The confirmation bias here would emerge by using more abstract language to describe the behavior, such as "that person was being dangerous or reckless." In contrast, if you liked the person (and the same negative behavior was, therefore, not confirming the initial impression), the language used to describe the behavior would be more concrete. You might say "that person drank too much and then drove." The more concrete description is easier to challenge with facts like "the person's blood alcohol level was not reliably over the legal limit" or "they waited before driving home." It is also seen as less stable—they acted this way this one time. Abstract descriptions of people, such as personality traits like "reckless" and "dangerous," are harder to disprove. They also suggest the behavior is caused by something more stable and thus is likely to persist over time. A linguistic intergroup bias predicts that we should see an increase in the use of personality traits (abstractions) to describe the behaviors of people acting in ways that support our first impressions. We use more concrete language when we see behavior that disconfirms our expectations. Wigboldus, Semin, and Spears (2000) show this increase in the use of stable personality traits to describe behavior that confirms a stereotype.

On the 20th anniversary of the September 11, 2001, attack against the United States, Serge Schmemann, writing for *The New York Times*, contrasted the abstract framing of the events from then-President Bush against an alternative framing of the same attack. The abstract framing used by President Bush described the events as arising from a stable form of evil worthy of rousing the spirit of war (e.g., "a far-flung, irrational Islamist hatred for freedom"). A more concrete description of the same facts could be used, for example: "the work of a band of Islamist radicals led by a Saudi and masterminded by a Pakistani as a response to American policies in the Middle East." While accurate, the concrete framing is less likely to invoke traits and stereotypes and passions for retribution and action as compared to the abstract framing (Schmemann, 2021). Abstractions (e.g., traits such as "evil") allow for attributes that describe a group's behavior to feel stable and long-lasting, and that stickiness helps us to remember and compels us to act when compared against concrete explanations that focus on the details. To confirm negative beliefs about groups we use abstract language in describing their negative behaviors, and are more concrete if forced to discuss their positives.

Confirmation bias in judgment is seen in online settings as well. In gaming, certain genres (such as first-person shooter games) are stereotyped as masculine. These stereotypes lead people to infer that when a player has an ambiguous username, or an ambiguous avatar, they are a man. These inferences then confirm the stereotype that men are more violent and that shooter games are masculine (e.g., Eden, Maloney, & Bowman, 2010). The same bias appears when people make gender inferences based on the social media site a person uses. For example, a feminine stereotype is associated with sites where diary blogs are posted, and a masculine stereotype with statistical and report-style blogs. Visitors to such sites whose gender is presented as ambiguous are inferred to have the gender stereotypical of the site. This leads to an overestimation of the number of women on stereotypically female sites, confirming the bias that women prefer such sites. The same is seen for male stereotyped sites and estimates of men (Bivens & Haimson, 2016).

Perhaps the review thus far has given the impression that confirmation bias in judgment is an effortless process. That people simply focus attention on the evidence that supports what they already believe to be true, and it is then confirmed. However, the bias to confirm a judgment is not always so easily attained. At times we may encounter information that directly disconfirms, or is inconsistent with, our first impression. That information may not be so easily dismissed or ignored. In those conditions we may either update the first impression to account for this new and discrepant information, or we may work to keep the first impression by finding reasons to dismiss the new information, or find ways to reconcile it with the first impression so that it no longer seems to contradict it (e.g., Sherman, Stroessner, Conrey, & Azam, 2005). There is evidence to suggest that people often do not update a first impression, but fight to keep it. Asch and Zukier (1984), for example, show that people exert effort to resolve any inconsistencies with a first impression, rather than change the first impression. Research participants formed impressions of a person who displayed traits that suggested one type of person. However, they also learned that the person possessed traits clearly antagonistic to that overall impression. The results showed that the research participants did not abandon the impression, but instead worked to resolve any inconsistency with it that the disconfirming information suggested—that is, they engaged in mental elaboration and effort to make those items seem less disconfirming; to interpret them in a way that would make them fit into a unified impression. One example of such effort is **"means-end" thinking** in which the inconsistent behavior is reinterpreted not as an inconsistent trait of the person but as a means by which some other goal is achieved. They shift their judgment of the quality from

> **Means–end thinking:** A style of thinking that dismisses information inconsistent with an impression as not truly inconsistent. The behavior is reinterpreted not as an inconsistent trait, but as a means by which a temporary goal of the person is achieved. For example, your polite friend is not labeled rude, but acting assertive.

being a (disconfirming) trait of the person to being a temporary goal of the person. Thus, the behavior can be explained as perhaps not really inconsistent at all because it helps the observed person to attain something else that is important to people of that type, thus making it fit. Another example of such effort is when attributions are used to "explain away" inconsistencies, such as when a behavior inconsistent with a stereotype is seen as externally caused (e.g., Sherman et al., 2005).

Confirmation Bias in Hypothesis Testing and Information Gathering

The way in which to gather accurate information is not to seek evidence on one side and to ignore evidence to the contrary but to actually seek out the contrary evidence. Or to ask questions that can at least uncover disconfirming information. Dozens of pieces of supportive evidence do not definitively prove an impression to be correct. You may see 100 white swans, yet this does not prove your belief that all swans are white. However, one piece of disconfirming information can be highly diagnostic that the impression is wrong, or at least needs updating. First impressions persist, in part, because we do not seek out such diagnostic information when engaging in **hypothesis testing** to see if there is support for our beliefs. Confirmation bias in hypothesis testing refers to seeking evidence in a manner that will yield answers in support of a hypothesis that is already believed to be true. With first impressions this means you have a hypothesis that a person has certain goals, traits, attitudes, or values and you seek to discover further information about the person that will support that impression. Unlike the examples reviewed above where the bias manifests in how one interprets the information that is presented, with hypothesis testing the bias manifests in how evidence is gathered and the type of information sought. Rather than attempting to accurately diagnose if a first impression is correct (and creating the possibility it may need to be overturned), a strategy is pursued in which confirming evidence is sought out.

Hypothesis testing: The process of seeking evidence that can shed light on the truth value of a belief or attitude. One can do this by focusing on asking questions that can diagnose whether the belief is true or false, or by asking one-sided questions focused on either its truth or falsity.

Evidence for this **confirmation bias in hypothesis testing** was first provided by Snyder and Swann (1978). Their participants were given a first impression that a person waiting in the next room was an extravert. Participants were then asked to test the hypothesis that the person in the next room is an extravert. To do so they were given a list of questions they could ask of the person to test the hypothesis, but from the larger list they could only select 12 to ask. The list included questions meant to provide confirming evidence that the person is an extrovert (e.g., "What do you like about parties?"), and included questions that would disconfirm the impression and suggest that the person was an introvert (e.g., "What factors make it hard for you to open up to people?").

Confirmation bias in hypothesis testing: Rather than attempting to accurately diagnose if a first impression is correct, a strategy is pursued in which confirming evidence is sought out. Accurate information is not gathered by such a strategy that seeks evidence on one side and ignores evidence to the contrary.

Although asking questions that could disprove the impression would allow for the most accurate test, people instead showed a tendency to ask confirming questions. Naturally, the answers provided to these types of questions provide evidence in support of the first impression and strengthen it. Confirmatory hypothesis testing was still present even when people were offered payment to ask questions that would best diagnose the person's true qualities.

Trope and Bassok (1982, 1983) make the point that we do not always simply seek out confirming evidence. This is a bias, not a rule. While people may avoid seeking evidence that proves the exact opposite of what they already believe (such as testing to see whether someone is an introvert when they are already believed to be an extrovert), they are capable of seeking such information. Additionally, they are capable of seeking information using what they refer to as a more **diagnosing strategy**, where the question would yield one response if the person had the quality presumed by the first impression, but would be answered another way if they did not. Such questions provide evidence that can distinguish between the hypothesis and an alternative. When given the choice between asking confirmatory questions or diagnosing ones, Trope and Bassok (1982) found that people prefer the diagnosing ones. However, Trope and Bassok (1983) found that preference for diagnosing questions emerges only when the questions were highly diagnostic and would easily distinguish how people in different categories would respond. In either case, whether asking diagnosing or confirming questions, the possibility exists to confirm the first impression. In one case the strategy is to prove the hypothesis true, and in the other (the diagnosing strategy) it is to determine the probability that it is true as opposed to an alternative. In neither is the goal really to disprove it, which makes the first impression hard to overturn.

> **Diagnosing strategy:** Hypothesis testing where the questions asked provide evidence that distinguishes between competing alternatives. The answer yields one response if the person had the presumed quality, another way if not. Such questions diagnose if the belief is true or false, rather than support it being true or false.

Subtyping: Resistance to Information That Is Stereotype Inconsistent

As seen from the previous examples, people observe behavior and often ask themselves whether that behavior can be seen as evidence in support of a hypothesis they already have. They ask whether it confirms a first impression of the person. Asking this question allows them to feel as if they have "justifiable evidence," even if the evidence is actually inconclusive. However, what if the evidence does not allow them to conclude this? What happens when they conclusively and unambiguously observe a behavior that violates the expectation for that person? We have already seen one way in which people respond in the work of Asch and Zukier (1984), reviewed above. They reinterpret the seemingly disconfirming information in a way that makes it fit.

However, a second way people might respond would be to dismiss the new evidence as untrustworthy or irrelevant. We might label it as "fake" or a lie. Or we might label it as true and relevant, but unusual or atypical of this person, and hence to be disregarded. When the answer to the question of whether the behavior confirms their expectation comes back negative, perceivers will often ask a follow-up question. This question takes the form "Do I have reason to conclude that this behavior is not representative of the person for whom I have an expectation?" If the answer to this is "Yes, the behavior is not typical," then the behavior can be disregarded, and the first impression once again remains intact. One reason first impressions stick is because when a behavior disconfirms it, we seek to see that behavior as atypical, not descriptive of the person. Kunda and Oleson (1995) propose that a similar question is asked when a perceiver observes a person whose behavior disconfirms a stereotype of a group to which they belong. The question takes the form "Do I have evidence for concluding that this person is unrepresentative of the group as a whole?" Again, this question allows them to maintain their stereotype even when a person's behavior clearly violates a stereotype. The stereotype persists by classifying the person who does not fit the stereotype as the exception to the rule—as a unique case that is

> **Subtype:** When a person is categorized as a group member, but their expectation-violating behavior does not alter the impression (or stereotype) of the group because they are labelled a special subcategory of the group. The stereotype persists by classifying exceptions to the rule as unique cases that are unlike the group.

unlike the rest of the group—a **subtype**. The first impression (in this case, a stereotype) persists, and we just "fence off" the cases that suggest it should not. We treat them as exceptions. They are atypical.

Confirmation bias at times takes this form of seeking information that justifies creating an exception: finding evidence to support fencing off those people whose behavior or qualities would undermine a stereotype. Kunda and Oleson (1995) suggest that if a person behaves inconsistently with a group stereotype, then one way to allow that stereotype to persist is by seeing the person as *generally atypical* from the rest of the group. By generally atypical it is meant that if a person is seen as unusual, not in just the one behavior that suggests the stereotype of the group is wrong but as being inconsistent with the group on other dimensions, it becomes easier to create a new category in which to place this person. A subtype of the group can form around the fact that some group members simply differ in so many ways from the typical group member. These people can be "fenced off" in this new category, leaving the stereotype intact. Kunda and Oleson show that perceivers cling to irrelevant information about the person to creatively use any evidence as support for the "many" ways this person is different and worthy of being treated as an exception. If a woman displays assertive behavior at work, the stereotype that women are passive could change. Or, the woman could be subtyped. To subtype her we might grab hold of another fact about her, such as that she has brothers, and become convinced that there is a subtype of women who are not representative of women generally: assertive women. Irrelevant facts, such as growing up around men, becomes a tool to label her an exception and serves as the foundation for fencing her off into the subtype.

In their experiment, Kunda and Oleson (1995) used stereotypes of lawyers as extroverts. Some people in the experiment (the control group) simply rated how extroverted/introverted lawyers are. Others rate lawyers on this dimension after they encounter a lawyer who is an introvert. Do they alter their stereotype of lawyers? Will having additional but irrelevant information about the lawyer stop them from altering it? To test this, some of the research participants were also provided with irrelevant information. Some were told an introverted lawyer works for a small firm, some were told they work for a large firm, others get no additional information (they just know they are an introvert and a lawyer). They found that people use the additional (but irrelevant) information to justify why this person was an introvert, and, therefore, not alter the stereotype of lawyers. The participants created a subtype—introverted lawyers—who are generally atypical in other ways, such as by choosing to work at small firms. (Or large firms.) Whatever the evidence is, they use it to see the person as generally atypical and to support the subtype. Treating people who defy a stereotype as an exception allows the stereotype to stick, rather than changing the stereotype.

Confirming versus Disconfirming Information: Which Is Really More Powerfully Recalled?

A perceiver often judges people in a way that confirms a first impression. Even when there is behavior that suggests they should not keep their first impression, they engage in the mental gymnastics of subtyping the person so that disconfirming information is dismissed and the first impression is not altered. Or of working to make it seem consistent rather than inconsistent. This does not mean people always dismiss and rationalize away disconfirming information. There are times they change the first impression. We end the book with a discussion of how and when this happens. However, our focus here is on the times when they do not change a first impression, consciously reporting that despite having learned information that disconfirms a first impression their judgment of the person is unchanged. It is confirmed.

Despite people consciously reporting a judgment that confirms what was already thought to be true, we have previously discussed (in Chapter 4) how memory can be used to more subtly detect an impression or judgment. Do people remember information in a way that confirms a first impression (which would provide a different type of evidence that the first impression sticks)? Earlier in this chapter we reviewed evidence that people have a bias to remember confirming information. However, in those experiments that we reviewed, the evidence merely showed that (1) people remembered a disproportionate amount of the confirming information relative to its actual numbers, or (2) people remembered the confirming information better than information that was irrelevant to the first impression. There was no *disconfirming* information. Is there a memory advantage for confirming information when it competes directly against information that disconfirms an expectation? In research on judgment we saw that the confirming information is victorious in that competition: that people work hard to dismiss and rationalize the disconfirming information as irrelevant. What about in memory?

Things that disconfirm our first impressions and stereotypes are surprising, challenging, and do not fit (e.g., Macrae, Hewstone, & Griffiths, 1993). We may need to wrestle with it to either try to explain it away or twist and spin it to make it fit (e.g., Asch, 1946; Asch & Zukier, 1984). Interestingly, the very act of engaging in the effort to try and dismiss the disconfirming information and to subtype it can make that information very memorable. The work required to try and rationalize it away to preserve our initial judgment makes that information salient. There is superior **memory for stereotype (expectation) disconfirming information**. This creates the unusual situation where despite having excellent memory for information that is inconsistent with a first impression, the impression that people report is still consistent with the first impression (e.g., Bargh & Thein, 1985; Hastie & Kumar, 1979; Sherman, Lee, et al., 1998). We process information that disconfirms our expectations more deeply as part of the act of excluding it from the impression. This greater depth of processing (e.g., Craik & Lockhart, 1972) makes the information more memorable, but it was made more memorable while in the service of protecting the first impression from these inconsistencies. Interestingly, sometimes we see a confirmation bias in the conscious judgment people report

> **Memory for stereotype (expectation) disconfirming information:** When people have enhanced memory for events that happened that are inconsistent with a stereotype (or any prior belief about a person). This can occur because such information stands out due to its distinctiveness, or because people expend effort trying to dismiss it as false, thus rendering it more memorable.

even when people have better memory for the facts that disconfirm the first impression. Does this suggest the first impression has actually changed due to the power of the disconfirming information, and that memory is a subtle way to reveal this? Or does it suggest the first impression is unchanged, as consciously reported, because of the power of the confirming information, but the person is simply left with unusually good memory for the information that violates and challenges that information as a side effect of fencing it off?

We explore the answer to this question in Chapter 13. For now, we end this section simply by pointing out that superior memory for disconfirming information need not be seen as at odds with the finding that people have formed judgments that rely on the (less well-remembered) confirming information. Nor does it call into question the existence of a confirmation bias. Sherman, Lee, et al. (1998) point out that even when we have great memory for details and specifics (such as recalling a large number of behaviors inconsistent with a first impression), this does not mean we use that information to form abstract impressions from it. I can note that a person acted in a way that violated my sense of the person as "intelligent" without changing my conception of the person as intelligent (such as when I recently ran around looking for my glasses earlier this week, only to find them 5 minutes later, on my face). That behavior could even be highly memorable (I am writing about it 6 days later) but still not impact my overall conception of myself. Encoding the details about a person means that those details were attached to a memory structure for that person, but it need not mean we change the abstract way we think about that person as a whole. It *could* trigger a change in the first impression, but it does not need to. Memory for inconsistent information can be memorable, yet inconsequential for the stickiness of our overall impression. I still judge myself to be smart even though I do very memorable stupid things, occasionally. Perhaps it is the contrast with the impression that makes such acts so memorable, even if not enough to restructure the impression. Confirmation bias can occur despite memory for inconsistent information, if it does not lead to a conceptual change.

Another way people can have strong memory for information inconsistent with an impression, yet still have the first impression persist, is to see the inconsistent information as more ambiguous and less clear-cut than consistent information. For example, my first impression that someone is a sensitive person can remain intact even after I recall them doing something insensitive (such as telling an inappropriate joke at a party), because the inconsistent behavior is remembered as being more ambiguous. Maybe it was a dumb joke (and meant to be dumb), or insensitive only to people who are extremely uptight about certain topics, or maybe the person was just drunk (and maybe I was also drunk and incorrectly remembered the behavior). These ambiguities do not erase the memory, but render it weaker as a form of evidence against the first impression. Jerónimo, Garcia-Marques, Ferreira, and Macrae (2015) had people rate the ambiguity of information that was inconsistent with a first impression and information that was consistent with a first impression. Research participants tended to see the inconsistent information as more ambiguous than the confirming information. This ambiguity made it harder for them to see traits in the inconsistent information, and therefore harder to see strong evidence that suggests the first impression should be changed. There were no new qualities to challenge and replace the first impression. They recalled the behaviors that were inconsistent, but their ambiguity made them less powerful. Ambiguity is less likely to be seen in confirming behaviors.

In summary, better memory for confirming information alone is not what causes a first impression to stick. Even when disconfirming information is better recalled, the impression can still be confirmed by (1) better recall caused by effort spent to dismiss the inconsistent behavior, or (2) not processing inconsistent behavior at a conceptual level and simply encoding its details, or (3) seeing the disconfirming evidence as ambiguous, not clearly suggesting an opposing trait. And, as we have reviewed, people do often simply have better memory for the confirming information because of biases in how they perceive and allocate attention, biases in how they gather information during hypothesis testing, biases to exaggerate the prevalence of consistent information, biases to describe consistencies abstractly, and biases to ignore inconsistencies.

MOTIVATED REASONING

With the confirmation bias, various types of cognitive processing were shown to be used to maintain an existing impression. This could at times be effortful (such as when working to explain away disconfirming information) or it could at times be rather effortless (such as pulling from memory only the supportive evidence). In either case it was described dispassionately. People have not been described as highly vested in confirming an impression but as simply having a processing bias to do so. If motivated, the motive was simply to maintain an existing belief because changing it might produce uncertainty, or be effortful. One was simply seeking to confirm what one knows, to see what one believes, because it is in our nature to know things rather than to abandon knowing things. Confirmation bias shows that once we have knowledge that is sufficient, we harness our cognitive resources to preserve and confirm it.

However, at times our cognitive processing is quite motivated. We may be motivated to have accurate information. At other times we are motivated to reach specific impressions, such as those that find an outgroup less desirable, or to see ourselves and fellow group members positively, or to produce a specific impression (to see your rival as arrogant, your partner as kind, etc.), or to defend an ideology. Chaiken et al. (1989) describe cognitive processing as motivated and as processing for a purpose. Impressions can be sticky because we are motivated to think and feel in ways that confirm or enhance them. Kunda (1987) referred to this very broad class of cognitive processes that are engaged in the service of helping one to achieve a specific goal as *motivated reasoning*. It occurs when one is desiring to reach and defend a particular conclusion and uses the cognitive processing system as a tool to make sure the conclusion is attained.

One does not need to be consciously thinking of one's motives for those motives to shape cognitive processing. Often our motives, especially when they are motives that we chronically pursue, operate as a filter for making sense of the world, a filter we are not consciously deciding to use in the moment. For example, liberals and conservatives do not need to be consciously thinking about the goals and values associated with their ideology for there to exist an influence on how they reason. Jonathon Haidt and his colleague introduced the **moral foundations model** (Graham, Haidt, & Nosek, 2009; Haidt & Graham, 2007; Haidt & Joseph, 2008) that proposes that there are five foundations, or "building blocks," of morality. These foundations then serve as a lens that biases how each person makes moral judgments of others and moral decisions about their own actions. Each foundation serves as a sort of taste bud contributing to one's liking or disliking of foundation-relevant information. The five foundations combine their influence when shaping one's moral response to a stimulus (Haidt & Graham, 2007). Each foundation varies in importance from person to person, receiving varying degrees of weight, shaping a person's moral judgment. Political ideology leads people to weight some of the foundations more strongly than others, and hence a way of reasoning about the world emerges. Regardless of whether one agrees with the particular five foundations they identified, the general point that ideological differences are caused by differences in underlying values, goals, and motives, and that these shape how we reason about the world, is consistent with what we mean by motivated reasoning.[2]

> **Moral foundations model:** A theory proposing that people are born with "building blocks" of morality that are arranged through one's social and cultural environment. That is, our groups shape how these foundational blocks are arranged. There are five foundations they identify through a literature review of various academic studies of morality.

Political ideology is just one example of a type of motivated reasoning, but a variety of theorists—not just those who believe in a moral foundations approach—have argued for basic differences in how conservatives and liberals think about matters. These can be matters that are not related to politics, as well as matters that relate to politics (e.g., Ditto, Scepansky, Munro, Apanovitch, & Lochhart, 1998; Graham et al., 2009; Jost, 2019a; Jost, Glaser, Kruglanski, & Sulloway, 2003; Skitka, Mullen, Griffin, Hutchinson, & Chamberlin, 2002; Wright & Baril, 2011). For example, liberals and conservatives use rationalizations and justifications in an effortful way to think about political and social issues that allow them to reach the conclusions they wish to reach. When asked to generate reasons for social problems such as poverty and income disparity, conservatives have been shown to emphasize personal accountability and liberals place greater weight on situational factors: what has been called an **ideo-attribution effect** (e.g., Skitka et al., 2002; Sniderman, Hagen, Tetlock, & Brady, 1986). They see causes they are motivated to see.

> **Ideo-attribution effect:** The finding that political ideology can shape the type of attributions made. Liberals and conservatives each have attributional biases used to support their views, with conservatives emphasizing personal accountability and liberals placing weight on situational factors when asked to generate reasons for social problems such as poverty and income disparity.

There are also examples of differences in how political orientation impacts reasoning about matters *unrelated* to politics. Using apolitical behaviors, and behaviors neutral with regard to moral issues, Olcaysoy Okten and Moskowitz (2020b) show that liberals and conservatives have the same pattern of judgment that emerges with political behaviors. Conservatives place greater weight on the person's own accountability in the outcomes observed, and liberals weight the impact of the situation more than conservatives. This suggests a general pattern of blaming and sense making in which conservatives and liberals place greater weight on different factors when understanding the world more generally (not just political matters). This brief foray into political ideology was merely to make the point that reasoning is biased by motives, and these motives are a lens through which we consistently see the world. Political ideology is just one example. This chapter's focus is not on the wide variety of motives that people pursue and that can bias us; Chapter 9 returns to explore the most common types of motives that impact our reasoning.[3] The focus in this chapter is on processing: *how* motives trigger processing that affirms a first impression. We explore a variety of ways motivated reasoning make first impressions stick.

Motivated Causal Explanations

In a first example, Kunda (1987) illustrated how people use a motivated form of hypothesis testing. The hypothesis being tested in this research is one relating to self-esteem motives. Many of us believe that the qualities that lead people (in general) to have a future filled with positive outcomes and happiness just happen to be the very same qualities that we happen to possess. In an attempt to maintain one's own self-esteem, and one's sense that one's future is under control and not random, one develops the hypothesis (even if implicit) that one will have a happy and positive future because the qualities that deliver such a future are the qualities that one possesses. Kunda argued that in the testing of this hypothesis, and when gathering evidence for such tests, people are motivated to use processes of causal explanation that confirm their hypothesis. For example, to test this hypothesis, you could gather information about when and why other people experience positive outcomes. You could do so using explanations or reasons during hypothesis testing that places the responsibility for the positive outcomes others experience in the personal attributes those others possess, but focusing on the attributes (such as personality characteristics and the behaviors they enact) that those others just happen to share with you. You could reason that good things happen and bad things do not because a person has the type of disposition, the specific qualities, that bring about those outcomes. By explaining others' good outcomes as caused by the qualities they share with you, the hypothesis is validated and confirmed.

In the experimental illustration of this, Kunda (1987) asked research participants to imagine a happy future where a person would have marital bliss. The divorce rate was said to be (accurately at the time) 50%, and participants needed to come up with explanations that would explain how to beat those odds. What qualities would make for a happy and lasting marriage? Because most people desire to have marital bliss as one of their own future outcomes, Kunda reasoned that people would generate a theory that explained the causes of a good marriage as residing in the personal attributes of the two partners. Moreover, as a way of affirming their own qualities as positive and desirable, research participants would explain that the attributes that make people successful at marriage are the very attributes that they themselves (the participants) already possess. Participants first read about a person who was described by either the qualities "introverted, independent, nonreligious, and liberal" or the qualities "extraverted, dependent, religious, and conservative." The person was said to be either happily married or divorced, and participants had to rate the degree to which each of these qualities might explain that outcome. Finally, the participants rated themselves on the extent to which they possessed these same qualities. The results showed that when a participant shared an attribute with the person, that attribute was seen as the one responsible for a happy marriage. It does not matter what the attributes are. The opposite attribute (e.g., religious or nonreligious) is seen as good for marriage if the participant has that attribute. But it was only seen as an attribute linked to marriage if the couple was said to have a good marriage. For example, if a participant read about a person who was "extraverted, dependent, religious, and conservative" and happily married, and the participant shared only one attribute with that person ("religious"), then they would generate a theory that religion is the attribute most responsible for a happy marriage. If that same person was divorced, the participant would no longer list their shared quality of religion as responsible for marital happiness. This process allows people not merely to be optimistic about the future but to see their impressions of themselves as the cause for that optimism. They not only affirm the first impression but imbue it with the power to control the positivity of future events.

Motivated Evaluation of Information

Kunda (1987) also illustrated that first impressions are confirmed by people being motivated to assess information such that they accept information that favors them and reject information with negative implications for the self. Research participants read a newspaper article reporting the negative consequences *for women only* of caffeine consumption, including a link (actually fictitious) to a disease that would cause painful lumps in the breast and to cancer. Consuming three or more cups of coffee per day was said to lead to an increased concentration of a substance called cyclic adenosine monophosphate (cAMP), and cAMP was the causal link between caffeine consumption, painful lumps, and ultimately cancer. Participants were asked to assess the evidence being reported on by the article. An interesting pattern of processing emerged, one where participants defended themselves from this potential threat. For men, the article is not threatening, regardless of the amount of caffeine they consume, because it describes a disease impacting women only. They should be, and indeed were, unmotivated to be biased in assessing the article. However, for women who drink three or more cups of coffee per day the article presented very threatening information, with less threat for women who consume less caffeine than this. Women for whom the article predicted a serious health threat *came to assess the article as providing unconvincing evidence*. Relative to people who were less threatened by such an outcome, women who face the most serious consequences rated the scientific evidence in the article relating caffeine to cAMP and cancer as unreliable. To protect their self-esteem from threat, they used cognition to deny a legitimate health threat, ultimately placing themselves at risk. Many examples of motivated reasoning reveal that people will make decisions that work against their best interests because they are motivated to use their cognition to deny threats rather than embrace the possibility of the threat, whether it be vaccine denial, climate change denial, support for policies that enhance inequality, or health outcomes. Motivated reasoning can lead to a defensive way of processing information aimed at embracing that which has positive implications for the self and trivializing and attacking information that has negative implications for the self. Even if behavior change can mitigate the threat in the long term, the immediate threat posed leads to evaluating the information to see it as illegitimate.

Ditto and Lopez (1992) similarly showed **motivated skepticism** in the health domain where people critically examine information they do not want to receive, yet information they are happy to receive is readily accepted. They had research participants receive health feedback. Some were told they were susceptible to pancreatic disorders because they lacked an enzyme, while other participants were told they had sufficient levels of this (actually fictitious) enzyme. Feedback about this threatening illness was provided by a test using a "chemically coated" paper that would turn color when coming into contact with saliva. The color would indicate whether the enzyme was present or lacking. People who received the threatening health feedback (the bad test result) responded with a defensive style of motivated skepticism, generating alternative explanations for the outcome other than it indicating a serious enzyme deficiency.

> **Motivated skepticism:** The process of evaluating information in a way that is aimed at supporting a desired conclusion by expressing doubt, defensiveness, and skepticism toward any person or evidence opposing the desired conclusion.

Compared to people who believed they had the enzyme, those who believed they did not defended self-esteem by (1) rating the enzyme deficiency as less serious; (2) being more likely to see the deficiency as a common disorder as a way to dismiss it as less worrisome; and (3) rating the saliva test as inaccurate, calling its usefulness into question. However, despite thinking the test was inaccurate, they also were more likely to retake the test to check its reliability. The self-threatening feedback triggered denial, skepticism, and a thorough cognitive analysis aimed at rejecting the result.

Vitriol and Moskowitz (2021) provide a similar example of defensiveness in one's reasoning about something that would be beneficial in the long run if heeded, but that would require facing a negative view of the self in the moment. Rather than information about their personal health, participants learned about their propensity to have prejudice. They were told (actually false feedback) they were significantly more biased than the typical person. For a person with strong internal motivations to be unbiased such feedback should allow them to become aware of their shortcomings so they can change their behavior. However, it is precisely people who are strongly motivated to be unbiased, and who would benefit from it, who evaluate the feedback defensively. As the motivation to see the self as unbiased and fair increases, their assessment of the validity of the tools used to measure prejudice becomes more negative. Reasoning processes are used to explain the poor feedback by criticizing the tools used to study bias (see also Howell & Ratliff, 2017; Howell, Redford, Pogge, & Ratliff, 2017). Feedback in this case is not simply a threat but a threat to one's moral fiber: an attack against one's character. To protect the self, one goes beyond just challenging the validity of the test, but one might challenge the validity of the entire enterprise (claiming the study of race and racism itself is wrongheaded), dismissing the science of bias altogether, being skeptical of the goals of the scientists who do such work (e.g., Moskowitz & Vitriol, 2022). When one is confident one is moral and unbiased, then if others disagree, it must be they who are biased.

The motivation to defend an impression does not only happen because people want to protect self-esteem. Any important goal can be defended from attack and bolstered by how one reasons. For over 25 years the psychologist John Jost (Jost & Banaji, 1994) has been studying the motivation—often at the unconscious level—to justify and defend the social systems that support the culture in which one lives, a phenomenon called **system justifica-tion**. These justifications are "used to explain some existing state of affairs, such as social or economic systems, status or power hierarchies, distributions of resources, divisions of social roles" (p. 3). People come to depend on a variety of social, economic, and political systems, and even when those systems place them at the bottom of the hierarchy or create personal disadvantage, people are still motivated to justify the systems that support their daily life (e.g., Jost, 2020; Jost & Banaji, 1994). They do this through seeing and remember-ing information that supports their ideology: motivated rea-soning. Much as threats to the self can cause defensiveness, even at the expense of one's well-being, negative feedback about the social system makes one defensive. The strength of the motivation to defend the system can vary across individu-als and situations. However, if the legitimacy or stability of a system is threatened, people are motivated to defend and justify that system. Whether it be a political system (a threat to democracy), a social system (a threat to White hegemony), an economic system (a threat to the fossil fuel industry), or a religious system (a threat to the legitimacy of religious leaders), embracing and repairing the threat may be what is rational. But motivated reasoning to defend the system and deny the threat is what is natural.

> **System justification:** The motivation to justify and defend the social sys-tems that support the culture in which one lives. People come to depend on a variety of social, economic, and political systems, and even when those systems place them at the bottom of the hierarchy or create personal disadvantage, people are still motivated to justify the systems that support their daily life.

The need to establish a socially shared view of there being a legitimate order and struc-ture is even internalized by members of a disadvantaged group so that they support and justify the very stratified system that disadvantages them, and to share in the negative prejudice of their group held by the dominant group (e.g., Jost & Hunyady, 2005; Jost, Led-gerwood, & Hardin, 2008). For example, research shows that people who endorse system-justifying ideologies become motivated to support policies that are not in their own best interest, such as support for unequal pay and the heightened perception of justified entitle-ment of a dominant group (e.g., Jost & Hunyady, 2005; Major, 1994). These motives can even be triggered in the moment, so that when women are given a motivation to justify the system during an experiment (by having them contemplate beliefs about meritocracy), they later indicate that they deserve less pay than men as compared to women who do not have system-justifying motives (O'Brien & Major, 2009).

Motivated Memory

Our discussion of motivated reasoning is next extended to memory processes. We continue with our discussion of system justification as the relevant motivation. Hennes, Ruisch, Fey-gina, Monteiro, and Jost (2016) examined how people distort memory when an economic system that they are motivated to see preserved is attacked. First, they needed to identify people who varied in their desire to justify the economic system to see how they reason about an attack to that system. Second, they needed a legitimate threat to that system to trigger the motivation to justify the system. Third, they needed a way to illustrate motivated reasoning in people's responses to this threatening information. To address the first two issues they examined the threat introduced to the economic system from man-made cli-mate change. The research participants learned about the findings of credentialed climate scientists (such as reports from Massachusetts Institute of Technology [MIT] professors to panels of experts). These reports argued that climate change was a serious threat (such as dangerous alterations in sea levels and global temperature) and that to deal with these threats required large changes to the economic system. To address the third issue, they examined distorted memory for the facts that they had read from the credentialed scientists about climate change. The results of this experiment revealed that as the motivation to justify the economic system increased (and hence the threat from the report increased), there was a greater tendency to misremember the evidence about climate change in a way that minimized its threat and increased skepticism about climate change. For example, when tested on the facts presented, people more motivated to justify the system were less likely to remember that scientists had reported three-quarters of carbon emissions to be man-made. They also remembered the evidence in a way that distorted changes in global temperatures, sea levels, and historical climate change data, all in a way to make the threat less severe and introduce skepticism about the science. They cherry-picked their memory for evidence to support the status quo and distorted the challenges.

As noted throughout this chapter (and this book), trying to avoid negative information about the self is a powerful motivating force. Instead, people strive to have a positive self-definition, even if it means twisting the facts to accentuate the positive and eliminate the negative (e.g., Campbell & Sedikides, 1999; Dunning, 1995; Greenwald, 1981; Sedikides, 1993; Taylor & Brown, 1988; Tesser, 2001). We forsake accuracy, if being accurate means admitting negativity. We favor an inaccurate, yet positive, sense of self. One way in which people are motivated to eliminate negative self-thoughts is to neglect such information when processing information about the self, including what one recalls about the self. Sedikides, Green, and Pinter (2004) called this **self-protective memory**, and they pose the

Self-protective memory: One way in which people are motivated to minimize having negative views of the self is to neglect negative information when recalling information about the self.

question "Will [people] remember negative information better than positive information?" (p. 162). They propose, and show, that the answer is "yes" when it comes to what we recall about others but "no" when scanning memory for self-relevant information. Indeed, as the information being learned poses increasing levels of threat to the self, the more likely that information will be neglected when processing it. This poorer processing results in negative information about the self being poorly remembered (e.g., Greenwald, 1980, 1981; Holmes, 1970). Recall is worse for increasingly negative information about the self.

To explore this question, Sedikides et al. (2004) gave research participants both positive and negative information to learn in the form of feedback from a personality test (the feedback was actually fabricated). Some participants were told the feedback was about the participant's own performance, while other participants were told the feedback was about another person (named "Chris"). Further, some of the feedback was about a quality that was central to the participant's identity, making negative feedback of this type very threatening if about the self, but not a threat if about Chris. They found that memory for these very threatening negative behaviors was poorer when they were about the self as compared to Chris. Memory was distorted to eliminate the negative, but only for very threatening information about the self. More peripheral qualities were not remembered in a distorted way that neglected the negative relative to the positive qualities.

Motivated Attention

Impressions are also protected by filtering out information that can harm them and attending to information that supports them. Thus, processes that determine what reaches conscious attention can shape the persistence of a first impression. Postman, Bruner, and McGinnies (1948) show this is motivated; they conducted an experiment that illustrates how information related to an important identity receives preferential attention, making it easier to be detected. Participants had words presented to them on a screen. The words were value laden, such as being related to the category of "political values" (e.g., politics, dominate, and govern) or the category of "social values" (e.g., loving, kindly, and friendly). The presentation speed for the words started with each word being subliminal. The speed was gradually slowed until a word could be consciously identified. Participants simply had to report when they could see a word. Prior to the task, Postman et al. determined what categories of words were central to each participant. They predicted, and found, that the more central a word was to one's core values and identity, the faster one could attend to it. Participants who valued politics "saw" words such as "govern" faster than "friendly." The reverse was true for people with strong social values. These lower thresholds of recognition for desired words suggest motivated reasoning prior to consciousness.

Roskos-Ewoldsen and Fazio (1992) similarly showed the motivated nature of attention by illustrating that people select items that are compatible with their attitudes from complex arrays. Research participants saw a visual display of six objects in a circle (e.g., backpack, airplane, squirrel, flower, umbrella, bicycle) that were flashed too quickly for all to be consciously attended. The results showed that items that jumped out from the stimulus array and captured attention were those for which participants had the strongest attitudes (as measured in a separate stage of the experiment). Attention was selectively directed to items people liked, even if flashed too briefly to detect all of the items (see Figure 5.4). As reviewed in Chapter 4, it is also the case that highly threatening information captures attention easily. This type of automatic attention allows first impressions to be made stable by the constant detection of reaffirming items in our environment. Detection of positive and negative stimuli allow those stimuli to reinforce the positive and negative attitudes already held toward those stimuli.

Balcetis, Dunning, and Granot (2012) provide another illustration of how attention is directed by motivation. They examined how an ambiguous set of stimuli during visual processing reaches conscious attention in an unambiguous way. To create visual ambiguity, they utilized the phenomenon of binocular rivalry. A perceiver has a different image presented to each eyeball, such as an image of a letter *G* presented to one eye and an image of the number 5 presented to the other. People do not see both images simultaneously and can

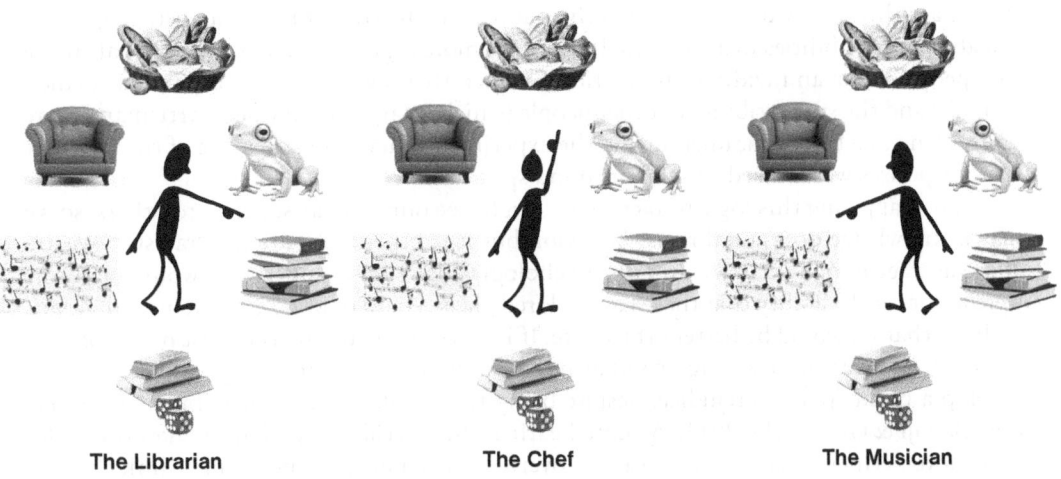

The Librarian   **The Chef**   **The Musician**

FIGURE 5.4. Motives guide attention.

report only one at a time (though it can rotate between them). Balcetis et al. found that the way this ambiguity is resolved is determined by people's motivations. Their attention was directed to the image on the eye that had been associated with a reward more often than to an image associated with costs.

The Illusion of Superiority

Most people see themselves as generally better than most others—the majority of people see themselves as more courteous, kind, and forgiving than the average person. For example, the psychologists Nick Epley and David Dunning found that people tend to see themselves as more moral than the average person. Naturally, a majority of people, mathematically speaking, cannot be above the median in morality (or any quality). While most of us acknowledge that we are capable of tripping and hitting the bar that sets the standard for poor behavior, few of us believe this makes us the type of person who can be described by this behavior. We see ourselves as highly moral (or kind, competent, courageous, decisive, etc.) with occasional missteps, and others as immoral (or unkind, incompetent, etc.). This bias of superiority could emerge because people have overly harsh assessments of their peers or because they have an overly positive self-view. The research of Epley and Dunning (2000) suggests that it is that people are motivated to have an overly charitable self-assessment that creates this bias.

Pronin, Lin, and Ross (2002) showed that even warning people about this bias does not eliminate it. In support of this they collected survey data from Stanford University students asking them about a series of biases in social judgment. After reading a description of the bias they were asked in one survey to rate how susceptible the "average American" was to this bias, as well as to rate how susceptible they were to this bias. A second survey asked participants to rate themselves and their fellow students (people in the same class as them). In each case the results revealed that participants saw themselves as less likely to fall prey to bias in judgment than other people. Most participants rated themselves above average as compared to others, replicating the illusion of superiority. However, when next told about the bias—that 70–80% of people see themselves as above average—participants denied they were susceptible to such a bias. The vast majority (63%) of the people claimed their prior ratings were accurate (they are indeed superior), and an additional 13% claimed that, if anything, they underestimated their ability in an attempt to be modest. People reason about their abilities in a motivated way to promote high self-esteem. Pronin et al. argue that people make an invidious distinction between their own susceptibility to bias (which is small) and the susceptibility of other people (which is large). Even when participants were performing in a biased manner during the experiment, they were not aware of the fact that their responses were biased—a self-bias blind spot.

When applying this logic to racism, we might see ourselves as superior to others, so we may acknowledge occasional racist behavior, but it is others who are the "racists." We are above average in our anti-racism. This psychological illusion of superiority would be funny were it not for the ability that these rose-colored glasses have to blind us to some dangerous realities that we would be better off to note. If I believe I am among the most moral of people, I will be resistant to seeing myself as having prejudice, even implicit prejudice. We thus develop a blind spot to prejudice, despite being readily able to recognize biases in others (e.g., Banaji & Greenwald, 2013). As noted earlier, this invisibility perhaps makes the influence more pernicious since it is harder to overturn. Even people who firmly think they are moral and unbiased may be influenced routinely by implicit prejudice being automatically activated. The belief that one is more anti-racist than others is an illusion when most people believe they are above average. This belief can contribute to the persistence of prejudice by making people less able to become aware of how their own responding needs to change (e.g., Moskowitz & Vitriol, 2022).

SOCIAL INFLUENCES THAT STABILIZE FIRST IMPRESSIONS

A final reason first impressions are resistant to change is that they can at times be tied to group pressures to keep them in place. This can take the form of conformity pressures that compel us to agree with a first impression, and it can take the form of more subtle forces that lead us to develop stronger inferences because of the impression being embedded in shared knowledge.

Extending Impressions among Individuals and Groups

Though we reserve more detailed discussion for Chapters 10 and 11, a **stereotype** is *information* about the characteristics, personal qualities, physical features, typical behaviors, and values that are associated with a social group. Stereotypes are our attempt to represent in our mind what the culture teaches us is a reality that describes (and prescribes the behavior of) a class of people in the world. A stereotype reflects an impression shared within a culture (and across members of that culture) about a group. By virtue of being shared among people we value, stereotypes in the culture create a type of social pressure to see the qualities ascribed to a group as true, and to also see those qualities to be true of any individual member of that group. This socially shared nature of the impression about the individual makes it more strongly held. It has inherent in it a sense of consensus that communicates the impression is correct; it takes on strength from the shared assumption within one's group that members of the stereotyped group share qualities. It is difficult for a perceiver to see the social pressure that impacts their judgment, or to recognize that their judgment of an individual is impacted by a culturally shared belief (a stereotype). Nonetheless, the shared nature of the stereotype exerts a subtle pressure to see an individual member of the stereotyped group in a way that confirms the shared impression of the group.

> **Stereotype:** Shared semantic knowledge about a group; *information* about the group's characteristics, physical features, typical behaviors, and value system. This mental representation describes (and prescribes the behavior of) group members. If triggered, this semantic knowledge impacts judgment and behavior, without one being aware of the stereotype's accessibility or its influence.

In addition to extending beliefs about the group to the individual, there is also social pressure to do the opposite, and to apply an impression formed about an individual group member to the entire group. By doing this, evidence to maintain a socially shared stereotype is constantly being provided by the perceiver taking the actions of an individual and, when those actions confirm a stereotype, using it as support for the culturally shared stereotype of the group. This greater generality gives the illusion of the quality being more common, more abstract, and thus harder to unseat. In each of these cases, extending the stereotype (either from the group to the person, or from the person to the group) roots the impression in a shared reality that makes the stereotype (as a first impression) stickier (e.g., Hardin & Conley, 2001).

An example of the extension of group qualities to individual group members is seen in the work of Hamilton et al. (2015). Their research is focused on demonstrating the ease with which people form impressions about new groups that they learn about. They do so spontaneously—without intending to do it or awareness of having done it. In their final experiment they illustrate that once such a first impression forms about the group, they then extend the same impression to an individual member of the group. This is true even when there is no information about that individual provided. A first impression formed about the group is extended to a new individual one encounters, simply because the person belongs to that group.

An example of the extension of an individual's qualities to the more general group to which they belong is seen in the work of Taylor et al. (2018). In this research they reveal a concern among members of a minority group that the behavior of another individual who is also a member of that minority group may reflect poorly on the entire group (and by extension, on the self). In their research, they create a situation where two people (one White, one Black) witness negative and stereotypic behavior by a third person, who is Black. When a Black person witnesses this stereotypic ingroup behavior, they then worry that the stereotype of their group will be inferred by anyone observing this third person, and that such observers will extend the stereotype to all group members. An innocent bystander, in this way, can have a negative impression associated with them because of their shared identity with an offending third party. In the situation created in their research, Taylor et al. demonstrate how the extension of a stereotype from an individual to the group can reflect poorly on other group members who have not acted stereotypically. A concern with having a negative impression extended to the self (as a member of the shared group) creates anxiety that makes one more likely to avoid cross-race interactions—that is, a Black person and a White person who observe the third person being stereotypic have their own interaction impacted by this social pressure. They become more avoidant of each other.

Stereotype threat: When knowledge of a stereotype about one's group creates worry that one's actions will be perceived as representative of the group. It is anxiety about damaging one's group by affirming the stereotype if one does not perform. This specific pressure reduces actual performance in stereotyped domains where one would otherwise excel.

Meta-stereotyping: Thinking about the stereotypic thinking of others. It is a contemplation of the stereotypes believed to be held by others, typically toward a group to which the person engaging in the meta-stereotyping belongs.

Work on **stereotype threat** reflects a similar concern. Stereotype threat is a phenomenon where individual members of a stereotyped group worry that their actions may be perceived by others as representative of the group as a whole. A member of a minority group is aware of the cultural stereotype and assumes that others hold an expectation (stereotype). It is these thoughts about the existence of the stereotype in others, and how one's own behavior might affirm that stereotype, that causes a bias. It is an anxiety about one's potential to be seen in the light of a stereotype and how that shines on the group. It is the product of an anxiety from the **meta-stereotyping** engaged—thinking about the stereotypic thinking of others. By considering how others might extend one's individual action to the group, one becomes anxious about how the group may be damaged if one does not perform well.[4] Steele (1997) defined stereotype threat as

the social-psychological threat that arises when one is in a situation or doing something for which a negative stereotype about one's group applies. This predicament threatens one with being negatively stereotyped, with being judged or treated stereotypically, or with the prospect of conforming to the stereotype . . . it is a situational threat—a threat in the air. (p. 614)

This anxiety or threat creates extra pressure that then actually interferes with performance. For example, Spencer, Steele, and Quinn (1999) showed that when a math test was framed as able to help *diagnose gender differences in math ability*, female college students who were equally skilled in math to male students did not perform as well as the male students on the test. The framing led to meta-stereotyping and stereotype theat. When no mention of gender differences was made when framing the test, women performed equally to men. Steele and Aronson (1995) showed a similar performance drop on highly qualified Black student test performance. Black students and White students of equal ability performed differently on the test, but *only if students were led to believe the test was relevant to race stereotypes.* When the test was framed in a way free of such concerns, Black students performed identically to White students. Performance is hindered by the pressure that comes from knowing a stereotype exists about one's group in a domain, and that one's own behavior could damage the group if one does poorly (since others will generalize one's individual performance to the group). Ironically, this is especially true if one is extremely skilled in the domain—where one has high achievement and the stakes are high. If it is a domain where one has great skill, and one is at the vanguard, the threat is felt particularly keenly if that domain is also relevant to a stereotype (such as women skilled at math). This may even lead to avoidance of the domain despite one's skill, so that the pressure from stereotype threat is never experienced. A female student might eschew a STEM field as a major, even if highly skilled, because a stereotype of women being poor in this domain creates stress; they do not want the anxiety of needing to constantly risk proving the stereotype through their behavior, and to do so in a hostile environment. Instead, they may avoid that environment altogether (e.g., Steele, 1997).

Thus, with stereotype threat there is a social pressure exerted by feeling as if one is being held up by society as an exemplar and standard bearer for the group as a whole. The threat of negatively reflecting on a valued group creates an enormous pressure to not let the group down. One can react to this pressure by disengaging altogether so that one is never held out as evidence. Or one can accept the challenge and need to act under conditions of greater pressure than others who are not subjected to stereotype threat. This can lower performance, and if it does (as research shows it often does), then one's behavior can confirm the stereotype (as feared), helping it to persist.

Social Groups Make Impressions Seem More Extreme

The social pressure to strengthen a socially-shared first impression is especially likely when people perceive their social circle to be more extreme in their stereotypes and beliefs than reality dictates. A **perceptual divide** can develop where one's perceptions of the norms and beliefs held by two opposing groups are more extreme than they truly are, leading those individuals to see greater polarization among the groups than really exists. This perceptual divide, or exaggerated sense of polarization, creates an even greater social pressure to agree with one's group, even if one privately disagrees with that group—one may agree with another group (or be indifferent) but say otherwise to gain acceptance with one's own group. Perceived extremity of group opinion serves as a pressure to confirm the first impression (or stereotype) offered by one's own group.

> **Perceptual divide:** When an individual's perceptions of the norms held by opposing groups are more extreme than reality dictates, leading one to see greater polarization among them than really exists. This exaggerated sense of polarization creates a pressure to agree with positions espoused by one's own group, even if one privately disagrees.

Robinson et al. (1995) illustrate how perceptions of one's own social group can be more extreme than the group really is, and this perceived extremity can pressure one to say that one's judgment is more extreme than it really is. They had conservatives and liberals read a story about an actual racially charged incident in New York City. This took place a few months after I first moved to New York and was a high-profile exemplar of the racism at that time. A Black man (Michael Griffith) and two friends were in a mostly White neighborhood (Howard Beach) because their car had broken down, and they were looking for a pay phone to call for help. Instead of help, they were greeted with racial epithets and were beaten by a group of White men who assaulted them for being in their neighborhood. In trying to escape, Mr. Griffith ran, and was pursued by the White men. He tried to cross a busy highway to avoid their wrath, where he was killed by a car. The story read by the research participants contained facts about this case—such as the White men deliberately chased Michael into oncoming traffic; Michael had been using cocaine that night; Michael was killed by a car. The participants made two types of ratings. The first was how a typical member of their ingroup (e.g., Conservatives) and a typical member of their outgroup (e.g., Liberals) would respond to this event. The second was their own evaluations of this scenario. They found that people expected their own group (and the other group) to be far more extreme than those groups actually were. For example, a Liberal participant believed that other Liberals would be more sympathetic to the victim and blame the racism of the White perpetrators than they personally did (even though they did see racism as the primary cause). They also believed that Conservatives would be more sympathetic to the White men from Howard Beach who did not intend to kill Michael (just beat him), and would engage in victim blaming. Conservatives were more likely to hold such views, but they were not as extreme as others believed they would be. This created an incorrect perception of the divide that separated the two groups, with one's own group seen as more extreme than it really was (see Figure 5.5). When social pressure is believed to be extreme like this, it can pressure one to exaggerate one's own view during self-report in order to fit in with the group. Perhaps today's media climate where people get "news" from partisan outlets fosters such exaggerated views of our groups, making such polarizing social pressure even greater (e.g., Rathje, Van Bavel, & van der Linden, 2021).

A danger of this type of social pressure is that if we all believe the group feels this way, but privately many people do not, nobody will speak out against it in fear of violating what is believed to be a shared norm. Prentice and Miller (1993) referred to this condition as **pluralistic ignorance**: one where people in a group misperceive the norms because everyone is acting inconsistently with their private beliefs because of a social pressure they believe exists. It may be that sexism is not as widely or as strongly held among men as men believe, but a social pressure exists because each man believes other men are more sexist than they

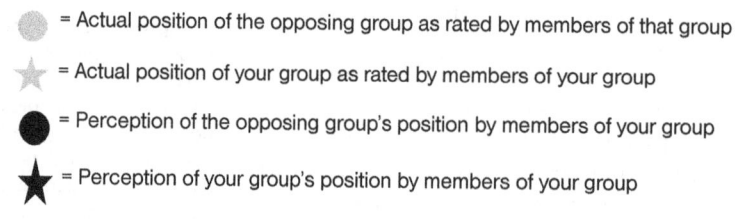

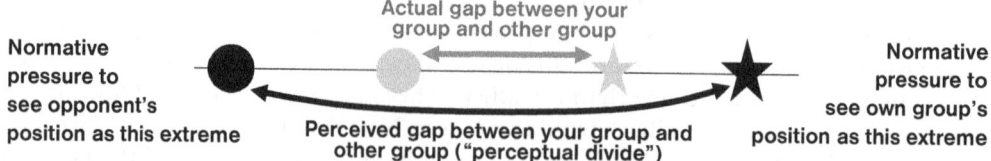

FIGURE 5.5. Normative pressure to affirm an impression from a perceptual divide.

really are. And when they look around they fail to see dissenting voices to alleviate that social pressure. This presumed norm leads them all to lie out of a social desirability concern, thus sustaining a system they could easily topple if they did not lie. This is one reason allyship is seen as important. It helps to communicate norms of anti-sexism and anti-racism. Social media bubbles can help reveal shared beliefs that allow people to break from such norms and shatter pluralistic ignorance.[5]

> **Pluralistic ignorance:** A type of social pressure where people believe the group feels a particular way and acquiesce to that belief, but privately many group members disagree and no group consensus exists. All people end up conforming to perceived norms and nobody speaks out in fear of violating that (perceived) shared belief.

Conformity and Dissent

Group membership contributes powerfully to one's sense of identity, and this connection of the group to the self creates strong normative pressures to follow the conventions, traditions, and beliefs of the group (e.g., Packer & Miners, 2014). When a first impression is one shared by an important social group, *rejecting that impression* means more than a simple update to one's attitudes and beliefs. Rejecting the impressions connected to a shared group reality have the power to invoke feelings of **dissent** and concerns with being shunned by the group. Since group members are expected to conform, if one does not, then one's lack of conformity can potentially lead to ostracism (e.g., Spears, Doosje, & Ellemers, 1997). As Packer and Miners point out, though dissent is often revered in the eyes of history (when it triggers an important social change), it is often personally difficult in the moment. Dissent becomes more likely as one believes that the dissenting actions will change the group for the better, and help to alleviate out-of-date, and no longer useful, norms (Packer, 2008).

> **Dissent:** When an individual publicly disagrees with their group. Though often revered in the eyes of history (when triggering social change), it is often difficult to do in the moment. Dissent becomes more likely as one believes the dissenting action is an expression of identification with the group, changing it for the better.

In this way, dissent from a group is seen by the dissenter as an expression of identification with the group, not rejection, and it is most likely to happen when the group benefits outweigh personal costs. One reason socially shared beliefs have particular strength is that it is easy to feel the confidence that consensus affords (and the costs to not conform), while simultaneously difficult to see the long-term benefits of dissent.

Of course, it is not impossible for group-level beliefs to be challenged. For example, despite strong norms to not question the role of police in American society, when police brutality occurs citizens will often see the benefits of challenging the notion that any police officer is unassailable, or that shared beliefs about supporting the police—no matter what—might benefit from dissenting voices that call for reform when needed. When one's group says "support the police," it may be very difficult to point out that there are instances when this impression of the police is wrong. A minority of police officers at times, just like all people, are criminals who should not be supported, but convicted. Such dissent helps a group by punishing those who sully its good name. Or it may be difficult to see that one way to "support" a group is to help them change when change is needed. For example, a research team I work with spent 2 years interviewing officers, many of whom felt they were frequently called into situations that required a mental health professional, for which they had no expertise. Adjusting the role of officers to remove them from such situations would be a form of support. Yet the officers were reluctant to speak about these concerns until they were in private and guaranteed anonymity.

As another example, social movements, such as the civil rights movement, are about far more than challenging a first impression, but breaking a destructive chain of disparity and harm that those beliefs engender. If a group member feels strongly that there are benefits to the group by breaking those links, then they will dissent. It is perhaps harder to dissent with a group when one is challenging what are seen as the group's incorrect stereotypes and negative attitudes. Whereas the would-be dissenter may see those shortcomings, the other group members may not. If such beliefs are harder for group members to see, they will be harder to challenge because the benefits to such a challenge will be difficult to see. Rather than helping the group via dissent, one might be seen as hurting it. These relationships between (1) the impressions we hold and (2) the power of norms to keep them in place, and (3) the difficulty in seeing a dissenting view as not a challenge to a group but an affirmation of the group, is not studied enough (e.g., Lin, 2017). Shared impressions that carry the weight of group norms should be more persistent and more difficult to change than are impressions less weighed down by those normative pressures. Impressions less tied to normative pressure should be less "sticky" because the person is not as strongly identified with the group and its shared reality, or because they are identified but the impression is not one strongly held by the group (making it easier to dissent).

Groupthink

There are times when terrible outcomes result from social pressures within a group to not challenge the authority or the prevailing impressions that seem to have consensual support. The Bay of Pigs invasion, the space shuttle *Challenger*, and the U.S. withdrawal after 20 years in Afghanistan all are examples of bad outcomes preceded by a shared consensus among people with authority. Janis (1972) described the phenomenon of **groupthink** as decision making that is marked more by a concern with group harmony and unanimity than with carefully deliberating and challenging prevailing beliefs. A shared impression can persist because of the unique condition posed by groupthink: one that does not exist when one is holding a private attitude or belief not tied to group pressures. Packer and Ungson (2017) argue that a concern with seeking consensus does not merely lead to a public expression of a common perspective but to the individual internalizing of that shared point of view. They go on to summarize three general categories of symptoms of groupthink that help to explain how this social pressure can strengthen an impression. Groupthink describes a group that is "(1) overly confident with regard to its morality and strengths (illusion of invulnerability, collective rationalization, perception of inherent morality), (2) derogating and simplistic about outgroups (stereotyping), and (3) exerting strong internal pressures on members to conform to shared opinions (illusion of unanimity, pressuring dissenters, self-censorship"; p. 184).

> **Groupthink:** Social pressures within a group to not challenge the authority or the prevailing impressions that seem to have consensual support. It is decision making that is marked more by a concern with group harmony and unanimity than with carefully deliberating and challenging prevailing beliefs.

CONCLUSIONS

When information is ambiguous, we have a tendency to see it in a way that confirms what we already believe. And much of social life presents us with ambiguous information. A confirmation bias strengthens those existing impressions and stereotypes by adding further evidence to support them. Confirming evidence can be produced by taking an ambiguous piece of evidence and seeing it one way versus another. Was the man holding a knife or a comb? Did the woman have a gun or a wallet? Is that person homeless or a hipster? This can happen at encoding (when making sense of new information), at retrieval (when recalling past evidence), and when gathering information and hypothesis testing. Confirming evidence can also be produced by the amount of evidence one thinks one sees. Do I recall a doctor as being more helpful than humorous? Do I attend to emotional behaviors from women more than honest behaviors? Do I see a Black suspect moving toward me to be moving faster or to be physically larger than a White suspect (as officer Darren Wilson perceived Michael Brown to be when explaining his reasons for shooting him dead in Ferguson, Missouri, in 2014). Whether we see *A* and not *B*, or see much more of *A* than reality dictates, we have a confirmatory bias that strengthens our initial impressions and helps to make them sticky.

However, it is not ambiguous information alone that is distorted to prop up our existing beliefs. Even when information is clearly presented, perhaps even when it clearly disconfirms a first impression, we still can produce confirmatory processing. It is true that when a first impression is strongly contraindicated by the data we can abandon a first impression. Such evidence may compel us to think more deeply and reassess our beliefs. Progress would never be made if a challenge to an erroneous belief never triggered systematic reevaluation of what we thought we knew to be true. But even such diagnostic information can be explained away. The cognitive toolbox is filled with devices to confirm existing impressions. Clearly inconsistent information can be rendered ambiguous, effort is exerted to dismiss or discredit contradictory evidence, we encode perceptual details but not conceptual information, and we render evidence more abstract and less concrete (or the reverse) depending on whether we want to stabilize it or render it mutable.

Let us not forget our motivational toolbox. In Chapter 1 myriad motives and goals were identified that can drive social cognition. This means that the energy and effort spent on thinking is not always used to gather the most objective data and form the most accurate impressions. We rationalize, spin, self-deceive, selectively attend and evaluate, and engage in mental gymnastics to prove what we want and desire to be true. While corporations, politicians, and media may try to persuade us by presenting biased information (even misinformation), our cognitive system misinforms itself to support and promote existing impressions that serve our wants and desires. Motivated reasoning can shape memory and judgment, distorting what we see and recall.

Finally, a glimmer of "good news" for fans of less bias in what we see. All of these examples of data distortion require data. If there was no behavioral evidence at all, and people were simply asked to make a judgment about "person 1 from Group *X*," would they still use stereotypes and first impressions? The aversive racism framework suggests no. When the situation is clearly one where norms about how to act are present (such as rules about not judging others), normative pressure and social desirability concerns keep us from acting inappropriately. Additionally, if there was absolutely no information on which to base a judgment, research on confirmation bias also suggests we would not stereotype. The bias emerges in how we assess the data we use to support an existing conclusion; in the absence of data one does not feel "licensed" to render an opinion simply relying on group membership. Darley and Gross (1983) said,

> If perceivers were asked for judgments at this point in the process, without any behavioral evidence to confirm their predictions, they would not report evaluations based on their expectancies. They would instead report that either they did not have sufficient information or they would make judgments consistent with normative expectations about the general population. . . . A teacher, for example, would be extremely hesitant to conclude that a (poor/female/immigrant/black) child had low ability unless that child supplied direct behavioral evidence validating the application of the label. (pp. 21–23)

Darley and Gross (1983) proposed a two-step process through which stereotypes bias people. In a first step, perceivers develop a hypothesis that might cause the behavior they are observing, and this is usually based on a stereotype. However, they do not just express this stereotype. Factors such as their goals of appearing unbiased, or the pressures of the situation to look unbiased, may cause them to want to express what appears to be a valid opinion. They must feel licensed to use a stereotype, and if they do not feel as if it is allowable to do so, they do not. Thus, people typically refrain from using their stereotypes until the stereotype can be tested against some evidence. If asked for a judgment prior to having engaged in such a test, they do not have an evaluation they are willing to offer in one direction or the other. In a second step, perceivers engage in such a "test" of the hypothesis, endorsing the stereotype and allowing it to bias judgment only after gathering supporting, hypothesis-confirming information. This suggests a somewhat happy conclusion: people judge other people according to a stereotype only if they feel there is evidence on which to base a judgment (what Yzerbyt, Schadron, Leyens, & Rocher, 1994, called a feeling that the target is worthy of being judged).

Despite this good news, two cautionary notes end the chapter. First, almost any type of behavior can be distorted and be seen as positive evidence for the first impression or stereotype. The amount of evidence it takes for a perceiver to decide the stereotype is correct is quite small, and can factually be ambiguous in its support. In the experiment of Darley and Gross (1983), the girl was judged in a stereotypic way when all that was provided was vague and mixed feedback about her ability. Second, while these steps that require one to test a hypothesis before expressing a judgment may govern an explicit impression, would someone be as careful when forming and expressing an implicit impression?—that is, if we do not know we are forming an impression, perhaps we will be willing to allow first impressions and stereotypes to shape that impression even in the absence of behavioral evidence. Is it possible to implicitly dislike a person simply based on their face, posture, gait, or skin color, with no behavior displayed at all? We turn to these issues in the next chapter.

NOTES

1. A variety of other cognitive processes give rise to illusory correlations other than people giving unusual attention to two distinctive pieces of information. There are simply too many to review for our purposes in this book, but Stroessner and Plaks (2001) has an excellent summary. All these various cognitive processes that can cause an illusory correlation to be seen illustrate that confirmation bias can occur without motivation to affirm a belief or attitude.

2. The first two foundations Haidt et al. specify are the *harm/care foundation* (which relates to beliefs about compassion and suffering), and the *justice/fairness foundation* (which relates to beliefs about fairness and equality). The next three foundations are *ingroup/loyalty* (which relates to beliefs about group obligations), *authority/respect* (which relates to beliefs about role fulfillment within a hierarchical social order), and *purity* (which relates to beliefs about physical and/or spiritual wholesomeness and chastity vs. feelings of disgust).

3. We can see that many of the best examples of motivated reasoning come from motives relating to *defending and enhancing self-esteem*. This is because when it comes to personal identity or social identity (derived from groups we align ourselves with), we are strongly motivated to preserve and enhance the positive impressions formed about the self by scrutinizing information in a selective manner. But many other motives also guide reasoning.

4. This is not a self-fulfilling prophecy, where a perceiver has an expectation and the perceiver actually behaves in line with that expectation, and the target person responds to the

behavior by acting consistently with that initial expectation. In stereotype threat there is no behavior from a partner to which one is reacting. It is a meta-stereotype—one's thinking about how others think.

5. Of course, this logic works to enhance sexism and racism as well! Perhaps sexism and racism grow because people had been perceiving norms of fairness to which they conformed. Yet, pressure to comply with these norms is lifted by authoritarian groups that social media brings together, groups that would otherwise not be seen, but now can provide a break to the pluralistic ignorance; one can see the hate that others share, making it seem OK.

CHAPTER 6

First Impressions Can Be Implicit, Making Them Even More Persistent

Imagine that you have been told that a person has spent significant time in prison, and that you are soon going to interact with them. This information may lead you to have stereotypes and expectations you associate with them, which may be quite specifically tied to the type of crime you think they committed. You may tell yourself you will be fair, and will withhold judgment until getting to know the person. Despite these explicit intentions to not form attitudes or judgments, we often do form such impressions without realizing it. They occur implicitly. We may not realize that we have evaluated and assessed the person, and this can shape how we treat them. You might further think that while a novice might fall prey to such bias, experts would not. Yet research in forensic psychology shows that such implicit impressions are formed and bias attitudes and judgments throughout the criminal justice system. Decisions rendered by judges are overly influenced by first impressions despite them knowing more relevant information and having heard conflicting evidence. Even impressions that form implicitly based on facial features (such as looking untrustworthy) can impact sentencing decisions (even rates of assigning a death sentence), the chance of being selected in a police line-up, and juror conviction rates for a person said to have a prior criminal record (e.g., Flowe & Humphries, 2011; Funk & Todorov, 2013; Jaeger, Todorov, Evans, & van Beest, 2020; Porter, ten Brinke, & Gustaw, 2010; Wilson & Rule, 2015, 2016). And once outside the justice system it may bias their opportunities for housing, employment, and loans.

The discussion in Chapter 5 of why it is difficult to change a first impression was focused entirely on first impressions formed explicitly. Explicit first impressions can be contrasted with impression formation processes that are routinized with experience and that occur without conscious intent or awareness. The example above was meant to illustrate one important domain in which implicit impressions form and have negative consequences for how we treat people. But we form such impressions easily and with consequence toward most people—criminality was just a dramatic example. For example, in Chapter 4 we reviewed methods for studying *spontaneous trait inferences* (methods such as cued recall following the encoding specificity principle, probe recognition tasks, "relearning" of traits that are paired with people, lexical decision tasks, false recognition tasks). In Chapter 4 we also reviewed methods for studying automatic attitudes as a type of first impression (methods such as the IAT, attitude automaticity measures, affect misattribution). Traits and attitudes are the most frequently studied types of implicit impressions, though other impression types exist (e.g., those built around goals). What makes implicit impressions sticky? The reasons that explicit impressions are sticky—such as confirmation bias and motivated reasoning—apply to implicit impressions, too. Yet, there are additional reasons implicit inferences are sticky that make them perhaps even more difficult to change than explicit impressions (e.g., Gregg, Seibt, & Banaji, 2006; Peters & Gawronski, 2011). Three such reasons are summarized next, and explored in detail in separate sections of this chapter.

First, the individual does not recognize having formed implicit impressions. It would be unusual to seek to change an impression one is not aware of (and did not intend to form). With an explicit impression one may see that it is irrational or wrong and make the effort to revise it. *When the impression is not seen, the motivation to alter it is obviously lower.* For example, Gregg et al. (2006) showed that even though people's explicit impressions were updated, their implicit first impression of two fictional groups remained the same even when people were told that the information about the groups had been accidentally reversed. With an explicit impression, being told the information received about the two groups had been flipped leads the participants to exchange the impression formed about each of the two groups. With an implicit impression there is no sense of anything that needs to be corrected. Peters and Gawronski similarly showed that when new information undermines the validity of the initial information, the explicit impression is changed but the implicit evaluation persists.

A second reason implicit impressions are especially sticky is that the invisibility and ease of the process allows for the impression to be *repeatedly reinforced each time the first impression is invoked*, without one knowing it. This silent strengthening of the impression makes it even more resistant to change. Consider the case of stereotypes. Stereotypes are inferences drawn about a person based on a group membership, and often take the form of traits believed to describe the group. For example, Bean, Stone, Badger, Focella, and Moskowitz (2013) show that health care professionals have a stereotype of Hispanic patients as noncompliant and unlikely to follow the medical advice that the physician recommends. These stereotypes can be triggered without one knowing it (in the case of the Bean et al. research, by flashing faces of individual group members subliminally). If a nurse or physician has the trait "noncompliant" unknowingly triggered each time they see a Hispanic patient, it would mean the first impression of the person, derived from the impression of the group, is repeatedly being supported through these invisible inferences. These inferences then serve as further evidence for the stereotype. This repeated formation of stereotypic inferences makes updating a first impression more difficult because the frequency with which negative traits (and negative feelings) are being silently tied to the person strengthens those associations. Repetition of associations strengthens them.

A third reason implicit impressions are especially sticky is that, because of the ease with which they are formed, perceivers feel they must be accurate. Greater confidence in the impression's accuracy reduces the motivation to want to change or update the impression (e.g., Chaiken et al., 1989; Wilson & Brekke, 1994). The phenomenal immediacy of an implicit inference allows the inference to form without any sense that one needed to work to form the inference. If it is experienced with ease and immediacy, without one needing to work at it, one concludes that this must be because the impression reflects the true qualities of the person to whom the inference refers (e.g., Tversky & Kahneman, 1973). And why change a true impression? The confidence in the impression is ironic since less work is engaged to produce it compared to when it is explicit. Thus, one might feel unmotivated to change an implicit impression not only because it is unseen but because it is confidently held and "feels truer" because of the ease with which it is made.

TYPES OF IMPLICIT IMPRESSIONS

Before examining what makes implicit impressions sticky, a review of the different types of impressions that are formed implicitly is in order. What is an implicit impression?

Impressions Built around Traits and Stereotypes

Ever since Asch (1946) described the importance of "central traits" in directing how people form impressions, the concept of "trait" has occupied a dominant place in the field of social cognition. Even before Asch, Heider (1944) laid the groundwork as to why traits can be so important in how we make sense of other people. Heider declared that with the inference of a trait, another person's behavior is understood in a clear and simple way, and that person becomes predictable because **traits** are enduring qualities of a person that cut across situations and time. They are characteristics of one's personality that are somewhat abstract (in that they can be expressed in a range of ways) that are believed to predict how a person will act in most environments, and as such satisfy the perceiver's need to have meaning and to experience predictability and control. With one simple inferential act the perceiver can explain the other person and understand what they are like, and likely to do. Winter and Uleman (1984) argued that trait inference is so routine and common that it happens "automatically," that we form trait inferences spontaneously. This focus on traits has also been extended to research on *stereotypes*, which are often treated as the traits characterizing an entire group of people (e.g., Hamilton et al., 2015; Hamilton & Sherman, 1994). While a stereotype can include more than traits, the power of traits in establishing a stable impression at the heart of the stereotype has been an assumption in place since Katz and Braly's (1933) pioneering work on the content of the various stereotypes that are held by Americans. Almost 100 years later, stereotypes are still described as manifesting as a set of traits associated with a group and the extension of those group traits to an individual because of that individual's association with a group. That association is sometimes made explicit, but is often simply an inference about the individual made from physical cues, such as facial features or skin tone (e.g., Chen, Quinn, & Maddox, 2022; Eberhardt, Dasgupta, & Banaszynski, 2003). Those cues trigger group assignment and invoke knowledge, drawn from the stereotype, that is applied to the individual (e.g., Eberhardt et al., 2006; Hamilton, 1981; Hamilton & Sherman, 1994).

The body of research on spontaneous trait inference (STI; see Uleman, Rim, Saribay, & Kressel, 2012, for a review) has provided converging evidence from multiple methodologies and cultures to support Asch's (1946) claim that impressions of another person's traits form in us immediately, easily. STI work goes a step further to show that our impressions about a person's traits occur without our intention, without our awareness, without us needing to be asked to form an impression, and despite conditions that limit our processing abilities (e.g., Newman & Marsden, 2023). For example, the process of forming STIs is an efficient one, undeterred by cognitive load. To illustrate this, Winter, Uleman, and Cunniff (1985)

Traits: Somewhat abstract (in that they can be expressed in a range of ways), enduring qualities of a person that cut across situations and time. They are personality characteristics that predict how a person will act in most environments. This allows perceivers inferring stable traits to experience having predictability and control.

used a procedure we reviewed in Chapter 4 that relied on the principle of encoding specificity. Participants read behaviors about a set of people and later in the experiment had their memory tested for these behaviors. During that memory test the participants were not only asked to freely recall all the behaviors they could, but were also provided with cues. Some of these cues were traits that had been implied by one of the behaviors learned about earlier and some were words semantically linked to the sentence. The logic is that when a trait appears as a cue, it should help memory for a behavior only if it is associated with that behavior in memory. And it would be associated with the behavior in memory only if it had been inferred spontaneously when exposed to that behavior. How do we know this happens spontaneously and happens with efficiency? In this experiment the participants were actually informed that their task was to memorize a string of numbers, repeatedly being presented with a new set of digits to learn. They were also told that to make this task difficult they would see a sentence after the digits, and that the sentence was meant to serve as a distractor to the digit-memorizing task. In reality, the opposite was true. The true purpose of the study was to see if people made inferences about the sentences, and the digits were a cognitive load. If the inference process occurs despite people thinking the sentences are distractors (to be ignored) and despite cognitive load, it is efficient and spontaneous. The results show that when a trait is presented as a cue, it helps people to recall the behavior it is associated with, and it only helps with recall of that specific behavior. This is true regardless of the amount of cognitive load. This would only occur if an inference spontaneously formed about a person from their behavior (see Figure 6.1). As noted above, this important process of spontaneous inference has been demonstrated in numerous ways, across many cultures, and reveals the ubiquity with which we use traits to make sense of the world. We like to see others as a "type of person." We later see (in Chapter 8) that these implicit first impressions that are built around traits are foundational for one of the most pervasive biases studied: the fundamental attribution error.

This tendency to spontaneously infer traits can be pushed up or down by one's goals (e.g., Uleman & Moskowitz, 1994). It can differ as a function of the perceiver's stereotypes (Wigboldus, Dijksterhuis, & Van Knippenberg, 2003), ideology (Olcaysoy Okten & Moskowitz, 2020b), and culture (Lee, Shimizu, Masuda, & Uleman, 2017). Because it can be brought under control in this way it is not fully automatic. Indeed, many researchers have shown that there are times people do not infer traits unless they are explicitly asked to

Behavior	Trait Cue	Semantic Cue
He left a 35% tip for the waiter.	Generous	Gratuity
She left the dinner party without thanking the hostess.	Rude	Meal
She always checks to see if her colleagues need anything before leaving for the day.	Considerate	Workplace
He usually drives to the newsstand, even though it is only half a block away.	Lazy	Car
He phoned for help while the others just screamed.	Calm	Emergency
She cheated on her partner whenever he was out of town.	Disloyal	Affair
He thought he did not deserve their award and praise.	Humble	Winning

FIGURE 6.1. A cued-recall procedure for examining spontaneous trait inference.

do so (e.g., Hamilton et al., 1980a). In such experiments research participants are provided with information that is not very informative about traits. For example, the information Hamilton et al. (1980a) provided to their participants were behaviors such as "read the newspaper," "cleaned up the house before guests came over." What is remarkable is not the fact that people do not form impressions unless asked, but that people are even able to form explicit impressions, when asked, to such nondescript and typical actions. Such research reveals humans to have a remarkable capacity to form a coherent impression of a person from very limited information if asked to do so. However, failing to do so without being asked merely tells us that forming an impression is not automatic—we do not do it simply because a person has appeared. The person must be transmitting some type of trait-relevant information. This does not undermine the fact that people infer traits and stereotypes frequently, easily, and without being aware. Research on implicit trait inference shows that when the actions of others even hint at personal causation, the implicit first response often involves inferring a trait, no asking needed.

The previous discussion suggests that vapid information does not lead us to impose traits on others. Yet, minimal amounts of information can encourage inference. And as the strength of the stimulus increases, the easier it will be to form inferences. The process can be pushed up or down by the qualities of the stimulus information, as is argued by an **ecological perspective** to impression formation, which is reviewed in detail in Chapter 9 (e.g., Gibson 1979; McArthur & Baron, 1983). The ecological perspective posits that stimuli differ in terms of how adaptive they are to the individual and the amount of information they carry relating to important goals. Attention is focused on instrumental stimuli that have utility or adaptive value. For example, mundane actions such as "the person read the newspaper" have little value. In contrast, actions implying that a person is a threat, such as "the person is violent," have adaptive value (and can be communicated by something as subtle as their facial features, facial expressions, and other nonverbal acts). Not only negative, but positive acts can have adaptive value, such as learning one has a role where they confer aid (such as nurse). Stimuli with such value are more likely to be attended to and have inferences readily drawn. For example, STI is enhanced if a person's *social role* informs a perceiver that the person has features with adaptive value (Person *X* is a nurse, a key feature of nurses is helping; e.g., Chen et al., 2014).

Ecological perspective: The view that people focus attention on stimuli with easily identifiable features and that have adaptive value. Rather than discussing the power of the perceiver to distort perception, it argues that stimuli grab attention and guide perception via being adaptive for people and inherently communicating information.

Some of the most compelling evidence for the implicit nature of trait-based impressions comes from the ability of these impressions to form around minimal amounts of information that have adaptive value. Much of the research has focused on how people form impressions from simple behaviors that they learn about. Yet, impressions form easily from much less information. In Chapter 3 it was reviewed that nonverbal cues are sent and detected "automatically." Here, we suggest that what is being communicated nonverbally is often the traits of the person being perceived. We form impressions from even short exposure to a person's nonverbal behavior.

Very brief observations of nonverbal behavior that range from 1 to 30 seconds are known as **thin slices of behavior** (Ambady, Hallahan, & Conner, 1999; Ambady & Rosenthal, 1992). Ambady and Rosenthal (1993) took videotapes of teachers from their institution's teaching laboratory and edited them down to 30-second clips with the audio removed (10 seconds from the start, from the middle, and from the end of class) to create such thin slices. Participants coded the videos to detect an

Thin slices of behavior: Very brief observations of nonverbal behavior that range from 1 to 30 seconds.

assortment of nonverbal behaviors (physical attractiveness, head shakes, smiles, nods, yawns, frowns, fiddling with an object, emphatic gestures, touching of the face, biting the lip, and walking around the room while talking). They also formed impressions of the teacher's traits, such as competence, enthusiasm, professionalism, and so on. As expected, their findings confirmed Dion, Berscheid, and Walster's (1972) classic finding that people have a stereotype about physical attractiveness: **What is beautiful is good**. The more attractive a person (in this case, the teacher), the better they are rated on a wide variety of qualities. More importantly, nonverbal cues other than good looks also shaped the impression. The ratings of the teacher that were based on the brief nonverbal cues watched in the thin slices of behavior in the video clips predicted ratings of the teacher's competence and skill. In fact, those ratings correlated highly with the ratings made of the teacher by students who took a course over an entire semester with that same teacher. The teacher is essentially rated the same by those with whom they spend months versus seconds. Each is apparently attending to the same nonverbal cues and using them to form the impression.[1]

> **What is beautiful is good:** A stereotype about physical attractiveness that associates good looks with a host of other positive traits such as competence and intelligence. It can also be thought of as a halo effect in which attractiveness leads to general positivity.

A further illustration that thin slices of behavior produce trait impressions (in this case, stereotypes) was provided by Ambady, Hallahan, and Conner (1999). Gay and lesbian students, as well as heterosexual students, were asked to help the researchers by recording a short video on balancing the many components of student life. They were not told that their sexual orientation was a component of the experiment. Using these recordings, the experimenters created three possible nonverbal messages to show to the research participants: a 10-second film, a 1-second film, and a still photograph (photographs included elements such as hair style, hair color, and fashion choices). Participants were asked to rate whether the person depicted was gay or straight on a 7-point scale. The gay men and lesbian women who were used in the video clips accurately received higher ratings on this scale when compared to the heterosexual men and women used in the video. Accuracy was greater in the 10-second than in the 1-second videos and photographs, but in all three forms of thin slices participants saw something in the nonverbal display to make them differentiate with some degree of accuracy the heterosexual versus homosexual students in the video. Rule, Tskhay, Freeman, and Ambady (2014) showed that participants made accurate judgments of sexual orientation from a still photograph (such as inferring the person was gay), even when the experimenters gave participants false information about the sexual orientation of the person in the photograph (such as telling participants the person was straight).

It may be surprising that trait impressions are made from still photographs alone. Kenny (1994) called these types of thin slices **zero acquaintance** conditions, where all a perceiver has to use for forming an impression are features such as posture, facial expression, skin tone, and physiognomy. Yet even under these conditions of zero acquaintance, perceivers are shown to have similar reactions to each other, often reaching a consensus in the impression they form, seeing the same traits from the impoverished conditions (e.g., Albright, Kenny, & Malloy, 1988; Kenny, Horner, Kashy, & Chu, 1992). A large and systematic research body now exists

> **Zero acquaintance:** The condition where all a perceiver has to use for forming an impression is a single image that communicates nonverbal features such as posture, facial expression, skin tone, and physiognomy.

showing the power of faces to communicate traits (see Johnson, Lick, & Carpinella, 2015; Shen & Ferguson, 2023; Todorov, 2017; Todorov, Olivola, Dotsch, & Mende-Siedlecki, 2015; Zebrowitz, 1997, for reviews).

Important studies starting in the 1980s illustrated a stereotype surrounding particular types of faces called **baby faces**. This describes adults who have features in their face—

Baby faces: Adults with facial features that resemble the structure of an infant's face—large eyes, high forehead, short chin, eyes toward the center of the face, short nose and ears. These characteristics trigger stereotypes that label the person as having child-like qualities—dependent, innocent, weak, loveable, flexible, and naïve.

large eyes, a high forehead, a short chin, eyes toward the center of the face (giving the illusion of a higher forehead), short nose and ears—that resemble the structure of an infant's face. The baby-faced facial characteristics trigger stereotypes that label the person as dependent, innocent, weak, lovable, flexible, and naïve (e.g., McArthur & Apatow, 1983; McArthur & Berry, 1987). Baby-faced people are also described as less dominant and more likely to acquiesce to the requests of others, and be gullible in accepting the far-fetched stories of others (McArthur & Apatow, 1983). Such a stereotype leads to differential treatment. For example, Zebrowitz and McDonald (1991) showed that people with baby faces were treated differently by the legal system. In cases involving negligence (which is compatible with the stereotype) they were more likely to be found guilty than less baby-faced adults. The opposite is true for cases involving an intentional offense (which is incompatible with the stereotype), where they were less likely to be found guilty than adults without baby faces.

Being stereotyped as weak, dependent, submissive, and intellectually inferior can lead to people repeatedly constraining your opportunities by constantly offering social support. This could make you weak (a self-fulfilling prophecy where the stereotypes of others lead you to act in accordance; e.g., Darley & Fazio, 1980; Snyder, Tanke, & Berscheid, 1977), or it could make you rebel against the patronizing behavior. Zebrowitz, Andreoletti, Collins, Lee, and Blumenthal (1998) show baby-faced adults rebuking the stereotype. For example, baby-faced adolescent boys were more likely to be delinquent than mature-faced boys, but only if they came from low-socioeconomic status (SES) backgrounds. Perhaps the stereotype is harsher in poorer neighborhoods, or punishment more severe, so people work harder to overcome that stereotype by violating it. Baby-faced students also achieved higher grades than a control group. Collins and Zebrowitz (1995) reported baby-faced American soldiers serving in World War II and Korea were more likely to receive awards for their military service. In all these cases it could be that baby-faced people are trying to disprove the idea they are weak, incompetent, and dependent (however, it is possible that these baby-faced people do not act any differently, and perceivers just hold them to lower standards. As seen with the phenomenon of shifting standards reviewed in Chapter 4, perhaps these soldiers acted no more bravely than anyone else, but had their actions seen as more brave because of the stereotype setting a low bar of expectations).

Alex Todorov and his colleagues extended the work on facial features from babyishness to how the face communicates specific traits such as competence and trustworthiness. In an amazing series of studies it has been shown that when voters know very little about politics, their voting choices, and a candidate's actual electoral success, were predicted by a politician's facial appearance. In an experiment where they used outcomes of real elections as the measure of interest, they found that a politician whose face better communicated competence beat an opponent whose face less adequately communicated competence (e.g., Ahler, Citrin, Dougal, & Lenz, 2017; Lenz & Lawson, 2011; Olivola & Todorov, 2010; Sussman, Petkova, & Todorov, 2013; Todorov, Mandisodza, Goren, & Hall, 2005). This occurs because a face clearly and easily transmits competence information that a perceiver detects and from which inferences form. They act on those inferences in the voting booth.

Similarly, faces can efficiently communicate information about trustworthiness. For example, Willis and Todorov (2006) showed impressions about trustworthiness formed after only minimal exposure to faces. Their participants saw faces for 100, 500, or 1,000 milliseconds, and the judgments they made about trustworthiness did not vary based on the timing (though longer exposures did yield greater confidence in the judgments). Subsequent studies found that as little as 34 milliseconds of exposure to a face is all that is needed for the trait of trustworthiness to emerge as one's first impression (e.g., Ballew & Todorov, 2007; Todorov, Loehr, & Oosterhof, 2010; Todorov, Pakrashi, & Oosterhof, 2009).

There is high consensus in how perceivers respond to faces, so there must be something in the face they are all detecting (e.g., Oosterhof & Todorov, 2008; Todorov & Oh, 2021). What is it about the face that can communicate the traits of competence or trustworthiness? Answering this question required an impressive series of studies using computational methods, where computer-generated faces could be altered in the tiniest ways. This approach is free of guesses about what features matter (Is it the shape of the mouth?, Is it the eyebrows?). It is also free of the limitations that manipulating such individual features could present (such as needing to know what features to manipulate, potentially leaving some out, or being unable to manipulate every possible combination—since even 10 manipulated features would produce over 1,000 combinations of features). Instead, Todorov and colleagues used data from an enormous number of facial stimuli (see Figure 6.2) so that the aggregated data reveal specific facial elements impacting a resulting impression (e.g., Oosterhof & Todorov, 2008; Todorov et al., 2011; Todorov & Oh, 2021; Todorov & Oosterhof, 2011). To quote Todorov (2023, p. 24):

> We used a statistical model of face representation, in which each face is represented as a 100-dimensional vector. The appearance of each face is determined by its coordinates in this multi-dimensional face space. Rather than manipulating features, we randomly sampled faces from the multi-dimensional face space, and asked participants to judge the faces on various trait dimensions. Given the average trait judgment, we can then build a model of this judgment that captures the variation in appearance that is important for the judgment.

The faces produced by these models invoke traits such as dominance, trust, and competence to varying degrees, depending on the model used to generate them, and they are

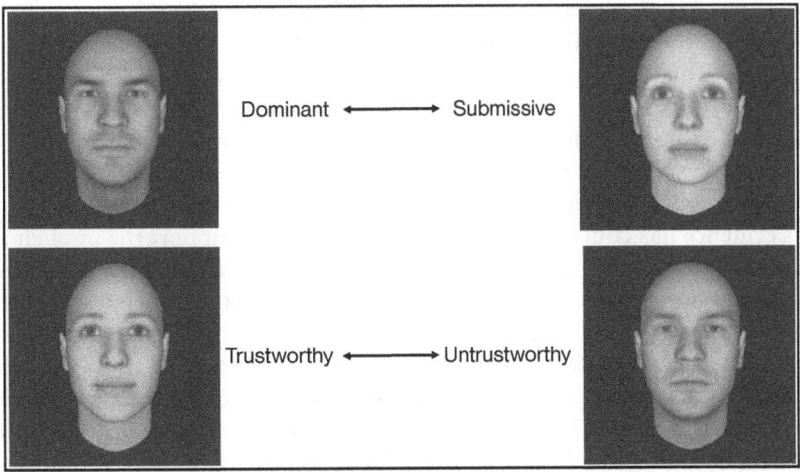

FIGURE 6.2. Sample faces produced by statistical models of face representation.

available for use to researchers interested in studying impressions from the face (Oh, Buck, & Todorov, 2019; Said & Todorov, 2011; Todorov et al., 2013).

The face is not the only part of the body that communicates important nonverbal information—research also has explored the meaning seen in a person's motion and gait (e.g., Freeman & Johnson, 2016). For example, people make categorizations about gender and sexual orientation by examining walking motions, such as swaying hips versus swaggering shoulders (Johnson & Tassinary, 2005). Swaggering of the shoulders leads people to infer the person is a man. Of course, other features typically overpower gait when making such decisions about a person's gender or traits. However, if other features, such as body shape, are ambiguous, then cues surrounding gait become highly informative. Researchers create such ambiguity in the lab (such as ambiguity about a person being male or female) by the use of in-point light displays: dark backgrounds with lights that approximate human forms (Johnson & Tassinary, 2007). These outlines of a human form made of light, alone, suggest no gender. However, when the ambiguous figures are made to display motion, perceivers infer categories and attributes (gender, sexual orientation) easily and spontaneously from the types of "body" motions (Lick & Johnson, 2016). Researchers manipulate the types of gaits the ambiguous images display, and gender is no longer felt to be ambiguous. Perceivers infer categories from the gait.

Another feature that invisibly promotes trait inference is the qualities of speech. As with the face, the voice can communicate socially shared information with adaptive value (e.g., Funder, 1995; Harris, 2010; Rim, Hansen, & Trope, 2013). Sands and Harris (2023) declare that **prosody** is central to helping perceivers form impressions about a person's traits. Developed over the lifespan, and stored in memory, they define prosody as "an index of prototypical vocal cues or acoustic parameters . . . a combination of acoustic parameters (e.g., pitch, decibels, shimmer) that helps the listener infer the mental state of the speaker" (p. 222). Just as nonverbal cues reveal something more than the content of what the person says, so too does prosody. And just as people learn to regulate some of their nonverbal behavior to try and communicate a particular quality, they also learn to regulate prosody as a way to facilitate their goals and manage the impressions other people form. Sands and Harris argue that the ease with which people express and infer traits through vocal qualities differs among the various traits. Some, which they refer to as baseline traits, attain this status of greater ease to communicate because of their adaptive value. Traits and emotions that signal threat versus opportunity to move toward a goal, and traits that signal deceit versus trust, are easier to express through, and to detect from, the voice. This converges nicely with the work on facial features reviewed above, where trust was identified as easily communicated and detected from the face. This is true of the voice as well.

> **Prosody:** The qualities or acoustic parameters of speech, such as pitch and decibel levels. Such qualities help the listener infer the speaker's mental state. Traits and emotions that signal threat (and deceit) versus trust (and opportunity to move toward a goal) are easy to express through, and detect from, the voice.

Just as evidence has converged across methodologies to support the implicit nature of impressions that are centered around a trait, a body of work now supports Allport's (1954) claim that cognitive processing gives rise to implicit stereotyping. When the people we form impressions of belong to social groups, the traits associated with the stereotype of that group are triggered (made accessible) in our mind. Those stereotypic traits are extended to the individual. Pioneering experiments in the 1980s illustrated the ease with which social stereotypes are triggered outside of awareness and without intent (e.g., Darley & Gross, 1983; Devine, 1989; Dovidio, Evans, & Tyler, 1986; Hamilton & Rose, 1980). And stereotyped impressions can form around these triggered attributes even when there is relatively little evidence to support using them, when behavior is at best ambiguous (e.g., Arndt &

Henderson, 2022; Chen et al., 2022). We later see (in Chapters 10 and 11) that these implicit first impressions are foundational for pervasive biases in the culture that contribute to disparity, inequality, and discrimination.

We end this section with a discussion of how facial features impact stereotypic impressions, as well as trait inference. Maddox (2004) described a **racial phenotypicality bias**. This is defined as a set of facial features being stereotypically associated with a group, such as the stereotypical features that American society associates with Black Americans: such as dark skin tone, broad noses, and full lips. Rather than a face communicating a single trait (like competence), it communicates group membership and stereotypes. Research from the lab of Keith Maddox shows that variation among Black Americans with regard to these specific features is associated with different degrees of stereotyping. People with more stereotypical facial features are stereotyped more, likely due to the inference that they possess the traits that characterize the stereotype to a greater degree (e.g., Adams, Kurtz-Costes, & Hoffman, 2016; Hinzman & Maddox, 2017; Maddox, 2004; Maddox & Chase, 2004; Maddox & Dukes, 2008; Maddox & Gray, 2002). Individuals stereotyped to a greater degree because of their facial features have a greater chance of experiencing the negative outcomes that are associated with the social stereotype.

> **Racial phenotypicality bias:** A set of facial features that are stereotypically associated with a racial group, such as the stereotypical features that American society associates with Black Americans, such as dark skin tone, broad noses, and full lips.

A variety of outcomes (police brutality, judge sentencing) are linked to this bias. Field experiments can show the powerful consequences of what appears to be a bias associated with the phenotypical features of a person's face. A growing body of research demonstrates that people more readily apply racial stereotypes to Black people who are thought to look more stereotypically Black, compared with Black people who are thought to look less stereotypically Black. Even with differences in defendants' criminal histories statistically controlled, defendants with the most stereotypically Black facial features served up to 8 months longer in prison for felonies than defendants with less-stereotypical features. Eberhardt et al. (2006) showed that the "stereotypicality" of a Black man's facial features was related to the actual sentencing decisions of judges. Using archival data from the city of Philadelphia, they found that racial phenotypicality bias influenced how likely one is to receive the death penalty. The researchers focused on the cases in which race was most salient—when a Black man was charged with murdering a White victim. They found that the defendants who had the most "stereotypically Black" appearance were more likely to receive a death sentence. Specifically, the defendants in the lower half of the distribution for looking stereotypically Black received a death sentence 24.4% of the time. Defendants in the upper half of the distribution for looking stereotypically Black received a death sentence 57.5% of the time—despite their crimes' similar circumstances.

Impressions Built around Positive or Negative Affective Responses (Automatic Attitudes)

The adaptive value of some types of impressions make them able to form efficiently and implicitly. Just as traits are adaptive in that they provide meaning, determining whether we should approach or avoid a stimulus is a twin psychological imperative to meaning making. It has been argued that detecting threats and opportunities is just as essential to human social cognition as is meaning making (e.g., Bargh, 2017; Fazio, 1986). Several decades of research have established that evaluations of positive and negative affect are among the first things we assess, happening within a half-second, and requiring neither the intent to evaluate the person or the awareness of having done so. This is consistent with the *ecological*

approach to impression formation reviewed above, where perceivers were said to focus attention on those things in the environment with adaptive value, such as opportunities and
threats—that is, aside from knowing what qualities a person or thing possesses, we need to
assess whether a person or thing is positive or negative. Such implicit affective responses
allow us to know whether a stimulus is a threat or an opportunity. When people are implicitly felt to be a threat because of a group membership, then implicit attitudes contribute to
prejudice and implicit bias (e.g., Banaji & Greenwald, 2013; Forscher & Devine, 2014). Chapter 4 reviewed methods for illustrating the implicit nature of impressions about individuals
and groups built around an attitude, such as the AMP and the IAT.

   With impressions based on implicit inferences about traits, the argument was that even
minimal amounts of information imply a trait. Implicit impressions form from thin slices
of behavior, still images, gait, vocal qualities, and faces. The argument put forth regarding impressions based on evaluative inferences is that *all* types of information trigger an
affective response; every person and object is associated with an attitude that is triggered
every time that person or object is perceived. It is for this reason that researchers began
to investigate the automaticity of attitudes (e.g., Bargh et al., 1992; Fazio, Sanbonmatsu,
Powell, & Kardes, 1986). *Automatic attitudes* were defined in Chapter 3 as positive or negative affective evaluations that are immediately triggered by the stimuli we encounter; the
mere presence of the stimulus leads to the activation of an evaluative response associated
with the stimulus. Automatically triggered attitudes differ from one another in a variety
of ways. For example, they differ in importance (some are tied to important goals or social
identities, others are not), extremity (some are very negative or positive, others only mildly
so), accessibility (the ease and speed with which an associated evaluation is triggered by an
attitude object), and ambivalence (some have a mix of positive and negative affect). An affective response is a basic element of impression formation.

   As with trait impressions made implicitly, an implicit attitude can be altered by one's
goals (e.g., Ferguson & Bargh, 2004; Lowery, Hardin, & Sinclair, 2001). The evaluative
response that is triggered can differ as a function of the perceiver's prejudice (Fazio et al.,
1995; Hausmann & Ryan, 2004), ideology (Ferguson, Carter, & Hassin, 2009; Nosek, Banaji,
& Jost, 2009), and culture (Greenwald et al., 1998). It can also be pushed up or down by qualities of the information; some contexts trigger affect more easily than others. Contexts with
counterattitudinal exemplars weaken the activation of implicit attitudes (e.g., Dasgupta &
Asgari, 2004; Dasgupta & Greenwald, 2001). Contexts that allow for practice at rejecting
the association can weaken the activation of implicit attitudes (e.g., Kawakami, Dovidio,
Moll, Hermsen, & Russin, 2000). Contexts that allow for evaluative conditioning can alter
the activation of implicit attitudes (e.g., Olson & Fazio, 2006).

   Several experiments were reviewed in Chapters 3 and 4 that illustrated the implicit
activation of attitudes. We provide one more example here, in the domain of prejudice. Not
all prejudice reflects a negative affective response. Many types of prejudice manifest as feelings of kindness and support being triggered toward a group, but these affective responses
arise from negative inferences about the group. Male biases toward women, and Imperialist
attitudes toward "colonized" peoples reflect the paternalistic belief that the "others" are
to be treated positively because they are inherently inferior and need support (e.g., Glick &
Fiske, 2001a, 2001b). One's own feelings of privilege and superiority require seeing others
as inferior, yet this perceived inferiority breeds implicit reactions of support and kindness
rather than dislike. This prescription of negative characteristics to others that allow them
to be seen as almost childlike, and thus breeding a positive evaluation, is known as **benevolent bias**. Glick and Fiske (2001b) said:

Although *benevolent sexism* [italics in original] may sound oxymoronic, this term recognizes that some forms of sexism are, for the perpetrator, subjectively benevolent, characterizing women as pure creatures who ought to be protected, supported, and adored and whose love is necessary to make a man complete. This idealization of women simultaneously implies that they are weak and best suited for conventional gender roles; being put on a pedestal is confining, yet a man who places a woman there is likely to interpret this as cherishing, rather than restricting, her (and many women may agree). Despite greater acceptability of benevolent sexism, our research suggests that it serves as a crucial complement to hostile sexism that helps to pacify women's resistance to societal gender inequality. (p. 109)

> **Benevolent bias:** A paternalistic response emerging when one's feelings of privilege and superiority breed reactions of benevolence, liking, support, and kindness (rather than dislike and fear) for those perceived as inferior. Even though the group is perceived to have objectively negative qualities, they are seen as almost childlike and thus positively evaluated.

Benevolent sexism allows people to express sexist attitudes in a manner that does not contradict their egalitarian and positive self-views, and in a way that does not conflict with societal demands of appearing to be unbiased. One appears to be expressing positive beliefs, but they are positive beliefs that will maintain and perhaps enhance a structural inequality. It is even possible that women may endorse such attitudes in a strategic attempt to not be seen as violating societal norms, especially in societies where there is a high threat of violence toward women from men.

In many modern societies, explicit attitudes are changing to reflect the endorsement of agentic roles for women. Yet the implicit attitude that women should not be agentic persists. Thus, despite the more modern explicit attitude, violations of the traditional prescriptions still held at the implicit level can lead to reactions of backlash to women who are agentic (e.g., Rudman & Phelan, 2008). A benevolent reaction to women can mask an implicit desire to see prescriptions held static. For example, Heilman, Wallen, Fuchs, and Tamkins (2004) found that when a woman was being considered for the position of vice president of a large corporation, the more agency that was seen in her portfolio, the more she was associated with negative attitudes. Even if bias against agentic women is not overtly expressed, overt benevolence can have harmful consequences. Heilman et al. found that the agentic woman was perceived as abrasive, pushy, and manipulative. Agentic women were less likely to be recommended for the promotion.

Is this paternalistic and benevolent reaction one that is triggered implicitly? Using an IAT, Oliveira Laux, Ksenofontov, and Becker (2015) provided an illustration. They developed two IATs to assess implicit attitudes to women that reflected the benevolent form, and the more traditional hostile form. In their IAT to assess benevolent sexism, Oliveira Laux et al. focused on the concept of paternalism (that women must be protected by men; that women are to be cherished by men). To assess benevolent sexism, one of the responses participants made was to see an image of a drawing of a man and a woman interacting. The task was to indicate who was the more agentic or active person in the image. Half of the images depicted an active woman and a passive man (such as a woman with a gun protecting a man; a woman helping a man to put on his coat), the remaining half used similar images with the roles reversed so that it depicted an active man and a passive woman. When a man being protective of women was paired with the same key as "pleasant" there was a compatible pairing for assessing benevolent sexism. Faster reaction times were found for the compatible versus the incompatible (agentic woman and positive paired) trials, revealing an implicit positive, yet sexist, response. And, the stronger the implicit attitude, the better it predicted explicit measures of benevolent sexism, but not explicit measures of hostile sexism. Additionally, the implicit measure was not correlated with a similar measure they developed for hostile (old-fashioned) sexism.

Impressions Built Around Goals

Traits, stereotypes, and attitudes are the most widely studied types of impressions people form. This is true for explicit and implicit impression formation. However, there are other types of inferences we make about people in a somewhat automatic fashion: inferences about their current state, inferences about their emotions, inferences about their preferences, inferences about how they are likely to act. We limit the review of types of implicit impressions to just one more type to bring under focus: inferences about goals. Linguistically, we use the same words to refer to a person's traits as we do to refer to their goals (e.g., Fiedler & Schenck, 2001; Fiedler, Schenck, Watling, & Menges, 2005). This makes it hard to distinguish among when people form a spontaneous trait inference versus when people form a spontaneous goal inference. Most of our implicit measures involve responding to a word in a reaction-time test, or using a word as a memory cue, or showing an association among words. Researchers have always assumed the words used in such tasks (such as "cautious") refer to the traits the participants inferred, but they could in fact assess goals that the participants inferred (Moskowitz & Olcaysoy Okten, 2016). For example, while the word "cautious" could refer to a trait ascribed to another person, it could also refer to the person's goals, without suggesting anything about the person's personality. Showing that a participant responds quickly to "cautious" after observing a behavior could mean the participant inferred that the person had the goal of being cautious, but not a trait.

Like traits, inferences about goals are about the person, but they describe a less stable and more variable quality of the person. A trait should be expected to emerge across situations (the woman is considerate with many people and in many different contexts), a goal should be tied to only certain situations or when interacting with specific people (the woman is considerate to her chief executive officer [CEO], or when at her daughter's school, but not when supervising her research team). Kruglanski et al. (2002) described goals by stating "they fluctuate from one moment to the next as we succumb to an assortment of distractions, temptations, and digressions" (p. 333). Further, because goals are dynamic and fluctuate, this implies that they are under the person's control and reflect something about why they have chosen to act in that moment. In contrast, traits are stable to one's character and not subject to control. For this reason, a trait tells you more about *what* a person will do in the future, while a goal tells you more about *why* the person acted as they did today. Finally, an impression that invokes a goal differs from one that invokes a trait regarding how we assign responsibility for the outcomes of behavior. With a goal, the person chose to act that way and we see greater culpability, but also a greater possibility of rehabilitation. With a trait, the outcome seems more determined by an uncontrollable force (even though it is a force of the person), and thus a greater chance of recidivism. In Chapter 5 we reviewed Asch and Zukier's (1984) research that showed how perceivers use these distinctions among traits and goals to confirm first impressions. If behavior is observed that is inconsistent with an impression, that impression may not change. Instead, people may use "means–end" thinking to reinterpret the behavior—it is seen not as an inconsistent trait of the person but as a temporary goal. Thus, the person has not truly acted inconsistently because the act is dismissed as a temporary goal unique to this one situation, not a trait. Such instrumentality, where a person is seen as pursuing a goal to attain something important to people of that "type," allows the seemingly inconsistent act to fit with the impression. Inferring a goal supports it, instead of inferring a trait that contradicts it.

It is true that Heider (1944) identified traits as a very powerful tool to use for making meaning out of the behavior we observe. However, Heider's larger point about meaning making is that *we tend to place emphasis on the disposition of the person*; we see behavior as being caused by something internal to the person and place less emphasis on the power of the situation. Heider (1958) quite clearly identified inferences about a person's goals, not simply their traits, as part of their disposition. **Goal inference** is also a dominant way we under-stand behavior. In the next chapter we focus on Heider's influence on social cognition and particularly on the attribu-tion theories he inspired. We will see that forming impres-sions about a person's goals plays a role in each of those theo-ries. However, it is only within the last 20 years that research has examined **implicit goal inference**, or the *implicit* nature of impressions built around goals.

Aarts, Gollwitzer, and Hassin (2004) illustrated goal inference in an interesting way. They reasoned that if a goal was spontaneously inferred from observing another person's behavior, then it would be more likely to be adopted for one's own behavior. This type of **goal contagion**, where one catches a goal from another person by inferring the person has that goal, can be used as a way to diagnose whether a goal infer-ence had occurred (in this case, making this inference about the person's goals implicitly). To strengthen the logic that goal contagion reflects an impression about the person's goals, they also explored whether the amount of contagion observed was moderated by the extent to which the perceiver person-ally valued the goal that they observed in the other person. As expected, they found that perceivers not only act consistently with the goals they implicitly infer in others but they do this to a greater degree if the perceiver values the goal.

> **Goal inference:** Perceivers' impres-sions of the goals a person is pursu-ing. Goals fluctuate from moment to moment as a function of opportunity, distraction, temptations, desire, and commitment. Thus, goal inference is about the temporary desires of the individual in relation to their context, not something stable about them (like a trait).
>
> **Implicit goal inference:** When a perceiver makes an inference about a person's goals without the inten-tion to do so or awareness of having done so, and despite conditions that limit processing ability. Perceiv-ers are skilled at seeing goals from the behaviors they observe without needing to be asked to describe the person's intentions.
>
> **Goal contagion:** When one "catches" a goal from another person. This involves first inferring a per-son has a specific goal, and then, because of the goal's activation, being more likely to adopt that goal for one's own goal-directed behavior.

Hassin, Aarts, and Ferguson (2005) showed evidence for implicit goal inference using a clever procedure in which par-ticipants read about behaviors that described a blocked goal. For example, a participant might read the behavior "Bill walked to the market, but the manager was locking up as he arrived (implying the blocked goal of "shopping"). Then, in a next phase of the experiment, the extent to which implicit inferences were made is assessed using the procedures reviewed in Chapter 4 to study STIs. For example, in one experiment they used the cued recall proce-dure reviewed in Figure 6.1. They found that participants made goal inferences from both blocked and unblocked actions. This shows the inference is indeed about a goal, and not just about what the person did, or a prediction about what they were about to do (shop). Since the inference is also made when the action was blocked, it must be an inference about what they were *trying* to do.

Of course, people can make both trait and goal inferences about the same person based on the same behavior (e.g., Ham & Vonk, 2003; Reeder, Vonk, Ronk, Ham, & Law-rence, 2004; Todd, Molden, Ham, & Vonk, 2011). This has led some researchers to wonder whether trait inference or goal inference is completed more quickly. For example, exam-ining activation in the temporo-parietal junction, neuroscience methods suggest that goal inferences are faster. Van Overwalle, Van Duynshaeger, Coomans, and Timmermans (2012) reached a similar conclusion using a reaction-time methodology to study implicit inferences about goals and traits. When reading behaviors, people identify words that are inconsistent with a trait after about 600 milliseconds, yet words inconsistent with goals are identified after 200 milliseconds (e.g., Van der Cruyssen, Van Duynslaeger, Cortoos, & Van Overwalle, 2009; Van Duynslaeger, Van Overwalle, & Verstraeten, 2007). Further, they showed that trait inferences are not only made after goal inferences but *only if goal inferences are also made*, suggesting that goal inference is necessary but not sufficient for trait inference.

With this summary of some types of implicit impressions now complete, we explore in more detail why it is that implicit impressions can be even harder to change than explicit impressions. Confirmation biases and motivated reasoning may make explicit first impressions sticky. But they are not "Krazy Glued" to a person. It is possible to change them. In the summary that started this chapter, there were several reasons reviewed to suggest extra stickiness for implicit impressions is to be expected. The reasons why implicit impressions should be even harder to change than explicit ones are:

1. People lack awareness an impression has even been formed.
2. Implicit first impressions are more efficient than the correction processes that might overturn them.
3. The impression is repeatedly reinforced (through repetitive priming) making the associative links and the memory trace stronger.
4. The ease of associations being triggered and impressions called to mind makes one feel confident in their accuracy and validity.

LACK OF AWARENESS REDUCES THE MOTIVATION TO UPDATE AN IMPLICIT IMPRESSION

Gregg et al. (2006) illustrated that implicit impressions about two fictional groups—Niffites and Luupites—are stickier than explicit impressions. Research participants learned information and formed first impressions about each group. Niffites were described as aggressors, authoritarian, barbaric, savage, ruthless, and brutal; Luupites were described as accommodating, benevolent, civilized, and constructive. After forming first impressions that Niffites are bad and Luupites are good, the experimenter announced a programming error. By mistake the computer mixed up the information, and information about the Niffites was actually about the Luupites; that participants "had been exposed to portrayals of the groups that were diametrically opposite to those intended . . . so in fact the Niffites should have been described as good and Luupites as bad" (p. 9). Wyer (2010) used a similar type of reversal to explore whether a first impression sticks. She had participants learn that a person was a skinhead and left them to infer that the person was in possession of all the anarchic and violent qualities a skinhead would possess. Then the participants learned this information was wrong and that the person's bald head was not an ideological choice made by a skinhead but a reaction to cancer medication. In each of these research examples, it was shown that research participants easily updated the explicit impressions of the person to reflect the correct, newer information. Awareness of having made an error when forming an explicit impression motivated change of that impression. Implicit impressions, however, did not change. Awareness that incorrect information was the basis for an implicit impression does not cause a change in the impression if one lacks awareness of the impression to start with. If the initial impression is invisible, then there is no motivation to alter it in light of new, better information.

Correction Neglect

In Chapter 12 we review an important set of theories that collectively are called *dual-process theories*. One common theme cutting across these dual-process theories was one of correction or "debiasing." Correction refers to the idea that consciousness (explicit processing) is used to overturn or fix errors that are produced by more uncontrollable and unconscious elements of cognition (implicit processing). Implicit processes operate easily, quickly, and invisibly, and explicit processes exert effort to monitor the outputs of the implicit processes (trait inferences, stereotypes, attitudes, etc.), overturning them when they are wrong, adjusting them when they are incomplete, and suppressing them if they violate one's intended goals, values, and actions. This is a **correction process**.

Across these different theories, awareness of bias is regarded as a critical element of the correction process. Whether it be the correction of an incomplete impression, updating a false stereotype, undoing a biased response or decision, or changing an attitude that is no longer confidently held to be true, awareness of the implicit impression is said to be needed to initiate change of the impression (e.g., Brewer, 1988; Chaiken et al., 1989; Devine, 1989; Gilbert, 1989; Martin & Tesser, 1996; Monteith, Ashburn-Nardo, Voils, & Czopp, 2002; Moskowitz & Skurnik, 1999; Strack & Hannover, 1996; Wegener & Petty, 1995b; Wilson & Brekke, 1994). Without awareness of a first impression, these models posit that it will persist. Why? These dual-process theories shared the assumption that people are not *motivated* to alter first impressions when the individual does not know that the impression exists. Awareness is regarded as essential because it triggers a second essential ingredient to the correction process: the goal to alter and fix a biased impression that they previously did not know existed. Awareness of the bias offers the possibility that we would then be motivated to address it. When a force has an invisible influence, then we are unlikely to detect it or be motivated to alter it. Because we do not see it, we neglect correcting it.

An example of this was shown above in people's failing to correct their implicit disliking of Niffites and liking of Luupites. Upon learning that the information provided was incorrect, they were motivated to change explicit impressions, of which they were aware. Learning that the information was incorrect did not impact implicit impressions that they did not know existed and were then not motivated to change. They neglected correcting those impressions. Todorov (2023) provided an example that takes us back to where this chapter started. If, as reviewed above, people make inferences from faces without realizing it (STIs), then those inferences will shape what we think without realizing it. Lack of awareness that we are inferring traits from faces can have a harmful influence when we are engaged in important decisions, such as judging a defendant's behavior in a criminal case (or a politician's trustworthiness). Our judgments of a defendant may be thought to be formed in an unbiased way, leaving us unable to combat the actual bias that exists from the implicit impressions formed (because we lack awareness that it exists). We may feel our reaction is based on evidence and not see the interpretation of the evidence is biased by a first impression.

Let us explore one additional example of lack of awareness of an impression being responsible for **correction neglect** (and the impression's enhanced stickiness). Bago,

> **Correction process:** When a person detects an error in their judgment and decision making, or suspects a distortion in how they have evaluated a person, they engage compensatory processes aimed at removing that bias. They attempt to correct the error and form what they feel will be a more accurate response.

> **Correction neglect:** Because first impressions are often not known to the individual, first impressions are unlikely to change even if they are biased. The person will be unmotivated to correct an impression they do not know exists in the first place, so any correction process will be neglected from being carried out.

Rand, and Pennycook (2020) provide a nice illustration while investigating people's susceptibility to fake news ("fabricated information that mimics news media content in form but not in organizational process or intent"; p. 1608). When people see information presented to them in a format that appears to be a legitimate media presentation, they will make an inference that the information is true. Without a thorough appraisal being conducted, they rely on theories and preconceived ideas about the style of the presentation as a substitute for deep thought. This "intuitive" or "gut" reaction leads them to accept fake news headlines as true. Even though enough information is provided to "debunk" the headline, the implicit impression is not corrected because people are not aware that there is a reason to doubt it. To illustrate this, Bago et al. used an experimental procedure where people read news headlines twice: first when responding intuitively and without deliberation, then again when prompted to think more deeply when assessing the headline. Some of these headlines were false and presented fabricated information, some were true. But all of them were presented in a format that mimics real news. When processing in an intuitive way, this "cue" that something looks like news led them to accept it as true, even if it was fabricated. It is important to note that they do not accept the false headlines as true as often as they accept the true headlines. Truth is still recognized more often. However, people still embrace fake news when responding intuitively because there are learned patterns of responding that tell us to intuitively trust information that has the look and feel of news based on the relevant cues. They never become aware of this bias, so they are unmotivated to correct it.

In contrast, correction does occur when people become aware of the possibility of bias. When prompted to deliberate, they can uncover the biases and inaccuracies that had riddled their "intuitive" response. Deliberation leads them to be more accurate in how they assess the information. This is especially true if they are motivated to do so out of a vested interest (such as when a news headline is relevant to the outcomes for the self or an important identity group to which one belongs). We do this when judging people as well: We rely on cues to tell us what to think, forming what feel to us as sufficient impressions based on shallow assessments. We correct such judgments when prompted to think deeply and to see the inaccuracies in simply relying on cues or preconceived expectations. Without awareness, we neglect to correct.

The Negative Feedback Loop

There are, of course, other steps required to change an initial impression besides becoming aware of a first impression. However, the starting point is posited to be awareness that an impression may need revision or correction—that is, feedback must be received (either delivered from others or through self-discovery) that the current response or impression is insufficient. As stated above, many theories posit that such awareness is needed because it *motivates* change and self-regulation (updating, correction, debiasing, modification). Why would it be that without awareness the first response persists and a correction process is neglected? The motivating properties of awareness rests in a model of self-regulation that emerged from research on goal pursuit (e.g., Carver & Scheier, 1981, 1982; Miller et al., 1960; Wicklund & Gollwitzer, 1982) known as the **negative feedback loop**.

Negative feedback loop: Self-regulation processes through which goals are pursued/achieved. First a desired end-state is specified, then operations aimed at achieving the end-state are initiated. Testing/monitoring assesses if the state was attained. If not, this negative feedback triggers further operations/responses. This loop repeats until the state is achieved or the goal is disengaged.

The term *negative feedback loop* combines two theoretical points. The first is that when an individual sets a standard or criterion they wish to attain when pursuing a goal, often that individual becomes aware that their current standing in the goal pursuit is not meeting that criterion (they receive negative feedback). The process of gathering feedback about whether the desired state is met (or approximates being reached), or if there is instead a discrepancy from where one stands currently and where one desires to be, is called **monitoring**. The second is that this negative feedback creates a sustained motivational drive to increase efforts, move closer to the standard, and to receive further feedback about how one is doing (steps that repeat in a loop until one reaches the standard). Awareness of *negative feedback*, that one's current response or impression is insufficient, is experienced as an **aversive tension** that creates a motivational state to remove the tension. The aversive state motivates new responding to compensate for the shortcoming (see Carver & Scheier, 1982; Moskowitz, 2009, for reviews). Self-regulatory **operations** are then engaged—both cognitive processes and actions—aimed at eliminating the aversive tension by compensating for the shortcoming. These compensatory responses move the person toward the desired goal. It is a negative feedback *loop* because this process of "monitoring-aversive tension-compensatory responding" is seen as a cycle that continues repeatedly until the negative feedback that causes the aversive tension is eliminated. If these self-regulatory operations do little to move one closer to the goal, and monitoring continues to deliver feedback that one is falling short, one may revise their commitment and desire to pursue the goal. The loop need not continue endlessly but can be exited. Lack of progress toward the goal can, eventually, lead to giving up on the goal altogether—what is known as **disengagement**.

Consider an example unrelated to first impressions: the goal of running 2 miles in 15 minutes as part of one's exercise regimen. You start to run. The goal then needs to be regulated or controlled through feedback about its status. Do you stop when you feel strained? No, you seek feedback or monitor your response. Have you run 2 miles? If the feedback is negative (you have run only 1 mile), then you continue to run. In this example you would monitor pace as well. Are you on pace to run a 7.5-minute mile? If the feedback is negative, then you alter the response and speed up. These activities loop until the feedback is no longer negative and 2 miles have been run in under 15 minutes. The loop can be delayed, since once this particular 2 miles has been run in over 15 minutes one can no longer achieve the goal in this moment. But one can continue the feedback loop at a later time, staying in this cycle of responding to pursue a goal, monitoring one's standing, feedback, and responding. The loop ends when the feedback is no longer negative (2 miles have been run at the desired pace) or when one decides to disengage from this goal altogether (7.5-minute miles are not for me).

Monitoring: Process through which one gathers feedback about one's standing in a goal pursuit and becomes aware (at some level, not necessarily consciously) that either the desired state is achieved (or approximates being reached) or that there is a discrepancy from where one stands currently and where one desires to be.

Aversive tension: When there is inconsistency among where one currently stands in a goal pursuit and where one desires to be this is experienced as dissonance, or an undesirable motivational state where one is driven to eliminate the negative affect engendered.

Operations: Responses aimed at eliminating the aversive tension that arises when monitoring yields negative feedback. These steps are aimed at compensating for not having achieved the desired end-state and are purposeful in that they move the person toward that end-state and address (and remove) the discomfort caused by the tension.

Disengagement: When negative feedback leads to lowered commitment, hopelessness, or feeling defeated, rather than an increased effort to attain a goal. The negative feedback "loop" is exited at this point, allowing the individual to shift to the pursuit of other goals that are now deemed to have greater value.

This same negative feedback loop logic applies to first impressions and their stickiness. The assumption is that people have the goal for their impressions to be accurate and not based on false or biased information. Awareness that the impression is not reliable, feedback that undermines confidence in that impression, will alert one that the goal is not being met. This negative standing that is delivered by the feedback, awareness of not having attained the goal, will motivate a change of that first impression. One will then respond in a way to eliminate the negative standing—one will seek to correct or update the first impression. To do so requires engaging the negative feedback loop. One monitors the goal to see if it is achieved. If not, one is motivated to respond. After having responded one needs to seek feedback again. And this repeats until the monitoring reveals that the bias in one's impression has been fixed (see Figure 6.3).

This example is predicated on the assumption that people have a goal to feel as if their impressions are accurate—that the meaning we make when observing the actions of others is not unreliable. You may not be aware that this particular goal exists but you may still be monitoring to make sure it is achieved. When you receive negative feedback that your impression is insufficient, that your goal is not yet reached (perhaps new and incompatible information has been learned; perhaps someone has told you that the impression is wrong, as with the Niffites and Luupites), the negative feedback will motivate you to initiate responses to produce the desired state (a sufficient impression). The loop ends only when the feedback is no longer negative—in this example, when the impression is felt to be sufficient once again.

As we saw in the previous chapter, negative feedback may not always initiate the motivation to update the impression. It is possible to retain the first impression by either convincing oneself that the negative feedback is wrong (motivated reasoning) or that despite the new information provided by the negative feedback, the original impression is still

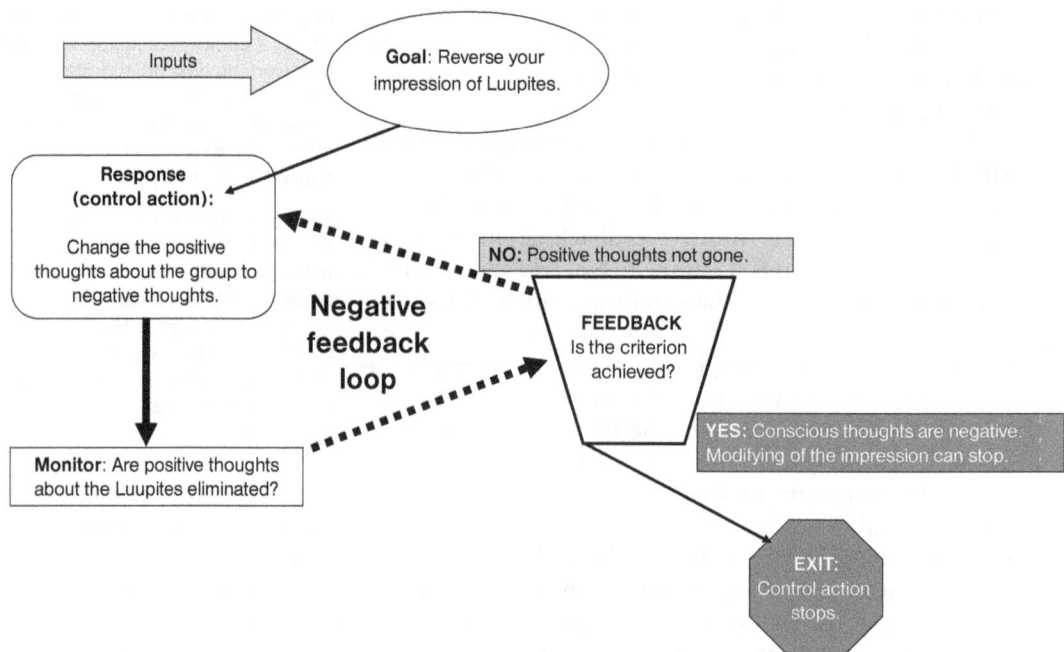

FIGURE 6.3. The negative feedback loop.

sufficient (confirmation bias). However, while awareness (feedback) may not be sufficient to produce a changed impression, it is necessary. Yet, if the impression is implicit, such awareness may not exist. Self-discovery of the insufficiency of the impression is unlikely because you have no idea an impression even exists. You cannot discover a bias, or provide the self with negative feedback about one's standing on whether one's impression is sufficiently accurate, if not aware one has an impression. Second, there is less of a reason to accept the negative feedback when it is discovered, such as when someone else tells you that your impression is wrong. If negative feedback is delivered by other people who report that your impressions are insufficient, this "awareness" will again often be met by incredulity, since one cannot see that an impression exists. How can someone else tell you to change an impression that you feel quite confident does not exist? While motivated reasoning and confirmation bias make all types of impressions sticky, implicit impressions have this extra layer of stickiness caused by their invisibility. It is hard to motivate the change of an impression if one is not aware the impression exists, let alone not aware that it is insufficient.

Bias Awareness as an Intervention Goal

Implicit impressions are "invisible" impressions and difficult to bring into view. However, a special class of implicit impressions will *resist* being brought into the light. There is motivation to keep them in the shadows and avoid awareness. This class of impression relates to information that poses a potential threat to the self. Implicit stereotyping and prejudice (aversive forms of racism and sexism) pose such a threat. Such individual-level biases can contribute to structural racism and racial disparities at the societal level (e.g., Department of Justice, 2016; Fisher & Borgida, 2012; Hansen, 2003). The very impressions that have the largest social significance, the impressions that people should have strong imperatives to change, may be the impressions that people are most motivated to keep invisible, creating an even larger obstacle to change (e.g., Devine, Forscher, Austin, & Cox, 2012; Greenwald, Poehlman, Uhlmann, & Banaji, 2009; Kaiser & Miller, 2001; Monteith, Mark, & Ashburn-Nardo, 2010; Moskowitz & Vitriol, 2022; Perry, Murphy, & Dovidio, 2015; Plant & Devine, 2009).

Why is there incentive to keep these particular implicit impressions outside of awareness (and thus increasing their stickiness)? Expressions of racial prejudice are socially unacceptable, so people become avoidant of having such a threatening impression exposed (e.g., Crandall, Eshelman, & O'Brien, 2002; Dovidio & Gaertner, 2000; Frantz, Cuddy, Burnett, Ray, & Hart, 2004). Indeed, people can be so motivated to see egalitarian goals as self-defining that their selective attention will filter out feedback to the contrary (e.g., Jost & Banaji, 1994; Moskowitz, 2002; Moskowitz, Gollwitzer, Wasel, & Schaal, 1999; O'Brien et al., 2010). And when others attempt to provide feedback that makes one aware of that bias, it is not accepted since it is diametrically opposed to one's self-image. One strategy that people use to avoid becoming aware of their implicit bias is to define racial prejudice as requiring deliberation and malicious intent; to focus on racism as caused by "bad people" like those in the Ku Klux Klan (KKK) who aspire to have terrible intentions. Such narrow definitions of prejudice make it impossible for one to become aware of it in the self, since the self does not fit the narrow definition (e.g., Bobo, Kluegel, & Smith, 1997; Kaiser & Miller, 2001; Norton, Vandello, et al., 2008; Sommers & Norton, 2006).

For all of these reasons, policymakers, CEOs, law enforcement, educational institutions, health professionals, and many other industries have invested substantial resources on interventions that hope to reduce implicit bias by making people *aware* of implicit bias. There are, no doubt, cynical reasons to introduce interventions: fear of legal action, window dressing to merely appear as if diversity initiatives are important, a cash grab in a burgeoning "diversity industry." But a well-intentioned reason to do so is to increase aware-ness of implicit impressions, with the operating assumption that such awareness will motivate compensatory responding in the form of lowered bias and behavior change. The goal is to get people in a negative feedback loop so that they seek to reduce their bias and hence remove the negative feedback that bias exists. For such interventions to work they must be able to convince skeptical people that there is an influence on them that they can-not see. For all of the reasons stated above, this can be more challenging than it sounds. People resist such information (since it is threatening), leaving a first impression not only unchanged but perhaps reinforced by such attempts at awareness raising, as people dig in (making a first impression stickier). This does suggest that interventions can easily back-fire. The conclusion, however, should not be to forsake interventions because science says they fail. A science-based approach would, instead, be to create interventions that do not make people defensive. What fails are poorly constructed interventions that threaten and engender backlash.

Defensiveness is one type of motivated reasoning in reaction to feedback about bias where the person resists the conclusions and consequences suggested by the feedback. A common type of reaction of resistance to manage the result-ing negative emotions and threats to self-image is (1) the dis-missal of the feedback itself as trivial and unimportant, (2) criticism of the methods used to provide the evidence or so-called facts provided by the feedback, (3) undermining the credibility of the entire field of study responsible for the feed-back and the "experts" who are the source of the feedback, and (4) derogating the deliverer of the feedback (the messen-ger) as purveyors of "fake news" or the "lamestream media." The defensive response manifests as derogating the informa-tion and questioning its credibility, perhaps even embracing conspiracy theories that devalue it. Resistance is a common reaction to feedback about unconscious bias, with peo-ple derogating the source of the information, questioning its credibility, and overestimat-ing the extent to which one is unbiased relative to other people (Czopp, Monteith, & Mark, 2006; Hillard, Ryan, & Gervais, 2013; Howell et al., 2013; Howell, Gaither, & Ratliff, 2015; Howell & Ratliff, 2017; Shepperd, Malone, & Sweeny, 2008; Spencer, Fein, Wolfe, Fong, & Dunn, 1998; Vitriol & Moskowitz, 2021). This is an unfortunate possible consequence, one where bias awareness has the opposite of the desired result: enhancing (rather than reduc-ing) a first impression by making people reduce (rather than increase) their motivation for prejudice regulation and strengthening barriers that protect the first impression (e.g., Duguid & Thomas-Hunt, 2015; Legault, Gutsell, & Inzlicht, 2011; Moskowitz & Vitriol, 2022).

Defensiveness: One type of motivated reasoning in reaction to feedback about bias where the person resists the conclusions the feedback suggests. This may take the form of (1) dismissing the feedback as trivial, (2) criticizing the methods and "experts" used to gather evidence, and (3) derogating the deliverer of the feedback.

There are many instances where instead of feedback creating the awareness of bias needed to motivate change of a biased impression, it creates defensiveness. Perry et al. (2015) explored this issue by identifying people who differed in their **bias awareness**. People high in bias awareness are those with a willingness to accept feedback about their own implicit biases. People low in bias awareness are those who become defensive to such feedback and reject it. These two types of people were provided with feedback that told them that they did poorly on a test of implicit bias. White participants high in bias awareness were found to react to the feedback by becoming motivated to pursue egalitarian goals and meet soci-etal standards regarding fairness and justice. They accepted the validity of the feedback and indicated a desire to change their biased impressions toward Black Americans. How-ever, participants who lacked bias awareness showed no such motivation to change their impression. They denied such an impression existed. Some have used the value-laden label "fragility" to describe such people and this set of processes (e.g., Ford, Green, & Gross, 2022). Rather than embrace a new term, we prefer to continue to use the more descriptive *defensiveness*. Identifying whether people respond with defensiveness versus heightened bias awareness is an important issue. If bias awareness is or is not heightened in an individual, it can impact the person's motivation to change their bias.

> **Bias awareness:** A heightened recognition in a person that they perhaps have acted in biased ways that are not temporary, arbitrary, or pressured by the situation. It is an awareness that their behavior is not always fair, and that this is worthy of concern, rather than being dismissed as trivial. This awareness requires acknowledging that one has goals and traits that cause one's inequitable responding—one has dispositional culpability. This might motivate one to not only change behavior, but see a disposition in need of change.

Rothman et al. (2022) explored this by providing feedback to research participants that they have implicit bias. Rothman et al. showed that some people react to the feedback with heightened bias awareness, others do not, consistent with Perry et al. (2015). In addition, when bias awareness does not exist, the first impression sticks and there is little motivation expressed to change it. Instead, people are defensive about it and show reduced support for policy initiatives that advocate for interventions to reduce implicit bias in law enforcement and organizational contexts (see the bottom path of Figure 6.4). However, when the feedback leads to heightened bias awareness, people express the intention to change their biased behavior. They feel guilty about their shortcomings in this domain, motivating them to accept that they must do better, and to align their policy beliefs with initiatives that will reduce structural racism (see the top path of Figure 6.4). There are many illustrations of how feedback about bias can successfully minimize bias, leading people to change an implicit first impression that has been brought into the light. This, however, is met with the reality that attempts to bring bias into the light can at other times create backlash and deepen/polarize biases. We suggest that practitioners should not conclude that attempts to reduce bias are just as likely to fail and worsen events as they are to make things better. Rather, the science is complicated and interventions can fail if left in the hands of people lacking expertise and if relying on strategies that are not tested. Feedback about bias has the potential to introduce threat and defensiveness, but this is not a necessity (e.g., Doriscar, Perry, & Gardner, 2024). Feedback can change implicit impressions, even implicit stereotyping and impression.

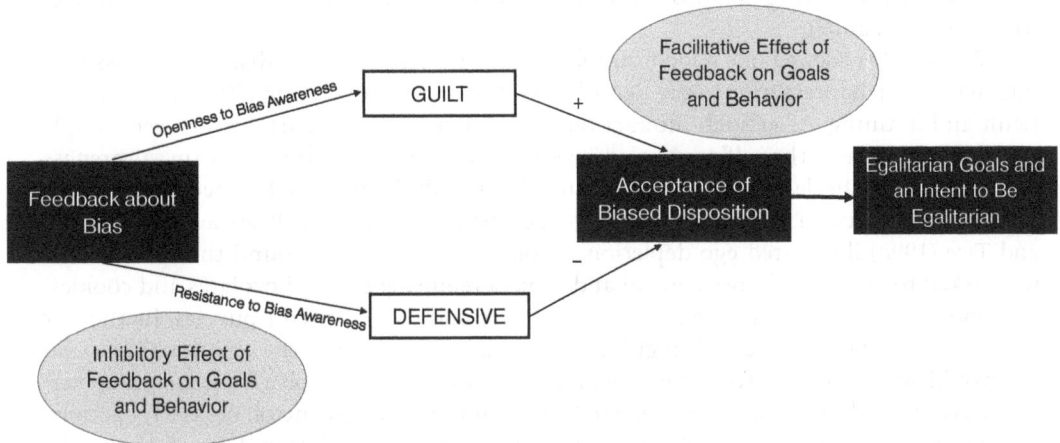

FIGURE 6.4. Feedback about bias can produce motivated change or motivated defensiveness.

THE BLOCKING OF EFFORTFUL PROCESSING
HELPS IMPLICIT INFERENCES TO STICK

Correction models start with awareness, and awareness creates motivation. However, it is often the case that even when a person is motivated and intends to act, they do not act. Even if motivated to exert the effort, we may not be *able* to exert the effort. The negative feedback loop model describes people as becoming motivated to initiate a compensatory response or control action. But what if one is unable to engage in that response? What if appropriate action is blocked? There are two dominant reasons one may fail to exert effort even when one wants to. The first is when one is feeling drained of the energy to do so. The second is when an external obstacle, such as cognitive load or time pressure, prevents one from doing so. Each can block correction, leaving an implicit impression intact because one cannot perform the desired response.

Ego Depletion

A first reason it is difficult to overturn an implicit first impression is that one may have exhausted the physical and mental energy in one's pool of regulatory resources; there are constraints to executive functioning, and these may get drained. When a person is so depleted that the resource for self-regulation has been usurped, then a temporary loss in self-control results that is known as **ego depletion** (e.g., Baumeister, Bratslavsky, Muraven, & Tice, 1998; Gailliot, Plant, Butz, & Baumeister, 2007; Vohs & Heatherton, 2000). A common metaphor used to describe this is muscle fatigue. We all have personal experience that using a particular muscle too much will result in the inability to adequately use it until the muscle is replenished and energy is restored. Though not a muscle, control also fatigues. Ego depletion is not restricted to the specific domain responsible for the depletion but is a general loss of self-control. For example, straining to monitor one's verbal and nonverbal behavior during an interaction can be effortful and this might impact one's regulatory ability in a totally different domain, such as controlling the desire to eat a tempting treat, or correcting an initially incorrect first impression (e.g., Richeson et al., 2003).

Ego depletion: The idea that resources for engaging in self-regulation are limited and can drain. One may exhaust the physical and mental energy in one's pool of regulatory resources so that executive functioning is tapped and resources for self-regulation usurped. This results in a temporary loss in self-control until resources can refresh.

We already reviewed one good example of this in Chapter 3 when discussing cross-race interaction. Such interactions were described by Richeson and Shelton (2007) as being difficult and draining. After such interactions were complete, their participants were simply less able to engage in the self-regulation processes that they wanted to perform. Awareness of a bias existed, the desire to correct it existed, but the ability to do so had been drained out of the participants. In a separate series of experiments, Baumeister, Bratslavsky, Muraven, and Tice (1998) illustrated ego depletion. In one experiment they found that people who were asked to exert regulatory control and avoid a tempting treat (chocolates and cookies) were more likely to give up when later asked to try and solve difficult puzzles. In another experiment they found that self-regulating caused by suppressing the emotional reaction one would ordinarily have to an emotional film led people to later solve fewer anagram puzzles (as compared to people who expressed their emotions). Self-control, or control actions taken during goal pursuit, can drain the resources for goal regulation. Even if drained by the exertion of effort when pursuing a control action on one task, this can leave one unable to control or correct on another task. The "tank is empty."

Cognitive Load

A second reason it is difficult to overturn an implicit first impression when motivated to do so is that one may be prevented from exerting the effort to do so by another task. While the first impression may be efficient, the correction process is not. Thus, the correction process can be constrained by other ongoing mental activity. A good example of this was provided in Chapter 3 when discussing automatic processes. Bargh and Thein (1985) had participants learn information about a person while under cognitive load. Their ability to use that information to form an explicit impression was prevented by the cognitive load. However, the cognitive load did not undermine the continued use of an implicit first impression. The implicit impression persisted despite cognitive load, while the effortful processing of information was disrupted.

Gilbert, Pelham, and Krull (1988) provided a clear illustration of how cognitive load contributes to first impression stickiness. They argued that people would form impressions that invoked a trait quickly and effortlessly (as shown by research on spontaneous trait inference). Next, they reasoned that if learning new information was more effortful—such as learning it when under cognitive load—then even if motivated to change the first impression, they would be unable to do so. In a clever experiment, they had research participants watch a video, with the audio turned off, of a woman in a conversation with a man. The woman is sending nonverbal signals of clearly being anxious. As expected, participants form a first impression that she is an anxious person. Next, participants learn new information that should invalidate the first impression. They learn that the conversation was about an extremely anxiety-provoking topic: The woman was asked to discuss her sexual fantasies with the male stranger. This new information should correct the first impression; she is not an anxious person but in an anxiety-provoking situation. Yet, this does not happen when the participant is experiencing cognitive load. Despite the clear existence of information that suggests correcting the first impression, it persists. Gilbert et al. argue that cognitive load prevents participants from including the new information into their impression. To correct the first impression requires effort, and the cognitive load disables the correction process. Despite awareness of the impression being biased and the motivation to change it, it sticks.[2]

Time Pressure

A similar illustration of first impressions persisting due to one being unable to correct the first impression is seen in research where there is a time constraint that blocks the correction process. A first impression forms easily, but then persists when time does not allow for the effort to update it. In one example, Jaeger et al. (2020) had research participants play a game where they needed to decide to trust (or not) a partner. They received pictures of the partner's face and a payoff scheme that told them how to maximize their earnings if they followed the scheme in a rational way. When the participants were placed under a time constraint, they were unable to use the rational decision rules. They were, however, able to form implicit impressions about their partner's trustworthiness from their face and made decisions about whether to trust them using this intuitive response. The rational and explicit decision was harder to make and disabled by the time pressure. The implicit first impression was able to persist despite the constraints. Another example was provided in an experiment using teachers by Kruglanski and Freund (1983).

Stereotypes, such as the example that started this chapter of people with criminal records being untrustworthy, form easily and implicitly. Part of the reason they stick is because we cannot correct them even if we want to. Kruglanski and Freund (1983) argued that teachers would be motivated to grade their students fairly, but would have first impressions guided by stereotypes, and might instinctively see a paper as inferior because of such stereotypes. Their motivation to do their job well and be fair might overcome this, but what if they were unable to engage the processing to overcome this? Time constraints while grading might make a teacher who is otherwise fair succumb to biases they do not even see that they possess. To test this, they asked teachers to grade papers that were either written by a member of one's own social group, or by a student from a disliked other group. The hypotheses were that (1) the implicit first impression would be that members of one's own group are superior to people from other groups; and (2) if given ample time, the teachers would overcome this bias and grade the papers correctly, but if under time pressure, their biased first impression would persist. Kruglanski and Freund placed half of their research participants under "time pressure" by asking them to grade essays within an extremely short time frame. The other half were not placed under time pressure. All of the teachers then were given the same essay to grade. Half of the essays were said to be written by a student who belonged to the same ingroup as the teacher, and half were written by an outgroup member. As predicted, when there was ample time to grade, the essays were rated identically regardless of what type of student wrote it. Teachers were fair. However, when time constraints existed, bias emerged so that the student from the teacher's ingroup received a higher grade. The implicit first impression was not corrected and the final grade reflected the biases that existed implicitly. A second experiment replicated this idea using primacy effects instead of stereotypes: when under time pressure the information learned first about a job candidate had a biasing influence on the decision to hire (if not pressured, employers considered all of the information appropriately).

REPEATEDLY REINFORCING AN IMPLICIT INFERENCE

Gregg et al. (2006) and Wyer (2010) each showed that after new information was learned, and an explicit impression was changed accordingly (the Niffites were now reported to be good), the implicit impressions formed based on the initial information were still intact. There were persistent negative associations to the person or group (the Niffites) who was originally learned to be negative (see also Petty & Briñol, 2010). Rydell and McConnell (2006) also showed that explicit impressions of a person could change quickly and easily from small amounts of contradictory information, but also showed that the implicit impression could change as well. However, it required learning an enormous amount of such contradictory information for the implicit impression to unstick. New associations can be forged if there is ample information.

The Associative–Propositional Evaluation Model

One explanation as to why implicit impressions are harder to overturn than explicit ones is that implicit impressions form through **associative learning** that allow an impression to develop ties to a person or group. As reviewed in Chapter 2, associations are links among related representations in memory, and these associations can vary in strength. Stronger associations allow the links to be traversed more easily, and for one representation in memory to be activated (or inhibited) more quickly once the other is triggered. For example, if the group Niffites is activated, it triggers the associated negative affect. Such associations are not only excitatory and cause the retrieval of the linked representation but can be inhibitory and block the retrieval of the linked representation (see Gawronski et al., 2018, for a review of associative learning). This network of associative links among related items in memory means that an implicit impression (such as negative affect) can be repeatedly triggered outside of conscious awareness each time an associated person or group is encountered (such as a Niffite) through processes of spreading activation among associations. This would serve to strengthen the association, reinforcing the link that binds the two together. This creates stickiness not

> **Associative learning:** When two constructs represented in memory are connected so that associative links form that tie them together. Associative links among related representations can vary in strength. Stronger associations allow links to be traversed more easily, and for one representation to be activated (or inhibited) more quickly once the other activates.

only because the association is reinforced, but because new information, especially limited amounts of information, might struggle to disrupt those strong associations. Even if the new information strongly contradicts the old learning (Niffites are actually good), it would be possible that the already formed association to negative affect would be triggered despite the new learning—that is, while being told that a Niffite is good can be consciously noted, at the unconscious level the exposure to the group "Niffite" triggers the association to the already-existing implicit impression (they are bad).

Gawronski and Bodenhausen (2006) proposed an important idea that moved impression formation away from this strictly associative learning model. They proposed an **associative–propositional evaluation (APE) model** that posits that impression formation is also driven by **propositional learning**. Propositional learning refers to the fact that more than an association between two constructs (such as a link that connects the construct "skin lotion" to the construct "rash") exists. There is also information about the *relationship* among the content that gets stored in memory (e.g., Gawronski & Bodenhausen, 2014; Hu, Gawronski, & Balas, 2017). One knows that lotion *soothes* a rash (a positive relationship exists among the two constructs in the association). Propositional learning contains information about cause and effect, or proposes a direction to a relationship among associated constructs. This is an important distinction. Association would mean that whenever one had a rash (a negative event) and one applied lotion, this would create a link between the negative outcome (rash) and lotion. The association would not capture the fact that the lotion was being used to alleviate the negative event. One would just associate a negative event with the lotion. Thoughts of lotion would then always trigger bad feelings (rash thoughts).

> **Associative–propositional evaluation (APE) model:** A model of impression formation that posits that attitudes and beliefs are driven not merely by associative links and spreading activation, but also by propositional learning.
>
> **Propositional learning:** When two constructs represented in memory are specified as having a relationship so that their representations contain information about cause and effect, or propose a direction to the relationship among the constructs. This refers to the fact that theories specify more than an association among two mental representations.

In impressions about people this would be the equivalent of associating feelings of discomfort or guilt or anxiety with a particular group (say police officers). This same association would exist just as strongly for someone who held the proposition that officers remove danger and crime (where the cause for the feelings of anxiety and threat is the crime that the officers prevent) as it would for someone who held the proposition that officers are the cause for one feeling anxiety and threat (because they abuse their power). An association alone would suggest both groups of people would have negative feelings triggered when encountering a police officer. A propositional model would suggest different reactions for one person versus the other person who held a different proposition. Stereotypes could work the same way. If we live in a culture that associates Black men with crime and violence, then these negative beliefs will be triggered when we think of Black men. One person could believe that Black men cause violence and are more threatening, and another could hold the proposition that society places Black men in more threatening and violent environments that are the cause of the association, and a third person could believe that the association between the two constructs is totally fabricated by the culture and is not real. Yet all three groups would have the negative association triggered equally despite their very different beliefs about the group. The groups would differ in the type of propositional reasoning in which they engage, not the associations triggered.

It has been suggested that propositional reasoning is far less likely for implicit processes, creating the possibility for associations to run amuck for implicit impressions. Associations would be constantly triggered and reinforced unknowingly, regardless of whether the evidence suggests a proposition that would shift the evaluation (such as lotion = good, or stereotype = wrong). This relatively greater associative processing and reduced propositional learning would make an implicit first impression stronger and more persistent than an explicit impression. Where the explicit impression could be reversed based on the propositional learning, the implicit impression would be bolstered based on the associative links. A contrast is being suggested between explicit impressions and implicit impressions, one in which the power of associations that are learned early is greater with implicit impressions. For explicit impressions it has been suggested that propositional learning has greater impact. Hu et al. (2017) provided a demonstration of this distinction between associations and propositions and their relationship to implicit versus explicit impressions. When a health product (lotion) co-occurred with a negative health condition (rash), the research participants made explicit judgments that reflected the propositional learning. When the lotion mitigated a rash, they had a positive impression; if the lotion caused a rash, they had a negative impression. But implicit impressions showed no such relationship to cause and effect (see Figure 6.5). The association "lotion–rash" led to a negative impression regardless of whether the association was caused by lotion curing or causing a rash.

This discussion is not meant to imply that implicit impressions reflect only associations and cannot be impacted by propositions, or that explicit impressions never are impacted by associative learning (e.g., De Houwer, 2014a, 2014b; Gawronski & Bodenhausen, 2018; Kurdi & Banaji, 2023). There is not a strict separation of processing systems (associative vs. propositional) for each mode of processing (implicit vs. explicit) being suggested. While implicit impressions are harder to change than explicit impressions (which are already hard to change), updating is not impossible, and in some cases can be quite simple to change due to propositional learning. We later (in Chapter 13) discuss how propositions and associations can promote the updating of first impressions, even removing some of the stickiness of implicit impressions. For now, our focus is on why it is that implicit impressions may be more difficult to change, or are relatively stickier. And the suggestion is that a greater impact of associations, and a lesser impact of propositions, can cause this. Associations are easy to trigger, are reinforced or strengthened once triggered, get frequently triggered, and do so without one realizing it. These properties of associations give an implicit impression extra strength relative to an explicit impression.

Ironically, it could even be the case that when propositional reasoning has the ability to weaken an explicit impression, it can at the same time strengthen an implicit impression. Telling a person "your stereotype is wrong" (as Gregg et al., 2006, did with Niffites and Luupites) can get them to reverse the explicit impression, but may serve to activate the original association and strengthen the implicit impression it was hoping to overturn. Galinsky and

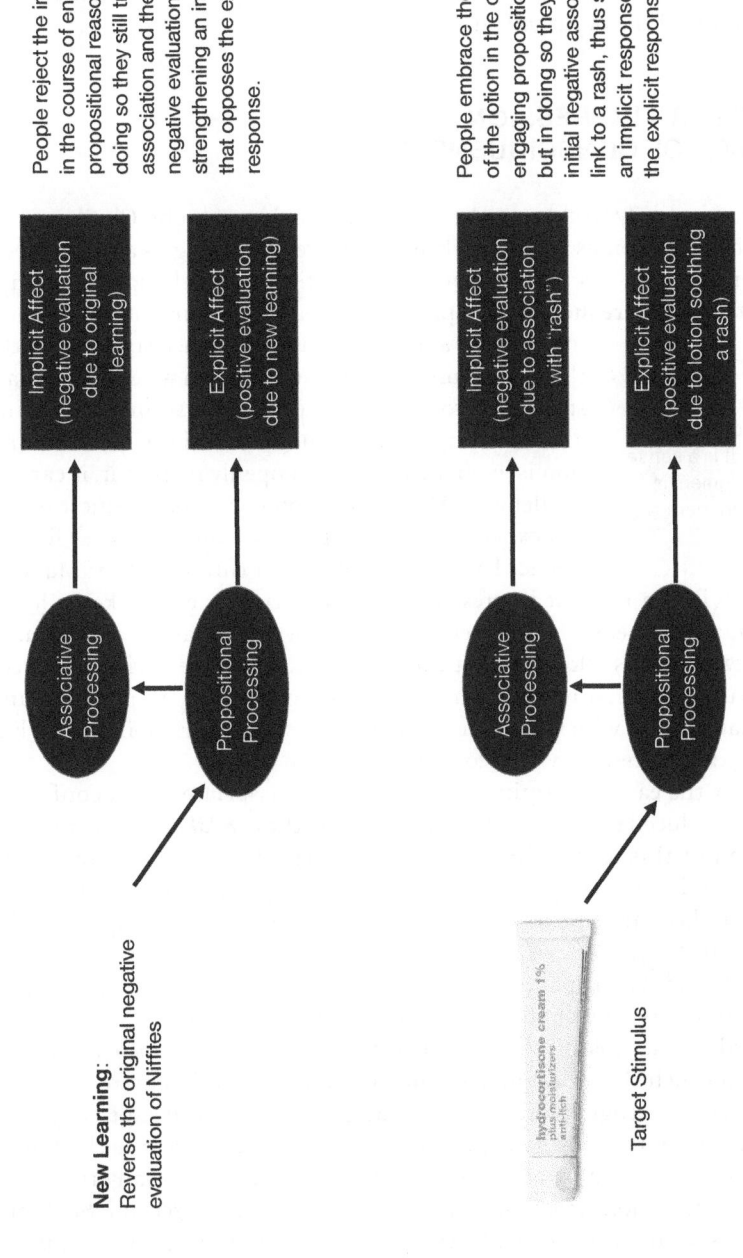

FIGURE 6.5. Two examples of the association–propositional evaluation model.

209

Moskowitz (2000b, 2007), as well as Macrae, Bodenhausen, et al. (1994), showed this with stereotypes. Across these several experiments the research participants were asked *to not use a stereotype* when forming an impression of a person (such as an old man). The explicit impression expressed was relatively void of stereotypic thoughts. However, the implicit stereotype was strongly activated. A lexical decision task showed heightened activation of words associated with the stereotype despite the cause for activation being a proposition to undo the association. The explicit act of not using a stereotype strengthened implicit associations and reinforced the negative stereotype of the group.

CONFIDENCE IN AN IMPRESSION
DESPITE A LACK OF CONSCIOUSNESS

Impressions are most likely to change when they are called into doubt. Chaiken et al. (1989) described a first impression as being unlikely to be altered as long as a person feels confident in the impression, and in the consequences resulting from relying on the impression. Imagine a **confidence threshold** that specifies a desired amount of confidence for an impression, and as long as confidence stays above that level, the first impression will stick. When we experience a sense of struggling to form an impression it seems less accurate than when the impression comes to mind easily. When an impression is explicit, and we can openly inspect it, it can be openly challenged. We can question it, others can question it, and we can experience doubt. There are opportunities for one's confidence level to slip below that threshold (e.g., Maheswaran & Chaiken, 1991). With an implicit impression, the inability to see it makes it less open to such inspection, and the ease with which it forms provides an air of confidence. Acting together, these two reasons allow implicit impressions to sit above this confidence threshold. Thus, a final reason that implicit impressions are more likely to persist than explicit impression is that the ease with which they form lends a sense of credibility; a lack of struggle in producing the impression yields confidence in it.

> **Confidence threshold:** The point at which one feels as if a judgment, belief, attitude, or decision is sufficient and valid enough. It is a sense of confidence that the judgment is sufficient and one need not perseverate on it any longer.

The idea that the ease of forming an impression is associated with confidence in its truth was first introduced in Chapter 4 when reviewing the *availability heuristic*. In an interesting illustration of this idea, Schwarz, Bless, et al. (1991) asked some research participants to describe a dozen examples from their past of a particular personality trait (e.g., being outgoing). Other participants were asked to describe only six examples. Logically, the more examples you can generate, the more the trait should be seen as true of you. Yet this is not what was found. Participants who listed only six examples were more likely to say the trait in question was true of them (e.g., they rated themselves as more outgoing than people who listed 12 examples). Why? Because 12 examples were *harder* to generate than six. The ease with which the six examples came to mind made them more confident it was a true impression than struggling to yield 12 examples. This logic is especially relevant for impressions formed from faces, where implicit impressions feel more true than impressions formed from propositional information that is objectively and rationally true. Recall that people form first impressions from faces in as little as a tenth of a second. Such processing ease makes the associated traits confidently held to be true, and exerts an impact on how a person is judged. Implicit impressions present no sense of struggle—the ease with which they come to mind creates a confidence that the information is true.

Implicit Learning Creates a Confidently Held Impression

Amodio (2019) makes the case for observational learning to be one manner in which implicit impressions form. We perceivers can observe an interaction between two other people, such as a manager favoring one employee over another. We then learn that association between the employee and competence even though it is based on the manager's actions, not any behavior on the part of the employee. We implicitly learn an impression held by the manager, and then we misattribute this learning to the employee and infer they are competent. This misattribution process in observational learning can occur even if the employee is not competent and the manager is simply biased in favor of this person. The actual qualities are deemed less relevant due to the implicit learning that we easily and quickly misattribute to the person. The perceiver's impression feels veridical about the target, even though it is a misattribution of the treatment of the person by their interaction partner. The implicit nature of the misattribution makes the perceiver feel confident that this quality is truly held by the target.

Schultner, Lindström, Cikara, and Amodio (2024) illustrate this in the choices made when the perceiver later has an opportunity to choose with whom they will interact. When the partner in the first interaction shows bias toward a target, the observer then shows the same bias to the target, even if more money would be earned in the perceiver's interaction with the target by avoiding this bias. So strong is their confidence in the judgment that it overrides a financial incentive to overturn it. They argue that this is one way in which prejudice develops and persists. Our impressions become biased in a negative way by the impressions we infer about a target based on how they are treated by others – we confidently perceive genuine group differences despite all that has occurred is implicit learning that some people dislike individual group members. Misattributing that inference to the group, implicitly, has the consequence of making that impression feel strong and unlikely to be changed (e.g., Amodio et al., 2008).

The Sufficiency Principle:
The Amount of Confidence in an Impression Must Be Sufficient

If it is true that implicit impressions persist because they are confidently held, at what point will confidence not be sufficient and the impression reassessed or changed? If there is a confidence threshold, why is it that implicit impressions often sit above that threshold? Chaiken et al. (1989) proposed what they called a *sufficiency principle*, which asserts that for whatever task a person is confronted with—whether it be forming an impression of someone, planning how to act toward someone, forming an attitude, making a decision, or simply comprehending information—there is a point at which one feels that the task has been sufficiently performed. Once they feel the task has been completed, they can move on to the next task at hand. This point is said to be achieved when the individual feels *confident that they have sufficiently performed the task* that was set before them. As noted above, this point of sufficient confidence that allows for a feeling of task completion can be conceived of as a threshold. We may not (in fact, we likely typically do not) desire to always have extreme confidence in what we say and do. The sufficiency principle allows us to conceive of the threshold at which we feel confident enough in our thoughts and actions to be set anywhere we choose, and is subject to change from situation to situation. We are sometimes happy simply to have moderate amounts of confidence in the judgments and feelings we possess, so long as we feel it is *enough* confidence to warrant relying on those judgments in our interactions. When evaluating a TV commercial or a stranger at the market we may feel relatively confident in the opinion we form despite barely listening to what is being said to us. Yet when evaluating a new love interest we may cling to the person's every word with an effort and detail that we might not have known we possessed. We seek to feel extremely confident that our responses to this person are accurate and appropriate, so we set a high threshold for deciding when our thoughts and feelings are sufficient.

The sufficiency principle asserts that people must exert *enough* effort in how they think about a target of judgment to reach the threshold. If people desire the feeling that their judgments are good enough, they will only rely on less effort in forming judgments if doing so delivers to them a sense of *judgmental confidence*. For the most part, first impressions, relying on what comes to mind easily or first, or fast evaluations will produce sufficient enough responses that allow us to navigate through social interactions. A judgment based on relatively little effort and implicit processing is good enough. To the degree that relying on such little effort leaves us feeling sufficiently confident that we have acted in a reasonable manner, then we do not need to engage in any further processing. However, if such processing is experienced as producing inadequate actions, judgments, or feelings—level of confidence in the judgments produced falls short of the threshold—one will exert more effort and continue

> **Confidence gap:** A state where the current level of confidence in one's judgment, based on one's current processing effort, is less than the desired level of confidence. This motivates one to engage in deeper processing, until effort yields a sufficiently good judgment.

working on the task until a feeling of sufficiency is achieved and the threshold is surpassed. This produces what is known as a **confidence gap**, where the current level of confidence in one's judgment, based on one's current processing effort, is less than the desired level of confidence. This motivates one to engage in deeper processing, until effort yields a sufficiently good judgment that eliminates the confidence gap by producing a judgment that rises above the threshold (see Figure 6.6).

For example, one may hold an implicit stereotype that people who are politically liberal do not oppose abortion. One may infer this quality simply when a cue—the other person's liberalism—is detected and feel confident it is true, even if one does not dedicate any conscious effort to thinking about it. This allows one to have inferences that seem reasonable enough, and that allow one to plan behavior that will yield a smooth and trouble-free encounter. Thinking "less" yields sufficient inferences that generate successful social behavior. This is depicted at Time 1 of Figure 6.6. However, if one's confidence in relying on this stereotype is made low when discovering new information about the person (e.g., when encountering a "pro-life" liberal), one's judgment will feel insufficient. This reduces confidence in one's judgment, creating a confidence gap that will lead to increased processing effort. This is depicted at Time 2 of Figure 6.6. One must now initiate more elaborate forms of evaluating until one has produced a judgment that feels sufficient (is reasonable enough to rely on). One's confidence in a judgment must catapult over the sufficiency threshold. This is depicted at Time 3 of Figure 6.6.

In this hydraulic-like model, the energy that drives the updating of a faulty first impression is a pressure to have greater confidence in the sufficiency of the judgment and to remove feelings of doubt. If an implicit first impression is one in which we have relatively little confidence in, this *confidence gap* is said to motivate the individual to increase processing effort and change the first impression. Some trade-off must be struck between the goal of exerting least effort and the goal of having judgments one is sufficiently confident in. However, if the first impression feels sufficiently good and if we have confidence in it, then it need not change and no trade-off needs to be struck. The argument is that an implicit first impression is often confidently held and is experienced as sufficiently good. Thus, no motivation to change it is generated.

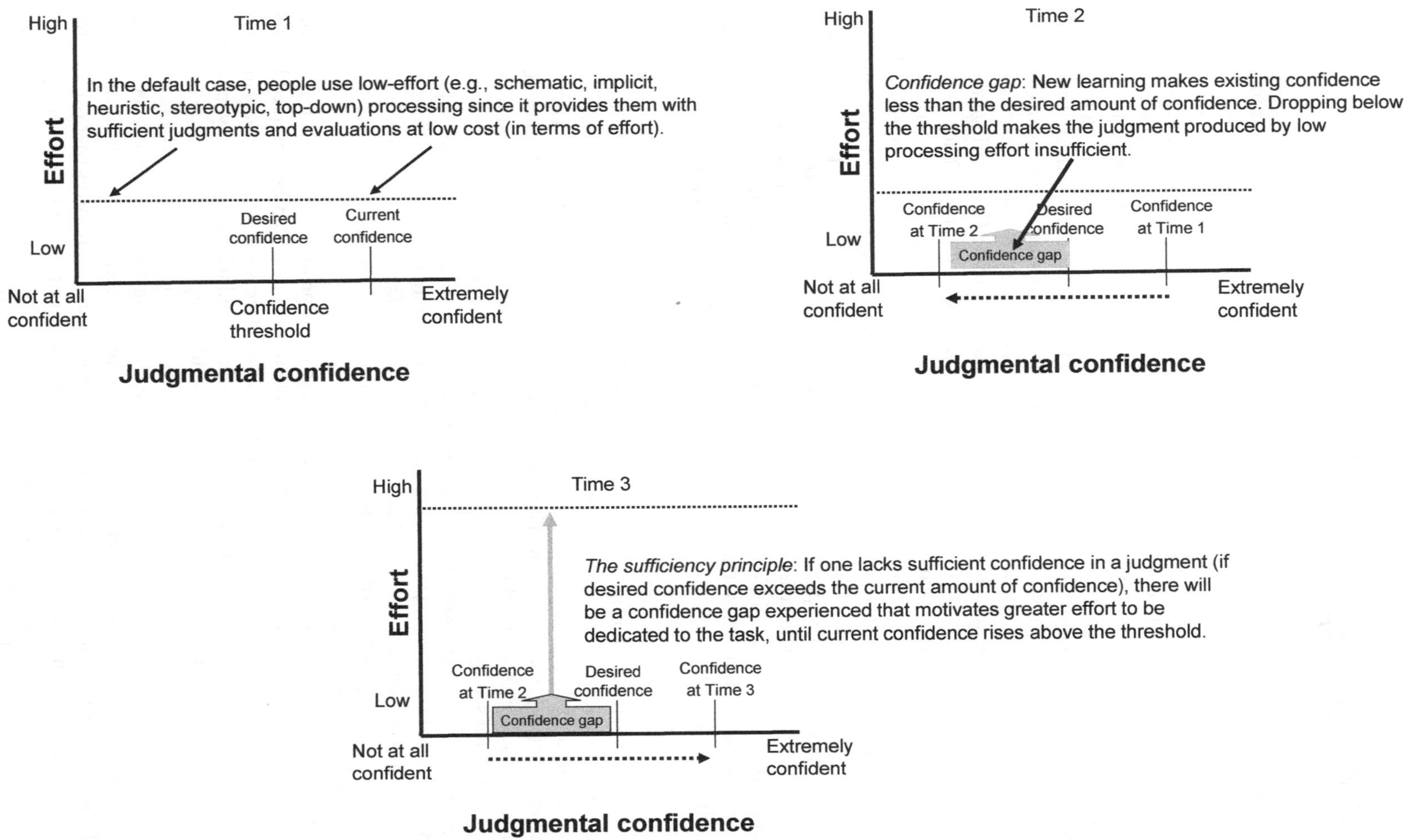

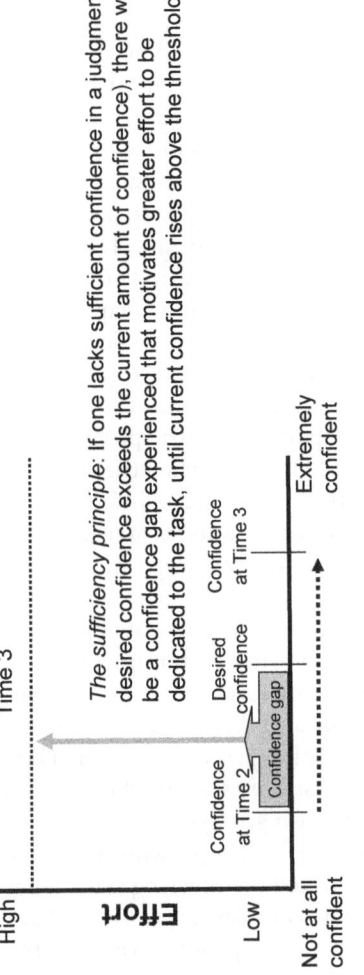

Time 1

In the default case, people use low-effort (e.g., schematic, implicit, heuristic, stereotypic, top-down) processing since it provides them with sufficient judgments and evaluations at low cost (in terms of effort).

Desired confidence — Current confidence

Confidence threshold

High — Low — Not at all confident — Extremely confident

Effort

Judgmental confidence

Time 2

Confidence gap: New learning makes existing confidence less than the desired amount of confidence. Dropping below the threshold makes the judgment produced by low processing effort insufficient.

Confidence at Time 2 — Desired confidence — Confidence at Time 1

Confidence gap

High — Low — Not at all confident — Extremely confident

Effort

Judgmental confidence

Time 3

The sufficiency principle: If one lacks sufficient confidence in a judgment (if desired confidence exceeds the current amount of confidence), there will be a confidence gap experienced that motivates greater effort to be dedicated to the task, until current confidence rises above the threshold.

Confidence at Time 2 — Desired confidence — Confidence at Time 3

Confidence gap

High — Low — Not at all confident — Extremely confident

Effort

Judgmental confidence

FIGURE 6.6. The relationship between judgmental confidence and processing effort.

CONFIRMATION BIAS AND MOTIVATED REASONING
WITH IMPLICIT INFERENCES

This chapter has focused on the reasons first impressions persist that are unique to implicit impressions. However, this does not mean that implicit impressions are not rendered sticky for other reasons, such as those that applied to the stickiness of explicit impressions. Rather than provide an exhaustive review, this chapter ends simply by providing an illustration that confirmation bias and motivated reasoning each occur with implicit impressions.

To illustrate confirmation bias, we can once again use stereotyping as an example. However, now the illustration must be of a wholly implicit process. A stereotype that gets triggered when group membership is detected (such as from body and facial cues) can influence an implicit impression, such as an STI or an automatic attitude, resulting in the qualities associated with the group being confirmed. For example, both Wigboldus et al. (2003) and Ramos, Garcia-Marques, Hamilton, Ferreira, and Van Acker (2012) triggered group stereotypes using occupations (such as professors and trash collectors). They found that stereotypes, once triggered, shaped the type of traits that were implicitly inferred from a behavior. The implicit impression that emerged confirmed the stereotype. Specifically, in both studies this happened by participants failing to form trait inferences from behaviors that clearly implied the trait if that trait was inconsistent with the stereotype. For example, some participants read "the professor wins the science quiz" and spontaneously infer the trait "smart." However, when they read "the garbage collector wins the science quiz" they do not make this spontaneous inference. The impression that they are smart does not form. The implicit impressions form in a way that does not merely make sense of the behavior but that coheres to the stereotype and confirms it. This despite the fact that both the triggering of the stereotype and the impression that is formed are implicit.

As an example of motivated reasoning, my own research on STI has always been concerned with showing such impressions to be governed by motivation. Even impressions we do not realize we form are shaped by our goals. This is true of stereotypic inferences (Moskowitz, 2010), and this is true of trait inferences about individuals. Moskowitz (1993a) posited that STIs happen for a reason: They allow people to attain meaning, knowledge, and closure. This suggests a straightforward prediction: If it is a form of motivated reasoning, then people with stronger motivations should engage in this type of cognitive processing to a greater degree. People who chronically desire structure are presumably more practiced at, and interested in, inferring traits from behavior, rather than in suspending judgment or forming more complex impressions that include situational factors. Moskowitz found that the extent to which people formed STIs was determined by their chronic needs for prediction, control, and structure.

More recently, my colleagues and I showed that the type of spontaneous impression formed (a goal vs. a trait) is motivated. Some people infer traits from an observed behavior, other people see the same behavior and infer that it reflects the person's goals and not their traits. Olcaysoy Okten and Moskowitz (2020b) examined whether ideology motivated different types of implicit impressions. Conservative ideology is known to value personal responsibility, and accordingly conservative participants should not make goal inferences, but should form trait inferences spontaneously when learning about behavior (they should place causal responsibility in the person, and should do so even in the implicit inferences they form). In contrast, liberals are known to value looking at social forces that can impact people, which argues for readily seeing pressures from the situation. As such, liberal participants should make spontaneous goal inferences when learning about behaviors. To explore this, Olcaysoy Okten and Moskowitz used the false-recognition procedure for examining implicit inferences that was detailed in Chapter 4 (and in Figure 4.5). If an inference was made when reading a behavior, people should mistakenly recognize the word that represents that inference when later shown the word and asked whether they had seen it before. Such false recognitions will occur more to these critical words than matched control words. Higher false recognition indicates the critical word (a goal or a trait) was inferred spontaneously. The results revealed that motives shape these low-level inference processes in the predicted ways. Conservatives easily infer traits in others, but not goals. Liberals easily infer both goals and traits. Each group produced motivated explanations. Conservatives and liberals each see what they are motivated to see, despite the inference being implicit.

CONCLUSIONS

The chapter began with a review of various types of implicit impressions, followed by an exploration of reasons why implicit impressions stick, or are hard to update. A first observation is that we make many types of impressions without realizing it, and this invisibility makes them more difficult to change. The motivation to change is less likely if one is unaware that an impression exists and if the ease with which it was produced creates a false sense of confidence that one's impressions are accurate. Explicit ratings reflect explicit learning, yet implicit impressions persist even when the explicit ratings contradict them (e.g., Gregg et al., 2006; Peters & Gawronski, 2011; Petty & Briñol, 2010; Rydell & McConnell; 2006; Wyer, 2010). An implicit first impression is invisible and beyond introspection, and it remains in place even after explicit learning and self-reported impressions argue against it.

A second observation is that these different impression types each have the ability to shape what we see, and thus can strengthen a first impression by (1) reinforcing the associations that link people and groups to traits/attitudes/stereotypes, and (2) producing evidence that reinforces a first impression (through confirmation biases and motivated reasoning processes). A third observation is that these different types of impressions can each impact the stickiness of the others. For example, an implicit attitude that a person is positive might lead to the trait inference that their behavior is persistent as opposed to stubborn, or confident as opposed to arrogant. In this way, ambiguous behavior (that could be seen as either persistent or stubborn) becomes clear evidence of a trait that supports the positive first impression. As another example, a goal inference could enhance (or suppress) a trait inference. Inferring that a person had a goal to socialize can enhance seeing the trait of extraversion. In contrast, inferring that the same person merely wanted to look like they were socializing to have their boss form a positive impression might not enhance an inference about the trait "extravert" and could suppress it. As a last example, as we saw with stereotypes, inferring a trait might lead you to assume goals that are consistent with those traits are present as well (if the trait criminal is associated with a group, the goal to steal might be inferred as well).

NOTES

1. It is worthwhile to contemplate whether such findings show accuracy (with the amazing finding being that people need exceptionally little information to correctly identify good teachers!) versus bias (with the amazing finding being that no matter how much time you give people, and effort they could devote, they still use relatively little information to label someone a good

teacher). The original paper is pitched more in terms of the former interpretation. However, it is important to think about it from both perspectives.

2. What is especially clever is that Gilbert et al. (1988) understood that for this logic to work, participants must be aware of the new (and impression-inconsistent) information. To make sure they were aware, the load was introduced by having participants memorize the topics in the conversation. Thus, the very thing that caused the cognitive load was also the thing that made the participants aware that their first impression was biased (that the topic was extremely anxiety provoking).

CHAPTER 7

We Follow Rules
When Asking "Why?,"
Acting Like Intuitive Scientists

Why, man, he [Caesar] doth bestride the narrow world
Like a colossus, and we petty men
Walk under his huge legs, and peep about
To find ourselves dishonorable graves.
Men at some time are masters of their fates;
The fault, dear Brutus, is not in our stars,
But in ourselves, that we are underlings.
— SHAKESPEARE's *Julius Caesar*, Act I, Scene II,
Lines 135-141 (emphasis added)

This book began with a discussion of *why* making meaning is so central to human cognition. It is useful; it is pragmatic. It is useful to help us to know how to act. Some theorists believe it is useful for survival—that we need to detect danger to cope with it, and to approach stimuli that afford us a chance to pursue important goals. However, a concern with survival is not what separates humans from other animals. Rather, it is our *high-level ability to process information about the causes of events and to produce reasons and explanations.* We are constantly assessing why events have happened—not just to survive but to produce meaning. And while it is likely true that other animals have some of these capacities—traits that appear in one species likely do not reflect an evolutionary leap but appear in an altered (different, less than) form in other species—humans have a complex capacity to reason (not to disparage chimps, who have been shown to have a theory of mind and can make inferences about the goals of others; e.g., Call & Tomasello, 2008; Hare, 2011; Povinelli & Vonk, 2003). A similar argument is made regarding what separates humans from artificial intelligence. Writing for *The New York Times* on March 8, 2023, Noam Chomsky described

> the most critical capacity of any intelligence: to say not only what is the case, what was the case and what will be the case—that's description and prediction—but also what is not the case and what could and could not be the case. Those are the ingredients of explanation, the mark of true intelligence. (Chomsky, Roberts, & Watumull, 2023, Section A, p. 19)

In other words, while computerized intelligence can predict and describe, it cannot offer causal explanation; it cannot (currently) offer "counterfactual conjectures" and explain why an event or action occurred using "but for" logic: "The apple would not have fallen but for the force of gravity."

Heider (1944) stated that each new event in our environment is experienced as a disruption that needs a reason to explain it. We attempt to discover "why" the change has occurred, and adjust our actions accordingly. Consider the individuals who escaped from the World Trade Center's two towers on September 11, 2001, in the moments after the first plane hit and before there was a second attack. It was only their ability to infer the possible cause of the initial damage (or someone else's inference that was then conveyed to them either through an order to evacuate the building, or a friend's encouragement to do so) that allowed them to attribute the chaos to a threat, thus leading them to flee (even people in the as yet untouched second tower). In the Shakespearean quote at the beginning of this chapter, Cassius asks of Brutus, "Why?" Why do we allow Caesar to walk like a colossus? Why are we underlings? Is it internally caused? Is it externally caused by Caesar imposing his will, or by an uncontrollable fate (the fault lies in our stars)?

This pursuit of answers to "the why question" is found in reaction to the smallest of changes to our environment (e.g., a piece of paper falls off the desk) to more complex changes (e.g., the building next to you is on fire following an explosion). For small changes the answer may be easily attained (the window was open and a gust of wind had blown the paper), for more complex changes we may wrestle with finding the answer (though there is no rule requiring that complex changes be effortfully analyzed). One of the most important and interesting types of changes to our environment that initiate the search for meaning are those produced by people (including the self). Social interaction is an essential part of human existence, and we need to understand the characteristics and motives of those around us. The person across the room is staring at you. *Why* has the behavior occurred? Is it faint recognition, sexual attraction, hatred, or a smudge on your face? A member of a minority group is denied entry to a party at the fraternity/sorority you just joined. Was this person the victim of prejudice, or were many people turned away for reasons unrelated to race, religion, or sexual orientation? A friend has failed to return a call. Why? A job interviewer seems to be acting friendly. Why? These examples illustrate that simple events, some that have nothing to do with you, are met with a search for explanation and meaning. In fact, it is not just the observation of changes in our environment that compel explanation,

Attribution: A reason/cause that is assigned by a perceiver to explain a behavior or event they either observed or learned about. It is an explanation aimed at answering the question of "why" the behavior/event occurred, and is typically produced through processing stages that allow for categorization, inference, and judgment.

it is also the expectation of changes that never occur. In such cases it is inaction that leads us to ask, "why." For example, if we observe a terrible event unfolding, and one person has the ability to end it with a phone call, yet the call is never made, it is their inaction we are compelled to understand. The processes through which we arrive at reasons and explanations to which behavior can be attributed is known as an **attribution**. It is the end result of classifying and explaining behavior (or the absence of action) to arrive at a decision regarding the reason or cause for the observed action (or inaction).

Developmental research shows this pursuit of meaning to be present early in life. Infants (as early as 10 months of age) are shown to be identifying actors' goals (Brandone, Horowitz, Aslin, & Wellman, 2014; Brandone & Wellman, 2009; Gergely, Nádasdy, Csibra, & Bíró, 1995). An infant will stare at a failed action (such as observing an adult reaching over an obstacle toward a ball, and failing to grasp it) *longer* than the same act that ends in success (the ball is lifted). This tells us that the infant attributes the action to the goals of the person (they intend to lift the ball) since they are "surprised" when the goal fails to be met (as indicated by their heightened attention). Infants understand that failed actions are guided by intentions that are not manifested in the action, such as knowing that a person who drops a ball was trying to pick up the ball (making an inference about the person's intentions and seeing those intentions as a cause for the action).

Chapters 2–6 highlighted the centrality of meaning making by reviewing that it happens easily, invisibly, and through processes that make first impressions (and stereotypes, schemas, and other forms of stored meaning) resistant to change. The concern now turns to *how* meaning is made—to the attribution process. Even when we are aware that we are trying to judge a person, evaluate their behavior, and reason about the causes for why they act as they do, we may not be aware of the rules we follow in doing so. The rules can follow shortcuts and heuristics. The rules can also be rational and follow what seem like intuitive use of the scientific method. We can be aware of the rules we follow, or can use them implicitly (even if a judgment or attribution itself is explicit). Operating in a seemingly rational way, as well as following shortcuts, can each produce serviceable judgments, and can each produce errors. Errors are the focus of Chapters 8 and 9. Here we explore the rules that are followed in producing meaning.

HEIDER'S COMMON-SENSE (OR NAÏVE) PSYCHOLOGY

Heider (1944; see also 1958) was the first to systematically specify general rules that govern how people generate explanations and make attributions. Heider first focused on identifying the broad dimensions that need to be considered for one to have explanations, reasons, and causes for an event. He identified the following set of forces that are essential for reasoning about "why?":

1. Determining the locus of the behavior—is it emanating internally from the person or is it externally compelled?
2. Determining intentionality—was the behavior unintended or intended?
3. Determining the stability of the behavior over time—is it variable or static?
4. Assessing a person's efficacy or capacity to produce the behavior—do they have the ability to produce the behavior or the outcomes of the behavior ("can" they do it?)?
5. Specifying social sanctions that facilitate or inhibit the expression of the behavior—do norms allow for it, or are there obstacles that prevent it? (As opposed to can they do it, this concerns may they do it?)

The Locus of Causality and Intent

Heider's (1958) analysis of attribution processes begins with a basic question: What *potential* causes exist? At this most basic level, he argued that a cause for an action can be due to only one of two determining forces: **personal causation** or **impersonal causation**. By use of the term "personal," Heider meant the cause emanates from a force within the person, which is similar to *intentionality*. When a perceiver attributes a behavior to personal causation they come to see that act as intentionally chosen by the person, and the perceiver's attributional task is to determine the reasons for that choice: Why did they intend to act as such? The answers typically involve dispositional causes such as goals, attitudes, emotions, and traits. By use of the term "impersonal causality" Heider meant that an act or event occurred *unintentionally*. With impersonal causes the perceiver sees a behavior as not intentionally chosen

Personal causation: An explanation for a behavior that attributes it to something internal to the person that was intended by the person. The reason or cause generated as part of the attribution process is one that focuses on the person's state, motives, and traits.

Impersonal causation: An explanation for a behavior that attributes it to something external to the person. The perceiver sees the behavior as not intentionally chosen by the person, and the perceiver's attributional task is to determine what would compel a person to act in a way they did not intend to act.

by the person, and the attributional task is to determine what would compel a person to act in a way they did not intend to act? The answers typically involve external forces in the environment such as social pressure, constraints imposed by nature, and the trappings of history. However, an impersonal cause can be an internal cause as well, as discussed below.

Heider (1958) assumed that traits were especially powerful in determining how perceivers assign a cause for intended behavior. Traits allow people to not only explain behavior but a trait explanation affords greater predictability and feelings of control than other types of explanations by "referring transient and variable behavior and events to relatively unchanging underlying conditions." On the other end of the spectrum, Heider argued that situational causes are subtle and hard to see. Whereas trait explanations come easily, situation explanations are perhaps harder for people to invoke.

Of course, people make situational attributions. Heider's point was that they tend to do so only if the situational force that pressures the person to act as they do is strong and clear—such as when a person is forced to lie at gunpoint, or compelled to lie when their newborn child's welfare rests on it. However, information is not always strong and clear. We infer situations to be causes less so under such less-clear conditions, but we infer traits easily (as the earlier review of spontaneous trait inference supports). Heider used the term **behavior engulfs the field** to describe this salience of behavior and subtlety of situations. The person performing the observed act, and by inference the person's traits, are what are figural in many contexts, allowing the situation and its pressures to slip into the background. For example, when you learn a professor will teach an extra course, it is easier to infer a trait as the cause (such as their dedication) and harder to see a situational pressure that may be compelling them (need for extra money, fear of their contract not being renewed if they do not take it on, etc.). Others have argued that situations are easily assigned the role of **enabling conditions** that, while necessary for the event to have occurred, are not likely to be seen as the reason (e.g., Einhorn & Hogarth, 1986; Kahneman & Miller, 1986; McClure & Hilton, 1997). In basketball, when a center fouls a shooter, the reason the shooter falls to the ground is not attributed to an external force such as gravity, which is necessary to enable the fall. But attribution is internal, to the center's hard hit.

Behavior engulfs the field: A person's behavior is often figural to a perceiver, allowing the situation and its pressures to slip into the background. The salience of behavior places the person at the center of attention, and with attention focused on the person the perceiver is likely to make attributions that invoke personal causation.

Enabling conditions: Factors that are necessary for a behavior/event to occur, but are not likely to be seen as the reason for the event. For example, a student cannot fail a test without the professor grading it, but the grading system is rarely invoked as the cause of the failure, even though its existence is necessary to enable it.

Identifying the locus as internal or external is not always straightforward. When a member of the police engages in a violent behavior, the perceiver needs to determine whether it was the act of "a bad apple," or the norms of a system that encourage that type of violence, or compelled by the presumed threat that is common as part of that heroic role the officer plays. In many cases, such determinations may be hard to make. Internal forces (a bad actor), external forces (a threatening situation), and forces with an element of each (deciding to comply with the normative pressures of a biased system) may all be present. If the situational force was greater, such as when a suspect threatens violence to others and brandishes a weapon, an external attribution could be made where the situation compelled the officer's violence. If the personal force was stronger, such as if an officer chokes and kills an unarmed person who has acquiesced, then the attribution could be internal to the officer. Finally, different perceivers can have different chronic tendencies: Some might typically place more weight on the situation, others on dispositions. One person's internal attribution might be another person's external attribution (see Olcaysoy Okten & Moskowitz, 2020b). Thus, internal versus external is not always easy to decipher.

Also, it is easy to mistakenly conflate the personal–impersonal distinction with the locus of causality. This would happen if you were to use the distinction between "internal" versus "external"—which characterizes the locus of the cause—to also refer to intentionality (equating internal with intended, and external with unintended). Heider meant these to be two factors that perceivers were believed to consider separately when forming an attribution. It is simplistic to equate an impersonal cause with an external cause because unintended actions (impersonal causes) are not always externally caused, and intended actions (personal causes) are not always primarily caused by internal forces (Malle, 1999). It matters a great deal when making meaning if we believe a person intended to behave as they do but was compelled by an outside force (such as extreme peer pressure) versus having a goal or trait. As an example, a person who is told to steal a particular item or else their kidnapped dog will be harmed has clearly intended to steal, but the reason is not something internal to the person. This distinction matters for unintended behavior as well, where the cause could be something internal to the person. Often an unintended behavior is caused by an accident, where the person is a victim of external forces, their behavior compelled by the situation. However, unintended behavior can also occur where a person is seen as responsible. One can close a door without the latch catching, leaving it open unintentionally, yet one would still be responsible for leaving the home in an insecure state. Locus of causality and intentionality are two separate dimensions of concern, and we should treat them as such. For example, the legal system asks jurors to make attributions by keeping these issues separate. A man who deliberately, with premeditated intent, shoots another person is treated differently under most nations' laws from a man who shoots another person unintentionally while showing off his gun collection (as with former National Basketball Association [NBA] player Jayson Williams) or while hunting (as with former Vice President Dick Cheney). An unintended shooting still has a personal cause, and the person is still culpable. But due to the lack of intent the person is not labeled a murderer.

Malle (1999) posits that perceivers use distinct types of explanations when a behavior with an internal locus is seen as intended versus unintended. He argued that **reason explanations** are used to describe intended actions. These are attributions aimed at describing the reason a person intended to perform an act. He argued that a different class of explanations, **causal explanations**, are used for describing what caused a person to engage in an act they did not intend. Malle's point was that these differences in explanations have important consequences: They lead the perceiver to very different conclusions about and reactions to the person. Consider an example: Imagine that you read that a person, Mr. Woods, was driving 25 miles over the speed limit when his car flipped. The reason for this event can lie within the person and be intended (he was trying to get somewhere as fast as possible) or the cause can lie within the person and be unintended (he failed to read the speedometer, or was texting and did not see a sign indicating the road curved). When research participants receive causal explanations, they react to the person very differently from when they

Reason explanations: A type of explanation used when a behavior with an internal locus is seen as intended. These are attributions aimed at describing the reason a person intended to perform an act.

Causal explanations: A type of explanation used when a behavior with an internal locus is seen as unintended. These are attributions aimed at describing what caused a person to engage in an act they did not intend.

receive reason explanations for the same behavior. The type of explanation alters the perception of the person's intent, just as the inference about intent alters the type of explanation.

The Stability of Action

Heider's (1958) attempt to uncover the rules that govern our attributional analysis next turned to examining the types of words we use in language to describe why people act as they do. Let us focus on three words in particular that Heider identified: what a person "can" do, what a person will "try" to do, and what a person "may" do. It is not just that people "do" things, but if we want to know the reasons why, we need to examine "can" and "try" and "may." Analysis of "can" and "try" points out another dimension along which attributions vary (to accompany the dimensions of locus of causality and personal causation). It is known as the **stability dimension**. Behavior may be attributed to either *stable* or

Stability dimension: A dimension used by perceivers when explaining a behavior that assesses if the behavior is unchanging/stable or changing/unstable over time. For example, aptitude is usually stable over time, whereas goals are often unstable and change as the opportunities and affordances of the situation change.

unstable forces. For example, when we say a person "can" do something, we may be referring to their aptitude or ability as a stable quality. When we say that a person "can" play soccer, or "can" do math well we mean that they have a stable and unchanging efficacy in the domain. It is an unchanging quality of who they are as a person. At other times we do not use "can" in this way, such as when it refers to something unstable, usually something unstable in the situation. For example, whether you "can" do math well may depend on whether

there is distraction in the setting (such as a loud noise, or stereotype threat). Whether you "can" modify a first impression could depend on whether your situation places you under time constraint, cognitive load, or in a state of ego depletion. You have the aptitude to do the work of updating an impression, but the situational pressure fluctuates such that at one point it can get done, and at other points it cannot.

This discussion is not meant to suggest that an internal force is always stable and a situational force is unstable. In the chapter's opening quote we saw an example of a stable situational force: Cassius entertains the possibility that the fault for his failings lies in the stars (fate). We have also reviewed many instances of an internal force that is unstable. Chapter 6 discusses how goal inferences are distinguished by the fact that they are unstable and change across time and situations (unlike trait inferences, which are stable). Heider (1958) explored how perceivers naïvely capture this notion of internal forces as unstable with the concept "try." "Try" refers to the goals one is pursuing at the moment, and these can vary within the same person over time and situations. Similarly, Heider explored how perceivers naïvely capture the notion of situational forces as stable with the concept "may." "May" indicates a social sanction that allows (or does not allow) a particular type of action. It tells us that there are stable forces in our environment, those that represent the rules of the culture and prevailing norms, that impact how we act. Further, Heider's analysis of the meaning of "can," "try," and "may" led him to this understanding that, totally separate from whether the behavioral force is impersonal or personal, or internal versus external, is the issue of whether the behavior is stable over time, or not.

Naïve Scientists

A simple categorization scheme from crossing these dimensions captures many of the types of explanations we use for making sense of human behavior. Take the two dimensions of stability and locus, and use them to examine how you might reason about a specific behavior—such as a bad performance on a statistics test. The scheme that emerges suggests four possible classes of causes for the behavior, and we attribute the cause for the behavior to one of these four (see Figure 7.1). The bad statistics test may be due to something stable and internal to the person, such as their low aptitude for math (ability). It may be caused by something unstable about the person, such as their lack of studying (effort), which can vary from test to test. The cause may be located within the situation, but to something unstable, such as a loud noise in the hallway during the exam (an instance of bad luck). Finally, the cause may be something stable in the environment, such as the extreme difficulty of the tests this teacher is known to give (task difficulty) or pressures from one's social group to get drunk the night before the exam (norms). Heider (1958) argued that, perhaps without realizing it, perceivers act like scientists in determining the dimensions of behavior that are central for attribution, and we see how behavior varies across those dimensions. The results of this naïve scientific analysis suggest a particular type of explanation.

THE RULES OF CORRESPONDENT INFERENCE

Heider (1958) specified dimensions we use when making meaning, but no formal rules for how we use those dimensions. Jones and Davis (1965) introduced the first model of attribution processes: one examining the specific rules perceivers follow when engaging in a systematic analysis of the behavior of others (attempting to make inferences about the traits, personality, and disposition of the observed person). The model is called the **theory of correspondent inference** because the basic question being examined is How (what rules are followed) does a perceiver infer that an actor's behavior corresponds with some underlying disposition? "Correspondence refers to the extent that the act and the underlying characteristic or attribute are similarly described by the inference" (p. 223). A correspondent inference asserts that the behavior of a person corresponds with an internal attribute of that person, such as an attitude, goal, or trait.

> **Theory of correspondent inference:** The first formal model of attribution processes. It examines the factors considered and rules followed when a perceiver explains behavior. It poses that the primary question asked by perceivers is: does an actor's behavior correspond with some underlying disposition? The theory details the rules perceivers follow to answer this question.

A perceiver's goal when making attributions for the intended actions that others have performed is to ascertain the reasons as to why that person behaved as they did. Jones and Davis's (1965) model focuses on one specific reason explanation: that the person has attributes that lead them to act in this way. For example, if a group of people march to a government building, armed with guns, and violently overtake police officers to enter the

		Stability	
		Stable	Unstable
Locus	Internal	Ability, Traits, Chronic Disease	Goals, Effort
	External	Norms, Fate, Task Difficulty	Luck, Cognitive Load, Time Pressure, Distraction

FIGURE 7.1. Four attributions that result from crossing the locus and stability dimensions.

building, perceivers will infer that these people have attributes that cause this action. The behavior corresponds with, or reflects, a trait, goal, or attitude. The goal for the perceiver is to figure out those reasons: What attributes correspond with these actions? Do they have attitudes reflecting a patriotic need to undo an injustice? Do they have attitudes that fascist displays are needed to restore their power? Are they violent people? Are they loyal people? Jones and Davis were concerned with identifying the rules people use to ascertain the attitudes and traits of the target actor that are the reason for the action.

Jones and Davis's (1965) model is based on a perceiver's analysis not only of the behavior they have observed but of the consequences that arise from the person having performed the behavior. An act can typically have many consequences, or in the language of the model, an act can have **multiple effects**. We know a behavior caused these effects, but the question of interest is why (for what reason did the behavior produce any given effect)? Was it an unintended consequence, or did the person mean to produce this effect? Not all of the effects that follow an action are intended; some even oppose what one intended to accomplish. For example, consider the multiple effects of storming a government building. It could produce the intended effect of giving one access to the building. It could produce the intended effect of delaying an important vote. It could produce the intended effect of supporters seeing the action as loyal. It could produce the *unintended* effect of a police officer having a heart attack and dying. It could produce the unintended effect of individual "marchers" being arrested and losing their jobs. It could have the unintended effect of creating sympathy for the lawmakers whose vote was being delayed. For every action, intended and unintended consequences (multiple effects) can be produced. Perceivers use the consequences of the actions they observe (the effects) to help them make inferences about the actor (the person who performed the behavior). A perceiver needs to first differentiate which from among the multiple effects were intended versus unintended. They then need to focus on the intended effects and determine which have causal weight (as not all intended effects reflect a reason for the action). For example, storming a government building may produce the intended effect of being seen as loyal, and it may also produce the intended effect of delaying an important vote. Each was intended, but one of them (delaying a vote) is a better explanation for the reason the march was initiated. It carries greater causal weight.

> **Multiple effects**—An act can typically have many consequences, and a perceiver not only examines the behavior observed, but the consequences that arise from the person having performed the behavior. This set of consequences that follow an action are the multiple effects, and they are essential for forming a correspondent inference.

We are unable to see into the hearts and minds of other people, yet we need to understand why they act. The theory of correspondent inference hinges on the idea that perceivers engage in an analysis of a behavior and its effects to determine the reasons for the behavior—perceivers make inferences about the reasons one would want a given effect to result. How do we carry this out?

Three Ingredients for Determining Intent

In agreement with Heider (1958), this theory stipulates that the first thing a perceiver must do is determine what was intended. To determine whether a behavior was performed intentionally, and to determine whether the effects that resulted from the behavior were intended, a perceiver needs to know three things about the person in addition to the consequences of the person's behavior. These three things were already hinted at in Chapter 6 when discussing a person's own intentions to change a first impression. Impressions were said to be difficult to change because perceivers are often (1) not aware an impression exists, so they would have no goal to change it; (2) not motivated to change the impression even if aware it exists; and (3) lack the ability to change the impression even if motivated to do so (because the impression is formed efficiently and changing it can be effortful and disrupted). These three ingredients are the same ingredients that perceivers use to determine whether other people intend their actions (vs. their actions being unintended).

First, to determine whether a behavior was performed intentionally, a perceiver needs to know whether the person they are observing was *aware* that their behavior would bring about the consequence that it did. To intend a consequence, one must be aware in advance that one's action could cause that outcome. If a perceiver believes that the person they are observing is unaware that their behavior would produce a particular effect, then the perceiver should be unlikely to assume the person intended that effect. As a perceiver, I may know that no protester could have foreseen that a police officer would die of a heart attack (the effect). So, I would not infer that they intended for that to happen. However, if a perceiver believes that the person they are observing is aware that their behavior would produce a particular effect, then the possibility exists that the observed outcome was intended. As a perceiver, I may know that each protester realized that storming the building would delay a vote (the effect). So, I would infer that they intended for that to happen.

Second, the perceiver must not only determine whether the actor was aware that their behavior would cause a particular effect, they must also have *desired or wanted* to bring about the effect. If one is not motivated for an effect to result from one's action, it makes little sense for a perceiver to infer that the effect was intended. As a perceiver, I may believe that each protester is aware that large gatherings, with guns, can yield unfortunate consequences, where someone may die. However, I may also believe that no protester *wants* that to happen. Thus, if someone dies, I could still label the effect as unintended because nobody desired it to happen. As a perceiver I may also believe that each protester is aware that violence can cause harm. If the protesters choose to turn violent against police, then I may now believe that the protesters wanted harm to happen, and the inference formed would change accordingly—harm was intended.

Third, the perceiver must not only determine whether the actor was aware that their behavior would cause a particular effect, and desired to bring it about, they must also have the *capability* to cause the desired effect. A person lacking either the capacity or efficacy to produce an outcome will not be judged to have intended that outcome. One may know a protest could lead to deaths, and even want some on the "other side" to die, but have no means to make that happen. We do not say death was an intent of the marcher if the person has no ability to kill another person. In the law, this is why an alibi removes culpability. One may have had motive and even stated that one wanted something to happen, but if one was in another country when that thing actually happened, one could not have had the ability to be responsible for it.

These three ingredients allow one to make a determination about intent, and thus suggest where blame should be placed. For example, is the person immoral, or was the outcome unintended and the person's disposition is not implicated as a reason? Imagine a department chair who receives a grant proposal from a faculty member as an email attachment. It is to be considered for the faculty member's promotion review. However, the faculty member attached the wrong file and sent a grant proposal they were reviewing from a very accomplished scholar at another institution. Since the faculty member has attached this work and indicated that it is their own, this is technically fraud, and could lead to the faculty member being brought up on charges of claiming another person's work as their own. However, it was an unintended act, and the (lack of) intent changes the morality associated with the action. The person simply attached the wrong file and was not aware of this and did not have the motivation to commit fraud. People act, at times by mistake. And at times with dire results. Determining whether an action is intended or unintended is essential, and we make determinations following rules.

People differ in the standards they use when applying these rules. One chair of a department might label the act of incorrectly attaching a file as unintended because the person was *unaware* of and lacked the *motivation* to attach the wrong grant. In response to that inference, they might just ask the person to replace the file with the one they intended to send. A different department chair could form a different inference. They might argue that the faculty member was engaged in a very important activity (submitting materials for promotion), where care to accurately present one's record is required. Doing so is seen as something they should be aware of, be highly motivated to do, and be able to do. Failing to do so could be seen as an intentional act. Such a department chair would report the intended act to the disciplinary committee, causing much stress and embarrassment for the sloppy faculty member. The point here is that even when people have different standards, *they are following the same rules, using the same ingredients* to infer intent. They assess the awareness, motivation, and ability of an observed person to bring about the effects caused by that person's behavior. These three ingredients allow for inferences about intent, allowing a perceiver to determine whether a correspondent inference should be made when trying to explain an observed action (whether the action reflects the person's disposition), changing how we designate blame and punishment.

Five Rules for Examining Effects

Of course, the important next question concerns how a perceiver uses these three ingredients to determine whether a correspondent inference is warranted. What rules govern this inference? The theory of correspondent inference proposes that one of the most common things we do as perceivers is make assessments of *the consequences of a person's behavior.* More than examining whether the person was aware and motivated to produce an individual outcome, we focus on comparing the many outcomes produced, the multiple effects, against one another. But we do more than this. We also consider the effects that would have occurred if the person had acted differently. We may not realize it, but we are constantly comparing the effects produced by a behavior against the effects that would have been produced if a person had chosen to act in a way that they did not. We engage in *counterfactual thinking* and imagine "What if the person acted otherwise, what would have happened?" How do those effects compare with the effects of the chosen act? These are complicated analyses, yet Jones and Davis (1965) argue that they are routine; so routine that a set of rules develop that guide our analysis and allow for inference.

Rule number 1 specifies that the **desirability** of the consequence of an action is inversely related to the probability that the perceiver will form a correspondent inference. The desirability of an effect is essentially the measure of how much the actor would enjoy it—whether they would derive pleasure or personally gain from the effect coming to pass. This rule may sound complicated, but the logic is simple. If an effect is one that is desirable, then knowing that an actor attempted to bring about that effect really tells us very little about that specific person's disposition. It does tell us one important thing about the person: that the actor intended to act in this way. We infer that the actor had the goal to bring about the consequences when those consequences are desirable. The more *desirable* an outcome, the more we can infer the person had the goal of producing that outcome, but the less we learn about the person's traits or

Desirability: A measure of how much the actor would enjoy a particular outcome or effect, deriving pleasure or gain from the effect coming to pass.

specific reasons for wanting that outcome (correspondent inference is less likely). For example, what if we learn that a person marched on a government building (an act) and enjoyed the camaraderie they felt with other marchers (an effect)? This would suggest that the person intended to produce that effect. After all, we intend to produce consequences we like. While we would know a feeling of camaraderie was intended, we would not learn whether this was *why* the person decided to march. Desirable effects are common, and the multiple effects of an action (delaying a vote, feeling loyal) are also likely desirable. We learn little about a person by knowing they perform acts that bring about desirable outcomes; this carries little causal weight. Knowing someone intended an *undesirable* outcome (such as getting arrested), however, is more informative about the reason for intending to act. It is easier to infer a trait, attitude, or goal (such as commitment to the people organizing the march) if the effect is not pleasant. If one is willing to suffer for an act, it carries causal weight.

Rule number 2 specifies that the number of **noncommon effects** is inversely related to the probability that the perceiver will form a correspondent inference. What is a noncommon effect? Noncommon effects are those consequences uniquely associated with one course of action, but not with another. We have already established that the behaviors we engage in have multiple effects. To know which of those effects is able to signal the real reason why someone acted as they did, people engage in a naïve analysis of what the effects were for the chosen course of action, and what the consequences would have been for *a nonchosen course of action*. When the consequences of one choice of action overlap with the consequences of another choice of action, these shared consequences are called "common effects." When the consequences of one choice do not coincide with those of other choices of action, those are *noncommon effects*.

> **Noncommon effects:** When the consequences of one choice of action do not overlap with those of another choice of action. A behavior has multiple effects, and a behavior not enacted would have had multiple effects had it been enacted. Noncommon effects are those consequences uniquely associated with the chosen course of action.

This second rule asserts that noncommon effects are useful in attempting to understand why a person acted one way versus another, as they tell us the different consequences that result for the person as a function of the different behaviors they could have performed. If there are only a small number of noncommon effects and a large number of common effects, then this means that there are many overlapping outcomes between the two courses of action. We are not able to distinguish why the person acted one way versus the other from the many common consequences they produce. However, it is very informative for making such a distinction if we examine the noncommon effects. If there are only a small handful of noncommon effects, it suggests that producing these specific effects distinguishes why the person chose to act as they did (as opposed to the alternative action). We can reason that the action was performed in order to bring about those particular effects that other actions would not have produced. As the number of noncommon effects increases, it becomes harder to determine why the person acted as they did. There are too many possible reasons that distinguish their behavior from another behavior. Too many noncommon effects make attribution less clear. For a first example, see Figure 7.2.

Consider another example: Imagine you are trying to understand the reasons that your friend from Parksville, New York, has chosen to go to one university (McGill) over another (Columbia). Let us list the effects your friend associates with each course of action (attending one university vs. the other). Columbia has the following consequences for the person: They will live in an urban setting, get prestige, be in a great academic environment, be linked to an only adequate tradition of athletic teams, and spend an extreme amount of money. Your friend decides attending McGill will have the following consequences: They will live in an urban setting, get prestige, be in a great academic environment, be linked to

Action X: Robin cheats on the exam.	(Nonchosen) Action Y: Robin does not cheat.
Effects of Action X:	Effects of Action Y:
• Robin gets to keep her scholarship. • Robin feels guilty. • Robin has her self-esteem threatened.	• Robin loses her scholarship due to poor grades. • Robin feels honest. • Robin has her self-esteem threatened.

Noncommon effects unique to the chosen Action X—Keep scholarship, guilt.

Analysis of which noncommon effects were *intended*—Keep scholarship.

A single noncommon effect provides a clear reason—We infer the reason was a *goal* to keep her scholarship.

FIGURE 7.2. The use of noncommon effects and desirability in causal reasoning.

an only adequate tradition of athletic teams, will spend relatively little money, and live in a foreign country with a multicultural setting. If we eliminate the common effects (excellent academics, urban settings, prestige, only adequate sports) and list the noncommon effects, we are left with the fact that attending McGill is less expensive and offers a multicultural environment. We would then assume that these noncommon effects correspond with the disposition of the person—your friend chose McGill because they have a goal to avoid debt, as well as to gain valuable experience in a foreign country with a different culture. Now consider the same task, but replace Columbia with the University of Florida. The effects listed for Florida include living far from home, having great weather, having only a subset of departments that are among the best in the country, spending relatively little money, and having an excellent tradition of sports. Once we eliminate the common effects we are left with numerous noncommon effects that are associated with attending McGill (urban setting, excellent academics, prestige, a multicultural environment, and adequate sports). Given all of these unique effects with going to McGill (increased number of noncommon effects), it is harder to make conclusions about what factor corresponds to the person's disposition. In summary, we make inferences about another person not merely by looking at the consequences of that person's actions but by examining how those consequences compare to consequences that would have resulted if the person acted in a different fashion. A few distinct noncommon effects unique to one course of action provide the clearest case for correspondent inference.

Rule number 3 specifies that "correspondence of inference declines as the action to be accounted for appears to be constrained by the setting in which it occurred" (Jones & Davis, 1965, p. 223). This third rule specifies the importance of examining the **situational constraints** that are placed on behavior. The perceiver asks, "To what extent does the situation

Situational constraints: Pressures, obstacles, and roles that a person experiences in a given context that limits what they are able to do.

promote the behavior performed and the effects being observed?" To the extent that the situation constrains what one is able to do, and reveals that there were no other options available to the actor, we would be less inclined to regard the actor's behavior as an indicator of their personal qualities. If the perceiver is free to choose among many courses of action, we are more likely to assume they intended the behavior they selected and that a dispositional cause is at the root of that intention. The roles we play in life create such situational constraint. Just because someone obeys orders as a member of the military does not mean the person is subservient by disposition. The role constrains action and dictates what one may do. Awareness of the power of such constraints should lead to a decreased probability of dispositional inference. This does not mean that the person is not subservient by disposition. The person may have chosen such a role because they like to follow orders. The degree of correspondence of an act cannot be solely determined by situational constraint. The rule simply states that if we know a person is constrained by the situation, then the behavior (being subservient) is less informative. However, if the person is free to act as they want, unconstrained by the situation, then correspondent inference should increase.

An excellent empirical illustration of this rule comes from Jones, Davis, and Gergen (1961). Research participants listened to a job interview. Some participants heard a tape where the person being interviewed was applying for a job on a submarine, others for a job as an astronaut. The ideal candidate for the job is described at the outset: The interviewer states that the submarine job requires one to be friendly, outgoing, cooperative, and obedient (the astronaut job is described with the opposite qualities). In each condition, the person being interviewed proceeds to respond in a manner that either makes it clear they possess the very traits that the job requires, or that they fail to possess the very traits that the job requires. So, half of the participants hear an interviewee respond in a way perfectly consistent with the role they were asked to play; they act in a way constrained by the situation. Half of the participants hear a person act in a way inconsistent with the role, unconstrained by the situation. The results showed that when the actions appear constrained by the situation, participants do not see the interviewee's responses as dispositional. If a job interview calls for you to be introverted, and you say you are introverted, then you are merely responding in line with the social pressure, and the perceiver learns little about your disposition. The situation offers a reasonable explanation for the behavior. However, if the same response is out-of-role, and is inconsistent with the situational constraint, a correspondent inference is formed and the interviewee is judged as having the traits claimed during the interview. If a job interview calls for you to say you are extroverted, and you say you are introverted, a perceiver will infer that you are indeed an introvert (see Figure 7.3).

Rule number 4 specifies that "correspondence increases as the judged value of the attribute departs from the judge's conception of the average person's standing on that attribute" (Jones & Davis, 1965, p. 224). The fourth rule is an analysis of how normative the behavior is. The more different your actions are from how the average person would act in the same situation, the more likely it is that your behavior will be seen as having been caused by your disposition. If you act in a normative fashion, then your action is not highly informative. Performing a behavior that most people would perform tells us little about your personality. However, when your behavior is distinctive and unique, unexpected relative to what others do, then it is more likely that the behavior corresponds to your underlying, stable disposition. An important distinction should be made about behavior that is surprising because it deviates from what other people do, and behavior that is surprising because it deviates from what that individual typically would do. As Kelley and Michela (1980) point out, behavior that is surprising because we have expectations about the person—provided by either a stereotype or a history of experience with the person—do not promote dispositional inference. Under those conditions we assume that something about the current situation has caused the person to act in the unexpected way (to violate what they normally do). However, if behavior is unexpected because it is not what most other people would do in that situation, then a dispositional attribution is likely. For example, Korman and Malle (2016) found that if a behavior was unexpected because it violated a script (or an event schema) that dictated how most people would respond, the perceivers used predominantly dispositional explanations to the person's mental states (traits and goals). We can return

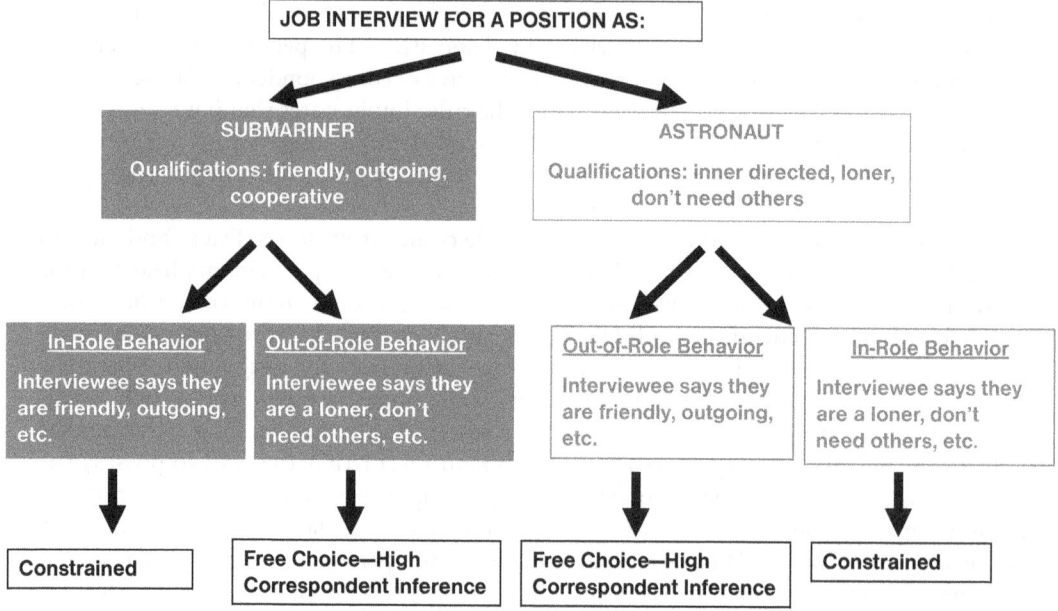

FIGURE 7.3. Situational constraint and correspondent inference.

to the example of an interview to work on a submarine. We might assume that most people would say whatever was necessary to get hired, even if it meant saying that one had a quality that one did not. If a person does the non-normative thing, and says they do *not* posses the quality in question, we might infer the quality they claim to have truly describes them—correspondent inference would be more likely.

The final rule we review is that perceivers analyze the **hedonic relevance** of an action. Hedonic relevance refers to the extent to which the behavior addresses the motives and goals of the *perceiver*. If an observed behavior helps to promote the values, goals, and desires of the person observing that behavior, then that action is said to have hedonic relevance for the perceiver. *Rule number 5* specifies that as hedonic relevance increases, so too does correspondence of inference. Why? Jones and Davis (1965) posit that when behavior produces its effects, perceivers for whom those effects are relevant will have experience with these types of outcomes (and behaviors) because they are so closely tied to the perceiver's own goals and wishes. This familiarity with the effects may lead the person to see two effects as being highly similar to each other (as both address one's needs). The same effects seen by a person for whom the effects lack hedonic relevance might be seen as very different from each other. Thus, for one person a set of effects is interpreted as essentially the same outcome, whereas for other people these effects are seen as several distinct outcomes. The consequence of this is that as hedonic relevance increases, the number of noncommon effects decreases. What to others may seem like many noncommon effects appears like a smaller set of noncommon effects if hedonic relevance is high. The result of a reduction in noncommon effects is an increase in correspondent inference.

> **Hedonic relevance:** The extent to which another person's behavior addresses the motives and goals of the *perceiver*. If an observed behavior helps to promote the values, goals, and desires of the person observing that behavior, then that action is said to have hedonic relevance for the perceiver.

DISTINGUISHING AMONG TYPES OF DISPOSITIONAL INFERENCE

Reeder and colleagues (2004) suggested that attribution research is too simple in its emphasis on a stable underlying attribute such as an attitude or trait. Reeder et al. describe attributions as "multifaceted, composed of inferences about goals, motives, and traits" (p. 541). This was certainly what Heider (1958) meant when he described dispositional inference as common. Of course, the fact that perceivers make inferences that refer to goals/motivation, as well as to traits, was not lost on Jones and Davis (1965) either. Their theory of correspondent inference, as just reviewed, highlights the importance of, in fact the primacy of, making inferences about whether a person's behavior was intended. The criticism is simply that attribution models often treat goal inference (when not ignoring it) as a step to what sounds like the more important stage of determining whether a trait or attitude is responsible. Does one have a goal to do X because they have a trait that compels them to intend X? The argument being made by Reeder et al. is that goal inference is not merely a step on the way to trait inference but an attributional end in itself.

Malle and Holbrook (2012) described a variety of attribution types that perceivers often use other than a trait or situation inference. Though dozens of subcategories can be created based on their analysis, there are several larger "meta-categories" of explanations that perceivers use. Internal states, such as beliefs (inferences about what the actor understands to be true), valuing (inferences about the attitudes and desires of an actor), and goals (inferences about the intentions of the actor), emerge as popular forms of causal explanation. In our own research (Olcaysoy Okten & Moskowitz, 2018) we find that when we ask research participants to make attributions to simple behaviors, the type of explanation they use—trait versus goal versus valuing, and so on—depends on the type of information we provide for them, as shown in Figure 7.4. There are times trait inference predominates (as in

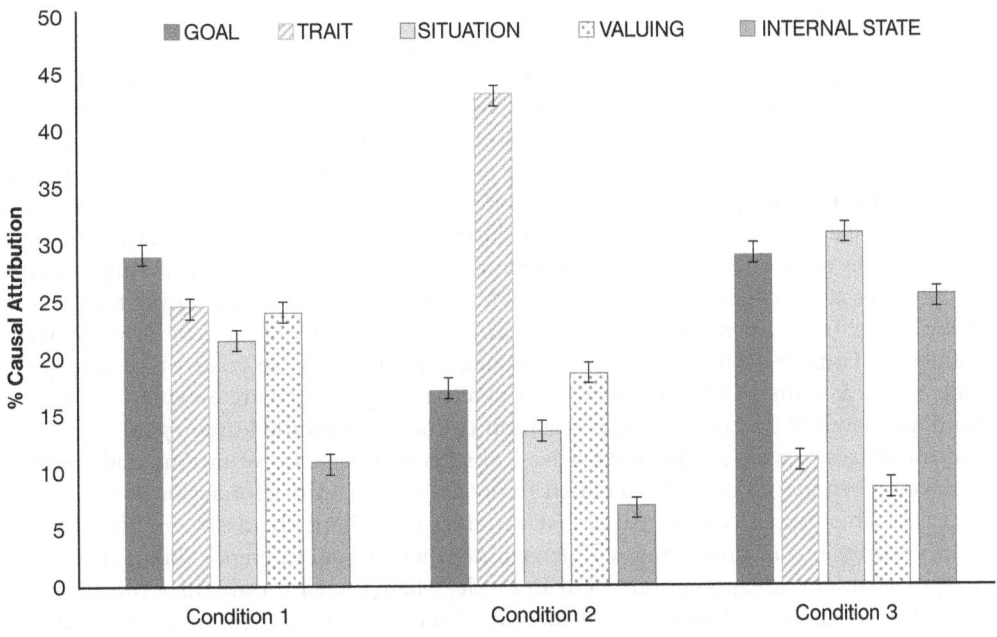

FIGURE 7.4. Attribution types under various conditions.

condition 2 of the figure), but times when goal inference is used most often (as in condition 1 of the figure). What those conditions are is explained shortly.

From both the theory of correspondent inference, and work on spontaneous inference (see Chapter 6), we see the proposition that *goal inference* happens before trait inference and is faster. Malle and Holbrook (2012) supported this conclusion. They compared the likelihood and speed of making a variety of inference types—not just traits and goals but inferences about desires and beliefs. They found that inferences about intentionality and desire are more likely to occur and faster to be made. Reeder et al. (2004) found that inferences about goals shape the types of traits people believe they will see in a person. They manipulated the goals of an actor and found that people rate that the actor had the trait that corresponded with that goal.

Reeder and Trafimow's (2005) **multiple inference model** argued that people infer both motives and traits in an actor simultaneously, but that goal attributions are the priority because they are necessary for making a trait attribution.

> **Multiple inference model:** A theory that argues that people infer both goals and traits in an actor simultaneously, but that goal inferences are the priority because they are necessary for making a trait attribution.

As reviewed earlier, goal inferences and trait inferences do not only differ in that one is more stable than the other. Goals provide more concrete explanations for a behavior relative to the more abstract language of a trait explanation (e.g., Malle & Holbrook, 2012; Read, Jones, & Miller, 1990; Reeder, 2009). This concreteness may be another factor that contributes to their primacy. Although there is much evidence to suggest that trait inferences should come *after* goal inferences, there is not yet an answer to the question of when and why goal inferences, once made, lead to trait inferences.

The Conditions That Promote Goal Inferences

Jones and Davis (1965) reviewed the rules that promote correspondent inference. Given that goal inference is perhaps an even more primary way of explaining behavior, and could be the final attribution (without leading to a trait attribution), it is critical to understand the rules that promote goal inference. Jones and Davis provide an essential starting point when reviewing the forces that shape an inference that a behavior was intended versus unintended. What dictates whether such an inference will push a perceiver toward seeing the reason for the intended behavior lying in a person's goals versus traits? Moskowitz and Olcaysoy Okten (2016) propose a set of factors that would be relevant. A first proposition is that the concreteness versus generality of the desired description should matter. If a perceiver requires their inference to predict what a person will do across a wide range of contexts, or to be abstract enough to explain a wide variety of behavior, they should form a trait inference. Traits are not *necessarily* bound to any specific entity (e.g., Winter, John, Stewart, Klohnen, & Duncan, 1998). They will be associated with multiple goals of an actor (e.g., Read, Jones, & Miller, 1990). However, if a perceiver requires concrete explanations that afford high levels of confidence and predictability, then they should lean on goal inferences. Goal inferences provide strong associative links between specific situations and concrete behaviors. They specify concrete acts tied to precise opportunities for action (e.g., Gollwitzer, 1993). This proposition suggests that variables that shape the desire for abstractness versus concreteness in processing will determine whether goal inference versus trait inference predominate in explanations.[1] For example, when a need for abstract thinking was induced in research participants, trait inference increased (Rim, Uleman, & Trope, 2009). And when research participants were provided explanations in terms of goals (vs. traits), a more concrete and cohesive memory structure emerged that produced better memory for specific behaviors (Hoffman, Mischel, & Mazze, 1981).

A second proposition is that when behavior is tied to a specific goal object, and repeatedly occurs with that object, goal inference is likely when that specific behavior is observed in response to that specific object. Bargh (1990) argued that goals have strong associations to mental representations of environmental properties, or goal objects. Research has shown that the mere presence of the goal object (the triggering of an environmental feature associated with a goal) will trigger the goal and goal-directed behaviors (e.g., Aarts & Dijksterhuis, 2003; Gollwitzer, 1993; Parks-Stamm & Gollwitzer, 2009). For example, when a perceiver sees a person in a library, that context triggers the associated goal perceived to be held by the person observed: that they intend to be quiet and studious. A perceiver can use this knowledge to infer that if a behavior occurs in response to a specific environment (the library), and does not occur in other situations or when exposed to other features (in their dorm), then there must be a goal that links their behavior (studying) to this goal object (library). Thus, goal inference is promoted by the specific association of a behavior with a unique or distinct person or situation—that is, goal inference is more likely when the observed behavior does not generalize across many contexts and people. Evidence for this is presented shortly, when we review "distinctiveness."

A third proposition is that goal inference is more likely when a person stands to gain from their behavior in a particular situation. Rather than the behavior suggesting the corresponding trait (kind behavior suggests a kind trait), a goal is likely to be inferred if the behavior also provides rewards for the actor. Under such conditions, a trait is less likely to be inferred than an **ulterior motive**—seeing the person as having a goal not directly tied to the most obvious implication of the behavior. As desirability of the effects increases, trait inference decreases. An increase in the desirability of an effect, as noted earlier, allows us to infer that a person intended an action and wanted to receive the positive consequences, but we do not infer what it is about them—the specific reason—that made them desire that goal. For example, if helpful behavior garners a favor in return, we do not learn whether they acted helpfully because they are a helpful person, or whether they had the ulterior motive of getting the other person to help them. If kindness induces a sense of indebtedness that results in the actor getting paid back in kind, then a goal inference is likely (we infer they intended to be kind), but a reason as to why is not known. We already reviewed one example from Jones et al. (1961), where trait inference was reduced when an actor behaved in a way on a job interview that was likely to result in a job offer. In that condition it is hard to differentiate a trait from an ulterior motive—is the person an introvert, or only saying so to get the job (see also Fein, Hilton, & Miller, 1990)? Reeder et al. (2004) showed that a perceiver is adept at making such goal inferences about an ulterior motive, and do so implicitly.

> **Ulterior motive:** When a person acts in a way that seemingly has one clear goal as an explanation, but there is in fact a goal not directly tied to the most obvious implication of the behavior that carries greater explanatory power.

A fourth proposition is that the amount of effort that is perceived to be involved in producing the behavior promotes a goal inference. In line with Heider's (1958) discussion of what one has the ability to do (the word "can"), traits should be seen as effortlessly producing a behavior due to it being derived from a stable and well-practiced attribute of the person. Heider's discussion of trying, on the other hand, is that from the perspective of the naïve perceiver, to learn that someone is trying to do something implies a lesser degree of natural capability and greater effort. As perceivers we feel that traits are easy and natural, whereas a goal should be more effortful to pursue. In support of this, Dik and Aarts (2008) found that perceptions of effort mediated goal inference. Higher effort in the actor's behavior made it easier to infer a goal.

A fifth proposition is that **entitativity** shapes inference type. Entitativity is a feature of a group that characterizes how cohesive it seems, the degree to which the members seem to hang together as a single entity with shared features. The "groupiness" of the group. The greater the entitativity, in which a perceiver sees abstract and enduring descriptors, such as stereotypes as shared characteristics of the group, the greater the degree to which people should infer traits in the groups (e.g., Hamilton et al., 2015; Spencer-Rodgers, Hamilton, & Sherman, 2007). Groups that are perceived to be less entitative and not possess a strong group identity, such as a group of colleagues at work, should be perceived to have causation for their acts as lying in malleable forces, such as situational constraints and shared group goals (e.g., Stroessner & Dweck, 2015).

> **Entitativity:** A feature of a group that characterizes its cohesiveness—the degree to which the members seem to hang together as a single entity with shared features. It is the perceived "groupiness" of the group.

THE RULES OF COVARIATION

Kelley (1967, 1972a, 1972b, 1973), similar to Jones and Davis (1965), was concerned with how we make decisions about a behavior's locus of causality: locating the cause of behavior as internal or external to the person.[2] Kelley used the term "person attribution" to refer to internal causes and the term **entity attribution** to refer to external causes. An entity is the particular place, object, event, or person (who is not the actor) that can potentially be seen as the cause of the action a perceiver is trying to understand. It is something or someone that draws out the behavior from the person, causing it to occur. The way people decide on the locus of causality in the Kelley model revolves around the notion of covariation. If two events occur in tandem (or fail to occur in tandem), they can be said to be varying together. Thus, the variance in one event is linked to the variance in another. The **covariation principle** asserts that an effect is attributed to the cause with which it covaries over time. The variance in the one event is linked via cause and effect to the variance in the other. For example, imagine a gift card to Starbucks is anonymously left on your desk every Wednesday (and not on anybody else's and not on any other day). The occurrence varies in when it occurs (Wednesday) and to whom (you, and nobody else). Imagine, as well, that only one person from among all in your company works remotely every day except one: Wednesdays. The presence of that person at work varies, and it is only that person whose presence varies (all others work at the office). You have noticed a covariation—the card appears on the same days that the remote worker shows up at the office; variance in the two events is linked. Using the covariation principle, most people at this point assume (attribute) the reason for the action (getting a gift) is the thing with which the presence of the action covaries (the remote worker). As Kelley (1967) stated: "the effect is attributed to that condition which is present when the effect is present and which is absent when the effect is absent" (p. 194).

Naturally, actual covariation is not required for an attribution. So long as the perceiver *thinks* two events covary, a causal link will be made between them. For example, one may think that an increase in vaccine use is covarying with an increase in hospitalization, when

> **Entity attribution:** An attribution to a situational cause. When an object, event, person (who is not the actor), or place can be seen as the locus of causality of the action. When something or someone is said to draw out the behavior from the person, causing it to occur.
>
> **Covariation principle:** A rule regarding how people associate events when making an attribution which asserts that an effect is attributed to the cause with which it covaries over time.

it is not. Even when two things do covary, the rules people use to determine the locus of that cause could still lead to error. For example, if hospitalizations and vaccine use did covary, a perceiver might incorrectly attribute this to vaccines causing hospitalization, when it may be that an increase in disease has led to both an increase in hospitalization and vaccine use. If the action we want to understand is hospitalization, and we see that it covaries with vaccine use, what rules do we follow when making an attribution? How do we determine whether the attribution should be internal to the target (vaccines) or to something external that compels the target (in this case, a disease or pandemic)? To Kelley (1967), a perceiver's processing of attribution-relevant information was similar to a scientist's use of the statistical procedure known as analysis of variance (ANOVA).

In using this metaphor, the first thing to note is that the action, and the consequences of the action (the effects), are akin to the dependent variable in an ANOVA. Additionally, just as in an ANOVA one would analyze several separate independent variables, in the attribution process a perceiver is said to weigh several different dimensions of information. Kelley (1973) identified three dimensions or types of information a perceiver weighs (the definitions of these dimensions will be reviewed shortly). These dimensions, just like the manipulated levels of independent variables, have levels associated with them; the perceived act could be described as either high or low on a given dimension. Perceivers analyze the pattern of outcomes when crossing different levels of these "independent variables" to calculate an attribution. When the action is high on dimension one, low on dimension two, and high on dimension three, this pattern would suggest to the perceiver a particular type of attribution (e.g., one with an external locus), which is likened to a main effect in an ANOVA. Foersterling (1992) adds that the strength of the attribution to a particular cause is like the F statistic in ANOVA, while the certainty of the attribution is akin to the significance level. While perceivers do not always follow this rational, *causal calculus* for arriving at attributions, Kelley argued that when perceivers are being rational, deliberate, and systematic in producing attributions, they follow these ANOVA-like rules. We start here, and define the three dimensions that are the independent variables in the calculus.

The Three Dimensions of the Causal Calculus

Consensus is one dimension of information that perceivers must consider to determine the locus of the cause for an observed behavior. **Consensus information** describes how people other than the actor would react toward the same entity, holding all else constant. As with all three dimensions of information that make up the causal calculus, there are two levels to the independent variable (dimension) known as consensus: high consensus and low consensus. *High consensus means that the action generalizes across other actors (is not specific to one person but is something that many other people would do). Low consensus means that few (if any) others act the same way the person being observed has acted.* Low consensus suggests that the entity did not cause the outcome (since it would have led others to act the same way). While low consensus does not rule out the possibility that the entity had something to do with drawing out the behavior from the actor, it suggests that the entity was not the primary cause. High consensus would lead you to lean toward concluding that the entity was responsible for the action. However, high consensus information alone does not rule out the possibility that it is something about the person. Other people may act similarly, but this does not rule out that there is something about the person we are examining that makes their disposition

> **Consensus information:** A dimension of information that perceivers consider to determine the locus of the cause for an observed behavior that examines how people other than the actor would react in the same situation or toward the same entity, holding all else constant.

the cause for their behavior. As one piece to the puzzle of making an attribution, high consensus suggests an external locus of causality, low consensus suggests an internal cause.

Whereas consensus is a dimension that gives us information about how other people respond to the same entity, **distinctiveness** is a dimension that provides information about

> **Distinctiveness:** A dimension of information that perceivers consider to determine how the actor reacts to different entities. High distinctiveness means the action does not generalize across entities; the actor behaves this way only in this specific situation (with this entity). Low distinctiveness means the actor behaves the same with many entities.

how the same person (the actor) responds to different entities. High distinctiveness means the action does not generalize across other entities but is specific to this particular entity. The actor behaves this way only in this particular situation (with this particular entity). Low distinctiveness means that the actor behaves the same way with many entities. Notice an important difference between high/low consensus and distinctiveness. Being able to generalize on consensus meant that lots of people did the same thing—this is high consensus. But generalizing on distinctiveness means that

lots of entities produce the same reaction—this is low distinctiveness. In other words, distinctiveness is about the distinct nature of the entity. Having similar reactions to many entities does not make a given entity very distinctive. For example, if Maria experiences true joy when visiting with Isaac, Benjamin, Cindy, and Joan, as she does with Joe, we cannot say Joe is particularly distinct when attempting to understand Maria's reaction. Distinctiveness is low. We would be less inclined to explain Maria's behavior with an external attribution to Joe after learning this. We would be more likely to make an internal attribution to her joyful disposition.

In the ANOVA model, one dimension of information alone does not provide for an adequate attribution. We need further information to engage in an ANOVA-like approach that considers the interaction among multiple dimensions. We can cross the different dimensions (the "main effects") and observe the pattern. Let us start by considering the interaction of the two dimensions discussed so far: distinctiveness and consensus information. What would the combination of *high consensus* and *high distinctiveness* suggest? For Maria and Joe it would suggest that many people besides Maria get joy from interacting with Joe, and that Maria is joyful only around Joe and not people in general. This would suggest there is something particular about Joe (the entity) causing Maria's response, and it causes this response in most others as well. We would make an external attribution to the entity (Joe). What would the combination of *low consensus* and *low distinctiveness* suggest? It would suggest that very few people get joy from interacting with Joe, and Maria experiences joy interacting with many other people other than (but including) Joe. This would suggest that there is something particular about Maria that causes the response. We would make an internal attribution to Maria.

So far, the ANOVA model only allows us to determine whether the cause is internal or external to the person. But Heider (1958) focused our attention on another dimension that

> **Consistency:** A dimension of information that perceivers consider to determine the stability or duration of the action—its ability to generalize across time given that the entity and the actor are held constant. High consistency suggests a stable attribution; the same action is produced each time the same entity was encountered.

helps determine causality and understand an action: stability. Kelley (1967) captured the stability dimension in his model of how perceivers form attributions using a causal calculus. This dimension was called the consistency of the action. **Consistency** refers to the stability or duration of the action—its ability to generalize across time given that the entity and the actor are held constant. High consistency means a recurring action by a person across time and with the same entity. High consistency suggests stability; the same action is produced by the same person when the same entity is encountered. Low consistency means there is instability in reaction to the entity over time. Using our running example, consistency information would allow us to know whether Maria gets joy from visiting with Joe each time she visits with Joe, or just this one time.

The dimensions of information (independent variables in the ANOVA) described by Kelley (1967) draw from, and can be traced to, the factors discussed by Jones and Davis (1965). For example, distinctiveness is related to Jones and Davis's notion of situational constraint. Low distinctiveness suggests no situational constraint, and high distinctiveness suggests strong situational constraint. Because high distinctiveness means that the behavior occurs only in a particular situation (it fails to generalize across entities), this could be because in the specific situation in which the behavior emerges one has no other options. Low distinctiveness, however, implies a person attribution because many situations would elicit the same behavior. This could only occur if one has the freedom to act as one wishes in those situations. Distinctiveness is also somewhat tied to Jones and Davis's notion of noncommon effects. A noncommon effect means that the consequences of a behavior occur only with one particular choice of action (it fails to generalize across other actions). This is a type of distinctiveness, one in which the consequences of an action are distinct to that action. Kelley took the concept of distinctiveness and applied it to the action being distinct to a particular entity as opposed to distinct to a particular action. Just as noncommon effects require perceivers to think about the other consequences that would have emerged if one acted in a different way (if the consequences of one's behavior generalize across other actions), distinctiveness requires perceivers to think about other actions that would have emerged if faced with a different entity. These similarities to the theory of correspondent inference might be partly responsible for why, as the story goes, Ned (E.E.) Jones found an early draft of Kelley's manuscript that crossed his desk to be one of the most important pieces of social-psychological writing that he had ever read. The story also has it that Jones thought the analogy to ANOVA to be so accurate and descriptive that he "kicked" himself for not making it himself.

What is hopefully clear is that both models argue that humans use principles of covariation for making explanations about why a behavior occurred. Jones and Davis (1965) focused on covariation among noncommon effects: how an actual behavior and its effects covaries with imagined effects that would have occurred if an alternative action had been taken (though it was not). If an action covaries with more than one noncommon effect, it reveals many possible intentions and ambiguity about disposition. Kelley (1967) was concerned with how two actual effects covary over time, people, and entities. In each model the information used includes considering what other people would do and how the behavior and its effects might generalize across time and conditions. Finally, you may have noticed that the types of answers to our "why" questions provided by the Kelley model are not very satisfying. The ANOVA model presents a rational account of how people deliberately and systematically locate cause as internal or external to the person. But it does not specify reason explanations (Malle, 1999). Intent is discovered, but specific reasons have not been.

Evaluating the ANOVA Model

For such an influential theoretical model, there is only a small body of research providing direct tests of the model, and attributions to specific combinations of consensus, distinctiveness, and consistency (e.g., Bassili, 1989; Cheng & Novick, 1990; Hilton, Smith, & Kim, 1995; McArthur, 1972; Olcaysoy Okten & Moskowitz, 2018; Sutton & McClure, 2001; Van Overwalle, 1997a, 1997b). This is also odd given how simple it would be to test—it is already set up as three-way ANOVA and specifies the variables to manipulate. McArthur provided such a test in which research participants were provided with distinctiveness, consensus, and consistency information relating to a behavior. Each dimension was manipulated to be either low or high. Overall, there are eight possible patterns or combinations of low and high distinctiveness, consensus, and consistency information. Thus, a research participant might get a description of a behavior that was said to have high consistency, consensus, and distinctiveness, while another would read a behavior described as having low consistency, consensus, and distinctiveness, with each possible pattern among the eight used. Particular patterns of information should lead to specific types of attributions. McArthur found that the actual attributions formed by research participants reflected the use of information in the manner described by the ANOVA model.

For example, when the person's behavior was said to be uniquely associated with the entity in question, and most other people were said to have responded in the same manner as the person whose behavior was described, as well as being consistent over time with that entity (the high-distinctiveness, high-consensus, high-consistency pattern), then research participants judged the cause of that behavior to be located in the entity. Imagine a perceiver who learns that an actor engages in domineering and violent action to protest an election result, but to *only one specific* election result (and to no others); many *other people* engage in domineering and violent action when marching to protest this particular election result; and this actor *always* engages in domineering and violent action when events to oppose this particular election result are organized. The perceiver should make an entity attribution, such as "the candidate who lost this particular election motivated the behavior in the person."

Consider another possible pattern produced by the McArthur (1972) experiment, one in which a person is described as behaving identically with many different entities, but their actions are dissimilar to how others act with this entity, and is described as an action that the person engages in consistently over time with this entity (a low-distinctiveness, low-consensus, high-consistency pattern). Under this combination of the three dimensions research participants judged the cause of the behavior to be located in the person. For example, imagine a perceiver who learns that this actor engages in a domineering and violent action to *every* election result that opposes their ideology; that *most other people* do not engage in domineering and violent action when marching to protest a particular election result; and that this actor *always* engages in violent and domineering action when events to oppose this particular election result are organized. The perceiver should infer personal causation to this low-distinctiveness, low-consensus, high-consistency pattern, such as "They are an authoritarian person." *This low-distinctiveness, low-consensus, high-consistency pattern is what is depicted in Condition 2 of Figure 7.4, where trait attributions predominate.*

Olcaysoy Okten and Moskowitz (2018) note that most research examining the covariation logic has focused on these two prototypic configurations that produce a clear trait attribution and a clear entity attribution. They argue that another type of dispositional attribution—to a goal rather than a trait of the perceiver—is also important. They show that goal attributions emerge from alternative configurations of Kelley's (1967, 1973) dimensions. What configuration of the dimensions produces a goal attribution? One such configuration is the low-consensus, high-distinctiveness, high-consistency (LHH) pattern. Olcaysoy Okten and Moskowitz show that an attribution is made to a goal of the person when: only this particular person acts this way (low consensus), they act identically over time when in the same situation (high consistency), the person only acts this way in this particular situation and not others (high distinctiveness). Consider an example: Imagine a person who is conscientious about excelling in a particular class that nobody else cares about, is not conscientious about excelling in other classes, and who is always conscientious in each session of this particular class. You would infer they have a goal to do well in this class. Plaks, Shafer, and Shoda (2003) also showed that perceivers make goal inferences when they learn that a behavior has high distinctiveness paired with high consistency. *This is what is depicted in Condition 1 of Figure 7.4, where goal attributions predominate.* McArthur (1972) and others (Hilton et al., 1995; Jaspars, Hewstone, & Fincham, 1983; Van Overwalle, 1997a, 1997b) have also provided tests of these alternate configurations, but did not describe them as producing goal attributions. Instead, people learning about behaviors with this LHH pattern are described as attributing the behavior to "something about the interaction of person and stimulus."

In addition to high distinctiveness and high consistency implying a goal, attributions to what McArthur (1972) called an interaction of the person and the situation emerge to behaviors with low distinctiveness and low consistency (e.g., Hilton et al., 1995; Van Overwalle, 1997a, 1997b). Olcaysoy Okten and Moskowitz (2018) also classify this pattern as a goal attribution. How can a behavior that is found to occur with many entities (low distinctiveness) be indicative of a goal, rather than just a trait of the person that leads them to act this way with many different people and in many different situations? This occurs when low distinctiveness is paired with low consistency. When there is low consistency in a behavior (it happens at one time with an entity, but not in other encounters with the entity) it suggests a trait is not the appropriate explanation since the behavior does not occur over time—it is not stable—which is a defining feature of a trait. This suggests a quality of the person that is not stable, a goal, as the cause. Finally, the addition of consensus information can help solidify this as a goal. If few other people respond the same way, it solidifies that the entity is an unlikely explanation. If cause is not in the situation, and it is something internal to the person that is unstable, the cause is a goal. *This is what is depicted in Condition 3 of Figure 7.4, where goal attributions predominate.*

Olcaysoy Okten and Moskowitz (2018) reveal two configurations of the Kelley (1967, 1973) dimensions that lead to goal attributions: low consensus, high consistency, high distinctiveness (Condition 1 of Figure 7.4); and low consensus, low consistency, and low distinctiveness (Condition 3 of Figure 7.4). However, a careful reader will have already deduced that these are two very different types of goals. The goal produced by the pairing of low distinctiveness with low consistency (depicted in Condition 3 of Figure 7.4) is an unstable and short-term goal of the person. In this moment they have a goal that can be met in a variety of situations or in interactions with a variety of people (low distinctiveness), but this behavior will cease at some point when the goal is no longer relevant. Traits are rarely invoked in the explanations generated since these behaviors are unstable and nonrecurring (low consistency). However, the pattern that pairs high consistency and high distinctiveness implies a long-term goal of the person. Though it is stable over time (high consistency), it is not a trait, since it emerges only in very specific circumstances or with very specific people (high distinctiveness). A trait would generalize across entities as well as across time. This reflects a goal that only certain people or situations afford an opportunity to act upon. This is why in Condition 1 people show a blend of traits and goals and states in their explanations—they seek to explain the behavior with something long-standing about the person.

Consider an example of how these distinctions matter in a simple interpersonal interaction. Imagine a teenager who has asked a teenage girl out on a date and she has said "no." Our devastated teenager wishes to understand the reason the girl has expressed rejection (the behavior) and engages in a causal analysis. A trait attribution would suggest that the girl has a quality that makes her not like our teenager (or perhaps anyone). An entity attribution would suggest that the situation (the place she was told would be the site of the date, the circumstances under which she was asked) or another person (a disapproving and controlling parent, a judgmental friend group) is the reason for the rejection. An attribution to a short-term goal would place the cause in an interaction of low distinctiveness and low consistency (another relationship that prevents her from dating anyone else, but that could potentially end with time, as most teenage relationships do). An attribution to a long-term goal would place the cause in an interaction of low consensus and high consistency (though most teenagers date, this teenage girl does not wish to date until she is 21). These various attributions have very different emotional consequences. Placing the cause in the fact that she wishes to date our teenager (has the ability and the desire) but her parents will *never* allow it, provokes a very different response than she wishes to date but will not cheat on a *current* relationship, which provokes yet a different emotional response than *not liking* our teenager. The reasons we arrive at matter, and are ubiquitous in daily life, pervading every behavior we see. Kelley's (1967) ANOVA model describes how we derive those reasons.

COUNTERFACTUAL THOUGHT: CONSIDERING WHAT MIGHT HAVE BEEN

Hilton and Slugoski (1986) argued that the rules of the ANOVA model do not adequately capture the way in which people make attributions. Rather than examining how consensus, distinctiveness, and consistency information covary, people instead were said to rely on "counterfactual and contrastive criteria of causal ascription, as unified in the notion of an abnormal condition" (p. 76). What do they mean by this? **Counterfactual thinking** is think-

> **Counterfactual thinking:** A style of thinking that imagines an alternative set of outcomes that would have emerged had a person acted differently. The perceiver asks: "what if the person acted otherwise, what would have happened in such an alternative reality?" Knowing how consequences change is essential for forming a correspondent inference.

ing that considers alternative realities—that which might have happened had one chosen some other path of action or inaction (e.g., Roese, 1997).This is similar to Jones and Davis's (1965) idea of chosen and nonchosen courses of action each having effects. For example, if one uncharacteristically yells at a loved one (causing tears), one might have counterfactual thoughts. One would ask, "What if I had acted otherwise and not yelled?" A consideration of counterfactuals means one considers alternative outcomes that might have emerged (no tears) if a different behavior (no yelling) was enacted.

Abnormal (vs. Typical) Conditions

The counterfactual (or abnormal conditions model) assumes that perceivers make attributions by considering such alternative realities. The perceiver examines a situation for what is atypical, or abnormal. One can assess what caused a behavior to occur by looking at what happens under *unique and* **abnormal conditions** *such as when a behavior that is usually absent has occurred.* The Hilton and Slugowski (1986) model further assumes that perceivers examine the normal conditions, or the conditions *usually found when a behavior is absent.* For example, when the behavior of yelling at a loved one is absent, we have the normal conditions, or

> **Abnormal conditions:** When a perceiver examines a situation for what is atypical or abnormal. One can assess what caused a behavior to occur by looking at what happens when a behavior that is usually absent (the abnormal condition) has occurred.

what is usually found. To know why a behavior occurred we simultaneously ask ourselves, "What would we expect if the behavior did not occur, and what is unique and unusual about the conditions when the behavior does occur?" By examining how conditions differ as we move from what happened (in this example, when one has acted atypically and yelled) to the counterfactual (if one had behaved typically), we can assess the cause for the behavior. We can likely attribute cause to those factors that are not present when the behavior is absent, but are present when the behavior is present.

It may very well be that the conditions that are typically present are *necessary* for a given behavior to occur, but without the addition of some atypical factors, the behavior would not have occurred. Thus, the typical conditions would not really be considered the cause. Only a consideration of the atypical would allow one to arrive at a reasonable attribution. For example, if a lawnmower catches on fire, it is necessary for a person to have first filled the machine with gasoline and turned on the machine. But these conditions (causes), though necessary for the fire to occur, are also typical of what happens even when a fire does not occur. The fire is dependent not only on the necessary and typical causes but on the necessary and atypical causes as well, such as the engine being in an excessive state of dirtiness.

Returning to the initial example, if one yells at a family member and causes them to cry, it is necessary that the family member has contacted you and has done something that is aggravating. These conditions, while necessary for one's outburst, are also fairly typical when one does not have an outburst. The yelling is dependent not only on the necessary and typical causes, but on the atypical causes—such as being extremely stressed about something important at work. When searching for the cause of a behavior, perceivers are believed to follow a process whereby they contrast the conditions that are typically found (the causes associated with a pleasant interaction with the loved one) with those abnormal or atypical conditions that are found when the behavior (yelling) occurs.

An example that Hilton and Slugoski (1986) borrowed from Hart and Honoré (1959) will hopefully make this even clearer. When a horrific accident, such as a train derailment occurs, people tend to immediately focus on the counterfactual reality—what if this did not occur? Why is it that it did occur now, whereas it has not happened in the past? What atypical or unusual conditions were in place that are not typically in place? These types of questions, that contrast the reality with some more typical alternative reality, are what people seek answers for in order to come to understand the cause of the event. In the case of a train derailment, there are many necessary conditions for the accident that, if those conditions had not been in place, the accident would not have occurred—the freight cars were excessively heavy, the train speed was quite high, one of the rails was damaged, regulations were repealed that govern the maintenance of the break system, and so on. How do we pick from among these necessary causes to determine our attribution? The answer is that perceivers are assumed to engage in a process of contrasting those necessary causes that exist under normal (no behavior) versus abnormal (a behavior has taken place that needs to be explained) conditions. Thus, when there is no train wreck (normal conditions), we typically find freight cars of excessive weight and trains traveling at high speeds. Although such conditions were necessary for the wreck to occur, the attribution is instead made to a cause associated with the abnormal event only (poor maintenance of the brakes).

Finally, an important point relating to this model is that the terms "normal" and "abnormal" are all relative. What is abnormal in one instance might not be considered abnormal if we altered what it was being contrasted against. This is particularly true in the more mundane types of behaviors that are the focus of person perception, such as when we are attempting to understand why a person got angry after a confrontation with a loved one, rather than why a train derailed. The manner in which we set up the comparison contrast will determine the type of attribution that is formed. For example, a person's psychoanalyst might contrast the person's anger toward the loved one with how other people might have responded in the same situation (thus highlighting consensus information as the relative comparison standard). However, the person's best friend might highlight how the person has responded with other entities (thus highlighting distinctiveness information as the relative comparison standard). If contrasted against conditions where consensus information is highlighted, a very different attribution might result than if the behavior is contrasted against conditions in which distinctiveness information is highlighted. In our example, if the comparison standard for determining what is typical is how other people would react (the standard established by the psychotherapist), then it might be that other people would not get angry with the loved one and the person would be seen as at fault for their anger. However, if we focus instead on how this person has acted with other people under similar circumstances (distinctiveness), we might learn that the person has not responded with anger in these situations. Thus, the first contrast for what is typical led us to expect the person is angry by disposition. The second reveals that they are not. It is the act of using what is defined as normal and abnormal to engage in a process of contrasting alternative realities that defines this model of attribution. And it is in this manner that the model suggests consensus, distinctiveness, and consistency information are important. Rather than being rationally covaried, the model says such information establishes contrast conditions. If consensus is high, then consensus information is used as a contrast, determining what behavior is normal and abnormal. But had consensus been low and distinctiveness high, a different focus for the contrast would exist, and suddenly what behavior seemed normal and abnormal (and thus received causal weight) would be altered.

Mutability and Mental Simulations

Spellman and Kincannon (2001) point out that, often, prosecuting attorneys take advantage of counterfactual reasoning, explicitly initiating it in jurors as a way of making sense of the defendant's behavior. They ask jurors to use counterfactuals to "undo" the action mentally. This strategy makes sense from the theories we have reviewed. If the juror can imagine the negative behavior of the defendant not having been done, and can imagine the negative consequences never having happened, it will fill them with regret over the fact that the victim need not have suffered. It also fills them with attributions of personal causality. If a defendant could have acted otherwise, it suggests that the defendant had freedom of choice. This focus on the choices made by the defendant reduces situational constraint. And as we reviewed above, trait inference increases as situational constraint decreases and perceived freedom to act otherwise increases. The prosecutor knows that if jurors can be led to think in terms of choice and alternative outcomes, they are pushing the jurors toward thinking in terms of personal causality. Obviously, the idea of personal causation is integral to the legal system. We punish people both on the effects they caused and on their intentions when causing those effects. Spellman and Kincannon quote the Penal Code: "Conduct is the cause of a result when: (a) it is an antecedent but for which the result in question would not have occurred" (p. 242). If you are a prosecuting attorney who wants to make a defendant appear to be the cause for the negative outcomes, get the jurors thinking "but for." The bad outcome for the victim would not have occurred but for the acts of the defendant, which could have been otherwise. There are two ingredients highlighted here. One is the ability to imagine another course of action. The ability to simulate other ways of acting highlights the choice that was made. The second is to realize that the outcome could change. This recognition that changing the antecedent action allows for a change in the outcome is known as **mutating the outcome**. The covariance of one's chosen and unchosen actions with one outcome versus another leads to the perception of culpability. With a juror, the ability to imagine a defendant

Mutating the outcome: The ease with which a perceiver can imagine different outcomes other than the actual outcome. Examining whether a different behavior would have prevented the actual outcome from happening (would the outcome come undone).

acting differently leads them to feel the negative event could have been avoided "but for" that choice. The ability to imagine a counterfactual act undoing an event is known as a **mental simulation**. This act of making the action mutable through a mental simulation of the counterfactuals leads jurors to see greater guilt in the defendant's actions. If a counterfactual reveals to a juror that an outcome was unlikely to happen, or other choices could have been made that would have not produced the outcome, the defendant is seen as more to blame. For example, on December 19, 2022, a Congressional committee examining the cause for the riots at the U.S. Capitol on January 6, 2021, concluded that "but for" President Trump's actions, the crowd would not have turned violent. The outcome (a riot) was mutable. When running a simulation, what did evidence suggest was responsible for undoing the outcome? The alternate possible actions of the (then) President. This suggested that Mr. Trump be culpable and indicted, which he soon was.

> **Mental simulation:** Imagining an alternative course of behavior that could have been enacted that would cause the outcomes of the behavior that had been enacted to be undone or changed. It is the mental act of simulating an alternative path with different results.

In research examining these issues, the research participants read a story with a bad outcome, such as a car accident. For example, the typical scenario used is very similar to what happened to my dear friend David Kramer. Mr. Kramer decides to drive home using a scenic route he rarely uses. At a yellow light he brakes hard and stops. When Mr. Kramer's light turns green again he starts to drive, but a car charges into the intersection through a red light and kills Mr. Kramer (in my friend's case, the car was driven by a retired police officer who was drunk). The participants who read stories like these are then asked to engage in counterfactual reasoning in one of two ways. They can complete an "if only" statement, such as "In such situations like Mr. Kramer's, family and friends often think, 'If only. . . .'" How did they continue the thought? Alternatively, they can be asked how the story could be changed so that the outcomes could be undone (e.g., Mr. Kramer could have taken his usual route home and not been in the wrong place at the wrong time).

Next, participants offer judgments about blame and punishment and the emotions of the people involved. Findings from such experiments show that people are more sympathetic to the family and harsher in judging the offending driver if the outcome can be mutated. The ease with which they imagine undoing the terrible act by considering a counterfactual alternative action (what if the other driver had stopped at the red light; what if he had not been drinking) creates greater causal impact. It is important to note (e.g., Mandel & Lehman, 1996; N'gbala & Branscombe, 1995) that even if it is the *behavior of the victim that is simulated* through a counterfactual (what if Mr. Kramer took his usual way home; what if he had sped through the yellow light rather than waiting until it next turned green), it can increase feelings of regret for the outcome, and increase blame for the offending driver. However, at times simulating the victim's actions can backfire and lead to victim blaming. This is likely when the simulation introduces potentially negative implications to the victim's choices, perhaps calling their morals into question. *This was not the case*, but what if the reason Mr. Kramer was driving home in an unusual way was because he was returning home from an adulterous affair? This would not change the fact that a drunk driver went through a red light and killed him. But a simulation—such as what if he had gone home after work and not met a mistress—might increase his blame.

Wells and Gavanski (1989) illustrated that mental simulation can have a strong impact on how we form impressions and reach conclusions about people. They presented research participants with a story of a paraplegic couple who were denied a cab ride. The couple then decided to take their own car, and the car ended up plummeting off a collapsed bridge, killing them both. What do participants think about the cab driver? The answer to this question depends on whether participants engage in mental simulation that can undo the accident or not. In one version of the story the cab driver was described as driving over the exact same bridge after denying them a ride, however, doing so moments before its collapse and hence avoiding any harm. In another version of the story, the cab driver's car met the same fate as the paraplegic couple's car, but the cab driver was able to swim to safety and did not die in the accident. In these two versions of the story the outcome for the paraplegic couple is the same: they are denied a cab ride, they take their own car, and they die. However, in one version of the story the outcome is highly mutable. It is easy to imagine the couple having survived if they had not been denied a cab ride because they would have made it over the bridge before it collapsed if the cabbie had just agreed to take them.

Mutability is essential to mental simulation. The couple would not have died if the laws of gravity had not been in effect, but the laws of gravity cannot be undone. However, the behavior of the cabbie is mutable and can be undone. What is the impact of being able to simulate the alternative outcome, or easily imagining the event being undone, on how you evaluate the cab driver? The driver is rated as more responsible and their decision to avoid driving the couple as more causal in their ultimate death when participants read a story in which the cab driver successfully navigated the same bridge on which the paraplegic couple met their untimely demise (as compared to a simulation in which the cab also crashes, and the mental simulation does not undo the horrible deaths). Despite the same outcome for the couple (they die) and the same behavior on the part of the cab driver (refusing to drive the couple) in the two versions of the story, the ease of simulating an alternative reality where the couple survives (in the story where the cab makes it over the bridge before it collapses) alters the way in which participants categorize, interpret, and assign blame. Consider the implication of such a finding for wrongful death lawsuits. A doctor might be seen as having greater culpability for a patient who dies (such as more responsible for the death) if mental simulations can produce alternative realities in which the patient lived. Preventing such simulations is a good defense strategy for the doctor's legal team. Promoting such simulations ("but for" the doctor's choices) is the prosecution's goal.

We blame people more when the actions are mutable, when we can easily imagine the alternative where the bad behavior never happened. Kahneman and Tversky (1982) called this the **simulation heuristic**. To make judgments, people run a simulation in their mind that asks "What if?" They simulate what if the person had acted differently. To understand if an antecedent action (taking an unusual route home) caused an outcome (a car accident), they imagine what if the antecedent had not occurred. They run a simulation of what would have happened. The easier it is to imagine that the simulation would undo the outcome, the more likely people will see cause in the antecedent action. In essence, the simulation heuristic, and the logic of counterfactual reasoning as a way to ascribe personal causation, is just a restatement of what Kahneman's colleague at Princeton, Ned Jones, had already said—noncommon effects from alternative actions are influential in causal reasoning. If one imagines several nonchosen courses of action, and in each of those counterfactuals the person does not die (or whatever the tragic event is, it does not occur), then the ability to mutate the tragedy in each simulation is a noncommon effect. The noncommon effect from the counterfactual that has been simulated makes the unwanted outcome seem mutable and unusual, or atypical, and hence we see greater blame in the person who performed the action that caused this outcome. The unwanted outcome also seems more controllable since we can imagine other possible actions the person could

> **Simulation heuristic:** To make judgments, people run a simulation that asks "what if" the person had acted differently; what if the antecedent action had not occurred. What would have happened? The easier it is to imagine the simulation would undo the outcome, the more likely they see cause in the antecedent action.

have chosen. This lack of situational constraint and greater perceived freedom of choice makes us, again, see greater blame in the person who performed the action that caused this outcome. If a person could have acted differently and prevented the outcome (e.g., Wells & Gavanski, 1989), this mutability provided by the simulation of alternative courses of action (counterfactuals) heightens blame.

Again, this is why prosecuting attorneys may get us thinking "Could the defendant have chosen to act differently?" This is especially effective because research shows that exceptional events are more easily mutated than more typical events, and immoral events are more easily mutated than moral ones. Unfortunately, defense attorneys can use this logic as well to try and get jurors to engage in victim blaming that makes the defendant (whom they represent) seem less guilty. If they can show that the victim made choices that are painted in a negative light, then the victim's actions and outcomes are the ones jurors are asked to simulate and mutate. For example, research participants who read a story about a rape were asked to mutate the behavior of the victim. When the victim's behavior is altered so that the outcome changes, people placed more blame on the victim (compared to mutations in which the outcome does not change). Defense attorneys use this logic to ask questions about what a rape victim was wearing, to imply that had she acted differently the outcome would change, thus shifting causal attribution from the defendant to the victim because of the mutability of the outcome and the simulation heuristic.

EVEN SHORTCUTS IN THE INFERENCE PROCESS FOLLOW RULES

In this chapter we have reviewed attribution occurring through rational processes that require the systematic and effortful examination of multiple pieces of information simultaneously. But, as we have seen throughout this book, people are at times not able to exert such effort due to limits in their cognitive processing. At other times we may have the ability to be rational, but there simply is not enough information provided to do so; we have no information about consensus or consistency or distinctiveness. Yet we still make attributions from limited information. How? Kelley (1972b) asserted that we have shortcuts, or heuristics, that he called **causal schemata** that specify rules for arriving at an inference with limited information:

> **Causal schemata:** Shortcuts or heuristics that specify rules for arriving at an inference when a perceiver is in possession of only limited information that is insufficient for a rational assessment such as that specified by the ANOVA model.

> The mature individual has a repertoire of abstract ideas about the operation and interaction of causal factors. These conceptions [enable perceivers to make] economical and fast attributional analysis, by providing a framework within which bits and pieces of relevant information can be fitted in order to draw reasonably good causal inferences. (p. 152)

Kelley details two rules used when observing a single action, to a single entity, performed by one person, and one must then attribute the cause for the action to one of several potential causes.

The Discounting Principle

When there are several potential causes that can explain an effect, this is said to be a state where there exist **multiple sufficient causes**. For example, imagine a father engaged in a strategy of helping a college-age son with "tough love." This takes the form of withdrawing

Multiple sufficient causes: When there are several potential causes that can explain an effect.

financial help. There are many causes a perceiver could generate to sufficiently account for the withdrawing of finances. The cause could be the father's (1) selfishness, (2) belief that support makes people weak, (3) anger toward the child for getting into trouble, (4) favoritism toward a daughter over the son, or (5) goal to help the child through their working things out independently. Multiple sufficient causes like these demand that one from among them be identified as the reason for the father's action.

Kelley (1972a) proposed that the case of multiple sufficient causes is similar to Jones and Davis's (1965) analysis of noncommon effects: "They have clearly stated the key idea of several versus one (many versus few) plausible reasons and have asserted that the case of one or few reasons permits more confident inference from behavior to person properties" (p. 10). Jones and Davis were exploring multiple consequences for a behavior, Kelley was discussing multiple plausible *causes* for the behavior. However, the rule invoked is similar. When there are fewer to select from among, an inference is made more confidently. "If [the perceiver] is aware of several plausible causes, he attributes the effect less to any one of them than if he is aware only of one as a plausible cause" (p. 8). This has come to be known as the **discounting principle**. In essence, a perceiver discounts the possibility of other causes if one stands

Discounting principle: When there are fewer plausible causes to select from among, an inference is made more confidently than when there are several.

out as sufficient. One can make a confident inference from limited information using this rule if one strongly associates one explanation, such as a trait, with a behavior. In the example above, we learn only that a parent did not provide financial support to a child. In the absence of more information, a plausible and common inference is to label the person who

fails to "give help" as selfish or unconcerned. The fact that such an inference happens easily and seems sufficient would be enough to discount other explanations and allow the perceiver to confidently assign a reason.

The discounting principle argues that what makes a cause seem more plausible and sufficient than others is if it is a **facilitative cause**. A facilitative cause is a cause that one

Facilitative cause: This is a cause that one perceives to be present (perhaps among other plausible causes) that by itself facilitates an observed action. It is sufficient to cause the action. Perceivers use a simple rule that says that in the presence of a facilitative cause, other possible causes will be discounted.

perceives to facilitate or promote the observed action; it is sufficient to cause the behavior. The perceiver uses a simple rule that says, "in the presence of a facilitative cause, all other possible causes will be discounted." Attribution becomes more difficult, as stated above, if multiple causes feel sufficient. Why should the reason be less confidently held with multiple causes, or even shift entirely if a different cause from among the plausible ones suddenly feels more sufficient? Imagine that one makes a trait inference that the father

described above is selfish, and that this is a sufficient cause to facilitate the tough love. How would the reason we use to explain the behavior change if we learn that the tough love was apparently not the strategy used with the student's sister? The father treats the daughter with support. The behavior (tough love) and the consequence (the son not receiving support) have not been altered at all. Now, however, with still limited information, the sufficient cause that seems more probable is no longer that the father is a selfish person. If the son is the perceiver trying to understand his father, he had a cause that facilitated the action: The father is selfish. The discounting principle ruled out other causes. However, once learning that his sister is being supported, "selfish" as the cause no longer facilitates the set of actions that need to be understood and is to be discounted. A new cause is facilitative: favoritism for the daughter. As Kelley (1972a) stated, "the role of a given cause in producing a given effect is discounted if other plausible causes are also present" (p. 8). With the more plausible cause now present, the son's attribution changes from selfish (and feeling angry) to being held in disfavor (and feeling sad).

The Augmentation Principle

Behavior does not always occur in the presence of a facilitative cause. In many instances a behavior occurs in the presence of some force that works against the occurrence of the behavior—what is called behavior occurring in the presence of an **inhibitory cause**. An external cause exists that can account for the behavior *not to be performed*. For example, consider a President of the United States who, while in office, has an adulterous affair. The act occurs despite (1) there being role constraints associated with leadership that demand heightened morality, (2) opponents are already scrutinizing them closely looking for scandals, and (3) there is heightened attention to their actions because they are running for reelection. These are obstacles that should inhibit adultery. When behavior occurs despite the existence of factors that should inhibit it, then a different schematic rule of inference is used than when there is a facilitative cause. If an inhibitory cause is present, but the act occurs anyway, then the behavior is perceived as having been enacted with great conviction (it was able to overcome the obstacles). Attributing the behavior to the person's disposition is heightened. This is called the **augmentation principle**. It describes a rule that says if behavior should be constrained, or would be expected to incur a cost, yet the behavior occurs anyway, it is attributed to the person even more than is typical. Kelley (1972a) stated:

> **Inhibitory cause:** When a behavior occurs in the presence of some force that works against the occurrence of the behavior. An external cause exists that can account for the behavior *not to be performed*.

> **Augmentation principle:** When behavior occurs despite an inhibitory cause, then the behavior is perceived as having been enacted with such conviction that it was able to overcome the thing blocking it. Reasons for the behavior that attribute it to the person's disposition are heightened.

> When an effect occurs in the presence of a plausible inhibitory cause, a reverse version of the discounting principle, which might be called the augmentation principle is required. This can be stated as follows: if for a given effect both a plausible inhibitory cause and a plausible facilitative cause are present, the role of the facilitative cause in producing the effect will be judged greater than if it alone were present as a plausible cause. (p. 12)

Probabilistic Inference

Cheng and Novick (1990) point out that inductive reasoning (such as that used when people use covariation information during attribution) may be rational in the rules it follows, but that people use additional rules to supplement these processes. They focus on people's use of probability estimates that go beyond the use of consensus, consistency, and distinctiveness information. Perceivers are said to use probability estimates of the likelihood that the presence or absence of some causal factors would result in an effect. In essence, we ask what is the chance that causes "that are psychologically prior to" an effect would have resulted in that effect. In estimating such probabilities, the perceiver is acknowledging the possibility that the relationship between the cause and the effect being arrived at is not necessarily a deterministic one, but one that occurs with some degree of chance (and a likelihood of the reason being offered being incorrect). For example, today I was giving an exam in my class (room 118 of Chandler Ullmann Hall), and a student I have never seen before sat down about 5 minutes before the exam was to start. Classes had been ongoing for 10 weeks at this point, and I had given two prior exams and felt confident that I knew every student in my class of 40 people. When I approached the student to ask who he was, instead of giving me his name he asked, "Is this room 218?" When I replied, "No, this is room 118," he got up and left. How do I reason about the event? I asked other students in the room and three reasons were generated: (1) this student was planning on taking the exam for someone else, and they hoped nobody would notice; (2) this student accidentally went to the wrong classroom that he has been attending for 10 weeks because he entered the building through a different entrance and got confused; and (3) this student had never been to his other class and did not know where the room was and entered my room by mistake. To make an attribution that explains this simple event could be done by running the causal calculus. But as a perceiver, we also use probability estimates. What is the likelihood a student never had been to their class after 10 weeks? What is the probability a student might cheat on a statistics exam by sending a mathematically gifted friend? What is the probability that in our admittedly confusing building with entrance doors on different floors, one might be confused about what floor one is on?

Cheng and Novick (1992) propose that our reasoning about cause and effect typically occurs through setting up contrasts. For Jones and Davis (1965), the contrast was between the noncommon effects of two behaviors (one chosen, one not). For example, if one wants to understand why there is a forest fire, then one sets up a contrast between the conditions when a fire started and the conditions that existed on other occasions when the forest did not catch fire (e.g., McGill, 1989). Cheng and Novick argued that the contrast is done by estimating probabilities for an effect given it was preceded by a particular cause. What is the probability that entering through the ground floor might lead you to be confused versus the contrast of entering through the first floor as usual? What is the probability that a fire would have started in the forest if campers had not been there, or if there had not been a lightning storm?

Cheng and Novick (1992) argue that to determine whether a particular factor is a cause for an effect, the perceiver needs to assess two probabilities. First, they must determine the proportion of times that the behavior produces the effect when the proposed causal factor is present. Next, they must determine the proportion of times that the behavior produces the effect when the proposed causal factor is absent. The perceiver then examines the difference among these probabilities. If it is zero, then the factor is not an effect. If it is not zero, then (like with a t test) the perceiver needs to determine whether the difference is large enough to conclude that the factor caused the difference. They used probability estimates in contrast to decide whether the effect follows the behavior reliably more (or less) when the factor is present. Cheng and Novick state:

> To illustrate our model with the forest fire example, assume that lightning struck the forest where the fire started immediately before it started. Applying our model to the focal set, we see that the proportion of cases for which fire occurs in the presence of lightning is greater than the proportion of cases for which fire occurs in the absence of lightning. Lightning is therefore a cause. (Notice that our model does not require that fire always occur in the presence of lightning to covary with it.) (p. 368)

CONCLUSIONS

Heider's (1958) book entitled *Interpersonal Perception* served as a rallying call and departure point for a generation of social-psychological research. Heider's approach was (with the benefit of hindsight) intuitively obvious—it assumes that to understand the manner in which we think about people in our social world we should analyze the language we use to talk about people. Through examining the words we use to describe why people act as they do we can get a sense of the types of reasons and motives that people use to categorize and explain others. Though contemporaries of Heider, such as Ichheiser (1943), Hart and Honoré (1959), and Michotte (1963), expressed extremely similar ideas, Heider's contribution to social psychology is a description of rules we all follow, derived from the common-sense language used by lay attributors to naïvely make sense of the actions of other people. The rules Heider established were vague (we seek to infer if an action was intended, if it was internally caused, and if the cause is stable), and have been more formalized by subsequent theories offered in models such as those of Jones and Davis (1965), Kelley (1972a, 1972b), and Hilton and Slugowski (1986).

For example, Heider (1958) stipulated that one dimension important to perceivers when trying to ascertain the reason for an event is its locus of causality—is it internally caused or compelled by something external to the person. This theme is repeated in many models of attribution and spelled out with greater detail. The counterfactual approach states that people run a simulation where they attempt to imagine whether the person could have acted otherwise. The theory of correspondent inference states that perceivers ask whether a situational constraint existed or whether the action is normative (indicative of how the average person would act). The ANOVA model states that perceivers try to discern the distinctiveness of the action, examining whether the action would generalize to other entities. All four approaches pose that the perceiver is trying to determine the freedom of the person to choose how to act versus having had that behavior compelled by forces external to them. All four approaches tell us ways that perceivers do this, and that when they see a greater role for the situation, they reduce blame. However, when perceivers see less situational pressure, and perceive greater choice, blame increases.

Using another example, Heider (1958) stipulated that perceivers attempt to ascertain whether there is personal causation. For a negative event we ask what if one had *tried* harder or had greater *ability*? For a positive event we ask what if one had *tried* less, or had less *ability*? The counterfactual approach states that people run a simulation where they not only imagine an alternative path of action, but ask whether the alternative action would have undone the outcome. The theory of correspondent inference states that perceivers ask whether the possible paths of action have common or noncommon effects. All of these approaches say that if the person could have acted otherwise, the perceiver wants to know what the effects are of doing so. Are the effects common, or would acting differently undo the effect and create a unique (noncommon) effect?

Looking at the final dimension Heider (1958) posed as important to attribution, perceivers are described as concerned with the stability versus instability of an action over time. The theory of correspondent inference states that perceivers ask whether the action has outcomes that are desirable for the person. On the one hand this allows us to know whether the behavior was compelled by the rewards the perceiver stands to gain (informing us about internal vs. external cause), but this question also allows us to learn about the stability of the behavior. Presumably the desirability of the outcome is a stable quality, so we also learn that if desirability is high, the likelihood that the behavior would occur again is also high. It should be more stable. The ANOVA model states that perceivers try to discern the consistency of the action, examining whether the action would (holding constant the entity) generalize over time. All of these approaches say that stability of an action over time is important for understanding the reason the action occurred, but it needs to be considered in combination with other factors. If it repeats simply because it is very desirable, then we learn little about the person other than they, like everyone, are compelled by rewards.

But if considered along with other information, such as how others would act, we learn whether the stability is due to a trait of the person.

Perceivers do incredibly complex analyses without necessarily realizing how they induce intent. They covary multiple dimensions of information. They consider counterfactual realities. They assess common effects and noncommon effects among two courses of action. They also use intuitive rules such as estimating probabilities associated with an effect occurring under conditions they can contrast, making use of inhibitory causal factors, and relying on assessments of facilitative factors. All this allows us to determine the reasons for an intended behavior and the causes that explain an unintended behavior—with such explanations for the changes to our environment being perhaps the most central task of social cognition.

NOTES

1. Variables such as construal level (Trope & Liberman, 2003), action identification (Vallacher & Wegner, 1985), and need for specific closure (Kruglanski, 1990)—are all reviewed later in this book.

2. Some researchers speak of an external attribution as the case where the cause for an act is in the situation. But the word "situation" is misleading, because in its common use we think of a geographic location: a place. If Paul gets drunk at a party, the party is the situation, and something about the party caused Paul to be drunk (a spiked drink, beer with high alcohol content). However, it is possible for *other people* to be a "situation" when making external attributions. When we learn Paul got drunk at the party because Andrew pressured him to drink heavily, Andrew is the situation. When we learn that Maria experiences true joy when visiting with Joe, Joe is the situation.

CHAPTER 8

Biases Are Common and Arise from Normal Cognitive Processes

By January of 2024 the United States had seen a tremendous drop in inflation, which had spiked during and after the COVID-19 pandemic. Yet, in surveys conducted late in 2023 and in January of 2024, the results revealed that Americans still perceived inflation to be a serious problem. Economists pondered why Americans failed to perceive the dramatic reduction in inflation that had occurred. One possible answer is that human social cognition is biased, and that humans do not always think rationally. One bias of social cognition implicated by economists is what is known as negativity bias, in this case manifesting as a greater focus on price increases (a threat) than price decreases. Another bias implicated by economists is a focus by perceivers on accessible (or frequently purchased) products such as groceries, which still had high costs, while most other products had largely seen inflation disappear. The accessibility of items that were still inflated in cost caused people to see the entire economic system as suffering, when it was not (Donovan, 2024). Donovan stated "In 2002, Italian consumers were convinced inflation was running at 18 percent year over year, when the reality was 2 percent. Further investigation revealed that an increase in the price of a cup of espresso drove much of this erroneous impression." People make sense of the entire economy by sampling from their highly accessible daily purchases and ignoring other data. They reason that "if my bagel or Snickers bar costs more, things must be bad."

Throughout this book it has been argued that people seek meaning that is sufficient for yielding appropriate action, rather than meaning that approaches maximal accuracy. Allport (1954) posed a "principle of least effort" to describe perceivers as seeking to maximize their judgments through the least amount of mental effort possible. Simon (1956) referred to this as *satisficing*, where perceivers arrive at adequate as opposed to perfect judgments and decisions. If satisficing and least effort are typical strategies that govern cognition, then it would be a necessity that errors or biases in cognition would frequently result. If we do not seek to be accurate, our cognition should not be expected to be error-free. This does not mean we never seek accuracy. Chapter 7 was dedicated to reviewing rules people follow when, like scientists, they try to produce rational judgments based on a systematic evaluation of information and the covariation of different dimensions of information types. Additionally, Chapter 5 reviewed evidence that people at times dedicate mental effort to processing the information that is inconsistent with their expectations and stereotypes, eschewing "least-effort" thinking (see Kashima, 2000; Sherman, 2001, for reviews). However, even when people seek accuracy they can fail to produce it:

1. As reviewed throughout this book, cognitive load and processing limitations disable the ability to engage in the pursuit of accuracy, even if highly motivated to be accurate.
2. Additionally, one can arrive at a false conclusion in deductive reasoning, even if using logical strategies of information processing.
3. It is also possible for inductive reasoning (of the sort people use when applying covariation information to inference formation) to follow rational processing steps and still yield biased conclusions. People deviate from normative inductive reasoning when using covariation information in a number of ways. For example, in McArthur's (1972) work there is a tendency for people to underutilize consensus information. Also, Cheng and Novick (1992) point out that when people are given a table crossing the presence and absence of a cause with the presence and absence of an effect, they do not reach accurate conclusions about cause and effect. They know the rules, but use them incorrectly.
4. Even if they use the rules correctly, the information they are fed can be misinformation and a logical analysis will still produce an inaccurate result because of inaccurate input.

A necessary first question is What is **bias** and how does it relate to being accurate? West and Kenny (2011) define a bias as "any systematic factor that judgments are being attracted toward, besides the truth" (p. 360). They describe biases as being characterized by a force and a direction (see also Wilson & Brekke, 1994). The biasing force reflects the idea that there are variables that predispose one to respond in a manner that does not reflect accuracy or truth, and that there is a degree to which one is attracted to this influencing agent. The directional nature of bias reflects the idea that the attraction is not only a matter of degree but a preference to a particular end of a judgment scale (e.g., Kunda, 1987), such as a positivity bias, or a negativity bias, or a bias to infer a communication is true (e.g., an illusion of truth). How a bias manifests is not just a matter of these two factors but *moderators* that help to determine the strength of each element of one's bias. As West and Kenny note, "a moderator variable does not influence the judgment directly (i.e., how perceivers 'see' the person or object being judged); rather, it influences the strength of the forces that do determine judgment" (p. 361).

> **Bias:** A systematic factor that moves cognitive processing away from objective/factual analysis with both a force and a direction. A biasing force predisposes one to such a subjective analysis to a specified degree. The directional nature of bias reflects the idea of preference to a particular end of a judgment scale.

Illustrating biases in cognitive processing has been an extremely productive type of research. The ways in which humans "fail" at arriving at rational judgments and decisions, and even misperceive basic facts at the lowest of levels, is documented in far too many ways to review in a single chapter. It has been the topic of an Academy Award-nominated film (*Moneyball*), a podcast series (*Freakonomics*), many books (e.g., Banaji & Greenwald, 2013; Eberhardt, 2020; Gilovich, 1991; Jones, 1990; Kahneman, 2011; Nisbett & Ross, 1980; Wilson, 2011), and cause for awarding a Nobel Prize (to Daniel Kahneman in 2002 and to Richard Thaler in 2017). What this chapter attempts to do instead is categorize the many biases that have been illustrated over the years into general types, with common underlying processes that help to produce each category of bias. We caution that this is a categorization scheme we are creating here simply as a way to illustrate the variety of biases, not to comprehensively catalog all biases, or to claim that these are all of the relevant categories.

Throughout this book there has been a distinction drawn between implicit and explicit processes (e.g., Corneille & Hutter, 2020; Gawronski, De Houwer, & Sherman, 2020; Jost et al., 2009; Kurdi & Banaji, 2019; Ma et al., 2012). Each processing type is capable of producing bias. In the categories of bias specified below there is no distinction drawn between implicit and explicit processes. Explicit and implicit processes can contribute to each of the categories of bias. This means that a separate category is not being created for implicit bias. The term **implicit bias** has come to be a proxy for—both in the vernacular and in the psychological literature—implicit prejudice and implicit stereotyping. We treat implicit bias more broadly than that, in keeping with West and Kenny's (2011) definition of bias, and just adding that bias, at times, happens implicitly. Rather than simply referring to prejudice and stereotyping, implicit bias is defined here as any systematic factor, other than the truth, that judgments are being attracted toward without one's conscious intention or awareness. The lack of intention and awareness can apply to either (or both) the judgment itself (as when one forms an implicit impression), or the influence exerted on it (as when one forms an explicit impression that is guided by forces one does not intend or see). The choice made here is to not specify stereotyping or prejudice as the only types of implicit bias. "Implicit bias" is defined here as a general term, and when bias exists in stereotyping and prejudice it can be referred to more directly as implicit stereotyping and implicit prejudice, respectively.

> **Implicit bias:** Any systematic factor, other than the truth, that judgments are attracted toward without one's conscious intention or awareness. The lack of intention/awareness applies to the judgment (such as implicit impressions) and/or the influence exerted on judgment (such as explicit impressions being guided by forces one does not intend or see).

Before this clustering of types of biases, by way of introduction to bias, and the many causes for bias, a single type of bias is reviewed in detail. This bias is one that has been touched on throughout the book: a tendency for perceivers to overattribute to disposition, at times called the fundamental attribution error, but originally dubbed the **correspondence bias**.

THE CORRESPONDENCE BIAS (FUNDAMENTAL ATTRIBUTION ERROR)

We have already mentioned one of the most widely studied biases in social cognition—the tendency for people to overattribute the cause of another person's behavior to that person's stable qualities (such as their traits) and to relatively ignore the role that the situation played in causing the behavior. Consider an example: Russ arranges to meet his cousin Cliff after having not seen each other during the entire COVID-19 pandemic. Russ decides that they should meet at a park so that Cliff's toddler can join him, knowing that the toddler can play while the men are speaking. During their encounter, Russ feels that Cliff seems distracted, inattentive to him, and unable to respond in what Russ considers appropriate detail to Russ's stories of his life situation. Russ concludes that Cliff has become rude and is disinterested in his friendship, and departs feeling neglected, hurt, and disrespected. Russ blames Cliff's personality and feelings toward him for the action that has occurred. The reality is that Russ, a person without children, does not appreciate the power of the situation. Cliff, while glad he was asked to bring the toddler, is now responsible for watching the child in a very busy environment. As a father, the situation dictates that Cliff's attention be divided. The fact that Russ specifically chose to meet at a park so that Cliff could simulta-neously monitor his toddler is somehow lost on Russ when he evaluates why Cliff is not paying adequate attention to Russ. The behavior is attributed to Cliff's qualities, even though an obvious situational pressure could be pointed to as the cause. The robustness of this tendency led Lee Ross, in 1977, to dub this tendency for overattribution to traits as the

Fundamental attribution error (correspondence bias): The tendency for people to over-attribute the cause of another person's behavior to that person's stable qualities (such as their traits) and to mostly ignore the role that the situation played in causing the behavior.

fundamental attribution error (Ross, 1977). A less dra-matic name, **correspondence bias**, arose from the work of Jones and Harris (1967). Earlier, Heider (1944) had already described this phenomenon: "changes in the environment are almost always caused by acts of persons in combination with other factors, the tendency exists to ascribe the changes entirely to persons" (p. 361). Heider (1958) identified this ten-dency as arising from the fact that *behavior engulfs the field.*

Research on this tendency has revealed that there are multiple ways that information processing can give rise to this tendency in addition to behavior engulfing the field (which is explained shortly). It is because this bias is multiply determined that it is our focus of detailed analysis here. After providing a sampling of cognitive processes that can serve as causes for this one type of bias, we then review how these categories of cognitive processes can give rise to other types of bias. Correspondence bias is a good starting point because it is contributed to by many of these categories of processing (hence its ubiquity, or status as a fundamental error).

Evidence for Correspondence Bias—Failure to See Situational Constraint

In Chapter 7, one of the rules of correspondent inference was that if a powerful situational constraint determines the behavior of others, then perceivers should not use traits to describe the person. The power of the situation to direct attribution was noted by Ichheiser (1943):

> The behavior of the individual is always determined by two groups of factors: by personal fac-tors (attitudes, dispositions, etc.) and by situational factors. The situation plays its part in deter-mining behavior in two ways: as a system of stimuli which provokes reactions, and as a sys-tem of opportunities for action (or obstacles to action). We cannot understand the underlying motivation of behavior without taking into account the dynamics of the situation involved . . . the importance of situational factors is often greater than the importance of personal factors: individuals endowed with different traits (attitudes), nevertheless, behave in the same way in identical social situations. (p. 151)

Jones and Harris (1967) sought to test the power of the situation suggested by Ichheiser (1943). Following the rule formalized by Jones and Davis's (1965) theory of correspondent inference, they proposed that as the freedom to act as one chooses is reduced (situational constraint is high), correspondent inference will be reduced. They expected to find, as the quote from Ichheiser suggests, that people use information about obvious situational pres-sure to discount personal causation as the reason for a person's actions. They were about to discover they were wrong!

Imagine it is the 1960s. The Cuban missile crisis has brought President John F. Kennedy and the United States to the brink of war with the Communist world. Martin Luther King Jr. is leading nonviolent civil disobedience rallies to change the civil rights laws of the United States and bring an end to segregation. Now imagine you are a student at a fairly liberal college during this point in history. It is safe to bet that you expect the average person in your college to be opposed to Castro's communist regime in Cuba and opposed to segregationist policies in the United States. How do you think you would react if you learned a fellow student was espousing the exact opposite views: they are pro-Castro, or pro-segregation? According to the theory of correspondent inference, there are two factors in this example that should shape your reasoning: (1) their presumed freedom to speak their mind (low situational constraint), and (2) the atypicality of their action; their opinion differs from how you expect the average person to act (given the norms at your liberal college, their behavior is unusual). Each factor, following the theory's rules, should compel correspondent inference. You should infer they have strong pro-Castro attitudes and strong segregationist attitudes: dispositional attributions. We now throw one more wrinkle into this example. Suppose you learn the person was asked to espouse these beliefs by a professor as part of an oral exercise that *was required* for a course. In this case, the deviant attitude expressed is no longer freely chosen but resulted from a pressure in the situation—if the student wants to get a good grade, they must attempt to espouse pro-Castro or pro-segregation beliefs in front of the class as part of the exercise. Now how do you suppose you would react? According to the theory, as situational constraint increases you should be less likely to attribute this set of beliefs to the person. Since they were required to make the comments (high constraint), you should assume their true beliefs are no different from the average student.

In a now classic experiment, Jones and Harris (1967) set up exactly this situation by constructing essays that were either in favor of or against Fidel Castro's political regime in Cuba (or pro- or antisegregation in the United States). Research participants were asked to read an essay either believing the person who wrote it was free to write about any position they chose, or were asked to write the essay as part of an assignment for a course (such as a final exam question asking them to make an argument supporting Castro's regime). The experimental design manipulates whether a person (1) has free choice or not, and (2) does something normative or not. Participants next judge the person's true beliefs on the matter; they rate the "pro-Castroness" of the person's true attitude. The expected and the actual results are presented in Figure 8.1.

The theory predicts that there should be more correspondent inference when there was choice, and the first finding that jumps out from the data collected is that the scores in the choice conditions are more extreme than those in the conditions where there is situational constraint. When a pro-Castro essay is freely written, the person is seen as extremely pro-Castro (59.62) and when an anti-Castro essay is freely written, the person is seen as extremely anti-Castro (17.38). Each response is more extreme than the responses provided by participants who believed the essayist was constrained in what they were to write (due to it being an exam). The second finding that jumps out is that the direction of the essay

Expected results from Jones and Harris		
	Essay direction	
	Pro-Castro	Anti-Castro
Choice	60.00	15.00
No choice	20.00	20.00

Actual results from Jones and Harris		
	Essay direction	
	Pro-Castro	Anti-Castro
Choice	59.62	17.38
No choice	44.10	22.87

FIGURE 8.1. Actual and expected results from Jones and Harris's (1967) attitude attribution experiment. Note that attributed attitude scores range from 10 to 70; higher numbers indicate a pro-Castro attitude.

played a huge role, regardless of choice. If the person supported Castro, they were rated as pro-Castro. If the person was anti-Castro, participants rated their true attitude as anti-Castro.

The clearest test of the theory of correspondent inference comes when people read an essay that espouses the unexpected, pro-Castro position. The theory predicts that the essayist should be seen as truly holding this opinion (is a Castro supporter) *if the essay was written freely.* The theory also predicts that there should be no effect in the no-choice condition. If a person *is forced to write an essay that violates group norms,* then your impression of that person's true attitude should not be influenced by the essay; the person was forced to say it! The theory predicts that you should just assume that the person's true attitude is the same as everyone else's—if they all hate Castro, this person should hate Castro. *This was not found.* Participants rated the essayist's true attitude as corresponding to the essay regardless of whether there was choice. Participants *should* adjust their ratings of the person's true attitudes to account for the situation—they were *forced* to write a pro-Castro essay—but they do not (see the number in Figure 8.1 in grey).

Now, this is a bit of an overstatement. People are paying *some* attention to the situation. When we expect them to be anti-Castro, but they are forced to be pro-Castro, the perceiver does seem to partially take the situation into account; the person's true attitude is rated lower (44.10) than when someone freely chose to write the same essay (59.62). But still, they do not give the situation enough appreciation, and they overattribute to disposition. This is indicated by the fact that the theory predicts that if the person had no choice, a perceiver should see that person's true attitude as just the same as (anti-Castro) everyone else, and to the same degree. But the ratings show this is not the case; the perceiver sees a pro-Castro disposition. A person forced to write a pro-Castro essay is not rated by the perceiver as having the same attitudes (with a rating of 44.10) as another person who was forced to write an anti-Castro essay (with a rating of 22.87). Despite being forced to write a pro-Castro essay, the person is seen as pro-Castro, as if the perceivers are not following the theory's rules; the obvious situational constraint is overlooked.

Jones (1979) reviewed several criticisms of this experiment that raise the issue of whether the bias to overattribute the cause of a behavior to disposition is something fundamental about how people interpret social behavior, or is an artifact of the way this experiment was designed.[1] One approach to dispel such alternative explanations is to run more studies using the same method that control for and address these potential methodological flaws—and such work was done. However, rather than review such efforts here, we turn instead to another approach that addresses this issue: one of convergent validity—that is, can we illustrate the same basic bias to overattribute to disposition using a totally different research design?

Evidence for Correspondence Bias—Failure to Appreciate Roles

Aside from lack of choice, another type of constraint that limits how we act is the social roles we are asked to play. Consider the roles played by the various people on a "game show." The host of the TV show enjoys the unique advantage of having a team of writers to research the questions and provide answers. Their role allows them to appear more intelligent than perhaps they are; by nature of the situation, their knowledge of the topics is superior to that of the contestants. Ross, Amabile, and Steinmetz (1977) conducted an experiment examining correspondence bias that takes advantage of this type of situational constraint. They manipulated the *roles* played by a person who would be judged, and observed whether research participants were able to adequately take into account the clear situational constraint imposed by these roles. They used the roles associated with a "quiz show." One participant was assigned to be a contestant in the quiz show who would be attempting to answer difficult questions. One participant was assigned the role of an audience member (the perceiver) whose job was to observe the behavior of the contestant. A third participant played the role of the "quizmaster" (the person asking questions), and was asked to construct difficult questions in some area in which they had idiosyncratic knowledge (that not many others would know). Thus, the participants in any given session were randomly assigned to play the role of questioner, contestant, and observer, and the behavior of interest was the contestant attempting (and most likely failing) to answer difficult questions in someone else's area of expertise. Do perceivers recognize that the questions in this context are difficult and would be almost impossible for anyone other than the person who composed the questions (and had the role of quizmaster) to answer? Or do perceivers instead assume that the contestants answering the questions (and assigned the disadvantaged role) are not too bright?

To highlight the situational constraint, the experiment was set up in such a way as to make it quite clear that the contestant in the quiz show would have relatively little chance at getting the answers correct. The person assigned to play the role of quizmaster was explicitly and clearly instructed to design questions that were in their idiosyncratic area of expertise (such as if a neuroscience major designed questions about electrophysiology or regions of the brain). They found that despite this clear constraint, observers did not adequately take the pressure of the situation into account when rating the knowledge of either the contestant or the questioner. A person unable to answer questions specifically drawn from the idiosyncratic knowledge of another person was seen as less intelligent, despite the fact that it is the situation that makes the person unable to answer the questions. They further rated the person assigned to the role of questioner as generally more knowledgeable than the person assigned to the role of contestant (since the questioner knew all the answers). They fail to take the roles into account adequately.

Evidence for Correspondence Bias—Heightened Inference from Strong Pressure

One last example providing evidence for this bias is now reviewed from the many that exist. Imagine that as part of a conference you were attending that "breakout groups" were formed in which you were asked to discuss extremely private matters about your sex life with a stranger. Such an event would likely make you feel anxious and nervous. Snyder and Frankel (1976) saw this as an excellent way to illustrate correspondence bias since it provided an exceptionally strong situational constraint and a strong behavioral response where—as Ichheiser (1943) had said—any and all people would show the exact same response of high anxiety if asked to discuss something so deeply personal with strangers. Do perceivers who observe a woman in such a situation take its obvious pressures into account? The theory of correspondent inference predicts that the woman should not be seen as an anxious person when the situation so strongly provokes anxiety. Snyder and Frankel found the opposite: a correspondence bias.

Male research participants watched a video (without the sound) of a woman being interviewed by a man she did not know. Some thought the interview topic was bland and uninteresting. Others were told the woman was asked to discuss her sex life. The assumption was that the discussion about sex would be seen as very anxiety provoking. Snyder and Frankel (1976) then predicted a confirmation bias would come into play that would cause the correspondence bias. When perceivers expect a person to be in an extremely anxiety-provoking situation, they would then interpret the behavior they observe as showing high amounts of anxiety. Other perceivers who thought bland topics were being discussed should not expect anxiety. Despite the fact that both of these groups saw the exact same video that depicted a woman showing equivalent amounts of anxious behavior, half of the participants were prepared to see her respond extremely anxiously. Therefore, the same behavior would be seen as showing a higher level of anxiousness, or the behavior seen as more extreme, when they believed the topic concerned sex. Even though the original expectation came from the situational pressure, once the behavior gets labeled as "extremely anxious" the participant can misattribute it to a characteristic of the person. It is not that they forget that the situation was anxiety provoking but that they fail to understand how the expectation created by that situation exaggerated their perception of the amount of anxiety being displayed and caused them to see extreme anxiety. The extreme anxiety "observed" is then attributed to her as a person (her trait anxiety). Rather than discounting trait anxiety as a cause for her feelings and behavior (given the power of the situation as a plausible alternate cause), participants instead made correspondent inferences. Ironically, an inference made strictly from an extremely powerful situation caused the behavior to be seen as more extreme than it really was, and that belief that an extreme response had been seen (that never occurred) was attributed to a trait.

We have now seen evidence for correspondence bias from different experimental designs. It is important to end this review of the fundamental attribution error with a caveat. While we perceivers see traits when observing others' behaviors more than we should, this "error" is less likely to appear when judging the self. One is more likely to see the role and situational pressures that impel one's own behavior, leading to a less frequent use of traits in self-description. Jones and Nisbett (1972) referred to this fact as the **actor-observer difference**. For example, in the "Quiz show" experiment, the participants assigned to ask the questions did not rate themselves as smarter than the "contestants," even though everyone observing them ask the questions rated them as smarter. Despite this caveat, the "error" has been demonstrated to be very robust when judging other people, and its robustness is contributed to by the fact that many different types of processes can produce an overreliance on traits. That is, there are different categories of processes that produce biases, such as correspondence bias, and at this point these various categories of bias will be reviewed.

> **Actor-observer difference:** A bias to over rely on traits when judging others is less prevalent when judging the self. When judging others we are less likely to consider the pressures from the outside that are far more evident to us when considering our own reasons for our own actions. The "actor" performing a behavior considers a wider variety of reasons for the action than a person observing them.

THEORY-BASED BIASES (CORRECTION BIASES)

There are times people develop an awareness (real or imagined) that they are being influenced in an undesirable way. Wilson and Brekke (1994) referred to becoming aware of, or holding a theory about, susceptibility to bias as **mental contamination**. When a person develops such a theory that their thinking is biased and their reasoning "contaminated," this motivates them to try to **correct or debias** their thinking to remove or adjust for the unwanted influence. To remove an unwanted influence requires having a theory about *how one is being influenced*. Ironically, bias can emerge if one has a poorly calibrated theory about how one's cognition is biased. To remove an unwanted influence also requires having a theory about *how one should respond to remove that unwanted influence*. Here, too, is another way that bias can emerge when one is attempting to not be biased: by having a poorly calibrated theory about how to best adjust for the bias. Such poor calibration in both knowing how one is biased and how to correct or debias is due to the fact that most cognitive processes are not open to inspection due to their implicit nature, leaving theories about bias untethered to actual processing. The best intentions to be accurate first require a person to have an accurate theory about how one is biased and an accurate theory about how to correct that bias. If either of those theories is incorrect, then the act of trying to debias can actually produce bias. People all too often hold such incorrect theories about correcting bias.

> **Mental contamination:** A theory about one's susceptibility to bias (real or imagined), when a person suspects that their cognition has been inaccurate, or produced an inaccurate output. Thus, those cognitive outputs need to be altered, corrected, updated, or changed to correct for this unwanted inaccuracy (contamination).

For example, in Chapter 6 we reviewed work by Alex Todorov and colleagues on how easily people form impressions from faces. When a perceiver receives information about a person from what they say or do, and also receives information from that person's face, the two may be at odds. Given the spontaneous and effortless nature of making inferences from faces people may choose to anchor on that information and rely on it more. They might recognize this as a bias, where

> **Correct (debias):** To remove or adjust for what is perceived to be an unwanted influence on judgment, with the goal of ultimately producing a judgment perceived to be free of contamination, fair, and unbiased. The impression is updated and altered to be bias free.

they emphasize the face too much, and what is said is insufficiently considered. They then develop a theory that inferences made from faces are too strongly influencing them and attempt to correct this. This can itself produce a bias in two ways. First, this theory might be correct, but they might have no precise gauge of how to correctly weigh what the person says versus what is communicated by their face. Second, the theory might be wrong, and they see a bias where none existed; information communicated by the face might be more trustworthy. Nisbett and Wilson (1977) illustrate this in an experiment. Research participants watched a film, some seeing it with a distracting background noise, others without. When asked whether the noise influenced their ratings, most reported that it had. However, the actual ratings of the film did not differ for these two groups. Their theory was incorrect; they perceived an influence by the noise where none existed.

Theory-guided corrections often work in a "do-the-opposite" manner—a theory about how one is biased develops that identifies the strength and direction of the bias, and the theory of how to correct it is to exert the same force in the opposite direction. If you became aware you judged a film negatively because an annoying noise was present (and you realized it was the noise that bothered you, not the film), then you would correct in the opposite direction and increase your rating of the film. If the noise truly had no effect, then you would now have a biased view of the film due to your attempt to correct for the nonexistent bias from the noise. As another example, if you became concerned that you reacted too sternly when judging a friend, then a correction would be to shift the judgment in the opposite direction and be lenient to the same degree (thus restoring judgment to "normal" and undoing the bias). Just as a theory of how one is biased can be incorrect, a theory about how to compensate for a bias can be incorrect. There are times where "do the opposite" is not how to restore an accurate response. There are times where it is correct, but the intensity or magnitude with which one does the opposite is incorrect.

The Flexible Correction Model

Wegener and Petty's (1995b) **flexible correction model** poses that perceivers will at times become concerned about mental contamination—that an influence in their context exists that compels an unwanted response. For example, one might develop a theory that the weather in exotic locations like Jamaica and Hawaii would impact ratings of how desirable a less exotic place (such as Indianapolis) is as a vacation spot. A common theory is that it

Flexible correction model: A model of how people correct for bias that assumes perceivers use naive theories of bias to generate a compensatory response that will remove bias. Their theory specifies a magnitude and direction of the bias and compensatory responses move in the opposite direction of the bias to correct for it.

would have a negative impact; that less exotic places will seem extra undesirable in comparison to Hawaii. Theories can also have a positive impact on judgment. One might develop a theory that the weather in exotic locations like Jamaica and Hawaii would impact ratings of how desirable it is to work in those places; that jobs in exotic places seem extra desirable because of the natural beauty and great weather. Once having identified these theories, we can now address the question of interest: Do theories about how to correct for these perceived biases introduce bias (either because the initial theory of bias was wrong, or the theory about how to correct it was wrong)? Wegener and Petty found that when a perceiver believed an exotic location would lead them to see Indianapolis more negatively, their judgments of Indianapolis were corrected so that it increased in attractiveness. This led to an unrealistic and incorrect assessment of how attractive Indianapolis is as a vacation spot. Participants saw the bias, tried to remove that influence from judgment, and this created a biased positive view of Indianapolis rather than a biased negative view. The more negative the theory of influence (such as theorizing one would harshly judge the Midwest after thinking about Hawaii), the more positive later ratings of the Midwest became.

Contrast Effects

Theories about how to correct bias also create a bias in how we think about people. Imagine you observe a man acting ambiguously, with elements of both bravery and recklessness. Your mind is full of positive thoughts, like "bold," "gutsy," "dauntless," fearless," and "daring." But your mind is also full of negative thoughts, such as "reckless," "dangerous," "crazy," "suicidal," and "rash." How should you judge this person—brave or reckless? Now imagine that just prior to seeing this person you had read an article about the astronauts who landed on the moon in 1969. You recall how brave and fearless you thought these men were. This creates a possible bias. Perhaps the only reason you see the ambiguous man as having any brave qualities is because you were just thinking about bravery in the astronauts. You develop a theory that the only reason bravery is in your mind is because of the astronauts, and you should not allow those thoughts to bias how you evaluate the man. To be accurate you attempt to correct your judgment and remove the unwanted influence. You deemphasize bravery and overemphasize recklessness. But this too is a bias—the behavior observed was actually ambiguous and had brave and bold connotations that you have now removed. The judgment has gone too far in the reverse direction, where you see the person as having less of the quality in question—what is known as a **contrast effect**.

Contrast effect: When a response is pushed away from, or made in a way that creates dissimilarity with, accessible standards or qualities. It is when the ambiguous behavior that is being judged, or any target stimulus, is seen as *dissimilar to* (pushed in the direction opposite of) a prime, theory, or standard.

Initial support for contrast effects emerging from theories of bias (and attempts to correct for it) came from experiments where the researchers made the possible biasing agent very obvious to perceivers, heightening awareness of a possible influence on judgment. Martin (1986) and Martin, Seta, and Crelia (1990) exposed participants to traits (such as hostile) in either a blatant way (where a theory that one might be influenced by this trait could develop) or in a subtle way (where a theory of bias would not develop). Participants then judged a person whose behavior was ambiguous regarding hostility. The results showed that when blatantly exposed to hostility, judgments of the ambiguous person were pushed in the opposite direction. They saw them as less hostile as compared to people subtly exposed to hostility. This contrast effect is a bias because the person's behavior was neither hostile nor kind, but the judgment gets pushed in the direction of "kind" because the perceiver has an incorrect theory of how to not be biased by the word "hostile" they had previously seen. This finding has been replicated in many different ways (e.g., Lombardi, Higgins, & Bargh, 1987; Newman & Uleman, 1990; Strack, Schwarz, Bless, Kübler, & Wänke, 1993). For example, Moskowitz and Roman (1992) created a theory of bias in half of their research participants by asking them to form an impression of a person after reading a behavior that implied the person was "cautious." Thus, people were blatantly asked to think about the trait "cautious." Next, the participants were asked to form an impression of an entirely different person whose behavior could be interpreted to be either cautious or reckless. They found that in order to not be biased by the influence from the first person, they rated the new person as reckless; they avoided describing that new person as "cautious," showing a contrast effect. The other half of the participants were not asked to form an impression of the first person but were instead asked to read and memorize their behavior. For these participants, without blatant exposure to the trait of "cautious," there was no theory that influence could be exerted, and no contrast emerged when judging the second, ambiguous person.

Theories of bias do not always produce a contrast effect as the form of bias—that is just a first example of how a theory of bias can produce error. For example, Wegener, Petty, and Dunn (1998) used violent and nonviolent people to establish a theory of bias. Research participants rated how violent a popular star of action movies was. Some participants made this rating after evaluating the Pope. Other participants made this rating after first making a similar rating about extremely violent people, such as Hitler and Stalin. Participants who first rated the Pope would worry they would be biased by the kind and nonviolent shadow cast by the Pope on their ratings of the action movie star. They would develop a theory that their rating of the actor as violent was too extreme because of being evaluated next to the Pope. Therefore, the bias is to recognize that a contrast with the Pope had already contaminated one's evaluation (making the star seem more violent) and that one needs to now adjust for this to restore an unbiased judgment. How does one respond to the theory that one was already influenced by a contrast effect and must correct for it? To be nonbiased one would have to make sure the movie star was rated as nonviolent—that is, to fix the initial contrast effect they believed was a source of bias, the person would need to see the star as more similar to the Pope as opposed to different, and adjust ratings accordingly. Participants who first rated Hitler (as opposed to the Pope) would worry they were being biased by Hitler's genocidal nature and would have underestimated the star's violence as a result. Thus, to be nonbiased these people would have to now increase their rating of the star's violence. This is precisely what was found. People correct for their theory of bias with another theory that accuracy will be delivered by adjusting the judgment so that the person being judged is not contrasted with the comparison standard, but seen as more similar to it (see Figure 8.2).

Thought Suppression

In Chapter 6 it was explained that interventions that are meant to reduce stereotyping will at times backfire if they cause the person to feel threatened by the intervention as opposed to desiring to correct their bias. However, such interventions can also fail if they leave attendees to their own devices regarding *how* to fix bias. If workshops raise awareness and motivate people to change, people still require a correct theory about *how to change*. Without such training in how to be more accurate, people will use their own theories, which are often wrong (see Moskowitz & Vitriol, 2022, for a review). As an example, an intervention

Theory That One Was Originally Biased by Contrast to the Pope:

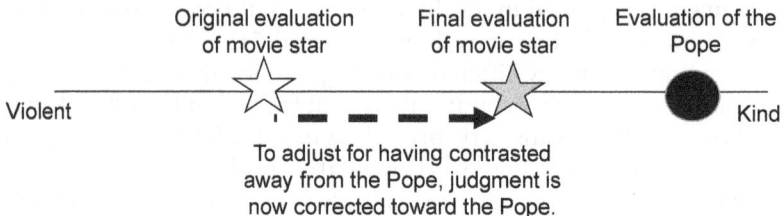

Theory That One Was Originally Biased by Similarity to the Pope:

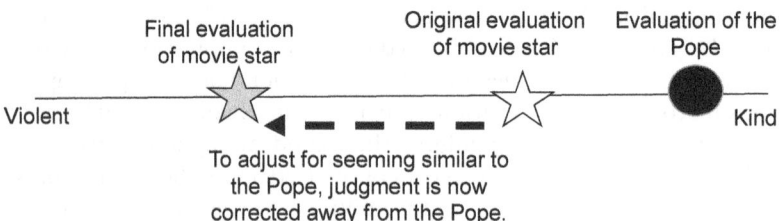

FIGURE 8.2. Flexible correction using a theory of how one is biased.

might raise awareness of implicit bias, and inform people that they stereotype without realizing it. Teaching them about implicit stereotyping and implicit prejudice is important, but if people are not also taught how to fix it, a common theory people adopt is to simply think to themselves "I must not stereotype. I must try to suppress all thoughts about stereotypes." Chapter 6 also described how such propositional reasoning may work to correct an explicit impression, but could ironically strengthen the implicit association. A person at an anti-racism workshop may consciously reject stereotypes during the workshop, but have stereotypic associations reinforced as a result, strengthening implicit bias.

This is exactly what research on **thought suppression** reveals (e.g., Galinsky & Moskowitz, 2000b; Macrae, Bodenhausen, et al., 1994; Monteith, Sherman, & Devine, 1998; Wegner, 1994; Wegner & Erber, 1992; Wegner, Schneider, Carter, & White, 1987). Thought suppression involves attempts to be accurate in one's impressions by not thinking about an unwanted thought (not just a stereotype but any unwanted thought). Suppression has the ironic effect of reinforcing the associations to that very undesired thought. Macrae, Bodenhausen, et al. (see also Wegner & Erber, 1992) argue that one might repeatedly trigger a stereotype simply through the act of suppression itself. They argued that to

> **Thought suppression:** A goal to avoid thinking about a specific unwanted thought. To suppress a thought requires, at some level, monitoring to be sure the thought is not present. For example, to correct for a perceived stereotypic bias, one might adopt the goal to suppress thoughts about stereotypes.

suppress a thought requires monitoring one's thoughts (as shown in the negative feedback loop of Figure 6.2 in Chapter 6) by scanning (even outside of conscious awareness) for the unwanted thought. To suppress something requires detecting whether it is present and correcting for this. This constant search for the unwanted item (in order to correct for it or suppress it) serves to repeatedly trigger the unwanted thought. To deny a thought's entrance into consciousness requires searching for it when relevant cues appear, which ironically strengthens the association.[2] For these reasons, a theory that one should suppress a stereotype to correct for its unwanted influence can lead to more bias. When a cue indicating group membership is detected, the search for the related stereotype (to suppress it) strengthens stereotypic associations, causing the stereotype to attain a state of **hyperaccessibility** (a similar reason for overattribution to traits and correspondence bias is provided by Yzerbyt, Corneille, Dumont, & Hahn, 2001).

> **Hyperaccessibility:** A state of acutely heightened accessibility of a construct that may arise following thought suppression. Suppression has the ironic effect of strengthening associations with the undesired thought because attempts to monitor for that thought require searching to see if the thought occurred (to then quash it), thus repeatedly triggering it.

Theories of Correction as Propositional Learning That Leaves Associations Intact

Even when we are told that information we have learned is false and a deliberate lie, it still might be hard to overturn a negative attitude that had already been formed. In Chapter 3 we defined an attitude as a structure represented in memory with not just an association among affective responses and an attitude object but additional associations to propositional learning and cognitive responses. In Chapter 6 we explored why such attitudes might be hard to overturn or correct. Using the example of a fictional social group (Niffites), it was reviewed that when research participants learned incorrect information about the group, the initial negative attitude was overturned if that attitude was explicit. It was appropriately corrected. But the bias persisted in the implicit attitudes—these correction attempts in response to the new learning did not alter the implicit association between the group and negative attitudes.

   Thus, even if aware of a bias, motivated to change it, and possessing the cognitive capacity to exert the effort to correct it, the bias is not corrected. Why? Richard Petty and colleagues (e.g., Petty & Briñol, 2010; Petty, Briñol, & DeMarree, 2007; Petty, Tormala, Briñol, & Jarvis, 2006) argue that an attitude, when stored in memory, receives a **validity tag**. The attitude's representational structure is not just a set of associations among an affective response and an attitude object. There are also posited to be associations to the *verity* of the attitude. Is it true or false? Is the information on which the affective response is based from a reliable source and is it trustworthy? If we form an attitude but later learn it is incorrect, then the attitude is linked to a "tag" that marks it as invalid and false. For example, during the fall 2021 semester a student told me that "the Lehigh football team has not scored an offensive touchdown in three years," which led me

> **Validity tag:** An association that labels an original inference as false, marking it as incorrect. While associations to such tags are initially weak and might not be strong enough to alter the existing impression, repeatedly learning information inconsistent with the first impression strengthens the tags and ultimately allows the impression to change.

to develop a negative attitude toward Lehigh football in 2021. When investigating this claim, I later learned that Lehigh scored an offensive touchdown against Lafayette College on November 23, 2019, which proved the original basis for the attitude as false. In the language of Petty and colleagues, a "false" tag would have been added to the representation of that attitude.

   How does this relate to correcting for bias? The false tag should negate the bias to associate negative affect with the attitude object. Often it does. If the association between the attitude and the false tag is strong, then the biased attitude can be corrected. However, this is not always the case. Instead, often the association among the attitude and the false tag is relatively weak. We may be told that the original information was wrong, but if that original information was told to us by a trusted news anchor, then our trust in the anchor would have led the initial attitude to be very strong. Later adding a tag that tells us that this "fact" was false is relatively weaker than the strong association initially made. We may consciously overturn the explicit attitude, but this weaker tag may be insufficient to correct the initial strong association, and the implicit attitude can persist (e.g., DeCoster, Banner, Smith, & Semin, 2006). Or it might be the case that the new learning that tells us to negate the initial learning is not vivid and memorable. Learning salacious facts about a group might be very salient, whereas a retraction is less so. With time, the validity tag might fade altogether so that one no longer recalls that propositional learning had been introduced that reversed the negative attitude. A validity tag might specify that it is incorrect to say "Niffites are bad," yet if this tag evaporates with time, then one is still left associating Niffites with negative affect. For these reasons, propositional learning might lead one to correct an explicit attitude, but in doing so it may trigger and reinforce the implicit association that was meant to be to corrected. This process can also explain why suppression attempts fail.

Suppression is often achieved by people believing they need to "try to think about something else," replacing the undesired thought with a distracting, unobjectionable thought. Macrae, Bodenhausen, et al. (1994) stated, "During suppression, perceivers are assumed to form associations in long-term memory between the unwanted item and each of the selected distracters. When these distracters are encountered on a subsequent occasion, they simply serve to cue or trigger the unwanted thought" (p. 812). This produces bias by creating new cues that can trigger the stereotype in the future. Just as the presence of features such as skin color or gender can trigger a stereotype because of a history of being associated with it, propositional learning that teaches one to replace an unwanted thought with a distracting thought allows the two to become associated. The presence of the previously irrelevant thought now comes to trigger the stereotype because of the newly formed association. For example, in 2008, a White person may have adopted a strategy of distracting thoughts of the stereotype of Black men with positive thoughts of President Barack Obama. Such a strategy may have caused President Obama to then trigger the unwanted stereotype due to having forged this association. For 8 years the person may have been explicitly rejecting the stereotype while implicitly strengthening associations to it (due to frequent exposure to Obama).

Anchoring Effects

As a last example of these "theory-based" biases, some of the earliest work on bias falls squarely in this category: **anchoring effects**. Anchoring reflects a final judgment or decision on a task that is biased by an initial estimate; where an initial judgment is tethered to a biasing agent and is insufficiently corrected (e.g., Kahneman & Tversky, 1982). When two individuals have different starting points in a judgment task (perhaps because the instructions to each person suggest different points at which work on the problem is initiated), they produce different final estimates, with final judgments biased toward the starting point. Two examples illustrate anchoring—the first was provided by Tversky and Kahneman (1974). They asked research participants to guess how many countries from the African continent are in the United Nations, a question to which they do not know the answer, and which is ambiguous enough that many answers might seem reasonable to the participant. The anchoring manipulation is simple. Prior to providing an answer, research participants observe the experimenter spin a wheel with numbers on it. People are to estimate whether the number of countries is higher or lower than the number on the wheel, and then provide the estimate. The wheel was rigged to land on either 65 or 10. Participants whose spin of the

> **Anchoring effects:** A bias in which a final judgment or decision on a task is overly influenced by an initial estimate that is insufficiently corrected. When two individuals have different starting points in a judgment or decision task, they produce final estimates/judgments biased toward their respective initial values.

wheel yielded the number 10 reported a substantially lower number of African countries in the United Nations relative to people who started with the number 65 as an anchor.

A second example comes from a different type of task. Tversky and Kahneman (1974) asked two groups to multiply a string of numbers in 5 seconds. The task could not be completed, and the logic of the experiment was that the initial computations would serve as an anchor on which the final judgment was based. The trick was that the exact same numbers were being multiplied in the two groups; what changed was the sequence of the numbers. The median response of people who saw $8 \times 7 \times 6 \times 5 \times 4 \times 3 \times 2 \times 1$ was 2,250; the median response of people who saw $1 \times 2 \times 3 \times 4 \times 5 \times 6 \times 7 \times 8$ was 512. An initial reference point serves as an anchor against which insufficient adjustments occur. Given an inability to provide an accurate answer (there is no time to multiply), one uses a theory to use initial thoughts as an estimate, and anchor to it if adjusting.

Applying this concept to correspondence bias, Jones (1979) proposed that if making an inference about a person's disposition and traits is the most immediate or viable hypothesis initially offered to account for the person's behavior, then trait inferences will act as a starting point, or anchor. The anchor then guides subsequent judgment (Park, 1989). Further, corrective inferential work may follow—one knows the initial impression is not final and needs to be adjusted. However, rather than starting out at a neutral point when subsequently evaluating causality, people start with an initial inference about the person's traits and attempt to adjust the inference from that anchor. Correspondence bias emerges from an insufficient adjustment due to anchoring (e.g., Quattrone, 1982).

Daniel Gilbert, a student of Ned Jones, extended this logic in a classic set of experiments. He started with the assumption that *behavior engulfs the field* offered by Heider (1958): "[behavior] has such salient properties it tends to engulf the total field rather than be confined to its proper position as a local stimulus whose interpretation requires the additional data of a surrounding field—the situation in social perception" (p. 54).

The salience of the behavior, and of the person performing the behavior, renders the situation more invisible, or hard to see; the role of the situation in causing that behavior goes relatively unnoticed, even though it could be extremely important. Instead, the causal weight goes to the salient item: the person. Heider (1944) further proclaimed that the aspect of the person that often gets the most causal weight is the person's traits. The behavior of the person and the traits of the person can be perceived as a perceptual unit, with traits being seen as a powerful cause that overwhelms the situational forces. Gilbert (1989) then noted that even if a perceiver tries to account for the role of the situation, correspondence bias still emerges. This is because the trait inference serves as an anchor, and adjustment away from it is often insufficient. They propose a **two-stage processing model** (see Figure 8.3) where traits are inferred at Stage 1, and the situation is considered at Stage 2 as an adjustment to (correction of) having overweighed the role of the person's traits at Stage 1. Why would this cause correspondence bias?

> **A two-stage processing model:** A model of how judgments are produced that posits an initial stage where implicit processes produce inferences/judgments about a person's disposition. In a second stage more effortful processing is engaged that can adjust the outputs of the first stage, such as by considering the role of the situation.

A first reason such a model could cause the bias is if the correction process at Stage 2 is blocked. In Chapter 6 we reviewed how attempting to adjust a first impression can be derailed by cognitive load that eliminates one's capacity to adjust an impression (e.g., Gilbert et al., 1988). The situation is prevented from being taken into account at Stage 2 because the correction process is effortful and disabled by the load. The trait inference that occurs at Stage 1 is unaffected because it is efficient, as already shown in Chapter 4's review of spontaneous trait inference. Traits are inferred quickly, without intent, and without

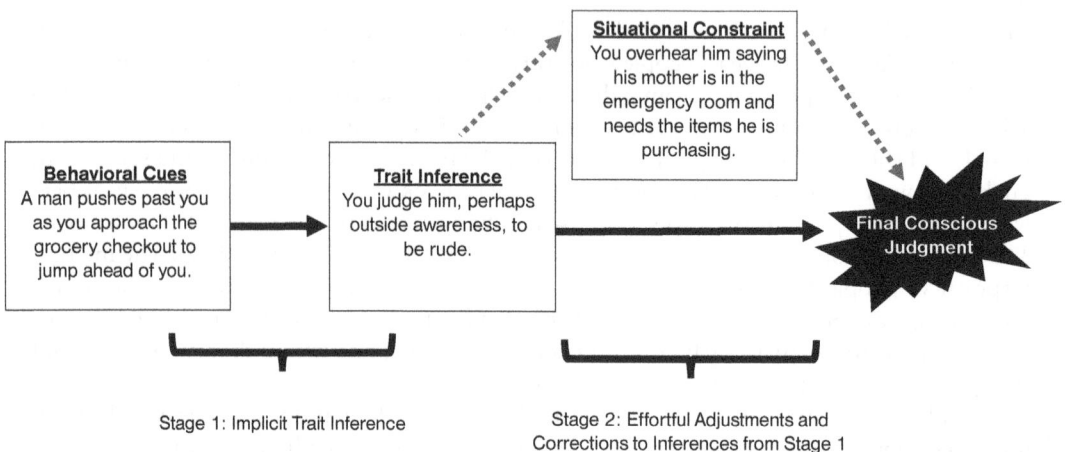

FIGURE 8.3. A two-stage model of correspondence bias: Trait inference followed by correction.

effort when we learn about a person's behavior. Gilbert (1989) said, "Perhaps it is only after we have drawn these erroneous, but effortless, inferences of disposition that we are afforded an opportunity to correct them through the labor of reason" (pp. 193–194). That opportunity is denied when cognitive load eliminates the labor, leaving only the already-formed trait inference that was unaffected by load. The dotted arrows in Figure 8.3 reflect this possibility that a correction process at Stage 2 of this processing model may fail to occur (despite the inference at Stage 1 proceeding unharmed).

A second reason that correspondence bias could emerge from this two-stage model has nothing to do with cognitive load. Even when a person has the capacity to correct at Stage 2, they may have a flawed theory about how to correct. In essence, to use the situation when forming attributions at Stage 2 one is essentially applying a theory that says "my reasoning has not sufficiently considered situational influences and has overly considered personal influences, and I need to correct or compensate for that." However, even if a situational constraint can be seen, it is often hard to see the *force* with which it hits the person. In the quiz show experiment reviewed earlier, a perceiver clearly knows each person is playing a role, and that the role of "questioner" conferred a strong advantage. They just failed to appreciate the strength of that advantage, or the power of the constraint. Therefore, when they adjust for its influence at Stage 2, the adjustment is small, and the power of the person's traits still has an advantage when explaining the behavior. Even though their theory about *how* the first impression was biased is correct (failure to consider situations appropriately), one lacks an accurate theory of *how much* the correction at Stage 2 needs to adjust the Stage 1 impression. The bias to disproportionately place blame on the person's traits remains (e.g., Gilbert et al., 1988; Gilbert & Osborne, 1989).

Identification, Inference, and Flawed Adjustment in Correspondence Bias

The explanation for the correspondence bias that was just reviewed focused on an inability to accurately gauge the power of the situation—having a flawed theory of bias. Yaacov Trope and his collaborators produced an alternative explanation for correspondence bias similarly grounded in a flawed theory and an incomplete correction process. Rather than focusing on not considering the situation enough, they considered an unusual way in which people consider the situation too much, and in doing so it has the unusual effect of augmenting the initial trait inference. In their work, the flawed theory is not about inaccurately gauging the strength of the situation, but failing to accurately consider the force of the initial bias to see a trait (e.g., Trope & Liberman, 1993). I confess it to be a complex model that I know Ned Jones considered to be his favorite explanation of the bias, and that when I took a course with Trope it took me several weeks to grasp the complexity of how it worked! But it starts with the example offered by Snyder and Frankel (1976; reviewed earlier in this chapter) in which seeing a person in a situation that is extreme—such as discussing their sex life with a stranger—leads the perceiver to infer that the person is reacting extremely in response. In this example, they infer extreme anxiety. This is what is meant by the initial inference being augmented by the situation. Snyder and Frankel showed that research participants who see a person in a terribly nerve-wracking situation formed an exaggerated sense of the person's dispositional anxiety (despite the person acting only mildly anxious). This exaggerated identification of the behavior as being anxious (because of their situation) led to the belief that the person had a stronger *anxious personality* than was warranted.

Trope (1986a) posited that this augmented initial attribution makes it hard for people to gauge the magnitude of their bias. One may realize that one has been biased by thinking about a trait, but if one does not realize *how strongly* that initial trait judgment was made, one will not adjust sufficiently. If the initial inference that the person has a trait is inflated, one's theory of how much to adjust that initial inference to consider the role of the situation will be inadequate. The magnitude of adjustment will be too small. Hence, the correspondence bias can be produced by an incorrect theory of how much to adjust an initial impression due to being unaware of how much the initial impression was exaggerated by the very situation one is trying to correct for.

Trope's (1986a) model (depicted in Figure 8.4) separates the processing that produces the correspondence bias in this way into stages. In the first stage, one observes a behavior in a powerful situation. As an example, one might observe a man with tears in his eyes at a

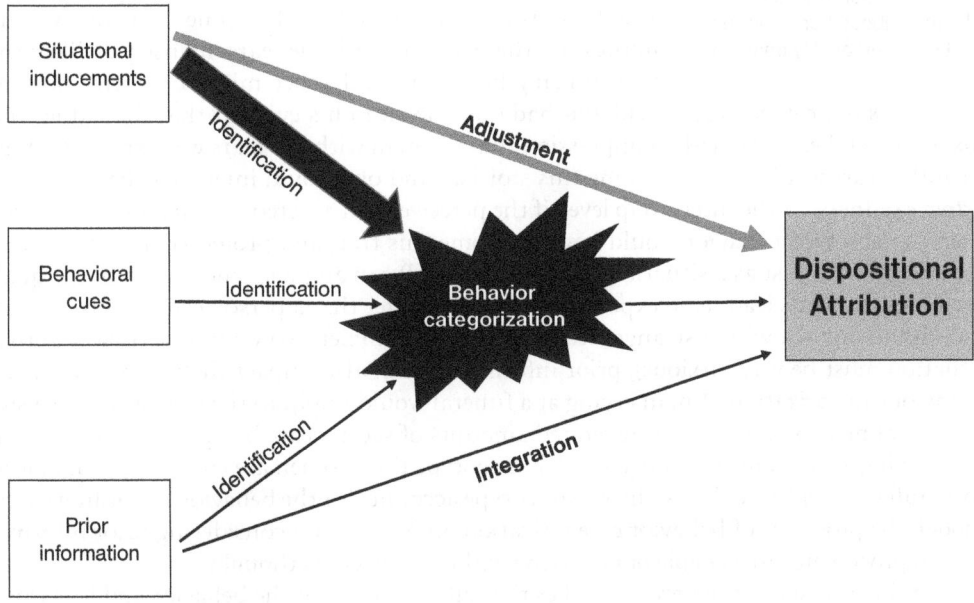

FIGURE 8.4. Trope's (1986) model of correspondence bias.

Behavioral categorization: Identifying the type of behavior that has been observed. Labeling the action and placing it into a category of similar actions (e.g., crying behavior, honest behavior, angry behavior, generous behavior, etc.).

Identification: An automatic process where attention is focused on a target stimulus, and analysis of the stimulus's features allows one to identify it as a member of a category or class. Without the perceiver's conscious effort, some form of information is perceptually salient enough in the stimulus to cue a social category.

Inferences: A stage of processing where one moves beyond identifying the type of action that has been observed to speculating about the nature of the behavior and why it occurred. That is, crying behavior is speculated to reflect sadness (in another context one might speculate that the crying reflects joy).

Prior information: A broad set of factors are perceived to be known about the person being observed which help define the behavior observed and motives for engaging in the behavior. These factors include knowledge about the person from past experience, stereotypic beliefs, gossip learned about them, information about their personality traits, etc.

funeral. In the next stage, one produces a **behavioral categorization** through a process of **identification**. This is where the perceiver identifies what sort of behavior was observed. In our example, the behavior is categorized as "crying." In the next stage, the perceiver makes **inferences** about why the behavior occurred, taking the context into account. The potential cause is, at this point, somewhat ambiguous. There are many reasons the behavior could be occurring. Inferences are made after one disambiguates the behavior through a process of eliminating potential alternative causes. In the running example, one may cry from joy, grief, or physical pain. Knowledge of the person's context is used to *disambiguate* the cause of the behavior. In this instance, the context is a funeral, and this allows for the inference that the man is crying because he is sad. Had the context been a wedding (or graduation, award ceremony, huge promotion, etc.) instead of a funeral, the inference would be that the tears represented joy. The *strength* of the inferences drawn about the behavior relies on both the behavior and the situation in which it occurs—that is, tears are not only ambiguous as to whether they indicate joy, pain, or sadness, but once identified as sadness it is ambiguous as to how strongly felt that sadness is. Being at a funeral would lead to an augmented inference about how sad the person is feeling.

The model further posits that once such initial inferences are made about the cause of the identified behavior, at a next processing stage the perceiver considers the **prior information** they have about the person—they take into account existing impressions and stereotypes (e.g., Trope & Alfieri, 1997). At the interpersonal level, if one had an existing impression that the man with the tears intensely disliked the person being buried, the inference might be altered so that the man is not categorized as sad, but had dust blown in his eyes. Or that the sadness on display was fake. If one had an impression that the man with the tears was extremely stoic, then the tears would have overcome this stoicism and one would infer that they represent *extreme* sadness. At the intergroup level, if the perceiver had a stereotype that men rarely cry, then the observed behavior would have overcome this trait and promoted an inference of *extreme* sadness. Just as a situation (such as a funeral) can augment the *amount* of the quality we see (funerals lead us to expect sadness, so we infer that a person crying must be very sad; discussing sex with a stranger leads us to expect anxiety, so we infer a person in that situation must be very anxious), prior information can also impact the magnitude of the behavior categorization. A man crying at a funeral would imply, to the perceiver with a stereotype of men as stoic, that exaggerated amounts of sadness are being felt. Had a woman been crying at the same funeral, a gender stereotype that women are emotional would lead to an inference of less sadness, since a stereotype accounts for the behavior. According to the model, the processes of behavior categorization, inference, and considering prior information in processing, are capable of occurring without conscious thought.

In the next stage, the perceiver takes the categorization of the behavior and its associated inferences and engages in the process of **impression formation**. Trope's (1986a) model describes this stage as more effortful and deliberate, where the initial inference is adjusted, modified, and updated to yield an attribution for the cause of their behavior. It is here where theories of correction can come in. One may develop a theory that prior information (first impressions and stereotypes) or the context in which the behavior occurred (situational constraint) needs to be used to adjust the inferences already formed. However, the perceiver, though clever enough to develop a theory of influence to consider these biasing agents at this stage, is usually not clever enough to realize *how strongly* those same forces were used in the earlier stages to augment or exaggerate the behavior categorization and the inferences. *The perceiver tries to discount the role of disposition in their final attribution about the person, but does not realize how the trait had been augmented by the context and by prior information, leaving the adjustment insufficient.* The theory of correction used by the perceiver does not take into account the degree to which context and prior information can exaggerate an initial trait inference (see Figure 8.4).

> **Impression formation:** Using behavioral information learned about a person along with prior information to form inferences that are combined into an overall judgment of why the person acted as they did. Where the earlier stages are typically implicit and can happen without awareness, the impression is often consciously realized.

For example, the anxious woman discussing her sex life was inferred to be excessively anxious because of the situation she was in. The perceiver may want to adequately recognize that anxiety-provoking nature of the situation, but does not realize how much it infiltrated the early stages of their thinking, exaggerating the amount of anxiety they see. Therefore, the magnitude of the bias the theory of correction assumes is incorrect, even though the direction of the bias is correct. Hence, an incorrect theory can help to produce the correspondence bias. Even though she is likely anxious only because of the situation, the situation leads us to infer much more anxiety than is actually present, and thus the adjustment for it will be insufficient. Even though a man is likely only crying because he is at a funeral, the funeral itself (and the prior information provided by stereotypes about his gender) lead us to see exaggerated amounts of sadness, and thus, still see a trait as being present even after adjusting for the role that being at a funeral may play. In Figure 8.4 this is represented by the two arrows emerging from the box labelled "situational inducement." The arrow leading to the categorization of the behavior is larger and more forceful than the one representing the adjustment for the situation's influence.

ACCESSIBILITY BIASES

Bruner (1957) discussed people as perceptually ready to respond to items of value and items that served important goals. Accessibility biases describe a similar **perceptual readiness**, but not because something is of value but because it is in a heightened state of **accessibility** relative to all of one's other **available knowledge**. *Available knowledge* is all knowledge known by the individual and stored in long-term memory. However, just because something is stored in memory does not mean that it is consciously known or easy to retrieve. Of the lifetime's worth of acquired knowledge available in memory, some of it is easier to retrieve than others; it is more accessible. Higgins (1996a) defined *accessibility* as "the activation potential of available knowledge. The term *potential* nicely captures several characteristics of accessibility . . . that

> **Perceptual readiness:** An older and alternative term for accessibility that refers to some knowledge, attitude, value, or goal having a state of mental preparedness that makes it more easily retrieved from memory, which gives it an advantage in meaning making. One is prepared or primed to see or recall something more readily than another.

> **Accessibility:** When a concept is not dormant in memory, but has a state of activation from recent or frequent retrieval; it has a heightened state of potential use. This gives it an advantage in meaning making—it will more likely be used when attending to and interpreting stimuli.

Available knowledge: All knowledge known by the individual and stored in long-term memory. However, just because something is stored in memory does not mean that it is consciously known or easy to retrieve. Of the lifetime's worth of acquired knowledge available in memory, some of it is easier to retrieve than others.

Misattributions of fluency: When construct accessibility is misattributed from the true source of the accessibility (the stimulus that primes the construct and makes it accessible) to a target that is being judged or evaluated that has nothing to do with the accessibility of the construct. Yet the perceiver mistakenly thinks it is responsible.

it is capable of being activated (and then used) but exists in a latent rather than in an active state" (p. 134; italics added). Bruner described accessibility as when a concept is not lying dormant in long-term memory but has a state of activation from having been recently or frequently retrieved. Accessibility means that a particular construct (such as a stereotype) has a heightened state of potential use, a perceptual readiness. This state of readiness makes it more easily retrieved from memory, which gives it an advantage in meaning making—it is more likely to be used when attending to and interpreting a stimulus. Accessibility biases are a class of bias that emerge when information influences cognitive processing due to its heightened state of accessibility. Some research characterizes these effects as **misattributions of fluency**, whereby the feeling of accessibility is misattributed from the true source of accessibility (the stimulus that actually makes the construct accessible) to the target that is being judged or evaluated (e.g., Jacoby & Whitehouse, 1989; Krieglmeyer & Sherman, 2012; Payne & Lundberg, 2014).

Priming Effects

The most studied form of accessibility bias is research on **priming effects in social judgment**. In such research, ambiguous information is interpreted in a manner that is shaped by accessible information. This occurs even if the accessibility arises from a source irrelevant to the ambiguous information being judged. Accessibility bias was introduced in Chapter 4 when reviewing misattribution procedures, and several examples were also provided throughout Chapters 5 and 6 as illustrations of confirmation bias (e.g., Banaji et al., 1993; Bargh & Pietromonaco, 1982; Devine, 1989; Fazio et al., 1995; Higgins et al., 1977; Moskowitz & Roman, 1992; Williams & Bargh, 2008). Accessibility can arise from a subliminal (or otherwise undetected) source (e.g., Bargh & Pietromonaco, 1982), or it can arise from everyday processes of which one is aware (e.g., Higgins et al., 1977; Moskowitz & Roman, 1992; Srull & Wyer, 1979). What matters is whether one has awareness of the influence of the accessible information on judgment (Bargh, 1992). When one is aware of the influence, then one attempts to correct for the influence, as described above, following a theory of how one has been biased. If one is not aware of the influence, then judgment of a new behavior is shaped by the accessible information. Because this bias is so routinely examined, and priming effects have become such a central concept in social psychology, we do not attempt to review it here. Rather, the entirety of Chapter 10 is dedicated to reviewing the nuance in this large research area in detail.

Priming effects in social judgment: The effect that accessible information has on the judgment made of new information, or on any cognitive process relating to a new stimulus. For example, ambiguous information is interpreted as behavioral evidence consistent with what is accessible, even if the accessibility arises from a source irrelevant to the behavior.

Additionally, the rise of stereotyping as a topic of intense focus in social cognition originated from seeing stereotypes as one type of priming effect, with the same power to implicitly bias judgment and memory as any accessible construct. Whether accessibility arises from a category label, perceiving group membership through salient features such as hair length, skin tone, or resemblance to a phenotype (e.g., Banaji et al., 1993; Devine, 1989; Dovidio et al., 1986; Maddox, 2004), the effect on cognition is powerful all the same.

For example, emotionally ambiguous facial features in men are interpreted as displaying more contempt when female research participants have stereotypes of men (such as their expected chauvinism) accessible (e.g., Inzlicht, Kaiser, & Major, 2008). As another example, a person is judged in a more stereotypic way after subliminal exposure to a stereotype (e.g., Banaji et al., 1993; Devine, 1989). Even perceptual experience can be biased by an accessible stereotype. Examples reviewed in Chapters 5 and 6 included skin tone being perceived as darker if the category "Black" was accessible (e.g., Levin & Banaji, 2006), faces being perceived as phenotypically consistent with a primed stereotype (e.g., Eberhardt et al., 2003), and Black children being perceived to be older than they truly are (Goff et al., 2014). Biases reviewed in Chapter 4 to more quickly detect (and respond to) stereotype-relevant objects, such as guns and weapons, are accessibility biases (e.g., Correll et al., 2002; Glaser, Spencer, & Charbonneau, 2014; Goff, 2016). The many ways in which stereotypes can be accessible and promote priming effects that bias judgment are reviewed in Chapter 11.

The Availability Heuristic

Perhaps the first example of an accessibility bias is the *availability heuristic* (e.g., Tversky & Kahneman, 1973), also reviewed earlier in this book in Chapter 4. This is a bias to associate the ease of retrieval of information with the frequency with which that information is encountered and the probability that this information is true. One example was provided in Chapter 6 when describing why people feel confident in their implicit impressions. Schwarz, Bless, et al. (1991) had some research participants generate *six* instances of their own assertive behavior; others participants were asked to generated *12* instances of their own assertive behavior. They all then rated their assertiveness. Those who listed only six assertive behaviors called themselves more assertive than participants who generated double the number of examples. This would sound impossible if it were not also revealed that generating six instances of a behavior is easier than the difficult task of trying to come up with 12 examples. Ease of retrieval is seen as reflecting something true. This is a bias because there are many reasons why we might easily recall something other than it being frequently encountered, of high probability, or true.

Salient information, familiar information, small amounts of information, and recently encountered information can all be easily retrieved. And this ease of retrieval can be irrelevant to what is most frequently seen or what is most accurate. Yet there is a bias to overestimate the frequency and accuracy of information simply because it comes to mind easily due to it being salient, familiar, or recently encountered. For example, in the immediate years after the September 11, 2001, attacks, U.S. citizens believed suicide bombings were far more prevalent than they really were. In reality, at that time more people died annually from animal attacks (or from falling down stairs, or from medical malpractice). However, terrorism was highly accessible and discussed regularly, both colloquially and in the media. Suicide bombings were highly accessible. That accessibility could have led to a bias in which the frequency with which suicide bombings occurred was overestimated. Ease of retrieval led to judgments of greater prevalence.

As reviewed in Chapter 4, the availability heuristic leads to bias because it creates a type of misattribution. Information is accessible in memory for one reason (such as recently seeing it, being personally more familiar with it), and this feeling of the information being accessible, or coming to mind fluently, is attributed to something else, such as it being true or being frequent. As noted at the outset of this section, many accessibility biases operate through processes of misattribution: where accessibility is attributed to one reason rather than the accurate one.

The Feeling of Familiarity and the False-Fame Effect

It is not only judgments of frequency and truth that are impacted by how easily information comes to mind. How easily something comes to mind also determines assessments of
how familiar it feels. What does it mean to say something feels familiar? Without explicitly being able to recall having seen something previously, one has the unshakable sensation that one has. Jacoby and Whitehouse (1989) argue that
"the feeling of familiarity" for some information relative to
other information is an attribution regarding the sensation
of increased *fluency* for that information. This fluency, or
heightened accessibility, is not typically detected consciously.
What people detect is a sensation that information has come
to mind easily, even if they do not consciously recognize this
sensation, and they are driven to account for it, or explain it.
When asking (preconsciously), "Why has this sensation been
detected in response to this information?," one attribution
that we make is that it is because the information is familiar. It comes to mind easily, or has
fluency and accessibility, because it is something we have encountered before.

> **The feeling of familiarity:** The sense
> that some information feels familiar
> even though one has no explicit mem-
> ory of having seen it before. Often
> this arises from information becom-
> ing accessible, or having increased
> fluency. And though not experienced
> consciously, this feeling leads to a
> sensation of familiarity that one then
> attempts to explain.

An illustration of this "familiarity bias" was provided in Chapter 4, where a study by
Jacoby and Whitehouse (1989) was described. Their research participants studied a list of
words for a memory test. They then later took a memory test that asked them to judge
whether "test words" they were now shown were from the list studied (old), or not from the
list (new). However, there was a trick that added a layer of complexity. Some of the time the
"test word" was preceded by a subliminally presented word that was the exact same word as
the test word. Some of the time the "test word" was preceded by the exact same word, but
not subliminally—it was clear and obvious that the same word was being presented twice.
When the test word was not on the original list, but was new, it would now have increased
fluency from having been seen twice at the time of testing—that is, it would be just as fluent
(or accessible) as words that were on the original list. If the extra fluency arose because of a
subliminal presentation of the word, the research participant would not have consciously
seen it. They would simply have a sensation that the word felt fluent, or was recognized easily when it appeared on the test. To make sense of this increased sensation of fluency they
would have no other logical explanation than to assume it is because the word was on the
original list. It must be fluent because it is familiar. They were correct—it *was* fluent because
it was familiar, they just misattribute why it was familiar. It was actually familiar because
it was subliminally flashed, but they are biased to think it was because they had learned it
earlier. Naturally, this bias disappears when the word is not presented subliminally. If the
word was shown in a clear and obvious way just prior to the test word, then the participant
knows exactly why the test word feels familiar. It had just been flashed at them moments
before. They are less likely to mistakenly call the test word an "old" word and more likely
to accurately label it as a "new" word. New words preceded by a subliminal flash of that
same word feel familiar because of its heightened accessibility. And because of this people
misattribute the feeling of familiarity to having learned the word previously. This bias to
misattribute accessibility to familiarity has been replicated many times using other ways to
create fluency besides a subliminal prime (e.g., Whittlesea & Williams, 2000, 2001).

As a further example, people not only attribute something feeling familiar to it recently
having been seen—they also attribute the familiarity to fame. The *false-fame effect*, also discussed in Chapter 4, is another instance of such a misattribution of accessibility to the
wrong source, where people try to link the fluency to a plausible cause and get it wrong.

Jacoby, Woloshyn, et al. (1989) showed that if one does not explicitly recall having ever seen a particular name before, or met a person with that name before, the reason the name feels familiar must be due to one knowing the name for another reason. One explanation would be that the person is of some fame. Banaji and Greenwald (1995) posited that if the false-fame effect represents an incorrect inference about the meaning of familiarity, then other factors that determine people's inferences about why someone might be familiar would impact on the false-fame effect. They argued that stereotypes about women would make it less likely for people to assume a woman is famous. If people have a stereotype that women are unlikely to be important enough to attain fame, then feelings of familiarity associated with a female name would be less likely to be attributed to the fame of the person relative to when it is a man whose name feels familiar. The results show both the basic false-fame effect (incorrectly attributing familiar names to the person being famous) and the gender effect that cancels this false-fame judgment—that is, the meaning of familiarity/fluency is different when one has stereotypic expectancies that impact on how that fluency is attributed.

The Mood-as-Information Framework

According to the **mood-as-information** framework, people sometimes evaluate an object of judgment by asking themselves how they feel about it, to assess their "gut reaction." They assume that their current feelings are a reflection of their reaction to the object of judgment, as opposed to arising from an unidentified source (e.g., Schwarz & Clore, 1983, 1996). Often, our current mood is totally unrelated to whatever it is we are asked about, but we misattribute our mood from its true (and unrecognized) source to the object of our current focus. For example, when people are asked to report about something as significant as their life satisfaction, Schwarz and Clore (1983) show that people report higher life satisfaction on sunny days than on cloudy days. They explain this finding by suggesting that people use their mood as information. In this example, people are in a good mood (or bad mood) due to the weather, but they do not realize that the weather has impacted their mood. They are not focused on it, or consciously thinking about it. When asked about their life satisfaction they assess their mood at that moment to tap their "gut reaction," and if it is positive, they attribute that positivity to the target of judgment: their life satisfaction. While one's actual life satisfaction is certainly a significant force in shaping what one reports, the judgment also reflects a bias to be influenced by one's current mood, which might have nothing to do with life satisfaction, but caused by the weather. But people do not correctly identify this influence and instead misidentify their mood as a reflection of life satisfaction. People incorrectly think that their mood and feelings at the time of judgment are diagnostic of the objective characteristics of the thing they are judging. The ease with which a mood state comes to mind has informational value that people use to help decide how they feel about a target object that is actually irrelevant to that accessible mood state (see Clore, 1992).

> **Mood-as-information:** When a perceiver unknowingly uses their mood to make an inference about a target. Mood can be a biased source of information when the source of one's mood is not the judgment target, but the mood is misattributed to the target from positive (such as sunshine) or negative (such as sewer odor) unrelated stimuli.

One way to illustrate that people are using such a "How-do-I-feel-about-it?" heuristic is to make people focus on the mood state that is the source of the bias. If aware they are being influenced by it, people should stop using it in their assessment, since rationally one's feelings about the weather (or whatever is the source of one's current mood) should not impact one's decisions and evaluations. People only use mood as information when unaware they are doing so. If helped to realize that a valid assessment process never occurred, and that their judgment is relying on a mood that was determined by an irrelevant factor, they stop using mood as information. This realization can occur by something as simple as reminding people about the weather, or whatever is the true source of their good (or bad) mood. Thus, Schwarz and Clore (1983) find that the pattern of reported life satisfaction is reversed when people were simply first asked about the weather that day. Once people realize that their mood can be attributed to a different source (other than resulting from one's life satisfaction)—such as to the weather—then the mood loses its informational value. If the true source of the accessibility is made salient, the accessibility effect disappears, and they no longer misattribute their feelings as information about a target object.

SHIFTING STANDARD BIASES

This category of bias emerges when a perceiver holds a standard against which new information is evaluated. As the standard of comparison changes, a different meaning is ascribed to the new information. **Social comparison** has long been seen as an essential element of meaning making, with the process seen as inherently biased by the standard of comparison used. Festinger (1954) stated, "there exists, in the human organism, a drive to evaluate his opinions and his abilities. . . . To the extent that objective, non-social means are not available, people evaluate their opinions and abilities by comparison respectively with the opinions and abilities of others" (pp. 117–118). Social comparison processes have bias built in; the type of meaning attained is relative to whether one engages a comparison to others who are upward or downward in ability (e.g., Gerber, Wheeler, & Suls, 2018), or who are extreme versus moderate in the qualities they possess (e.g., Herr, 1986). One might experience a feeling of loss or inferiority when comparing against one person, but the same outcomes might be experienced as relative gain or superiority when compared against someone else. As the standard shifts, a different judgment is arrived at, introducing possibility for bias. We sometimes engage in **upward social comparison** with someone who is superior to the self. Such comparisons may leave us feeling badly as we pale in comparison to the achievements of the standard. However, these comparisons are useful because we learn about our own ability, where we need to improve, and what goals to strive for. And on occasion we do not pale in comparison to revered others, and this feedback can boost self-esteem (however, it is also true that if one expected to match up well with an elite standard, and one does not, this feedback can feel crushing and create feelings of impostor syndrome). At other times we engage in a **downward social comparison**, which is a comparison to someone whose performance is likely inferior to our own. Such comparisons typically yield a positive view of the self. This can produce bias if we go too low with our standard, delivering false feedback about our ability since we are comparing against a person with very low ability. We cannot help but look good.

Tesser (1988) proposed a **self-evaluation maintenance model** that suggests that people are systematically biased in

Social comparison: A foundational process through which humans evaluate information by examining its standing relative to a standard that has been selected. It is a drive to evaluate one's beliefs, feelings, and abilities against other people to see where one stands in relation to others.

Upward social comparison: The process of evaluating the self against someone who is superior to the self, because such comparisons, although they may leave us feeling badly about our own ability, can set standards to strive for. Additionally, such comparisons can at times provide surprisingly positive results that can boost self-esteem.

Downward social comparison: The process of evaluating the self against someone who is inferior to the self, which will typically yield a positive view of the self. This can also produce bias if we go too low, delivering false feedback about our ability because we are comparing against an unreasonably low standard.

how they evaluate the self, and others, by their shifting use of "comparison standards." We select people whom we expect to be similar enough to yield useful information about our abilities. However, the information we seek about our abilities will change dependent on whether we are motivated by concerns about feeling threatened by another's accomplishments, versus basking in the glory of another's achievements, versus getting accurate feedback, versus verifying an existing belief about the self. These different motives will determine whom we select as an appropriate comparison standard, hoping that the social comparison will then yield the desired result. An assessment of how one is doing in school can shift based on whether one uses a high-achieving friend as a comparison standard (which can be a threat to self-esteem), or an oft-drunk friend (against whom one's own academic performance might shine). A high-achieving relationship partner may not be seen as a threat if used as a comparison standard because one sees a shared identity with the person, and their achievements reflect positively on the self, even if they outperform the self. For example, Pinkus, Lockwood, Schimmack, and Fournier (2008) found that when people do an upward social comparison to a friend they feel a threat—if the friend is better, this reflects poorly on the self. Surprisingly, they found that if the standard for evaluation shifts to a person with whom one shares an even closer relationship, a long-time romantic partner, that threat is removed. Instead there is a rise in positive affect and increased relationship satisfaction. Rather than envy, we bask in their success.

> **Self-evaluation maintenance model:** A theory positing that people use social comparison in a strategic way to manage a particular impression of themselves. People shift who they use as appropriate "comparison standards" allowing them to avoid threat and boost self-esteem if desired or to embrace potentially negative feedback if ready to face it.

Framing Effects

Kahneman and Tversky (1979) provide an excellent example of how meaning changes when the standard of comparison used to assess information shifts. **Framing effects** are a bias in one's decision to pursue an outcome, or in one's judgment of a person, that arises when the standard shifts from considering the gains being posed by a particular course of action to the losses being posed by that same course of action. Imagine a disc jockey (DJ) who is involved (but not hurt) in a car crash. A police officer at the scene determines that the other person is to blame. Audio and video equipment that is no longer under warranty was in the trunk and destroyed, and will cost $15,000 to replace. Now imagine that the DJ's attorney has arranged a settlement that the other driver will accept for sure (100% chance). In this settlement the DJ gets only $9,000 of the $15,000 to replace the equipment, but will definitely get this $9,000. If he goes to court, there is a 40% chance that the judge will decide against him and he will get nothing, and there is a 60% chance the judge will decide in his favor and he will get the full $15,000. Based on this information, which of the two options should he choose: settle, or go to court? Now, imagine this settlement again. This time, the attorney arranges it so that the DJ will lose $6,000 of the $15,000 spent to replace the equipment, but will definitely not lose the full amount. If he goes to court, there is a 40% chance that the judge will decide against him and he will lose the full $15,000, and there is a 60% chance the judge will decide in his favor and he will lose nothing. Based on this information, which of the two options, depicted in Figure 8.5, should the DJ choose?

> **Framing effects:** A bias emerging when the exact same situation is framed either in terms of what one stands to lose versus what one stands to gain. As the standard of comparison for assessing an action's outcomes shifts from considering its gains to its losses, the decision on how to act appropriately shifts (from risk aversion to risk seeking).

If you are astute, these settlements should sound pretty similar. In fact, they are exactly the same in terms of outcomes. There is a sure thing that results in the DJ having $9,000

276

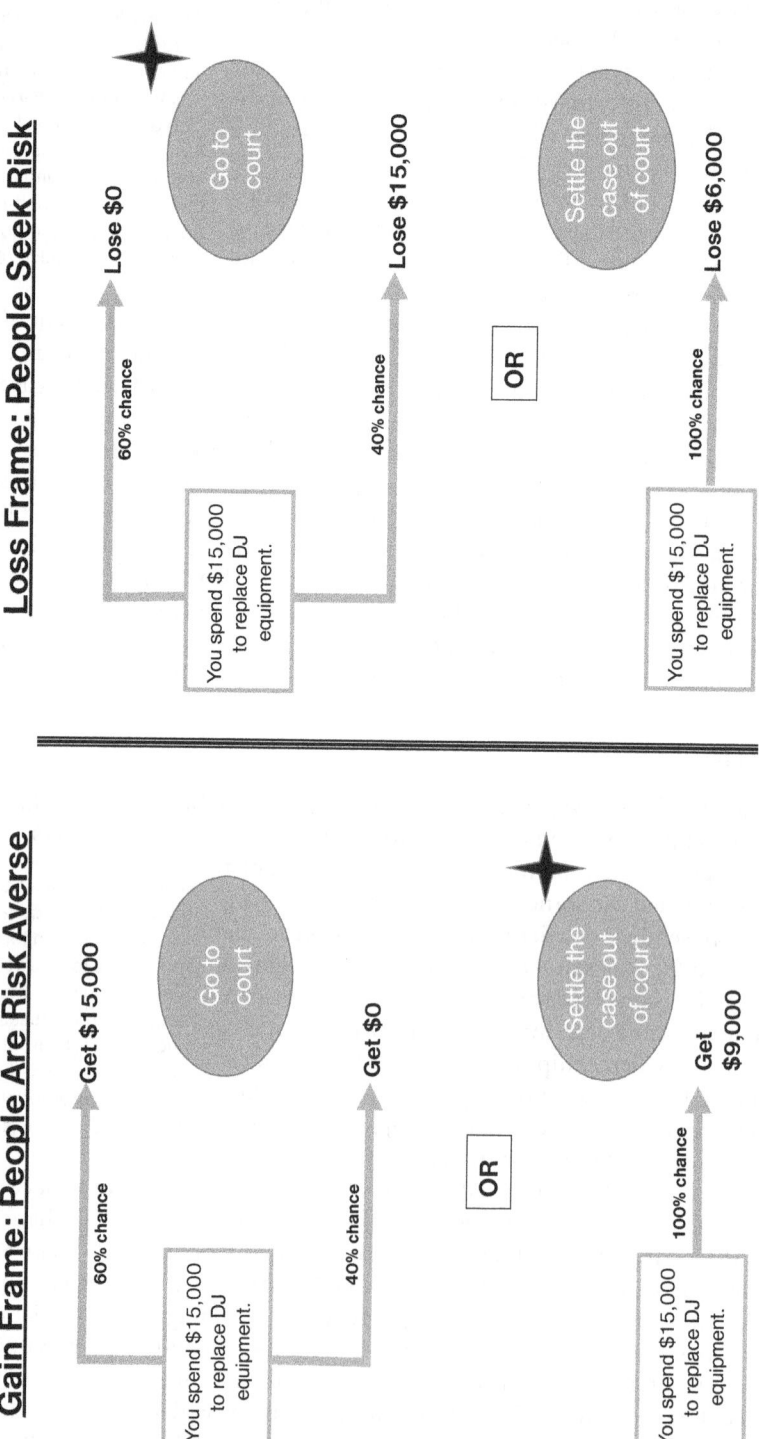

FIGURE 8.5. Framing effects.

returned, and there is a risky choice that presents a 60% chance of having $15,000 and a 40% chance of having nothing. Therefore, these are the same outcomes just described in two different ways. One is framed as a gain, the other as a loss. Tversky and Kahneman (1981) presented research participants with scenarios similar to the one just described. Despite the outcomes being the same, the framing altered the choice. Remarkably, people are less likely to take risky choices when framed as a gain (they take the sure thing, as depicted on the left side of Figure 8.5), and more likely to take a risk (in this example, going to court, as depicted on the right side of Figure 8.5) when the exact same outcome is framed in terms of what they stand to lose. Why?

> **Risk aversive:** Biased toward being cautious by choosing actions that protect, rather than threaten, one's gains. When a situation is described in terms of what people have to gain from it, people are placed in a state where they try to keep what they have.

> **Risk seeking:** A bias toward taking chances to allow one to meet the goal of avoiding a feeling of loss. Where one becomes riskier in their selected actions if it might mean avoiding loss. When a situation is described in terms of what people stand to lose, they become more willing to take chances to seek opportunities.

When a situation is described to people in terms of what they have to gain from it, people are placed in a state that has been called **risk aversive**—they try to keep what they have for sure. This is why when a team has a lead close to the end of a game, in every sport, the coaches often get conservative, cautious, and enter "prevent" mode. The focus on the win that is so close makes them risk averse. When the same situation is described to people in terms of what they stand to lose (such as for the team that is trailing with little time left), people are placed in a state that has been called **risk seeking**—they are willing to take chances in hopes of preventing loss. This is a bias because the exact same result is preferred when framed in terms of the gains and is avoided if framed in terms of the losses. The point is that a subtle shift in the standard used for evaluating the information influences how people respond by altering the way in which the data are interpreted. We come to see choices as more or less risky with one standard versus the other.

The way in which we interpret the qualities of a person can also depend on framing shifts. Shafir (1993) demonstrated that the same person (in this case, a child's parent) could be seen as either more desirable than an alternative (a child's other parent) or as less desirable than the alternative, dependent on the framing. For example, participants were asked to assume the role of a judge who was to decide which one of a child's two parents to award custody to following a divorce. One parent was described with average features, such as having decent working hours and a good rapport with the child. The other parent was described in a more enriched way that had more extreme positive information (having an extremely close relationship with the child) and more extreme negative information (having a job that required being away from home often). When the case was framed in terms of awarding custody, the participants wanted the child to be with the "enriched" parent. However, when framed in terms of loss—which parent should be denied custody—the participants wanted the child to be with the "average" parent. Presumably, the decision to award custody made salient the positive features of the enriched parent more strongly than the negative features. In contrast, the decision to reject custody made salient the negative features of the enriched parent. Similar reversals in preferences as a function of how questions are framed was shown by Ganzach and Schul (1995) for making decisions regarding whether to cancel a trip, postpone taking a course, and voting for a political candidate.

Regulatory Focus

Another way a shift in standards can change judgment and behavior is through one's **regulatory focus**. Regulatory focus is a strategy for pursuing a goal where the individual

Regulatory focus: A strategy for pursuing a goal where the individual chooses standards focused on either approaching a desired end state or avoiding an undesired end state.

Promotion focus: A regulatory focus strategy in which the person sets a standard of approaching a desired state.

Prevention focus: A regulatory focus strategy in which the person sets a standard of avoiding an undesired state.

chooses standards focused on either approaching a desired end state or avoiding an undesired end state (e.g., Higgins, Roney, Crowe, & Hymes, 1994; Liberman, Molden, Idson, & Higgins, 2001; Shah, Higgins, & Friedman, 1998). A standard of approaching a desired state is called **promotion focus**, while a strategy focused on avoiding an undesired state is called **prevention focus**. With a prevention focus people are concerned with being careful, vigilant, and not experiencing a loss—this creates strategies aimed at being safe, preventing mistakes, and preserving security. With a promotion focus people are concerned with maximizing advancement and gains—this creates strategies aimed at self-realization and a concentration on one's aspirations, ideals, and hopes. Higgins et al. argue that whether one has an approach versus an avoidance regulatory focus will alter how the goal is pursued (and whether you are successful at attaining it). For example, regulatory focus should influence the types of investment choices people make by making them more sensitive to risks of loss versus chances at gains. Zhou, Pham, Mick, Iacobucci, and Huber (2004) found that when research participants were placed in a prevention focus they were more likely to make conservative investment choices (such as investing in bonds over stocks). Under the exact same conditions, people with a promotion focus made the opposite investment choices. Crowe and Higgins (1997) used a signal detection logic to make a similar point. When asked to perform memory tasks where a list is memorized, and then later one sees a new list and needs to decide whether items are old or new, one can focus on what are called hits versus correct rejections. A hit in this example is when an item that was previously presented is accurately identified as such, whereas a correct rejection in this example is when an item that was not previously presented is accurately identified as such. Research participants with a promotion focus had a bias to focus on hits, so they develop a strategy to say "yes" to the question of whether an item is old. Participants with a prevention focus, instead, have a bias to say "no," trying to maximize the correct rejection of an item that is to be avoided (and minimizing false alarms as well).

In another illustration of the power of regulatory focus, Förster, Higgins, and Idson (1998, Experiment 2) manipulated promotion standards in some participants and prevention standards in others and used a far more subtle measure of the impact. They had research participants pursue a very easy goal: they were asked to press a button. But they were asked to either press the button by pushing their arm forward toward a button that was in front of them and away from their own body (arm extension), or by using an arm movement in which they moved their arm toward their own body in order to press the button, thus flexing their arm in a drawing-toward motion (arm flexion). Their logic was identical to that used when we described the experiment of Chen and Bargh (1999) in Chapter 3—arm flexion is compatible with the goal of approach, because to approach something means to bring it closer to one's body; arm extension is compatible with avoidance goals, because to extend one's arm is to engage in a pushing-away motion. They found that people with a promotion focus pressed the button with greater force when they were flexing their arm, while people with a prevention focus pressed harder when they had to extend their arm. Participants not only lacked awareness that a regulatory focus was being used as a standard, they were not aware of how this determined the strength of their button press.

These examples show that information that is compatible with a regulatory focus is processed differently from information that is not. It is better encoded and has a greater impact on judgment. It is also preferred (e.g., Avnet & Higgins, 2003; Cesario, Grant, & Higgins, 2004; Higgins, Idson, Freitas, Spiegel, & Molden, 2003; Lee & Aaker, 2004; Pham

& Avnet, 2004). Regulatory focus affects the value people derive from the fit between their regulatory focus and their goals. For example, Sassenberg, Jonas, Shah, and Brazy (2007) found that when a promotion focus was the standard being used to pursue a goal, research participants liked high-status groups as compared with research participants with a prevention focus, who favored the low-status groups. They reasoned that high-power groups more typically employ approach strategies to pursue their goals and low-power groups more typically use avoidance strategies. This describes instances of what is called **regulatory fit**, where there is a match among the standard being used by the participant (their regulatory focus) and the qualities of the thing being judged. In the example of high- and low-status groups, a group with risk-aversion strategies fits a prevention focus, while one with risk-taking strategies fits a promotion focus. In instances where fit exists, the thing being judged seems to have greater value and feel more desirable. Thus, people with a promotion focus like the high-power group better because they perceive such a fit.

> **Regulatory fit:** The match between a person's chosen regulatory focus and the qualities of the person/thing being judged. Qualities relating to security, caution, and vigilance fit prevention focus; qualities relating to aspirations, achievement, and advancement fit promotion. When fit exists, the thing being judged seems to have greater value and be desirable.

In another example, growth-related information is more convincing to people with a promotion focus, whereas safety-related information is more convincing to people with a prevention focus (e.g., Aaker & Lee, 2001). Such regulatory fit leads to better evaluations of consumer products. For example, buyers who had a prevention focus were concerned with a product's dependability; buyers with a promotion focus were concerned with the product's ability to innovate (Chernev, 2004; Freitas, Liberman, & Higgins, 2002; Higgins, 2002; Werth & Foerster, 2007)—that is, dimensions of the product that were associated with prevention were better able to fit the consumer's prevention focus, and were more heavily used in the consumer's assessment of and liking for the product (and the same is true for the fit to a promotion focus). In a final example, students were willing to pay more for a mug with their university's name on it if the purchase was described in a way that had regulatory fit. Students with a promotion focus paid more for a mug when it was described as the best choice as opposed to the correct choice, but students with a prevention focus paid less for the same mug when it was described as the best choice, seeing more value in making the right decision (Higgins et al., 2003). Regulatory focus and fit can be applied to the pursuit of any goal. Ending with a socially relevant example, the goal of being unbiased could be pursued through a promotion focus, such as using a standard of trying to be fair or egalitarian. However, the same goal could be pursued through a prevention focus, such as trying to avoid thinking in a stereotypic way. When constructing bias-reduction workshops, practitioners need to be careful not only of the goal (to mitigate bias) but the standards used when framing the goal (Moskowitz, 2010). We can use fit to increase the effectiveness of our attempts to change attitudes and behavior (e.g., Cesario, Higgins, & Scholer, 2007).

Latitudes of Acceptance and Rejection

Perhaps the oldest research on the impact of shifting standards is in the attitudes literature. Sherif and Hovland's (1961) **social judgment theory** applied the principles governing contrast effects with perceptual stimuli, such as the Ebbinghaus illusion, to social perception. Social judgment theory asserts that attitudes are represented in memory using a reference scale that specifies what they called latitudes of acceptance and rejection. A latitude of acceptance is the range

> **Social judgment theory:** A theory that attitudes are represented in memory using a reference scale that specifies latitudes of acceptance (the range of acceptable beliefs) and rejection (the range of unacceptable beliefs). These beliefs establish standards against which new information is judged—is it seen as similar or dissimilar to the standard.

of the scale where the beliefs a person finds acceptable are contained; a latitude of rejection is where the beliefs a person finds unacceptable are contained. These latitudes establish a reference point, or a standard, against which information is judged. Just as perception of a circle's size changes with the size of other circles around it, they believed that a judgment of a person's beliefs is influenced by one's own standards on the issue as established by their latitudes of acceptance and rejection. A prior attitude serves as a standard against which new information is judged.

For example, if one has an initial attitude, such as being anti-vaccination, this attitude establishes a standard against which information about a new vaccine is judged. If the initial attitude is a moderate one, or a mildly anti-vaccine view, it establishes a standard that falls in the middle of the latitude of acceptance, where many other views might seem compatible with it. If one then receives information from another person that is neutral toward vaccines, one's own standard will allow the other person's attitude to fall within the latitude of acceptance. This information about the person's views would be seen as more similar to one's own, or **assimilation** to the standard occurs. Since one's position is anti-vaccine, the new information is also seen as anti-vaccine. However, if the initial attitude is an extreme one, such as strong opposition to vaccines, then very few other views would fall within the latitude of acceptance. Most would fall within the latitude of rejection. Since the anti-vaccination attitude is a strong one, it sets an extreme standard. If one then receives information from another person that is neutral toward vaccines, then one's own extreme standard will make the other person's attitude seem more provaccine than the evidence actually suggests. When one is receiving information relevant to one's existing attitudes, and this information falls within the latitude of rejection, a process of **contrast** will result, where the effect of comparing the newly received information against one's existing attitude result in the reaction to the new information being polarized (seen as especially different from the existing attitude). As Eagly and Chaiken (1993) say, "the statement or position is perceived to be farther from the person's own attitude than it truly is. Within this contrast range true discrepancy is overestimated, and the magnitude of overestimation grows larger as true discrepancy increases" (p. 367).

Assimilation: When a response is drawn toward, or made in a way that creates similarity with, an existing standard or quality that is accessible. It is when ambiguous behavior that is being judged, or the target stimulus to which one is responding, is seen as *similar to* a primed construct.

Contrast: When new information is pushed away from, or seen in a way that creates dissimilarity with, accessible standards or qualities. It is when the ambiguous behavior that is being judged, or any target stimulus, is seen as *dissimilar to* (pushed in the opposite direction of) a prime, theory, or standard.

In Chapter 5 we reviewed a hostile media effect, where people with extreme views that were pro- and anti-Israel heard a moderate news report and saw it as more extreme than it really was, and in a direction opposite to their own view. Their extreme view caused the neutral news report to seem dissimilar to their own, and judged to be extreme. Political partisanship similarly reveals people with extreme views to see moderates as opponents. These examples illustrate how the moderate and extreme views of the perceiver set standards against which the attitudes of others are judged. The views of a person are perceived differently as the standard used by the perceiver shifts, determining whether the attitude falls within the latitude of acceptance or rejection. A similar logic of shifting standards is seen in research on forming first impressions, where people use whatever information is available at the moment to serve as a standard for evaluating a person. Behavior seen in the light of one standard could be seen totally differently in the light of a different standard, just as with attitudes using moderate and extreme standards.

For example, Herr, Sherman, and Fazio (1983) exposed research participants to ferocious (e.g., grizzly bear, shark) and nonferocious (e.g., dove, kitten) animal names. They then were asked to judge the ferocity of some new, ambiguous animals (animals that did not really exist, whose ferocity was unknown). If an extreme standard for ferocity had been set ("shark"), the ambiguous animal was seen as not very fierce; if an extremely nonferocious standard had been set ("kitten"), the same animal was judged as fierce. Herr (1986) showed that if an extreme standard exists, the target being judged against it will seem to have less of the quality in question, resulting in contrast. The moderate behavior of others will fall into the latitude of rejection. In another experiment, Herr exposed some research participants to an *extreme standard* for the quality "hostility," such as "Dracula," and exposed others to an extremely nonhostile standard, such as "Gandhi." Participants were then asked to form impressions of a person (Donald) whose behavior was ambiguously hostile. Donald was judged to be hostile if people used Gandhi as a standard, but saw Donald as nonhostile if they used Dracula as a standard. Donald was judged as either friendly or hostile despite performing the exact same behavior. All that changed was the standard of comparison. However, if a less extreme (moderate) standard is used, new behavior will be assimilated into that standard due to it falling within the latitude of acceptance. Herr found that *moderately hostile* standards, such as "Robin Hood," and "Joe Frazier," led to assimilation and higher ratings of Donald's hostility. Moderate standards share many features with ambiguous behavior and create a perception of similarity (assimilation). More extreme standards share fewer features with a target, creating judgments of dissimilarity (contrast; see also Moskowitz & Skurnik, 1999). If the standard shifts, judgment shifts (see Figure 8.6).

Shifting Standards and Stereotyping

In the above examples, a shifted standard caused a perception of more versus less similarity. In research on stereotyping we see how stereotypes can specify **shifting standards** that change the meaning we arrive at. This research was already reviewed in Chapter 4, where we saw that using "tall" as a dimension on which to evaluate people results in shifting standards of comparison when judging women versus

> **Shifting standards:** A bias where a construct's meaning changes as the standard it is compared against changes. For example, the meaning of "tall" changes when the standard is a man versus a woman because what one thinks is typical for each group is used as the standard against which "tall" is compared.

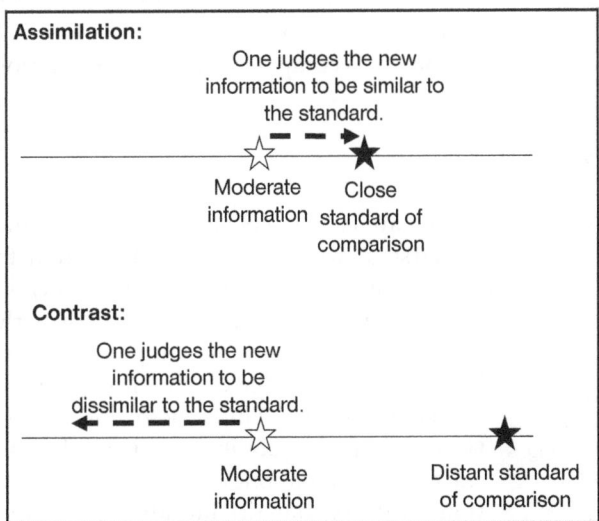

FIGURE 8.6. Shifting standards and assimilation versus contrast effects.

judging men. Since men are, on average, taller than women, the standard being used to represent "tall" is different. This shift in the standard of comparison has been shown to be a form of bias that facilitates and maintains stereotypes (e.g., Biernat & Manis, 1994; Biernat & Thompson, 2002). A woman who is objectively the same height as a man seems to be tall, where the man is not, due to a lower standard.[3]

Self-Discrepancy Theory

Finally, a large literature exists on the shifting standards that people use during self-evaluation. We see important emotional consequences when a standard of comparison shifts from an internal expectation (what one would do if acting according to one's ideals, or what one would hope to accomplish in the best possible case) to an external expectation (what one ought to do to meet the expectations of others, or what one should do). In work on **self-discrepancy theory**, it is hypothesized that how one actually behaves is often discrepant from a standard against which that behavior is compared. The theory identifies specific types of standards responsible for determining how the resulting discrepancy is experienced. **Ought standards** are reference points that specify how one should act to meet the expectations of important others. **Ideal standards** are reference points that specify how one hopes to behave if acting according to one's ideals and wishes. A discrepancy with an "ought standard" leads to agitation-related emotions (such as anxiety, fear, and guilt), which over time (if chronically experienced) can lead to fearfulness (e.g., Strauman & Higgins, 1987, 1988). A discrepancy with an "ideal standard" leads to dejection-related emotions (such as disappointment and sadness), which over time (if chronically experienced) can lead to depression (e.g., Higgins, 1987, 1989). The same behavior that fails to meet a standard leads to different emotional consequences dependent on the standard being used. One might be dejected or angry for doing poorly on an exam when considering one's ideals, but guilty or ashamed if considering parental expectations. Shifting the standards against which a behavior is compared changes the emotional experience.

Self-discrepancy theory: A theory that posits that there are multiple standards against which to evaluate the self, and that the evaluation, and the emotional response to that evaluation, can shift as the standard being used shifts.

Ought standards: A self-standard used in self-evaluation that specifies who one should be, or what one ought to do to meet the expectations of others who are important to one's self-definition (such as spouses and parents).

Ideal standards: A self-standard used in self-evaluation that specifies who one would be if acting according to one's ideals, or if striving to meet an idealized and aspirational version of the self.

MEMORY BIASES

Mandler (1980) proposed that there are two independent types of memorial information (see also Jacoby & Dallas, 1981). First, something might look familiar to you, so you recognize it as something you have seen before. This type of memory is called **familiarity**, or a vague signal of "pastness" or prior contact. Second, you may distinctly recall the information, not merely recognizing it as feeling familiar to you, but having knowledge of what it is, where you saw it, and its associated details. This type of memory is called **recollection**, or a specific ability to retrieve elements of the memory trace. For example, one often encodes more than the information itself (its content), but also something about the original *source* of the information, as well as something about its

Familiarity: A type of memory where one has only a vague sense that the information was previously experienced, or has an unspecified feeling that one had come into contact with it at some prior point, but no explicit memory for having seen it before.

context of acquisition (e.g., Johnson, Hashtroudi, & Lindsay, 1993). Accurate recollection of any given piece of information we have encountered in the past depends on the amount and quality of the information that was encoded in the first place. The encoding of any of the individual elements of a memory can be interfered with—such as the prevention of thorough

> **Recollection:** A type of memory where one has the ability to retrieve detailed information such as the context of encoding and the source of the remembered information.

initial encoding of the source of some information—producing memory traces that are not well formed. When this occurs, it is difficult for people to accurately recollect where and when they learned that information, or whether it was true or not (e.g., Gilbert, Krull, & Malone, 1990; Gilbert, Tafarodi, & Malone, 1993). Imperfect recollection for prior learning can also be caused by memory decay. The passage of time can reduce the likelihood of recollection, as a memory trace fades with lack of use.

In the absence of perfect recollection, or when only experiencing feelings of familiarity, people attempt to fill in the gaps in their memory. This can be done in a biased manner. In fact, many of the biases already described above can be characterized as *memory biases* because at their core is an inability to accurately recollect prior events. Guessing biases (e.g., Sherman, 2006), stereotype-confirming memory biases (e.g., Cantor & Mischel, 1977), false-fame effects, the illusion of truth, misattributing feelings of fluency (e.g., Jacoby, Kelley, Brown, & Jasechko, 1989), and the feeling of familiarity are all examples of perceivers being directed by a bias when recollection fails. The lack of accurate recollection renders one open to the influence of misattributed fluency and guesses that are informed by stereotypes and theories.

Gilbert et al. (1993) show how disrupted memory encoding leads to imprecise recollection, and hence bias. They had research participants learn translations for dozens of words in a language they did not know, and were told at the time of learning that some of the translations were true and some were false. For example, they might read "A Monishna is a star" followed by "This is a true statement," or "A Gurflet is a child" followed by "This is a false statement." After learning many such statements, they are then tested by being asked whether a statement was earlier said to be "true," or earlier said to be "false," or is a new item not learned previously. There is one additional component of the experiment: half of the participants were interrupted while learning the initial list so that encoding could not happen with as much depth or accuracy. They found a bias to misremember false information as being true (relative to calling true items false or to calling new items true), but only for participants who had encoding interrupted. Why does this bias to remember things as "true" happen? There are several possible explanations. The one suggested by Gilbert et al. is that when we learn information, our "automatic" response is to encode it as "true," and to next (in a separate stage of processing) correct this by tagging it as "false." The interruption prevents that "false" tag from being applied, or from being applied in a strong and clear way, leaving the participant with an inaccurate memory trace. This is essentially the same model depicted in Figure 8.3 to explain correspondence bias—an automatic first process, and then a corrective second process that gets disrupted. The memory trace is degraded so that precise memory of its falsity does not exist, leaving a bias to call it "true."

Gilbert et al. (1993) showed how this memory bias could impact important decisions, such as the way in which crime is judged and punished. They asked research participants to play the role of a judge and make sentencing decisions of what they believed to be an actual criminal case. The "judges" were provided with information about a defendant that was said either to be proven true (written in black font) or false (written in red font). The false information varied so that some participants read false statements that exacerbated the seriousness of the crimes, and others read false statements that attenuated the seriousness of the crimes. Critically, half of the people were interrupted while receiving this information, half were not. They found that if interrupted while reading *false information*, participants (1) misremembered the false items as true, (2) exaggerated their ratings of how serious the crime was to align with the false information, and (3) meted out punishment that was more or less severe to align with the false information. The inability to accurately recollect what information was true or false led to a bias in judgment.

The Feeling of Familiarity and the Illusion-of-Truth Effect

An interesting line of research helps to illustrate how misinformation or "fake news" can spread through incomplete recollection. As noted above, people are often able to recollect they heard something, but not the details of where they heard it, whether the source was credible, or whether it was true. When recollection fails, people can still have the form of memory defined above as familiarity. And as we learned when discussing the availability heuristic, when something feels familiar we have a bias to call it true. This is why repeating something, even if wrong, can help people to strengthen the associations that help that "fact" feel familiar, and familiarity makes it feel more trustworthy or true. Begg, Anas, and Farinacci (1992) called this specific case of the availability heuristic the **illusion of truth**: a tendency to label familiar information as true. This bias would not emerge if people had clear and accurate memory for the information (since under those conditions they would also recall it was false). It occurs when people are instead forced to rely on a theory that familiarity means truth (e.g., Begg, Armour, & Kerr, 1985; Hasher, Goldstein, & Toppino, 1977).[4]

> **Illusion of truth:** A tendency to label familiar information as true. If people do not have clear and accurate memory for information, they still have some recall, such as a memory that the information is familiar. Theories about familiarity are typically that it means something is likely to be true.

In fact, people can be explicitly told something was *not true* at one point in time, but later be left recalling only that it feels familiar, not whether it was true or false (Hasher et al., 1977). In fact, telling people that information is false while they are learning it can have the opposite effect: It can make them more likely to later misremember it as true (Skurnik, Yoon, Park, & Schwarz, 2005). A person might be more likely to remember a rumor or lie as true if they were told the rumor explicitly for the purpose of informing us it is wrong or ridiculous than if they had never been told about it at all—especially if it is repeated often enough. For example, Allport and Lepkin (1945) performed a study examining rumor transmission during World War II. In this study the strongest predictor of belief in wartime rumors was simply repetition of the rumors. Of course, repetition of information from independent sources can be good grounds for belief—but in this case, sometimes the source of repetition was a special newspaper column designed precisely to warn people of unfounded, false rumors. People seem to tell themselves, "I think I've heard this information before," and then once having determined simply that it feels familiar, they decide "so it's probably true." Such inferences are not irrational (Grice, 1967; established rules we assume govern most communications, such as a norm that dictates that information a person has chosen to share and communicate is likely to be true information). Ironically, a person attempting to argue against a lie, by providing evidence that it is false, can make the original misinformation feel even more familiar. If the perceiver later forgets that a credible source told them that the original information was false, but still has left the vague feeling of the original information's familiarity, then their theory that familiarity is equated with truth will still lead them to bias (e.g., Skurnik et al., 2005). If an attempt to counterargue against misinformation is complex, it can potentially backfire and lead people to favor the simpler (incorrect) misinformation (e.g., Sanna, Schwarz, & Stocker, 2002; Schwarz, Sanna, Skurnik, & Yoon, 2007). For several reasons, harping on someone else's lie might ultimately make people remember it as true.

Even a retraction, where a person confesses that an original report was fictitious, fails to have the intended effect of undermining belief in misinformation (e.g., Johnson & Seifert, 1994; Wilkes & Leatherbarrow, 1988). For example, a trusted source tells us a certain politician has molested children, and a strong association forms linking the politician to molestation. However, if we later learn this is a conspiracy theory started deliberately to discredit the politician, we might still implicitly associate the politician with molestation since the association is strong, and we might later forget the propositional learning that tells us this was just a lie, a false rumor (e.g., Skurnik et al., 2005). A lie can be reinforced even by the act of telling us it is wrong because it strengthens the original association. When explicit memory for the fact that the original information was "fake" is no longer present, all one has left is the feeling of familiarity and the strong association among familiarity and truth. This is one reason people are especially susceptible to rumors and lies that are started by a source that they trust.

There are many empirical illustrations of the illusion of truth that can be applied to the social media example. Hasher et al. (1977) showed research participants a list of unfamiliar trivia statements, some of which were true and some of which were false (e.g., Zachary Taylor was the first U.S. President to die in office). They had the participants return 2 weeks later to rate the truth of a mix of trivia items—some from the original list and some new statements. They found that the trivia items from the list 2 weeks earlier were more likely to be rated true. This is not a bias if those statements were in fact true. However, people are more likely to label as true those items that were explicitly labeled as false when first learned, as compared to new items. The old items felt familiar, and familiarity was mistaken for truth. In another example, Begg et al. (1992) also had research participants study trivia items that were clearly identified as true or false. Later, they saw a second list with a mix of new items (not seen before) and items from the old list, some of which had been true, some false. They rated each item on this list as true or false. Participants were more likely to rate "false" statements from the original list as "true" than they were to rate new and unfamiliar statements as "true." These types of experiments help us to see that a person's theories about why information is familiar (such as it being equated with truth) can have a negative impact if those theories are incorrect (see Greifeneder, Jaffé, Newman, & Schwarz, 2020). This is a danger of social media. Any lie can simply be told as if it were true, and the spread of that misinformation across a social network would make it feel familiar to a large number of people. The mere familiarity that comes from its repetition across social media platforms, and from multiple "friends" within a platform, makes it feel true. This bias makes it very difficult to change misinformation (e.g., Lewandowsky, Ecker, Seifert, Schwarz, & Cook, 2012).

Moskowitz (2001) suggests one way to do so. It is argued that since the bias is caused by theories about familiarity, then changing the theory could change the bias, even if labeling a fact as false cannot. If one is led to believe that familiar information is mostly false (rather than true), then the tendency to call things that seem familiar "true" would be reversed. Skurnik, Moskowitz, and Johnson (2001) provided evidence for this. They trained participants that an old list had mostly false information (as opposed to mostly true, or 50–50). Thus, participants developed a theory that familiarity (in this case) means something is likely false. The illusion of truth bias typically seen was reversed, and became instead an illusion of falseness bias. In the social media example, this suggests that if a theory developed that information shared on Facebook (or Instagram, or TikTok, etc.) is largely rumor and speculation, it might eliminate the threat of misinformation disseminated over social media being accepted as true. It would instead lead to a theory that familiarity from learning something on social media means "the something" is likely to be false.

Source Confusion

Johnson et al. (1993; see also Johnson, 1988; Johnson & Raye, 1981) describe a bias they called **source confusion**. With a source confusion a person has difficulty in determining whether the source of information they learn about is real versus imagined. Consider the case of the eyewitness who believes they remember having heard the accused suspect say something that is considered to be damning evidence by the prosecution. It is possible, however, that what is being recalled is a news report claiming the person said the damning statement rather than the eyewitness having heard the information. People may also label something that was imaginary as having really happened (perhaps mistaking a dream from 2 weeks ago for a real event, or a rumor heard from a gossip as an item seen on the news). They confuse who said what.

> **Source confusion:** When one mistakenly identifies where one's recalled information was originally learned (its source), such as when one misremembers (confuses) something imagined as real (and vice versa). For example, an eyewitness may believe she remembers overhearing an accused person having said something damning, when in fact the eyewitness actually heard an anchorperson on the news make this claim about the accused having said the damning quote.

How do such errors occur? According to Johnson et al. (1993), remembering the source of information may be simple (and automatic) if it is stored as part of the memory for the event. When memories do not have tags that indicate their source (such as real vs. imagined, or reliable vs. unreliable), they infer the source at the time of retrieval by evaluating the stored aspects of the memory trace along with its compatibility with prior knowledge, which could be a more effortful process. This allows people to be accurate in remembering *that* they have seen information before, but unable to identify the *context* in which they acquired the information. This is because memory for context can be selectively impaired by things such as divided attention, time delays, and aging. In sum, people may be very accurate in believing they have seen a piece of information before, but be confused about the source of the information or the context in which it was learned. These factors can determine whether memory is accurate and detailed, or false, or even something else—vague and unspecified, or a "context-free" memory trace (Mandler, 1980). Above we reviewed the illusion of truth, where information that feels familiar is labeled as true. Here we identify a separate impact of familiarity where the result is a source confusion. Just as with the illusion of truth, this memory bias can result in the spread of misinformation, this time by allowing people to confuse an unreliable source with a reliable one. If one cannot recall the correct source of information, familiarity may lead to an error.

This type of source confusion can exacerbate gender bias in the workplace, where a good idea expressed in a meeting by a woman is confused for having been said by a man (e.g., Bohnet, 2016). Another form this bias can take is when excellent contributions made by women can be forgotten altogether, whereas the contributions made by men are accurately recalled and attributed to the correct source. For example, Lamer, Dvorak, Biddle, Pauker, and Weisbuch (2022) illustrated that **intersubjective norms** can influence memory in this way. Intersubjective norms are beliefs about what other people think is true, or essentially one's knowledge of a cultural stereotype held by others that can serve as a norm prescribing what one is expected to think. When women believe that there is a norm that minimizes the competence of women, it creates

> **Intersubjective norms:** These are beliefs about what other people think is true, or essentially one's knowledge of a cultural stereotype held by others that can serve as a norm prescribing what one is expected to think.

gender-based memory omissions.[5] People with strong knowledge of the norms (especially normative beliefs that women lack competency and agency) have a greater tendency to forget statements made by women relative to statements made by men. Thus, in addition to women having their contributions falsely recalled as having been made by men, their contributions can also just be omitted from memory.

Directed Forgetting

Most of the research on memory biases reviewed above reflects *unintentional* processes (the decay or weakening of associations, the loss of detail creating incomplete recollections) where changes to a memory contribute to bias. Research on **directed forgetting** (e.g., Sahakyan, Delaney, Foster, & Abushanab, 2013) shows that people can *intentionally* control the information that gets committed to and omitted from memory, which can also result in bias. Directed forgetting explores the issue of whether people can intentionally forget the behaviors of others. Research findings show that memory for a word list is worse following a postlearning instruction to "forget" the list as compared to no instruction, or an instruction to recall the items on the list. Memory is not only reduced for the items in

Directed forgetting: A phenomenon where people intentionally forget the behaviors of others. Research findings show that memory for a word list is worse following a postlearning instruction to "forget" the list as compared to when no instruction is given or an instruction is given to recall the items on the list.

the original list but is biased in favor of other information learned. If a second list is learned simultaneously, the instruction to forget the first list improves memory for the second list (e.g., Hupbach, 2018; Scully & Hupbach, 2020). This memory bias can impact how we evaluate other people. Scully and Hupbach show that when a person intentionally tried to forget the negative behaviors of a fictional character, this skewed their judgments of the character. As memory for negative behaviors was reduced, the character was explicitly judged to be both warmer and less dominant. However, Hupbach, Olcaysoy Okten, and Horn (2022) show that intentionally forgetting the behaviors that imply traits does not eliminate from memory the *traits* that were initially inferred. Even if explicit judgment shows a bias to use more positive evaluations, implicit memory shows the original negative traits are still stored.

Reactivation and Reconsolidation

Bias also arises from memory structures being updated and reconsolidated, with new information altering the original memory (e.g., Hupbach, Gomez, & Nadel, 2015). When a stable (i.e., "consolidated") long-term memory is reactivated, it can enter a state of plasticity where it is no longer stable but able to be modified. The memory is made flexible. Once in this state, a memory can have its content changed. It can be strengthened, weakened, or erased. It is susceptible to interference from other information that is irrelevant to the original memory, thus changing the memory to include new components that were not part of the original learning episode (e.g., Hupbach, Gomez, Hardt, & Nadel, 2007; Hupbach, Gomez, & Nadel, 2009). **Reconsolidation of memory** refers to the processes that restabilize reactivated and plastic memories (e.g., Dudai, 2012). Hupbach (2013) suggested that such processes happen naturally when new information related to an existing memory reactivates the memory, and in

Reconsolidation of memory: When a stable ("consolidated") long-term memory is reactivated, it enters a state of plasticity where it is modifiable and its content is changed, strengthened, weakened, or erased, thus changing the memory to include new components that were not part of the original learning episode. Reconsolidation refers to processes that restabilize these altered memories.

so doing alters the old memory to conform with the newer information. Reactivation makes memories more vulnerable to intrusions from competing memories, allowing for the intrusions to be reconsolidated as part of the original memory. This suggests that memories can be altered once reactivated and have new, perhaps incorrect, information added to the memory. To the individual the memory seems to reflect only the original learning episode, but, in reality, it has been modified to include later learning.

This is one reason biases emerge in eyewitness testimony. The memory has been unknowingly distorted and updated. For example, Chan and LaPaglia (2013) found that critical details of an event could be changed in memory if a consolidated memory was first reactivated and then the individual was presented with misinformation about those details. Consider the implications when a police officer illegally obtains a confession through pressuring a suspect. Kassin and Kiechel (1996) found that people can be convinced by authorities that they committed crimes (when they had not), especially when the defendant's memory for the event is vague and the authorities present false evidence. Once having forced the person to admit to the behavior (using tactics such as misinformation and deprivation of food, sleep, lawyers, etc.), it is now possible that the person's memory has been altered so that they recall the false events as having happened. It is hard enough, based on what we learned about correction processes being biased, to ask a jury to disregard a false confession. It is even more difficult if the defendant's memory is altered so that their false confession feels real to them (e.g., Kassin & Sukel, 1997).

This overview of memory biases will end by returning to the correspondence bias. The bias may arise due to memory decay. Even if a strong situational constraint is salient when information is first learned, it may become relatively less salient as time passes. Perhaps the advantage of using dispositions over situations to categorize and understand behavior may increase over time because the behavior is salient and has a stronger memory trace stored in episodic memory than the situation. As with source confusion, it may be that the context is not accurately recalled, leaving only memory for the behavior itself, not where it happened or under what conditions. Thus, correspondence bias could be caused by forgetting (as opposed to not seeing) the situation. This explanation would be particularly useful when explaining past behavior, as many times our judgments of others occur after time has elapsed, and we are asked to reflect on their behavior. For example, consider how faculty members evaluate graduate students (or how managers evaluate employees). Graduate students are attempting to juggle their research interests along with their teaching assignments. However, some graduate students are released from the responsibility of teaching (usually due to no work of their own, but to their research advisor having received research funding—this allows the student to be paid by a grant to do work they would also need to do if teaching). If some students focus only on their research (without the distractions of teaching), they have a clear advantage in how productive they are in this domain. And it is this domain that typically dictates how well they are evaluated by the faculty. Over the course of a semester a faculty member may attribute the student's relative lack of research productivity to their teaching load (which may be salient during the semester, especially if the student is helping the faculty member to teach a course). But months later, during the evaluation period, this situational constraint may have waned in its salience. As students are now evaluated side by side for research productivity (and perhaps determining nominations for awards), those who worked for their money are now seen as less successful than those who were assigned to be free of teaching. The relative superior productivity of one student over another is attributed to traits. A similar fate may impact women and other minorities at work who are often assigned extra tasks as a service to the organization (tasks relating to their identity, such as mentoring other members of their minority group) that impeded productivity. At the time that these service tasks are performed they are valued, but perhaps that value is forgotten when the employee is later evaluated. At such evaluations it is productivity that is emphasized. The power of the situation to limit productivity, though obvious at the time, may seem invisible in the future.

CONFIRMATION BIASES

In Chapters 5 and 6 an extensive review of confirmation bias was provided. It was shown that memory for old information, and judgments of new information, are drawn to existing beliefs, hypotheses, theories, attitudes, and expectations that get confirmed repeatedly through their use as a lens through which information is seen. In that earlier review the focus was placed on first impressions as the thing to be confirmed, and subsequent judgment and memory about the same person or group as what was being biased. Given that this type of bias has been reviewed, we simply provide here a few illustrations of confirmation bias outside of the domain of person perception, since the previous examples all concerned first impressions of people.

Functional Fixedness

Research on performance during decision making and on creativity tasks has found that people have a bias to rely heavily on existing knowledge and known examples, even when instructed explicitly to "think outside the box." This proclivity has been described as **functional fixedness**, or a tendency to lack innovation and to instead use objects in the way they are traditionally intended, and to make decisions relying on accepted and standard ways of approaching the problem (e.g., Marsh, Landau, & Hicks, 1997; Rubin, Stoltzfus, & Wall, 1991; Smith, Ward, & Schumacher, 1993; Ward, 1994). For example, Rubin et al. (1991) asked research participants to generate names for a new pasta product, and found that the generated names resembled the names of existing pasta products. The examples of "new" names had similar word endings (using "Italian-sounding" word endings such as "etti," and "ini") and similar numbers of syllables to existing pasta products. Surely if explicitly instructed not to use old names as a reference point, and to try to be creative, this fixedness on existing names would disappear. This is not the case. Smith et al. found that instructing participants to "not copy" any features of old pasta names led to *more* rather than less reliance on the old names (see also Marsh, Landau, & Hicks, 1996; Sassenberg et al., 2022). The new ideas confirm the examples already established. Having a hard time going beyond existing examples and typical associations is not limited to conscious examples. Marsh, Bink, et al. (1999) found that unconsciously triggered knowledge had a similar "fixing" influence on idea generation.

> **Functional fixedness:** A tendency to use objects in the way they are traditionally intended and to make decisions relying on accepted, standard ways of approaching problems, with limited ability to see beyond traditional functions. This tendency can cause a lack of innovation and a fixation on existing ideas and solutions.

Duncker (1945) provided a classic illustration of functional fixedness with the **Duncker candle problem**. This is a task where participants are shown a candle, a book of matches, and a box of thumbtacks and are told to problem solve—the task is to affix a lit candle to the wall so that wax will not drop onto the table or onto the floor. To solve the problem requires seeing one of the objects taking on an *unusual function*. The box holding the tacks needs to be seen as something other than a box, but as a base for holding the

> **Duncker candle problem:** A task where participants receive a candle, matches, and a box of thumbtacks and must figure out how to affix a lit candle to the wall without wax dripping to the table/floor. The solution requires seeing the box of tacks as able to take on the unusual function of a base for holding the candle.

candle (after emptying out the tacks). In this way it can be both tacked to the wall and catch the dripping wax. The encoding of the box as having its usual function is the critical factor in preventing the problem from being solved (Glucksberg & Weisberg, 1966). Participants become fixed on this one function (a repository for tacks) and see the box as having uses consistent only with this function. Problem solving is enhanced if atypical uses for the box are embraced (e.g., Galinsky & Moskowitz, 2000a; Higgins & Chaires, 1980).

Hindsight Bias

If hindsight is 20–20, there is a cost to seeing things so clearly after the fact. It leads to a bias where the outcomes seem obvious (since now they have already happened) and a belief that because they were so obvious, you knew to expect those outcomes all along. This is known as the **hindsight bias**, a tendency to say that an event that had been unpredictable (or at least difficult to predict in advance) was obvious and predictable after one has the benefit of seeing how things turned out. We overestimate our ability to have predicted the outcome of an event. We see an outcome and we confirm that our expectations prior to the event match the outcome that materialized—I knew all along the candidate would win, or that Steve would divorce his wife, or that the Yankees would win the division, or that the levees would break in the storm, and so on.

> **Hindsight bias:** A tendency to say that an event which had been unpredictable (or at least difficult to predict in advance) was obvious and predictable after one has the benefit of seeing how things turned out. We overestimate our ability to have predicted the outcome of an event.

This phenomenon is different from the phenomenon of **paradoxical knowing**, where people believe they know the outcomes of unknowable events before they happen (e.g., Gollwitzer, Olcaysoy Okten, Pizarro, & Oettingen, 2022). Whereas with paradoxical knowing a candidate might honestly believe "I know the election was rigged" without any evidence to support it, with the hindsight bias an election would actually turn out to be rigged, and a person who had not thought this was a likely outcome before the event now says, "I knew it was rigged all along" (e.g., Fischoff & Beyth, 1975; Roese & Vohs, 2012). It is possible that hindsight bias helps to give birth to paradoxical knowing, since one consequence of hindsight bias is overconfidence in the ability to know how things will turn out. This tendency to retroactively overestimate our ability to see the implications of our choices and actions may lead us to eventually believe we know the outcomes of unknowable events. This overconfidence can be contributed to by a memory distortion where the hindsight bias causes a confirmatory bias in memory. We distort recall for past events to fit or confirm the outcomes we just learned to be true, allowing us to remember that we always thought the outcome would emerge. This emerging overconfidence from confirming that the outcome was one we knew all along can have the danger of leading us to make riskier choices than are warranted, secure in our belief we know they will turn out fine. In essence, a confirmatory bias in memory to see your thoughts prior to an event as being consistent with the outcome of the event allows you to overestimate your skill at assessing probabilities of outcomes. This false sense of making high-probability decisions can lead to a false sense of skill, and hence bad decisions. Carli and Leonard (1989) argue that hindsight bias can partially explain the tendency to blame victims, especially in legal cases such as victim blaming seen in rape cases. The prevalence of hindsight bias in one's own life, where one thinks "I knew it all along," can lead a person to blame another person who has been victimized by saying "they should have known it all along and not chosen to be in situations that so clearly would harm them."

> **Paradoxical knowing:** A phenomenon where people believe they know the outcomes of unknowable events before they happen.

CONCLUSIONS

Unfortunately for perceivers, they often do not know they are biased. And when they do suspect an influence, the theories they have about what might be influencing them may be incorrect (e.g., Nisbett & Wilson, 1977). And even if the theories were correct in identifying the appropriate type and direction of the influence (e.g., Wegener & Petty, 1995b; Wilson & Brekke, 1994), they may still incorrectly gauge how much they are being influenced (e.g., Martin et al., 1990; Moskowitz & Skurnik, 1999; Trope, 1986a). This chapter reviewed many illustrations of bias, across different categories of bias, and focused on correspondence bias (where perceivers blame behavior on the person doing the behaving, often at the expense of considering external pressure that forces that person to behave). Whereas correspondence bias is an interpersonal problem, many of the biases we reviewed extend beyond interpersonal dynamics and impact groups and social problems. Researchers have illustrated the implications for issues such as the blaming of rape victims, the ability to judge the cause of a crime, evaluation of a police officer who illegally obtains a confession, and impressions of stigmatized group members.

This chapter clustered biases by the common underlying cognitive process from which they arise. There was no distinction drawn between implicit biases versus explicit biases. One might prefer such an organizing scheme. If using that rubric, it may be useful to think of bias in terms of a two-by-two ANOVA design. One factor is the implicit versus explicit nature of *the processing* through which the bias is expressed (such as explicit trait judgments vs. implicit trait judgments). The second factor is the implicit versus explicit nature of *the influence exerted* on processing. This produces four cells that are each a type of bias. One can engage in an explicit process, such as impression formation or a hiring decision, that is biased in an implicit manner by a stereotype one does not detect (e.g., Dovidio et al., 2002). One can engage in an implicit process, such as impression formation (a spontaneous trait inference) that is biased in an implicit manner by a stereotype one does not detect (e.g., Otten & Moskowitz, 2000; Ramos et al., 2012; Wigboldus et al., 2003). One can pursue explicit processes that are explicitly influenced, such as when one engages in motivated reasoning to produce a desired outcome (e.g., Kunda, 1987). Finally, one can engage in implicit processes that are influenced by an explicit bias. For example, one can adopt an explicit goal to form an impression from a set of behaviors (vs. a goal to memorize the behaviors) that influences the types of spontaneous inferences one forms (e.g., Uleman & Moskowitz, 1994). Or one could adopt an accountability goal that influences implicit stereotyping or accessibility effects (e.g., Neuberg, 1989; Thompson, Roman, Moskowitz, Chaiken, & Bargh, 1994).

NOTES

1. One criticism is that even though not explicitly asked to do so, research participants are implicitly told by the experimenter to make correspondent inferences. If given an essay to read by an authority figure and told the task is to determine how well it reflects the true attitude of that student, one might assume the information provided is to be used (if not, the experimenter would not have provided it). Another criticism concerns the essays themselves—perhaps they were written in such a way as to suggest the person was truly an expert. The research participant might think "Who else but a true advocate of Castro could construct such clear arguments?"

2. Similar to trying to suppress a stereotype is the goal of trying to be colorblind (to avoid thoughts of race). This has been shown to lead to heightened pro-White bias on implicit

measures of negative affect (e.g., Richeson & Nussbaum, 2003) and to the increased use of race (e.g., Norton, Vandello, et al., 2008). Rather than correcting the bias, this theory about how to correct bias can enhance it.

3. As another example, men and women described using the same trait (e.g., "analytical") can be judged very differently. Analytical means something different as a standard when judging women relative to judging men. Since stereotypes suggest a typical woman is less analytical than the typical man, the standard used for judging women is "lesser" than that for judging men.

4. Consider an interesting use of this phenomenon by the 45th President of the United States. Trump, as part of a routine medical exam, was given a cognitive test that he claimed to do very well on. Soon afterward, he took many opportunities to report how well he had done on the test, and to use it as an opportunity to prove how intelligent he was. He repeatedly told people of his amazing performance, and even showed his ability to remember (many weeks later) one of his answers on the exam that showed how smart he was (he was able to still recall five words he was asked to generate for the test: "person, woman, man, camera, TV"). By repeatedly reporting his belief in his mental acuity the media was helping to strengthen the association between Trump and intelligence. This is a good example of the phenomenon of familiarity breeding truth since, in actuality, the test he was given was *not an intelligence test*. It was a test designed to detect whether a patient is suffering from cognitive degeneration and diseases such as dementia. Yet people do not remember this fact. The repetition of the conclusion offered by the President—of his mental superiority—made most people very familiar with the feeling that Trump had done well on an intelligence test, but no recollection of the detail that its source was a dementia test. And people do not recall that the test actually asks for one to generate five *unrelated* words and remember them, and his list did not contain even one word that is unrelated to any of the others.

5. It also leads women to feel a lack of fit at their organizations and universities, and be less likely to voice opposition to bias.

CHAPTER 9

Biases Are Common and Are Often Motivational in Nature

In 2003, the United States invaded Iraq (Operation Iraqi Freedom). Most Americans were prepared to think of their country as a force of freedom and goodwill and viewed the attack as one intended to topple a tyrannical force that posed a threat to Iraqis, and to the world. However, American troops were not greeted in Iraq as liberators. The Iraqi press, and the media across the Arab world, saw an act of American aggression, sending the message to the public each day that American troops are killers. President George W. Bush was depicted (falsely) in an Egyptian newspaper in a Nazi uniform. The two groups saw and described two different events, with opposing understanding of the war's goals and the meaning of specific interactions between U.S. troops and Iraqi civilians. This is a form of *naïve realism* described in Chapter 1: seeing information in the exact opposite way as a competitor. What causes such a bias? One answer explored in this chapter is the propensity to see people and events through the lens of our motives. We assess them in a manner that makes certain the conclusions we reach support our motives. In Chapter 5 we called this *motivated reasoning*.

Even implicit cognitive processes—such as the tendency to overattribute to traits, the tendency to have stereotypes triggered upon categorization, the directed focus of attention, selecting one category over another, and so on—can be biased by one's motives. Let us focus momentarily on the tendency to overattribute to traits. Why infer a trait over other ways of making meaning? Why make meaning at all? One could simply observe the behavior and form no inferences about why it happened. The reason is because perceivers have a chronic *goal* to impose meaning on stimuli and to do so in an efficient way (e.g., Moskowitz, 1993a; Uleman, Newman, et al., 1996). As explained earlier, traits afford one a rather complete explanation that allows for prediction and a feeling of control. Despite people not realizing they are inferring traits, this lack of awareness does not mean the process is not being directed by a goal or serving some purpose. Individuals differ in how strongly they possess a goal to make meaning quickly and efficiently (Moskowitz, 1993a). They may belong to a culture that stresses ways of making meaning other than traits, thus shifting the nature of how meaning is made in the service of those chronic goals (e.g., Newman, 1993; Newman & Marsden, 2023). They may possess self-esteem goals that lead them to see fellow group members differently from outsiders (Otten & Moskowitz, 2000). They have ideologies that shift their styles of meaning making (Olcaysoy Okten & Moskowitz, 2020b). The specific task one is pursuing (such as memorize the text, or scrutinize it for typos) can alter how meaning is made (Uleman & Moskowitz, 1994). All of these examples show that when we infer traits we are doing so for a reason: We are motivated.

Let us now focus briefly on the implicit triggering of a stereotype. We saw in Chapter 6 that merely seeing words relating to a group subliminally (such as the label "woman") can trigger the stereotype. Why do we have stereotypes so ready to be used? Is this purely a cognitive process beyond control? In my own research I have shown that stereotypes are a tool people use to *achieve an end* (e.g., Moskowitz, 1993a, 2001, 2010, 2014); the triggering of a stereotype is motivated, even if the processes involved happen quickly and outside of awareness. A stereotype is activated *because* it serves a goal of the perceiver and is not just an automatic and mechanistic associative response. Many goals encourage us to use stereotypes—a goal to compete with other groups of people, a goal to enhance self-esteem, a goal to dominate others, a goal to promote the distinct identity of a group to which we belong, or a goal to efficiently impose meaning on stimuli. These goals are often invisible to us. Since we do not see the goal, it makes the stereotyping perhaps seem automatic—an unmotivated triggering of a chain of cognitive processes. However, just because a goal that motivates stereotyping is invisible, this does not mean stereotyping is unmotivated. To illustrate that the activation of a stereotype is in the service of a goal, we could demonstrate that altering one's goals will reduce its activation. If one has a goal other than those listed above, such as a goal that requires a stereotype to be inhibited, stereotype activation is controlled. For example, adopting a goal to be egalitarian and fair eliminates (and even inhibits) stereotype activation (e.g., Moskowitz, 2001, 2002; Moskowitz et al., 1999; Moskowitz, Li, Ignarri, & Stone, 2011; Moskowitz & Li, 2011; Moskowitz, Salomon, & Taylor, 2000). We explore the issue of reducing stereotyping later in this book. The point here is that what may appear to be a purely cognitive response is in fact motivated.

We have reviewed in Chapters 5, 6, and 8 the types of motivated cognitive processes that produce bias: perception, attention, categorization, judgment, and hypothesis testing. The focus was on the reasoning aspect of the perceiver's *motivated reasoning*. However, we have not yet reviewed the categories of motivations that are capable of biasing us. Let us focus here on the motivations themselves. Throughout this book we have seen that important motivational states have the capacity to bias cognitive processing, whether those motives relate to survival concerns, threat avoidance, self-esteem promotion, identity concerns, a need to belong, epistemic needs, or vested interests. This chapter does not provide a complete review of all motives that guide people but instead focuses on the major classes of motivations that have been of interest to social cognition: consistency motives, epistemic motives, motives to avoid threat, self-esteem motives, and group-enhancing motives.

CONSISTENCY MOTIVES

Confirmation bias was described as a class of cognitive bias in which information that confirms an existing belief was preferentially processed. In the cases of confirmation bias explored in Chapters 5 and 6, the biases observed were not motivated. Either an expectation existed and served as a lens for remembering and judging information, or a standard had been set against which new information was evaluated. Here we explore a similar bias to confirm an existing belief, but *because one is motivated* to defend an existing belief: a goal to see information as consistent with what is already known. This class of motivation is about

consistency seeking. When an expectation exists, people may be *motivated* to affirm that expectation when evaluating evidence. Why? We are motivated to affirm existing beliefs because the mere experience of inconsistency is unpleasant; it is an aversive state we are motivated to eliminate. To eliminate that aversiveness we seek evidence consistent with what we already believe and feel.

> **Consistency seeking:** The motivation to be consistent with existing beliefs or prior actions and to ward off inconsistency (which is experienced as aversive). Consistency seeking often results in affirming prior beliefs when evaluating new behavioral evidence, searching memory, and testing hypotheses. The motivation to be consistent is especially powerful when inconsistency also threatens self-esteem.

Cognitive Dissonance

Consistency biases are perhaps most famously seen in **cognitive dissonance**. Festinger (1957) described cognitive dissonance as an unpleasant negative tension state experienced when people realize they hold two competing or inconsistent cognitions. The experienced state of tension is so aversive that people are motivated to resolve the inconsistencies that give rise to it, particularly if the failure to be consistent compromises self-esteem (e.g., Stone, 2001). Rather than referring to the inconsistent cognitions, as implied by the name "cognitive dissonance," the term refers to the unpleasant psychological tension state that one is motivated to eliminate (e.g., Vaidis & Bran, 2019). To resolve the inconsistency and remove the discomfort (the dissonance) one can use two broad classes of strategies: (1) one can change an existing belief or behavior so that consistency among the cognitions is produced, or (2) one can bolster one cognition while minimizing or discrediting the other through rationalization, trivialization, denial, and distraction.

Dissonance is most aversive, or produces the greatest drive to reduce it, if there is **insufficient justification** for the lack of consistency. By insufficient justification it is meant that there is no alternative explanation that can explain the dissonance-arousing act. If I am free to act in any way I choose, or espouse any attitude, and I choose to be inconsistent with my prior actions or beliefs, that inconsistency cannot be justified and will cause dissonance. However, if my inconsistent actions or attitudes can be justified, such as I was forced or paid handsomely to do it, it will be less likely to create dissonance. If one can see that a person was compelled to act by being made "an offer they couldn't refuse" then the inconsistent response is perceived to be justified, attributed to the situational constraint, and no dissonance is aroused. Interestingly, this conception of dissonance produced a prediction that was counterintuitive at the time the theory was introduced in the 1950s, given the dominance of behaviorism

> **Cognitive dissonance:** An unpleasant psychological tension-state experienced when people realize they hold two competing or inconsistent cognitions. The tension is so aversive that people are motivated to resolve the inconsistencies giving rise to it by restoring consistency among the cognitions. This can be achieved through attitude change, behavior change, rationalizations, and trivializations.
>
> **Insufficient justification:** When a person is not compelled to act/think/feel in a way that creates dissonant cognitions but, rather, feels as if they have freely chosen to do so. The dissonance cannot be justified by feeling as if one had no choice.

and conditioning theories. Dissonance theory predicts that the more one is paid to perform an act that is inconsistent with existing cognitions, the *less* one should feel compelled to report liking it. Attitudes need not change to align with the "inconsistent" behavior just performed (and eliminate the dissonance) because the money serves as sufficient justification for the act. One can keep the original attitude that the action is disliked. Behaviorism, in contrast, says one should like an act as one associates reward with it. At the time dissonance theory was introduced, it was a revolutionary idea to suggest that the way people reasoned about rewards (and the dissonance reduction motivation that such reasoning introduced) was more important than the laws of reinforcement.

Festinger and Carlsmith (1959) famously showed that by changing one's attitude to align with an inconsistent behavior, dissonance reduction is achieved, and consistency among one's cognitions is restored. However, the experience of dissonance, and hence the amount of attitude change needed to resolve the inconsistency, is strongest when a person has been paid less to perform the behavior—that is, whereas a behaviorist would predict one would like a behavior more *the more* one was paid to engage in that behavior, dissonance theory predicted one would like the behavior more *the less* one was paid. To test these predictions, and establish that dissonance motivation depends on how one reasons about an inconsistency, Festinger and Carlsmith had their research participants perform an extremely boring task, repeatedly, for a long period of time. They had to load spools of thread onto a tray slowly, then when the tray was full, dump them off and start all over again. They were then asked if they would go to the waiting room and report to the people waiting that the task was exciting and enjoyable. They were free to say no, but most participants comply. Some of the participants were paid $20 to tell this dissonance-arousing lie, an enormous amount of money for a student in the 1950s. Others were paid a relatively trivial amount to tell the exact same lie. In each case the lie was inconsistent with their true belief about the task, but for half of the participants there was an insufficient justification for doing so—they were not handsomely rewarded. Finally, participants report their true attitudes for the task. The findings revealed that the people who change their private attitudes to say they liked the task are not the people who were paid well to lie to others and say the task was fun. It was the people paid very little to lie to others and say the task was fun. Insufficient justification for the act (low pay) led to a stronger experience of dissonance compared to sufficient justification (high pay), and the way to resolve its aversiveness was attitude change—to convince oneself the task was enjoyable.

Insufficient justification is not the only factor that determines the **strength of the dissonance**, and the drive to restore consistency. As the importance of the inconsistent cognitions increases, so too does the cognitive dissonance aroused. If a topic is central to one's daily activity (such as drinking, smoking, having a personal connection to the dissonance-arousing event, or having a strong attachment to it) or is an important element of one's identity and sense of self, then dissonance in that domain can be particularly strong. Given that dissonance is greatest when inconsistent cognitions are important, inconsistencies that involve the self-concept can create powerfully motivating states of dissonance arousal (e.g., Aronson, 1968; Cooper & Fazio, 1984; Stone, 2001; Thibodeau & Aronson, 1992). Additionally, if the incongruence has no **aversive consequences** (no harm caused), dissonance will be weaker. Yet, when harm is caused by the dissonance, or it produces shame or guilt (e.g., Gosling, Denizeau, & Oberlé, 2006), then the drive to eliminate the inconsistency will be particularly acute.

> **Strength of the dissonance:** The drive to restore consistency can fluctuate in strength as the importance of the cognitions in competition increases. If a topic is central to one's daily activity or is an important element of one's identity and sense of self, then dissonance in that domain can be particularly strong.
>
> **Aversive consequences:** When harm is caused by the inconsistent actions or cognitions that create the dissonance then the drive to eliminate the inconsistency will be particularly acute. The strength of the dissonance increases as the negative effects increase.

The most often-studied dissonance reduction strategy is attitude change. This is partly because of its practical importance. If you hope to persuade another person, Festinger and Carlsmith's (1959) experiment suggests you just need to make them feel dissonance relating to the topic and they will gladly change their attitude. Creating dissonance in others with the hope they will change their attitudes is used by politicians, marketers, and anyone who needs to shape others' attitudes about a topic (e.g., Cialdini, 2007). However, changing an attitude is at times difficult to do. Especially if the inconsistency, as just noted, involves something important to you. To a supporter who has been aligning their political identity with Donald Trump since 2013, Trump's indictment for a crime in 2023 (a cognition inconsistent with their attitude) might not lead them to reduce this dissonance by concluding, "I no longer like Donald Trump." An alternative means to resolving cognitive dissonance is to alter one's behavior instead of the attitude (e.g., Stone, Aronson, Crain, Winslow, & Fried, 1994). One could work to find sufficient justification for the indictment (such as Trump's opponents abusing the justice system), and this behavior would resolve the dissonance. Attitude change as a strategy of dissonance reduction is especially unlikely when one has been reminded of one's attitudes on an issue (such as by making a public statement, or answering a survey question).

If confronted with one's inconsistency immediately after being reminded of one's true attitudes, an acute form of dissonance that we know by the term **hypocrisy** will be triggered. Hypocrisy is when one detects a discrepancy between how one should act and how reality reveals one acts. In such instances the attitude that has been undermined by one's hypocritical behavior is hard to change, so one turns to behavior change to alleviate the dissonance. Stone et al. (1994) illustrated this in one experiment by making people aware of the hypocrisy in their use of condoms. Participants recorded a message that the experimenter said would be

> **Hypocrisy:** Detecting a discrepancy between how you should act and how reality reveals you do act, especially when the domain in which the discrepancy occurs is important, and the attitude about how you should act is difficult to distort and change.

shown to others, about the importance of using condoms during sex to prevent the spread of AIDS. In some research participants' hypocrisy was aroused by making them aware of their discrepant behavior with the position just espoused. They have at times not used condoms. The attitude is hard to change—one has publicly stated support for condom use. The dissonance is resolved, instead, by behavior change. Upon exiting the lab, participants made aware of their hypocrisy were more likely to purchase condoms than people who were not made aware of their hypocrisy. Stone et al. find that hypocrisy is an especially powerful inducer of cognitive dissonance when it occurs in a domain that is self-relevant.

Of course, just as it can at times be difficult to resolve dissonance by altering one's attitude, it can also at times be difficult to alter behavior. One cannot undo the lie about the boring task in the Festinger and Carlsmith (1959) experiment. One might not be able to engage in behavior to help prove Trump's opponents abused the judicial system. One may not have an opportunity to purchase condoms when feeling hypocritical about it. What happens to reduce dissonance if, as may often be the case with important beliefs and behaviors, both attitudes and behaviors are hard to change? Festinger (1957) described several other strategies that people use to eliminate dissonance aside from changing an attitude or changing a behavior. He argued that one can either reject/change one of the inconsistent cognitions, or one can add a new cognition that could explain away the seeming inconsistency among the competing cognitions (see Harmon-Jones & Mills, 2019; McGrath, 2017; Stone, 2001, for reviews). The addition of such new cognitions will either rationalize the inconsistency or trivialize the inconsistency (e.g., Brock & Balloun, 1967; Cotton & Hieser, 1980).

Consider a person who smoked cigarettes in the 1960s. At that time, smokers were being made well aware of the dangers of smoking by publicity campaigns led by the Surgeon General of the United States. The cognition that smoking was a health concern stood firmly inconsistent with a smoker's enjoyment of smoking and the belief that they personally are unlikely to be a cancer risk (e.g., McMaster & Lee, 1991). Their positive attitudes toward smoking were also supported by relentless advertising campaigns by the tobacco industry. It seemed unlikely that changing attitudes about smoking was likely to be the chosen dissonance reduction strategy of smokers. Smoking also is a very hard habit to break, making behavior change also very difficult. Thus, the hope of the Surgeon General was that creating dissonance would change behavior, but perhaps this backfired among smokers, who could not find the strength or desire to change their attitudes and behaviors. Instead they might rationalize their actions or trivialize the consequences.

Rationalization involves restoring consistency among discrepant cognitions by adding a belief that will resolve the inconsistency. This can include new cognitions that label the source that produced the inconsistency as untrustworthy, or the evidence on which the inconsistent cognition is based as illegitimate. It can also include adding new thoughts that are consistent that can counterbalance or offset the inconsistency. For example, if one wanted to rationalize smoking, one could add the cognition that the research that says smoking is dangerous is flawed. Or one could argue that the health risks will happen to someone else, not me. Or that the government is too intrusive in trying to regulate personal behavior.

> **Rationalization:** Reducing dissonance by adding a belief that will resolve the inconsistency among discrepant cognitions. This can include labeling the source of the inconsistency as untrustworthy, or deciding evidence on which the inconsistency is based is illegitimate. It also includes adding new consistent thoughts that can offset the inconsistent thoughts.

It can also include adding positive thoughts about smoking such as it is relaxing, or helps one stay thin. In exploring the dissonance-reducing strategies of smokers, Fotuhi et al. (2013) found that both functional cognitions such as "smoking helps me concentrate" and risk-minimizing cognitions such as "the medical evidence that smoking is deadly is exaggerated" were used by people who smoked. They found functional cognitions are especially likely to be endorsed because they are harder to scrutinize and disprove.

Consider an example of rationalization introduced by Festinger, Riecken, and Schacter (1956). They described a charismatic cult leader in the 1950s who claimed to be receiving messages from aliens that Earth was going to be destroyed on December 21. The leader's further claim was that a select few individuals could be saved and transported off the planet. The leader set about recruiting a small band of people to be saved, demanding a high price: They had to sever all ties to the world, renounce all their relationships and worldly goods, and move to a compound to await their time to be saved from the Earth's impending destruction. These people had sacrificed everything to be a small and fervent group of followers. Festinger and his colleagues pondered about what happens to such people after they realize the prophecy had failed and the world did not come to an end on December 21. Their dissonance would be overwhelming, but they could not change their actions. They had already given up all of their possessions, and this could not be undone. On the next day, will they accept their poor decisions and simply change their attitudes? This too seems unlikely given their sacrifices in the name of that attitude. Cognitive dissonance suggests that they should rationalize to resolve the dissonance. Cognitive dissonance theory suggests that the group would now become even more fanatical, not less. Rather than admit their error, they should become more dedicated to the cause, increasing efforts at proselytizing and trying to recruit new members. This is precisely what happened to this particular cult. They added new beliefs such as "the world was spared from disaster because of the unwavering faith of our small group." Rather than keeping to themselves, as they had prior to December 21, they now sought publicity and proclaimed they had saved us all. They sought to recruit others to their ranks. They dug in to their beliefs, adding consonant cognitions and actions as rationalizations.

It hardly takes joining a cult for dissonance to motivate people to engage in (what seem to others) extreme rationalizations. Even something as ordinary as smoking cigarettes can be rationalized. Devotion to a political candidate, for example, can lead one to rationalize what to others seems like obviously poor behavior. Let us return to our supporters of Donald Trump. A Trump supporter could rationalize the inconsistency of his being indicted with a focus on one element of the alleged crime not being perceived as illegal at all: paying a person to conceal an adulterous affair. If one could rationalize that many people cheat and try to conceal it, one can assume an indictment over payments made to conceal an affair is a sham and a "witch hunt."

Another way to achieve consistency and reduce dissonance is to use a strategy of **trivialization**. This involves dismissing the consequences of the inconsistency, or minimizing the importance of the inconsistent cognition. Simon, Greenberg, and Brehm (1995) reasoned that when changing one's attitude as a means of dealing with dissonance is hard (such as when the attitude is important or salient), a strategy for dealing with the threat is to trivialize the importance of the domain. For example, if one receives negative feedback that is inconsistent with the positive view one has of the self, dissonance can be reduced by denigrating the person providing the feedback. It can also be achieved by minimizing the importance of the domain the feedback is targeting. To illustrate this, Simon et al. reminded some participants (in this case, students) of their attitudes against a policy proposing that there should be a university-wide comprehensive exam as a requirement for graduation. Other students were not reminded of their attitudes toward this policy (but held them just as forcefully). To induce dissonance, they had students volunteer to write essays that favored implementing comprehensive exams. Participants who were not reminded of their attitudes changed those attitudes; they were more in favor of the exams. However, people reminded of their attitudes removed the aversive arousal caused by the inconsistency of their action via trivialization. Instead of changing their attitudes about whether comprehensive exams were good, they rated the issue of comprehensive exams as less important.

> **Trivialization:** A strategy for reducing cognitive dissonance in which a person restores consistency among discrepant cognitions by minimizing the importance of the threat, or rather than dismissing the threat, convincing oneself that it does not matter or is trivial.

When the dissonance arousal is associated with shame or guilt trivialization is an especially useful strategy (Elliot & Devine, 1994; Gosling et al., 2006). An example of this was provided in Chapter 5 in the domain of prejudice feedback. Vitriol and Moskowitz (2021) had research participants receive feedback about their propensity to have prejudice. Did they react to this inconsistent cognition with a changed attitude ("I am more biased than I thought") or changed behavior (working harder to be unbiased)? No. Instead, many people reacted with trivialization. Their assessment of the research methods, the usefulness of the feedback, and the goals of the scientists who do research on bias became more negative.

Dissonance is so aversive, that people even take proactive steps to preempt the experience of dissonance. They attempt to block the receipt of inconsistent cognitions and augment the presence of consonant cognitions. When a person makes a choice between two options (such as do I prefer taking a course with Professor A or Professor B?), that choice involves deciding that one option is preferable to the other. There is an attitude formed that one likes one of the choices more than the other. Once the choice is made for option A, one is motivated to expend cognitive effort to maintain the impression that A is better than B. Especially once a behavior has been enacted in support of that decision (such as registering for a course and spending a large amount of money to do so), the exposure to information that undermines that impression is dissonance arousing (e.g., Harmon-Jones & Mills, 2019). To avoid that threat they can rationalize the choice they made and trivialize the unchosen options (McGrath, 2017). Reducing dissonance and feeling consistency is maintained is also easily achieved through distorting memory about the choice alternatives. This leads to a **spreading of choice alternatives**, where one distorts memory of how positive the chosen item was and how negative the unchosen item was, increasing the perceived discrepancy among them to make the chosen alternative seem better. Attitudes become polarized through one's memory of the features of the respective choices, thus protecting, even bolstering, the positive feelings about the choice one had made. For example, negative attributes of a chosen item may be misremembered as belonging to an unchosen item, and positive attributes of an unchosen item may be assigned to a chosen one (e.g., Mather & Johnson, 2000).

> **Spreading of choice alternatives:** When, following a decision, one is motivated to support one's choice and derogate unchosen alternatives, often manifesting as biased memory. Distorted, polarized memory of how positive or how negative the chosen item was prevents dissonant thoughts by enhancing the choice's perceived value relative to unchosen options.

It is important to note that not all forms of inconsistency are unpleasant and motivate people to seek to resolve the inconsistency. This is only true when there is a logical or motivational incongruence that means holding one "cognition" makes holding another "cognition" incorrect, hypocritical, or threatening. However, it is possible for two attitudes, ideas, or acts to be inconsistent in a manner that does not create such tension. For example, one can hold strong positive feelings and beliefs about one's home (it is a source of great positive affect, it is where the kids were raised, it is where many holidays were hosted, it was where we became a family, etc.). Simultaneously, one can hold strong negative feelings and beliefs about one's home (it is where the dog died, it creates such large amounts of unpleasant work in the yard, it constantly needs to be cleaned, it requires so much of our monthly income to maintain, etc.). Such thoughts and feelings that are inconsistent with one another, but not oppositional in any other way, do not create dissonance. They create **ambivalent attitudes**, as reviewed in Chapter 2 (e.g., Rothman & Melwani, 2017; Rothman et al., 2022). Ambivalence, in such conditions, rather than creating an aversive state, can have the benefit of opening a person to a wider range of influences. When presented with positive and negative information about a stigmatized person, ambivalent people showed greater responsiveness to this information than unambivalent people (MacDonald & Zanna, 1998). Similar to attitude ambivalence is what Rothman and colleagues defined as *emotional ambivalence*: the nonthreatening experience of emotions that are both positive and negative in any given moment (e.g., Rothman & Melwani, 2017; Rothman, Pratt, Rees, & Vogus, 2017). Emotional ambivalence has a similar motivating quality of opening people up to a variety of perspectives and greater cognitive flexibility (e.g., Kleiman & Hassin, 2013; Rees et al., 2013; Rothman et al., 2022). It is not aversive.

> **Ambivalent attitudes:** Having both positive and negative attitudes toward a particular attitude object simultaneously. This can be aversive or arousing, unless this opposition poses no threat. Such mixed feedback can be even be sought out, rather than eliminated, when uncertainty is desirable to an individual.

Self-Verification

> **Self-verification:** Motivated by a need to see self-concept stability, one seeks and gives preferential treatment to information that supports existing beliefs about the self, labelling it as diagnostic. Verifying beliefs thought to be true about the self also helps to enhance the important perception that the world is predictable and controllable.

Swann (1990) argued that a specific type of confirmation bias exists where one is motivated to maintain the views held about the self. He called the motivation to seek consistency and ward off inconsistency when making self-relevant judgments **self-verification**. To promote verification of self-beliefs, people use implicit processes of attention, encoding, retrieval, and interpretation to seek out information that supports existing beliefs about the self, giving it preferential treatment and labeling it as more diagnostic than other types of information (e.g., Swann, 1983; Swann & Read, 1981). The self-concept strives to fulfill a need to confirm or verify itself. The reason Swann believed the motive to self-verify is so important is because having stability in the self-concept creates a perception that the world, more generally, is stable—it is predictable and controllable.

Swann (1990) argued that people would prefer self-verifying information above self-enhancing information. That it is better to confirm what one believes about the self than embrace something positive that is inconsistent with what one believes. One example is provided by Swann, Pelham, and Krull (1989). Research participants were first asked to identify their worst quality—such as "I am bad at spatial reasoning." They were then informed that two observers had been watching them over the course of the experiment and that the observers had rated them on performance dimensions, such as the quality they had just listed as their worst quality. The participants then learn that one of the observers had rated them positively on this bad quality, while the other observer rated them negatively. Participants were then asked to pick one of these two observers to interact with in the next part of the experiment. Rather than choosing the person who saw one positively on the negative dimension, people instead chose the person who verified their own views about this negative quality. They were more motivated to verify than enhance their self-concept.

ADAPTIVE VALUE

Some information has a special power to grab attention and be preferentially processed. This can create a bias where such information is overrepresented in one's processing. While some information is preferentially seen, by extension some information is less likely to be seen and, therefore, underutilized in one's social cognition. In Chapter 6, an ecological perspective to social cognition was introduced (McArthur & Baron, 1983) where stimuli in the environment were described as differing in terms of the **adaptive value** they provide for the individual. People focus attention on the more adaptive type of information and easily draw the inferences they imply. For example, stimuli that are relevant to threat have such adaptive value (we review threat as a separate category later in this chapter). Heider (1944) argued that stimuli that easily suggest traits have such adaptive value because they promote the need to have meaning. Several theorists have, across many years, argued that stimuli that suggest two traits in particular (as reviewed in Chapter 1) have such adaptive value: competence and warmth (e.g., Asch, 1946; Fiske, Cuddy, Glick, & Xu, 2002; Osgood, Suci, & Tannenbaum, 1957; Todorov, 2023). Finally, some information leaps out from the background and grabs attention relative to other less prominent stimuli in the context. Such information is salient, or has increased **salience**. The properties of objects that make them salient are well-known in the study of object perception, and include suddenness, bright colors, intensity, novelty, luminosity, repetition, complexity, movement, and unit formation (e.g., Postman et al., 1948, Snowden, 2002). These features of the people and things that we observe, the "data" in our environment, have more power at directing attention and impacting our responses than others. McArthur (1981) claimed that in "person perception, as in object perception, perceivers selectively attend to intense,

Adaptive value: Stimuli that afford an individual the opportunity to pursue goals that are essential to their survival. This can include survival needs that promote avoiding aversive and approaching appetitive stimuli, but can also include psychological imperatives such as seeking belonging, finding meaning, and promoting self-esteem.

Salience: When a stimulus's features have the power to direct attention and thus exert a greater impact on responding. Perceivers selectively attend to features of stimuli that make stimuli attention-grabbing. Such features include a stimulus that is intense, sudden, changing, complex, novel, repetitive, in motion, luminous, bright, loud, and unit-forming.

changing, complex, novel, and unit-forming stimuli" (p. 202). We are motivated to see stimuli that afford us an opportunity to survive and those that serve as threats to our survival. The perceptual system is geared to detect change in the environment and render it meaningful and constant. Thus, complex, novel, sudden, and changing features in behavior stand out and capture attention.

Salience

Salient people and objects have featural prominence—they seem to leap out from other stimuli in our environment for the reasons listed above (novelty, brightness, fast moving, etc.). This prominence can be inherent to an object or person. An exceptionally tall person will always stand out for their height. Featural prominence can also be momentarily achieved. What is novel in one context (such as being the only man in a psychology class with 30 women) can be mundane in another (such as being a man in an engineering class with 30 other men out of 40 students). Whether the salience is a permanent or temporary feature, it is attention grabbing. Taylor and Fiske (1978) asserted, "Causal perception is substantially determined by where one's attention is directed within the environment and that attention itself is a function of what information is salient . . . salient information is then overrepresented in subsequent causal explanations" (pp. 253–256). McArthur and Ginsberg (1981) manipulated salience using a relatively *novel* feature of people in their context—having red hair. Participants watched a video of two men, one with red hair, the other with brown hair. Behind each man was a black-and-white photograph that was unrelated to the conversation the men were having. If red hair was salient, people would be attending to that man more closely and be more likely to detect and analyze other elements in his immediate context. As expected, they found that the picture behind the red-headed man was better remembered. How do we know it is not the picture that is salient, rather than hair color? Better memory for the picture behind the red-headed man only occurred when the video was in color, as opposed to black and white (since red hair was not detected in a black-and-white video).

As noted above, what makes a person or object salient can change from situation to situation. One's features may be salient and attention grabbing only in certain contexts. Taylor, Fiske, Etcoff, and Ruderman (1978) state that

> instead of perceiving a group of persons as a set of unique individuals, the perceiver may . . . select salient social or physical dimensions to use as discriminating variables for grouping and managing person information. If this is true, certain variables such as race or sex would be likely candidates for such categories, since they are physically salient as well as useful social discriminators. (p. 779)

Physical features such as gender and race, however, are salient only if the context places that feature in isolation. We would not argue that women are salient by virtue of their gender alone, because approximately half of the population is female. Similarly, Black citizens may be a minority in the United States, but they are hardly surprising to encounter. But contexts can make members of these groups rare and surprising—salient. Novelty within a context is one factor that can determine which from among our many categories is salient. Women were unique and rare at the last three technology jobs at which my wife worked as a programmer, or in the engineering departments in which her closest female friends were receiving their PhDs, and this might make gender something that is attention grabbing in those settings. Even self-categorization is shaped by solo status making some features salient. My identity as a Jew was never more salient than when I moved to Munich,

Germany, where my religious affiliation was a fairly novel one. My identity as a Gen Xer is made salient when I co-host a social cognition conference that is more populated by millennials and members of Gen Z. Qualities such as race and gender (as well as others) attain heightened salience when the context places them alone.

Does this overemphasis on a person because of their solo status lead to a bias in which that factor is seen as responsible for their actions? If race or gender is what grabs attention and shapes how others categorize you, does this mean that race or gender is overemphasized as what causes you to act and speak? If race or gender makes you salient, will more focus be placed on you, and greater causal weight assigned to the things you say (relative to other people)? Taylor et al. (1978) found support for this in that the solo woman in a group was presumed to have more stereotypic features and play a more stereotype-prescribed role in the group than the same woman in a gender-mixed group. Taylor et al. manipulated salience across situations by making gender temporarily salient in a particular context. Participants listened to a dialogue between six members of a group. Each time a person from the group spoke their picture appeared on a screen. Participants later rated how influential, talkative, and prominent a particular group member was. Participants in the different conditions of the experiment did not hear different things; the person they were evaluating spoke exactly the same number of times and said exactly the same things. What differed between participants was whether the person's gender was salient in the context or not. Some participants saw and heard a group that had one woman and five men. Others saw and heard a group with three women and three men. Finally, others saw and heard a group with one man and five women. Despite the exact same words being spoken, evaluations of the person's contributions to the group differed as a function of whether the person was salient in that context. In a group with one man, his novel gender made him salient, and hence he was perceived as disproportionately more influential and prominent than in the condition with three men and three women. Identically, the solo (novel) woman was more influential and prominent versus the condition when there were three men and three women.

Another factor that determines whether a person will be salient within a situation is their physical position within the context. Position in a context can make one momentarily salient because they are located in a position where all eyes happen to be focused. The impact of where a perceiver's physical gaze is focused was examined by Taylor and Fiske (1975) by manipulating the seating arrangements in a group of research participants. Two confederates working for the experimenter were asked to engage in a scripted dialogue while six research participants watched. Among the six, two were seated so their gaze was focused on one of the confederates and two seated so their attention was directed toward the other confederate. The final two participants were seated so that both confederates were equally visible and gaze was not directed more strongly toward either one. The participants later made judgments about who was more responsible for directing the tone and topics of the conversation. Focus of attention had an impact. The person who was salient by virtue of being momentarily the recipient of visual focus was seen as playing a greater causal role in shaping the interaction. Similar results were found by Storms (1973) using video recordings of speakers shown to participants. Whomever the camera was focused on was seen as more responsible for how the discussion unfolded. They further found that a physical change in perspective that alters who is salient also altered the causal explanations provided. When rating a person's influence, it is greater if the person is the focus of attention, and less when they are not.

McArthur and Post (1977) similarly manipulated the salience of one person relative to other people in the context to study the impact on judgment and attribution. Salience was created by placing a person under a bright light. When a person had salience by virtue of being more brightly lit, they were seen as a central cause for the events that transpired, despite the fact that the same behavior, when not well lit, was not seen as causal. A famous example of this effect was the first U.S. Presidential debate between Richard Nixon and John Kennedy in 1960. The typical description of this debate is that listeners on the radio heard no advantage for Kennedy relative to Nixon in terms of how well he handled the questions asked. However, those who watched the debate on television heard a different debate; they heard a stronger performance by Kennedy. Afterward, he moved from trailing in the polls to leading. Given that most people were aware that Kennedy was the more attractive man, something salient in the TV context is a likely explanation for the extra weight given to Kennedy's performance (not his good looks). Kennedy and Nixon were equally well lit. But Nixon wore a suit that blended into the background, and Kennedy's darker suit contrasted with the background; it made him more salient. Perhaps this salience gave him causal weight. By the time of their last debate each man wore a dark suit.

Utility

Stangor, Lynch, Duan, and Glass (1992) propose that what makes a particular feature salient to a perceiver depends not only on the novelty of that feature within the context but the utility that feature has for the perceiver within that context. It is the feature that has the most information value for the perceiver that provides them with a useful basis for making inferences. Hair color is usually not very informative—there are few useful stereotypes about hair color that would allow one to make inferences and plan appropriate behavior. However, gender is a fairly useful and inference-laden social category. The utility of this category makes it the more likely one to capture attention and become salient (thus making perceivers more likely to pigeonhole the person according to that feature). To examine what grabs attention, Stangor et al. showed research participants a series of photographs of people and an accompanying text of statements made by each one. The people in the photographs varied on several dimensions or features that could potentially have captured attention. After having examined a stack of such items, a surprise memory test was given in which the participants had to try to match which people had made which statements. One way to assess what types of features were capturing attention is to look at the types of errors people make: Do they routinely confuse people with particular types of features? If women are routinely confused for having made statements made by other women, but are rarely confused with statements made by men, it would suggest gender was salient and attention grabbing as a feature than another feature, such as shirt color or race. They predicted that a more utilitarian category, one that carries meaning for the perceiver, will capture attention.

To test this hypothesis, Stangor et al. (1992, Experiment 5) pitted a utilitarian category against one that is not particularly informative to see whether errors in memory were more likely to align along the utilitarian dimension. The photographs contained pictures of people who differed from one another in terms of race (the utilitarian category) and clothing color (a noninformative and not very useful category). The photographs were of four White women and four Black women. Two of the White women and two of the Black women wore a white shirt, while two of the White women and two of the Black women wore a black shirt, thus creating two features, each presented an equal number of times. The number of within-race errors and the number of between-race errors were computed, as was the number of within-clothing errors and the number of between-clothing errors. While there was no difference between how many errors were made within one clothing color (mistaking a white-shirted person for a different white-shirted person) as there were between clothing colors (mistaking a white-shirted person for a black-shirted person), such differences were in fact found for race pairings. People were more likely to make errors that confused a person of one race with something said by a person of the same race than they were to confuse something said by a person of one race with something said by a person of a different race. They concluded that salience is not determined by novelty alone but by the value a feature holds for the person. Some features, such as race and gender, have natural informational value because of a rich history of stereotypes and beliefs that perceivers are motivated to lean on.

Unit Formation

A person belongs to many categories: a gender group, a generation (baby boomer vs. Gen X vs. millennial vs. Gen Z), an occupational group (academic or medical professional), a race (Black or White), a religious group (Jew or Muslim), a nationality (American or Canadian), a social subculture (Goth or punk), and so on. Potentially any of these categories can be made salient, and as such have the power to capture attention and bias impression formation. Utility and solo status are, of course, not the only ways a feature can attain salience. Unit formation is another. By unit formation it is meant that specific features are isolated and linked to the person so that they are more salient than other qualities also possessed by the person. For example, a great deal of media attention was focused on Joe Biden's age during the campaign for the 2020 Presidential election, and again in the 2024 campaign, despite many qualities he possesses that could be used to form a salient unit with him. Donald Trump, who is about the same age (one began college in 1961, the other 1964), opposed Biden in each election; rarely has age been mentioned as people focus on other features (see Figure 9.1).

Macrae, Bodenhausen, and Milne (1995) illustrated how the salient features of the social environment can be used to form a unit with a person. They showed research participants a videotape of a Chinese woman, but varied which of these two categories was salient. Some participants witnessed a Chinese woman eating noodles with chopsticks, thus allowing the woman's nationality to form a unit with the behavior and seem salient. Other participants saw a Chinese woman putting on makeup in front of a mirror, thus allowing her gender to form a unit with the behavior and seem salient. When the same woman is seen putting on makeup or using chopsticks, what becomes salient is altered, and the concept that forms a unit with the person shifts. In each case a feature of the person has the potential to be salient, but unit formation determines which will eventually gain prominence. They further found that salience determined processing. When gender was salient people

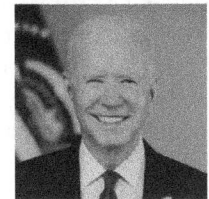 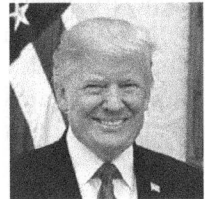

Two presidential candidates in 2020 and 2024, each about the same age (their college years overlapped). How can unit formation be used to try to focus voters on some aspects of their identity (such as age vs. wealth) so that it is this quality that is salient when thinking about each man?

FIGURE 9.1. Salience of Presidential candidates.

were likely to have gender stereotypes accessible, but not stereotypes of the Chinese (which instead were now inhibited). However, if the Chinese category had been activated by the process of unit formation, it was the stereotype associated with this category that was most accessible, and gender stereotypes were inhibited.

THE MOTIVATION TO AVOID THREAT

Affordance biases specify that some stimuli have the capacity to afford us an opportunity to pursue a goal. However, stimuli are adaptive not only because they help us to move toward desired goals. Equally important is avoiding threats. One of the earliest biases examined in social cognition is linked to the human need to detect threats. The fear of threat and the need to avoid threat leads negative information to have great affordance value. It is detected easily, and, as we saw in Chapter 4, the ability to detect threats quickly allows us to avoid engaging with threatening stimuli (e.g., Bean et al., 2012). Thus, one class of motives that guide social cognition are motives to detect threatening and arousing stimuli. One bias that is caused by threat that we have already discussed is that people become avoidant when they feel threatened, perhaps even avoiding people and situations it would be advantageous to approach. An excellent example of this was introduced in Chapter 5 and the discussion of stereotype threat. Steele (1997) describes stereotype threat as leading stigmatized people who excel in a domain that is stereotyped in the larger society to become avoidant of that domain. For example, stereotypes of women as bad in science, technology, engineering, and mathematics (STEM) fields may lead women who excel in math and science to avoid these majors when in college. Pietri et al. (2019) showed that if women are told gender biases are pervasive in STEM, they feel less welcome in settings where such norms exist. Another example was provided in Chapter 3, where it was shown that cross-race interactions lead to arousal. Blascovich et al. (2001) show that among many White research participants, interracial interactions induce a malignant form of cardiovascular reactivity (see also Mendes, Blascovich, Hunter, Lickel, & Jost, 2007). Such arousal is communicated through subtle signals such as gaze avoidance, physical distancing, speech errors, body lean/posture, verbal dominance, language style matching or synchrony, abstraction in word use, and general distraction due to excessive need to self-regulate the expression of one's arousal (e.g., Dovidio et al., 2002; Maass et al., 1995; Richeson & Shelton, 2007; Semin & Fiedler, 1991; Trawalter, Richeson, & Shelton, 2009; Vorauer & Kumhyr, 2001).

   Desire to avoid this type of arousal can lead to avoidance of such intergroup interactions. And if one is in such an interaction, one may wish to exit the encounter expeditiously. For example, research shows that perceivers avoid (or prematurely exit) interactions with partners from outgroups who are perceived to be arousing or threatening (e.g., Hebl et al., 2002; Kawakami et al., 2009; Peck & Denney, 2012). Hebl et al. found that fewer words were spoken in a job interview to gay than straight applicants. Also, the length of the interview was shorter with gay versus straight applicants (M = 245 seconds vs. 383 seconds, respectively). Let us next explore some more subtle ways in which people show a bias in their avoidance of threat.

Perceptual Bias

As noted above, when race is introduced to a context it can be very arousing to some people. The more one is threatened in this way by race, the more aroused one should be. One consequence of this just discussed is that it may make one avoidant. A far less obvious consequence is when a social threat produces high levels of physiological arousal and distorts perceptual experience. One such bias is when the experience of time is distorted (slowed) in the presence of arousing stimuli. Time perception research shows that drugs associated with arousal and with sedation can cause time distortion (e.g., Fortin, Rousseau, Bourque, & Kirouac, 1993). Haloperidol (a dopamine antagonist) is a sedative that slows the internal clock and makes the experience of the outside world move faster than reality dictates (e.g., Meck, 1983). Methamphetamine (a dopamine agonist) speeds up the internal clock, slowing the passage of time; arousal creates the perception that time slows (e.g., Marciq, Roberts, & Church, 1981). By time perception slowing it is meant that any given duration of time is overestimated. It feels like 5 minutes has passed when it has been less. A given duration (10 seconds) is perceived as having arrived in less time (after 7 seconds), making the actual duration feel longer to arrive. Time seems to drag.

Does social arousal cause the same **time perception bias** seen from physiological arousal? A small body of research exists showing that time slows when seeing taboo words, emotional faces, and emotionally arousing films (e.g., Gil & Droit-Volet, 2011; Tipples, 2010). For example, an angry face is arousing, and research participants perceived angry faces to be present for a longer duration than reality dictates—time slows when viewing emotionally arousing faces. In research from my own laboratory we examined whether the threat of being seen as prejudiced will be arousing and cause this bias to emerge. We reasoned that if arousal makes time slow, and triggering race makes some White people threatened and aroused, such people should have a time perception bias when viewing faces of Black men relative to faces of White men. Our research (Moskowitz, Olcaysoy Okten, & Gooch, 2015; Moskowitz et al., 2017) shows time, for White participants, seems to move more slowly when perceiving the duration of Black versus White men's faces. But, this is only true if participants are aroused by race due to the threat of appearing biased (have high external motivation to avoid prejudice). In this research, the participants are exposed to faces of White men and Black men (as well as to images of geometric shapes) repeatedly over multiple trials. Each trial of the experiment shows one such image that is first preceded by an image of a geometric shape (triangle, square, etc.). They are asked to perceive whether the duration of the second item was longer or shorter than the first item (see Figure 9.2). Our results showed that the duration of the Black man's face on the screen was perceived as longer than a White man's face shown for the same duration. This pattern emerged only for participants with high external motivation to control prejudice. This suggests that arousal from one's implicit prejudice causes a time perception bias.

> **Time perception bias:** When physiological arousal induced by either drugs or emotional reactions slows time perception so that any given duration of time is overestimated. A given duration (10 seconds) is perceived as having arrived in less time (after 7 seconds), making the actual duration feel longer. Time seems to drag.

Recall that in Chapter 1, we discussed several ways in which the perception of stimuli from our environment is altered and twisted in the perceptual process. One was through motivation, in what was referred to as a "New Look" at perception that emerged in the 1940s. What was new about this approach was that it argued that perception was guided by the needs and goals of the person doing the perceiving. Information that was relevant to the self and that could potentially enhance self-esteem if detected efficiently was shown to have a biasing effect on low-level cognitive processing (e.g., Bruner & Goodman, 1947; Bruner & Postman, 1948; Postman et al., 1948). Stimuli relevant to the individual's important needs and values can be detected because the self is chronically ready to capture such stimuli, scanning the world and biasing one to preferentially process self-relevant and self-enhancing stimuli. This power to facilitate the detection of information that promotes one's motives relative to information that is irrelevant to one's motives is referred to by the term *perceptual*

Is Target 2 Duration > Target 1 Duration? "Yes"/"No"

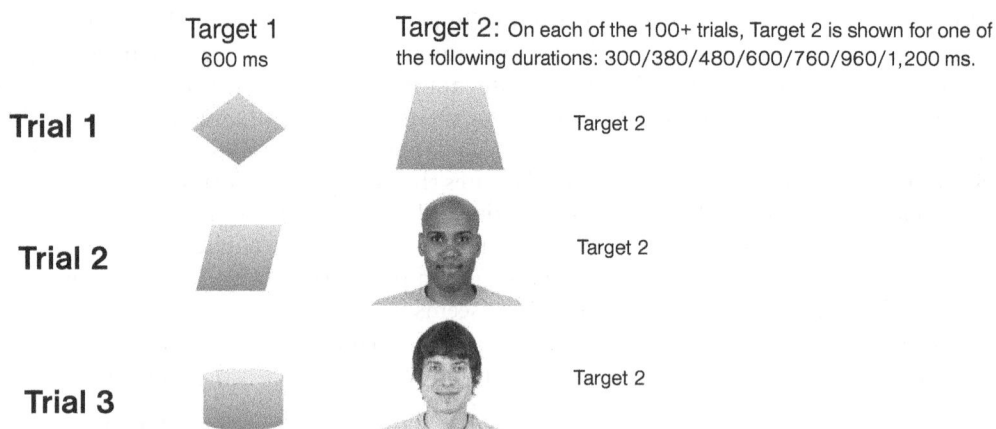

FIGURE 9.2. Procedure to assess time perception bias (faces are from the Chicago face database). From Ma, Correll, and Wittenbrink (2015). The Chicago Face Database: A free stimulus set of faces and norming data. *Behavior Research Methods, 47*, 1122–1135.

readiness. However, at times our motivation is to avoid threatening information, people, and events. When this is the case, motivation does not facilitate the detection of such information but disrupts the detection of such information. This type of preconscious defense system, in which we prevent ourselves from consciously seeing concepts that are threatening (or at least delay the recognition of such concepts), is known as **perceptual defense**. As Postman et al. stated: "value orientation not only contributes to the selection and accentuation of certain percepts in preference to others, it also erects barriers against percepts and hypotheses incongruent with or threatening to the individual's values" (p. 152).

> **Perceptual defense:** When motives, goals, and values do the opposite of heightening selection of certain percepts as with perceptual readiness, and instead block perception and attention to stimuli incongruent with or threatening to the individual. Perception is guided by one's needs/goals, resulting in unwanted information being detected efficiently and blocked from consciousness.

To illustrate this implicit protection from threat, McGinnies (1949) conducted an experiment in which people made verbal responses (report when they could see a word) to threatening and disliked stimuli: "taboo" words. In Chapter 5 an experiment by Postman et al. (1948) was reviewed in which people responded faster to words they were ready to see because they were relevant to their motives and values. McGinnies predicted the opposite—that people should take *longer* (have higher thresholds of recognition) to identify words that they are motivated to avoid because those words are threatening. Such words were further predicted to not only affect verbal reports but cause autonomic arousal. To test this, McGinnies assessed physiological arousal (through the use of galvanic skin responses), as well as verbal reports of word recognition. The verbal report measures were taken similarly to Postman et al., where a taboo word was initially flashed so quickly that it can only be subliminally detected. The presentation speed was then gradually slowed until a participant could consciously report being able to recognize the flash as a word. The presentation speed at which this verbal report occurs is then registered. It was found that it took people longer (slower presentation speeds) to recognize the taboo words relative to control words.

Additionally, it was found that emotional reactions to taboo words were registered by galvanic skin responses when such words were *not yet being consciously detected*. The preconscious was apparently detecting these words and defending the conscious mind from them, delaying recognition (raising the perceptual threshold). Although alternative explanations for these early studies can be generated (and perhaps you are rushing them to mind now—such as people effortfully suppress speaking words they do not wish to speak, even if they really can see them; or perhaps the effort to suppress the speaking of such words causes changes in galvanic skin responses). Subsequent, more thorough research, with compatible findings, helps us to keep hold of the idea that there is preconscious analysis of stimuli in our world that is guided by things such as perceptual readiness (see Erdelyi, 1974, for a review). More importantly, any interpretation of the findings still reveals a bias to avoid threatening stimuli.

Negativity Bias

A **negativity bias** refers to the preferential treatment afforded to negative information in forming impressions and in remembering information due to its value for detecting threat and conveying information about potential harm (e.g., Anderson, 1965b; Baumeister et al., 2001; Carlston, 1980; Hess & Pullen, 1994; Reeder & Spores, 1983; Rothbart & Park, 1986; Skowronski & Carlston, 1989; Wyer & Gordon, 1982). For example, negative information has been shown to carry extra weight in impression formation because it captures attention easily. Pratto and John (1991) performed an experiment in which research participants showed heightened attention to negative stimuli. Negative items were presented as distracters to a focal task. When the negative items were shown at the same time as the focal task they caused a slowdown in the task relative to when positive items were present. The negative items were more likely to capture and keep attention. Despite wanting to place attention on the focal task, the negative information—despite being a distractor—was hard to ignore. It kept pulling attention away.

> **Negativity bias:** The preferential treatment afforded to negative information in forming impressions and in remembering information due to its adaptive value for detecting threat and conveying information about potential harm.

A similar attentional pull to a threatening stimulus was reviewed in Chapter 4. Bean et al. (2012) found that when faces of Black men were presented with their face appearing to gaze directly at (perceived as a threat) a White perceiver, the gaze of the White perceivers was directed toward these images to a greater extent than when the faces were presented with an averted eye gaze (reduced threat). This effect emerged for faces presented at a speed of 30 milliseconds, which is too fast for participants to consciously choose to direct their attention (measured via eye gaze) to the face. The threatening stimulus captured attention. Another sign that this is a threat, is that a threat-avoidance pattern emerges when people have more time to respond—attention is grabbed then averted. White perceivers who attended to faces at 30 milliseconds, show avoidance of the same faces of Black men when presented for 500 milleseconds (when there is sufficient time to exert control). Trawalter et al. (2008) also showed that White participants had attention diverted to the faces of Black men relative to White men. This was evidenced by flashing a face of a White man and a Black man side by side on a screen and showing there was interference with locating a dot when it appeared in the place where the face of the White man had been (see Figure 9.3).

Mogg, Bradley, and Williams (1995) used a similar procedure in which words relating to threat and neutral words were shown simultaneously, one above the other. Of these two words, one was quickly followed on the screen by a dot, and people had to indicate where

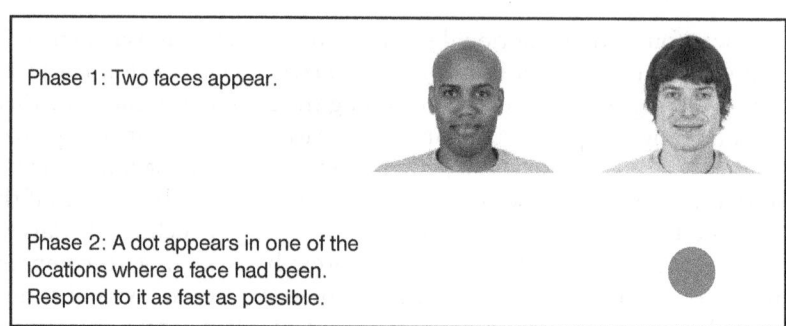

FIGURE 9.3. Dot probe task to detect racial bias in attention (faces are from the Chicago face database). From Ma, Correll, and Wittenbrink (2015). The Chicago Face Database: A free stimulus set of faces and norming data. *Behavior Research Methods, 47,* 1122–1135.

the dot appeared. There were faster responses to the dot when it occupied the spot where the threatening word had been. Mogg and Bradley (1999) modified the task to include threatening versus nonthreatening faces. Again, threatening faces capture attention and facilitate responding to the dots (relative to happy and neutral faces) when the dot appeared where the threatening face had been.[1]

Fiske (1980) illustrated that greater attention is given to negative information and that greater causal weight is assigned to negative information as a result. Research participants saw pictures of people performing a behavior, and each behavior varied in how negative it was (from extremely negative to moderately negative to moderately positive to extremely positive). Participants made judgments of the likability of the people involved for every type of behavior observed. Fiske found that both the negativity and extremity of the behavior shaped the rating given. Negative and extreme behaviors garnered more attention. Fiske concluded:

> Perceivers must ration social attention or be overwhelmed. In this instance, people seem to allocate processing time in an adaptive manner. Rather than equally weighting whatever comes along, social perceivers apparently attend to the most unusual cues—the nonmodal ones (p. 904).

In Chapter 5 there was a discussion of information that disconfirms an expectation or stereotype, and how such information is at times ignored and at other times captures attention. Skowronski and Carlston (1989) identified a bias in how people attend to, and are influenced by, such information. When the initial expectation is positive, and the disconfirming information is negative, attention is more focused and the initial impression is more easily updated than when a negative first impression is followed by a newly learned positive behavior. They refer to this as a negativity bias because they argue that negative behaviors are perceived to be more diagnostic of a person's genuine characteristics than positive behaviors (which are more normative, and hence less informative). Positive actions could represent an ulterior motive, or be enacted out of social desirability concerns, thus clouding their implications. Negative behaviors are not limited by such alternative possibilities and can be more easily taken as something true (e.g., Carlston, 1980). The change from a positive first impression to a negative impression is more prevalent and robust for this reason (e.g., Anderson, 1965b; Rothbart & Park, 1986; Skowronski & Carlston, 1992; Ybarra, 2001). This is especially true of immoral behavior, where a single immoral act can overturn an impression that someone is moral, whereas a single moral act is unlikely to change an impression that someone is immoral (e.g., Brambilla, Carraro, Castelli, & Sacchi, 2019; Brambilla & Leach, 2014). This negativity bias in how existing impressions are updated is seen in implicit impressions as well (e.g., Cone & Ferguson, 2015; Olcaysoy Okten & Moskowitz, 2020a; Petty & Briñol, 2010). Even though the initial impression is implicitly formed, negative information that is inconsistent with a positive first impression is highly diagnostic. The new information is associated with the person, just as the initial impression is. Yet, the diagnosticity of the new, negative information could make its association to the person stronger and more durable than the initial positive impression. The negative information, though learned later, is the one the perceiver associates with the person due to the strength of the association that negativity creates. This allows for an implicit first impression to be overturned. We review this in more detail later in the book.

The negativity bias is not only seen in how people revise an existing impression, but in forming impressions (Baumeister, Bratslavsky, Finkenauer, & Vohs, 2001; Hess & Pullen, 1994; Skowronski & Carlston, 1989). A perceiver is more likely to infer traits from negative behaviors than from positive behaviors (e.g., Reeder & Spores, 1983; Rothbart & Park, 1986). Alves, Koch, and Unkelbach (2017) show that this is perhaps because positive behaviors are not as distinctive as negative behaviors. Positive behaviors can be perceived as similar to one another and lumped together as one piece of information. Negative behaviors are encoded in a more distinctive fashion, treating them as separate from one another, and creating a sense of each piece of negative information being more diagnostic of a trait than any piece of positive information. The greater use of negative information is observed with implicit impression formation as well. Carlston and Skowronski (2005) found that people made spontaneous trait inferences to negative behaviors more than they did to positive behaviors. (It should be noted that each of the examples of negativity bias illustrate principles of the theory of correspondent inference, reviewed in Chapter 7, such as correspondent inference increasing as desirability of a behavior decreases.)[2]

Social Desirability Threat

Chapter 3 introduced the arousal associated with social desirability concerns; an arousal over how one will be viewed by others, creating concerns with not meeting expectations, being evaluated negatively, and not behaving appropriately according to norms (e.g., Deci & Ryan, 2000; Fazio & Dunton, 1997; Schlenker & Leary, 1982). What types of consequences do people fear from social disapproval (or being seen as shamefully inappropriate)? They worry about being seen as less likable, being devalued, being alienated and ostracized, being denied opportunity, being "canceled," and being seen as immoral (if not criminal). For example, if one has an external motivation to avoid prejudice, one is focused on the threat posed by other people thinking you are biased, their negative evaluation and disapproval, and the consequences for the self of being viewed in this way (e.g., Plant & Devine, 1998, 2003). These fears relate to the consequences of one's violation of **prescriptive norms**. Prescriptive norms specify how a person *ought to act or should act* according to culturally accepted standards. Also known as *injunctive norms*, prescriptive norms specify goals and plans on how to behave relating to gaining and maintaining social approval. These prescriptions pressure people to act accordingly, or face the threat of suffering the consequences. Relatedly, prescriptive stereotypes specify how a person should act based on expectations that exist as a member of a cultural or identity group (e.g., Eagly & Karau, 2002; Fiske, Cuddy, Glick,

> **Prescriptive norms:** Also known as injunctive norms, they specify how a person *should or ought to act* according to culturally accepted standards and expectations for members of an identity group. Additionally, they specify goals and plans dictating how one should behave for gaining and maintaining social approval.

& Xu, 2002; Goodwin & Darley, 2012; Janoff-Bulman, Sheikh, & Hepp, 2009). As Prentice and Carranza (2002) stated: "The stereotypic belief that women are warm and caring is matched by a societal prescription that they should be warm and caring" (p. 269).

Descriptive norms specify what the cultural beliefs are regarding how people *typically act* (and descriptive stereotypes list the qualities of the group that socially shared beliefs identify). Unlike *prescribing how people should act*, descriptive norms are sources of informational influence that specify expectations regarding *how people actually behave* or, in the case of descriptive stereotypes, what qualities to expect based on what is known about a group. While descriptive stereotypes often do inform prescriptions, the two do not always align (e.g., Devine & Elliott, 1995; Hudson & Ghani, 2021). Descriptive norms might change even as prescriptions linger. For example, although descriptive norms and stereotypes are changing to accept more agentic and powerful women, prescriptive norms and stereotypes may not change as quickly

> **Descriptive norms:** The culturally specified and socially shared beliefs regarding how people *typically act* (e.g., descriptive stereotypes list qualities of the group that are socially shared). Rather than prescribe how people should act, they serve as sources of informational influence specifying how people actually behave or, with descriptive stereotypes, what qualities to expect.

(e.g., Eagly & Revelle, 2022). Although lack of agency may no longer be prominent in how people describe the typical woman, agentic tendencies that are seen as normative in men are seen as incompatible with how a woman *should* act. This means that while an organization may be able to point to there being no gender bias in how it defines what is appropriate, women may still be subject to different standards of how they *should* act. Descriptive and prescriptive norms do not fit.[3]

When such prescriptions exist, such as when gender is associated with ways a person is expected to behave, it creates a threat that if one violates the prescriptions, there will be disapproval. In the current example of women at work, this disapproval or threat is that one will be seen as less promotable, desirable, and likable. If a woman were to try to ascend the corporate ladder using the same behavior a man would use, this could be seen as a violation of how they should act. This is a threat because the penalties for such violation of prescribed gender stereotypes can be harmful to the advancement and promotion for competent women (e.g., Fiske et al., 1991; Heilman, 2001). That is, women fear being penalized for (directly or indirectly) violating the norms and expectations that the stereotype says should be appropriate. There is a bias to perceive a lack of fit between the prescriptive stereotypes that characterize women and the characteristics that are required by upper-level managerial positions (e.g., Eagly & Karau, 2002), resulting in agentic women being derogated as unlikable, lacking social skills, and less desired as bosses (Heilman et al., 2004; Rudman, 1998; Rudman & Glick, 1999, 2001). The bias is to see the traits that are required for leadership in organizations as overlapping with the traits associated with men, while women's traits and roles are seen as opposing what is required for leadership (e.g., Glick & Fiske, 2001a, 2001b; Rudman & Glick, 2001). Social skills are highlighted when research participants evaluate female job applicants rather than competence, yet the reverse pattern is found when evaluating men (Phelan, Moss-Racusin, & Rudman, 2008). These prescriptive norms about gender are shared among both men and women (e.g., Rudman, Moss-Racusin, Phelan, & Nauts, 2012).

Women are placed in a double bind—they face a threat of not advancing if they conform to prescriptions (since those behaviors are not seen as typical of leaders)—but they face a threat of not advancing if they violate prescriptions to act in ways expected of leaders. This form of threat experienced by women at work is known as a fear of **backlash**. It refers to being devalued for displaying counterstereotypical behavior, such as being agentic and assertive, as opposed to communal (e.g., Rudman, 1998). Williams (2014) called this a situation of women needing to walk a "tightrope," stuck in a dilemma of needing to balance likability and competence, of expressing too much agency versus too much warmth. With the "right" balance, agentic women are less likely to face backlash and are rated as more influential; this requires moderating displays of agency with simultaneous communal displays (e.g., Carli, 2001; Carli & Eagly, 2007; Heilman & Okimoto, 2007; Rudman & Glick, 2001; Schock, Gruber, Scherndl, & Ortner, 2019). However, these gains are incurred with extra effort spent managing the threat of backlash and engaging in impression management, effort that men do not exert and could be used more productively in other endeavors.

> **Backlash:** Reacting negatively to feedback that a prescriptive norm was violated. If the feedback is about others it often manifests as devaluing them for their counterstereotypical behavior. This serves to encourage conforming to the prescriptions. If feedback is about the self, it often manifests as devaluing the feedback and its source.

What type of impression management does this threat compel? One example is that it influences concerns about **voice**. Employee voice refers to how women speak in organizations, especially expressing opinions and suggestions to one's boss, or to other people with power. Raising problems with an approach or suggesting improvements to a strategy is not only good for the organization (preventing groupthink and promoting innovation) but good for the employee. Withholding one's voice can be detrimental to the employee, and there is a bias for women to be motivated to be silent. Brescoll (2011) found that women in organizational settings reduced their talking time out of fear of backlash; also, female CEOs who talked longer, but for equal amounts of time as men, received lower ratings of competence and leadership ability.

> **Voice:** Speaking up at work, especially by expressing suggestions to one's boss and people with power. Withholding voice is detrimental to employees, yet women are often motivated to be silent in employment settings for fear of backlash. Women worry about seeming confrontational and dominant, succumbing to prescriptions of modesty and withholding voice.

Due to the threat of seeming confrontational and dominant, women succumb to prescriptions to be modest. Tenney, Coll, Bain, and Kreps (2021) report that women are especially likely to withhold voice in employment settings that are marked by *incivility*, such as those where coworkers are disrespectful, condescending, and rude (e.g., Porath, Overbeck, & Pearson, 2008; Schilpzand, De Pater, & Erez, 2016). These types of workplaces perhaps make fear of backlash more salient, increasing the motivation to keep silent, and leading to a bias whereby women are less likely to voice opinions. This is true of not just women at work but for any stigmatized group in a power structure that signals one's group is vulnerable to violations of prescriptions. They will feel compelled to stay quiet out of fear of being ostracized or punished. Whether it be offensive language used by a coach (such as the emails of Jon Gruden released in 2021), a dismissive joke made by a plenary speaker to a complicit audience, or signals of incivility by coworkers, a bias to inhibit one's voice can emerge when a vulnerable person experiences threats signaled by the norms of the power structure.

In a final example that normative threats compel a change in how we behave, we can look at the expression of prejudice. Stangor, Sechrist, and Jost (2001) illustrate that learning about the prejudiced attitudes of others is a biasing agent—people become less prejudiced if norms reflect this, and more prejudiced if that is what the group seemingly endorses. This impact is dependent on how strong the consensus is among the people in the group, suggesting that it is indeed the threat of not fitting in that compels the change. In a prejudice-ameliorating condition the participants learn that a large percentage of people in their ingroup had more favorable racial attitudes than those initially expressed by the participant. In a prejudice-enhancing condition the participants learned that a large percentage of people in their ingroup had less favorable racial attitudes than those initially expressed by the participant. The results revealed that endorsement of positive attitudes increased in the prejudice-ameliorating condition, and endorsement of negative attitudes increased in the prejudice-enhancing condition. Thus, an individual's attitudes about a group can be changed by learning about the norms of ingroup others.

In a second experiment Stangor et al. (2001) found that when the norms are expressed by a group with which one *highly identifies*, the impact is more pronounced as compared to a group with which one is less strongly identified. Haslam et al. (1996) also found evidence for people becoming more nonprejudiced when they learned that less-prejudiced norms were held by the members of a desirable ingroup. Yoshida, Peach, Zanna, and Spencer (2012) argued that while attitudes allow for personal expression and prepare one to know how to behave, norms prescribe what is expected of one—how one should behave. Thus, when we identify with a group there is also a threat to adopt the attitudes of the group and to conform to its norms (e.g., Hornsey, 2008; Turner, Hogg, Oakes, Reicher, & Wetherell, 1987). The prejudice of others could create a pressure on us to show similar prejudice, or else fear being ostracized.

Fear of Death

Another way in which a motivation to avoid threat can lead to bias is revealed by a line of research on the biases that arise from thoughts about death. Thinking about death (whether consciously or not), particularly thinking about *one's own mortality*, is known as being in the state of **mortality salience**. Mortality salience creates an existential threat for the individual, and research shows that people have a motivation to regulate this threat because thoughts about death are aversive to most people. Mortality salience creates a threat to our very existence, and we are motivated to reduce this aversive form of arousal through a set of processing strategies that is referred to as **terror management** (e.g., Arndt, Greenberg, Pyszczynski, Solomon, & Simon, 1997; Greenberg, Solomon, & Pyszczynski, 1997). This means that even when not aware of it, unconscious thoughts about death can motivate people to manage this aversive state (terror). One successful way to manage this terror is to identify or link the self with institutions, groups, and values that have a sense of permanence and positivity. Thus, a bias emerges in the face of mortality salience to ward off the threatening thought of the fleeting nature of existence, which is accomplished by linking the self to time-honored traditions and cultural worldviews. This bias has been shown to manifest as increased positive evaluations of people who (or objects that) share one's belief system, negative evaluations of (and aggression toward) those who threaten one's cultural worldview, reluctance to violate cultural norms, physical distancing from outgroups, and increased personal and group-level esteem (e.g., Greenberg et al., 1990; Greenberg, Pyszczynski, Solomon, Simon, & Breus, 1994).

> **Mortality salience:** When thoughts about death (whether conscious or not) are accessible.

> **Terror management:** Mortality salience creates a threat to one's fleeting existence that is threatening and unpleasant, a terror that must be regulated or managed. Terror management is the term given to this motivation to manage this existential fear of death. Terror management occurs through linking the self with institutions, groups, and values support one's belief system and have permanence and positivity (and also a reluctance to violate norms and aggression/avoidance toward those who threaten one's worldview).

For example, Jonas, Fritsche, and Greenberg (2005) did an experiment outside of the lab, where German research participants were interviewed either in front of a shopping mall or in front of a cemetery that was a few blocks from the same mall. They found that the people interviewed by the mall reported feeling equally favorable to German products versus foreign products. However, Germans interviewed in front of the cemetery strongly preferred German products. In doing so they were aligning themselves with their national identity, linking the self to something larger and more enduring. Arndt et al. (1997) showed that terror management processes can happen without conscious awareness. Participants from the United States were subliminally shown words that either increased mortality salience (e.g., *death*) or did not (e.g., *field*). Next, the participants performed an ostensibly separate experiment that measured the expression of pro-American sentiment. Do they align themselves with the shared worldviews of their national identity? Arndt et al. found that with unconscious increases in mortality salience came greater favorability toward the United States. They also found that increases in death-related thoughts not only promoted nationalism but that subsequent expressions in defense of one's worldview served to reduce thoughts of death back to baseline levels. It succeeded in managing the terror.

SELF-ESTEEM MOTIVES

While research on motivation waned in the early days of social cognition, one line of work on motivation held steady: research on self-serving and group-serving biases. Researchers have argued that self-esteem enhancement is among the most important drives of human responding (e.g., Allport, 1937; Fiske & Taylor, 1991; Gilovich, 1991; Sedikides, Gaertner, & Toguchi, 2003; Sedikides & Hepper, 2009; Taylor & Brown, 1988). Allport claimed that the person's "most coveted experience is the enhancement of his self-esteem" (p. 169). People tend to adopt and pursue a positive conception of self. This tendency has gone by many names: *positivity bias, ego protection, self-esteem enhancement,* and *positive illusions*. The desire to hold positive self-esteem is related to many biases where people evaluate information through egotistical glasses. The motivation to hold one's identity in positive regard has been shown to bias (to name just a few variables) group preference (e.g., Tajfel & Turner, 1979; Van Bavel, Packer, & Cunningham, 2008), attributions and explanations (e.g., Sedikides, 1993; Taylor & Jaggi, 1974; Zuckerman, 1979), the expression of prejudice (e.g., Fein & Spencer, 1997), perceptions of one's well-being/future/personal control (e.g., Taylor & Brown, 1988), self-assessment (e.g., Tesser, 1988), judgments of distance (e.g., Xiao & Van Bavel, 2012), selective attention (e.g., Erdelyi, 1974; Riccio, Cole, & Balcetis, 2013), and overestimation of abilities relative to a typical person (e.g., Alicke, Klotz, Breitenbecher, Yurak, & Vredenburg, 1995; Dunning, 2011).

Self-Affirmation

Our earlier review of dissonance theory illustrated how people are motivated to maintain consistent views of the self. One way to conceive of cognitive dissonance is as a discrepancy among two specific "cognitions" (such as between an attitude and a behavior, or an inconsistency between two beliefs). However, it is also the case that in many instances such discrepancies arise because a positive cognition about the self (such as "I am generally healthy and do not engage in risky behaviors") is discrepant with another more negative cognition (such as "I eat many unhealthy foods," or "I smoke cigarettes"). In such cases dissonance is not merely experienced as a specific type of inconsistency between two cognitions in a given domain (such as health) but as a threat to the **integrity of the self-system**. Many scholars have proposed that the self is best described as a system or set of interconnected (mostly) positive beliefs and attitudes that produces a coherent

> **Integrity of the self-system:** The belief that consistency striving is not necessarily about inconsistencies between two specific attitudes or beliefs, but an inconsistency with one's global sense of self. That what one desires is a coherent self-image as a good and moral person, with consistency among interconnected sets of positive beliefs about the self.

self-image of a good and moral person (e.g., Baumeister & Leary, 1995; Lyubomirsky, 2022; Markus, 1977; Steele, 1988). If dissonance is aroused from inconsistent cognitions about the self, the self-system as a global set of mostly positive beliefs is placed at threat. This is because the inconsistency in cognitions that is introduced comes in the form of suggesting something negative about the self. In addition to a specific cognition being challenged, the positive affect associated with the global self-system is challenged. If true, a motive to be consistent is accompanied by a motive to restore self-esteem, or perhaps consistency strivings take the form of self-esteem promotion.

For example, in the original dissonance experiment by Festinger and Carlsmith (1959) the inconsistency involved lying about one enjoying a task one had actually experienced to be boring. It is not simply that there are two inconsistent cognitions—experiencing the task as boring and declaring the task enjoyable—but that being a liar is inconsistent with a positive view of the self. At times dissonance is induced by highlighting a lie. At times dissonance is induced by spotlighting a dangerous habit such as smoking, or not using sunscreen. Other times it is induced by making one face their hypocrisy, such as holding egalitarian ideals yet acting in a biased way (e.g., Moskowitz et al., 2011; Stone, 2001; Stone et al., 1994). Dissonance often involves such threats to self-esteem from feedback about negative or hypocritical responses. Perhaps the motivation is actually to restore self-esteem.

Steele (1988) asserted that when cognitive dissonance is aroused by cognitions that challenge self-esteem, the dissonance arousal can be reduced, and the integrity of the system restored, by **self-affirmation**. Self-affirmation is a process of retrieving memories about, or engaging in behaviors that highlight, positive aspects of one's self-concept. The affirmations need not be in the same domain as the threat, but can be any positive aspect of one's identity. While the logic of cognitive dissonance is that it produces a motivation to restore the violated sense of consistency by addressing the specific source of the inconsistency (changing attitudes about one of the inconsistent cognitions), the logic of affirmation suggests something different. It suggests that that the dissonance can be removed with a more global approach of restoring the integrity of the self-system: by any affirmation of a positive aspect of one's identity. For example, Steele and Liu (1983) had participants act in a way that violated their attitudes. They found that people changed their attitudes so that their attitudes became more consistent with the behavior that was performed, as dissonance theory would predict. However, other participants were allowed to affirm an important component of their self-system before having attitudes measured. They reasoned that this self-affirmation would restore the threat to the self-system. Such people should no longer feel compelled to change these attitudes since the dissonance would have already been resolved through the affirmation of the global self-system. This is what was found. The threat to the self-concept was already handled through self-affirmation, so the negative behavior that had been engaged in no longer motivated consistency seeking. Consistency was already restored.

Self-affirmation: A process of retrieving memories about, or engaging in behaviors that highlight, positive aspects of one's self-concept. If done as a response to threat, affirmations need not be in the same domain as the specific dissonant cognitions that caused the threat, but can be any positive aspect of one's identity.

At times, restoring the integrity of our own self-system, our own affirmations, come at the expense of others. One way we feel better about ourselves is by putting other people down. This can be done through a direct comparison, where we say, "I am better than person X," or it can be done more indirectly by simply seeing others negatively, or stereotyping them in a negative way. As with a positive self-affirmation, affirmations achieved through negative assessments of others do not have to happen in the threatened domain. Self-esteem may suffer from feedback that one lacks intelligence, but derogation of others does not need to be about intelligence. It is esteem enhancing all the same to simply stereotype others. For example, Fein and Spencer (1997), as well as Spencer et al. (1998), show that when self-esteem is threatened, people respond by derogating a minority group. Further, derogating the minority improves one's own self-esteem. Their research participants received either negative or positive feedback on a bogus intelligence test, thus either affirming or threatening their self-esteem. They next reviewed a description of a woman as part of a job application. Her name either implied she was Jewish or non-Jewish. The experiment examined whether self-esteem threat created a drive to denigrate a stereotyped outgroup by having participants assess the job applicant's qualifications and personality. They found that when self-esteem was threatened people rated the Jewish applicant more negatively on both job qualification and traits. This stereotyping effect did not emerge among participants who had received positive feedback about their own intelligence. This effect of increased stereotyping of a minority following self-esteem threat was replicated using a different minority group: gay men. Additionally, self-esteem was measured after participants completed the evaluation of the target. The opportunity to derogate a minority seemed to repair self-esteem. Participants who received negative feedback and had the opportunity to derogate showed a larger increase in self-esteem after having evaluated the job applicant than other participants. Putting others down is affirming.

Self-Completion

While both positive affirmations and affirmations achieved through negative assessments of others can restore the threat felt to the more global sense of self, does it address the more specific source of the inconsistency (e.g., Galinsky, Moskowitz, & Skurnik, 2000; Moskowitz et al., 2011; Stone, Wiegand, Cooper, & Aronson, 1997)? It is true that Steele and Liu (1983) showed that when self-esteem is raised through an affirmation, dissonance appears to have been resolved. People no longer feel compelled to change their attitude, even though the affirmation had nothing to do with the challenged attitude. But does this global sense of feeling good simply mask the fact that the underlying inconsistency is still there? Is it lurking below the surface, ready to be reinstated? It remains possible that some types of dissonance are indeed threats to the integrity of the self-system, but that only addressing the specific threat to the self will fully remove the dissonance.

This is precisely what has been argued by the **theory of symbolic self-completion**, which was developed as a way to explain goal pursuit. The theory argues that when shortcomings with respect to the pursuit of a goal are encountered, the individual experiences self-definitional *incompleteness*— that is, failure at achieving a goal one has set for the self will result in an important aspect of one's sense of self having been undermined. This is aversive, and one is then motivated to reduce that sense of "incompleteness" in the domain of the self that has been undermined. An aspect of one's identity has been threatened and one's behavior is shown to be inconsistent with an important aspect of the self-concept. To restore a sense of "self-completion" and eliminate the inconsistency to this aspect of one's identity (to make the identity complete, or consistent), people acquire symbols that suggest one possesses the qualities associated with the goal. People attempt to display to themselves and to others that they are not inconsistent by acquiring symbolic evidence that will "undo" the apparent inconsistency (e.g., Gollwitzer, Wicklund, & Hilton, 1982; Wicklund &

> **Theory of symbolic self-completion:** A theory arguing that when shortcomings with respect to the pursuit of a goal are encountered, the individual experiences self-definitional *incompleteness* that is aversive and that one is motivated to reduce. To restore a sense of "self-completion" people acquire symbolic evidence that suggests one possesses qualities associated with the goal.

Gollwitzer, 1982). The theory argues that when people realize a discrepancy (or inconsistency) exists between their current state of responding and a goal they have set, they experience this discrepancy as an arousing tension. This discrepancy/inconsistency (or negative feedback) motivates the person to remove the discrepancy by attaining the goal. Goal-relevant behavior is initiated as a response.[4]

For example, Sciara, Regalia, and Gollwitzer (2022) hypothesized that social media platforms are especially well suited to self-completion strivings and that posts on platforms such as Instagram and Facebook are often tailored so that the people posting can restore completeness to a threatened aspect of their identity. If a threat to a valued identity creates a need to establish symbols of success in the domain, what better way than reaching many people at once through self-aggrandizing posts about achievements in the domain that will help restore the challenged identity? Sciara et al. established this by studying the social media posts of medical students and law students. She found that when these students experienced incompleteness concerning their professional identity, the students took to social media to compensate for the incompleteness by posting symbols that attach their identity to the threatened domain—that is, they do not simply affirm by saying positive things about themselves in such circumstances (with photographs of a great dinner or fabulous trip or cute children and dogs) but they specifically post images that tie their identity to the threatened domain (e.g., such as wearing their white medical coats). They show an increase in such posts of indicators of their goal attainment in the domain only when a threat in the domain has occurred, and not when a threat to that identity has not occurred. Further, they engage in self-symbolizing only when the incompleteness they experience refers to their specific career goals and aspirations (e.g., medical success for medical students, legal success for law students) and not to identities that are irrelevant to them (e.g., lacking legal skills for medical students, lacking medical knowledge for law students). Not to say media posts do not allow one to affirm the global self, but they are especially useful for self-completion of a specific identity.

In another example, if racism has caused the incompleteness, people should seek to acquire symbols that they are not racist—such as contributing to social justice causes, attending a bias-reduction workshop, and remembering anti-racist actions from their past. However, one needs to acquire symbols that reassert success in the *specific domain* that has been challenged. Affirming the self in an irrelevant domain, such as acquiring symbols that point to one being a good family member who has helped siblings in a time of need, will not compensate for the incompleteness of being a racist. The evidence acquired must restore completeness in the domain that has been threatened. Moskowitz et al. (2011) used precisely the type of situation just described to illustrate the point. Research participants with egalitarian goals were asked to contemplate a time in which their behavior had led to a racist outcome. The participants were then allowed to affirm their sense of self. Some did so using a global affirmation that addressed their positive qualities in a domain unrelated to racism. Other participants affirmed the self by addressing the specific source of the incompleteness—by affirming their egalitarian goals. If any affirmation of the self-system can reduce the "dissonance," then both groups of participants would no longer feel incomplete. To assess this, Moskowitz et al. used an implicit measure of the participants' motivation to pursue egalitarian goals. Do both types of affirmation result in the restoration of one's sense of completeness in this domain, as measured by the goal to be egalitarian being less strongly activated? They do not. Only the affirmation that specifically addressed racism led to the reduction of the aversive state. The results show that even if people no longer consciously experience a sense of incompleteness after self-affirmation of the self-system globally, the motivation to restore the specific inconsistency is still present at an unconscious level. Goals to be egalitarian (a motivation to address the challenged identity) are still accessible despite the global affirmation. Only nonracist behavior, addressing the specific domain challenged, restored identity. The goal of being egalitarian was no longer accessible; it had been addressed.[5]

Self-Esteem Enhancement

Taylor and Brown (1988) identified a set of biases that serve the purpose of promoting a positive sense of self. In fact, they called this positive conception of self that people seek "illusionary," as most people see themselves positively when reality defies this inference. Taylor and Brown review several types of processes that people use to achieve heightened self-esteem. One is to hold **unrealistically positive views of the self**. Attaining and maintaining positive self-esteem is accomplished if one can assert that they possess mostly positive traits and that there exist mostly positive causes for their action. One example is the **better-than-average effect** in which we display the ability to see ourselves as being better than others across most domains in a way that defies logic (at least in domains that are self-relevant; e.g., Tesser, 1988). For example, in Chapter 5 we described research illustrating an illusion of superiority, where people have a tendency to see themselves as more moral than the average person (e.g., Dunning, 2011; Epley & Dunning, 2000; Sedikides & Strube, 1997). They also have a tendency to see themselves as less prejudiced and more objective than others (e.g., Pronin et al., 2002). Naturally, not all people can be above average in morality or objectivity. Some of us have to be below average. Despite this relentless fact of life, most people maintain above-average views of their ability, traits, behavior, and attitudes. We have an exaggerated sense of positivity regarding the self. Alicke (1985) found that when asked to judge how self-descriptive a set of adjectives are, the research participants overwhelmingly choose positive over negative traits.

> **Unrealistically positive views of the self:** When self-relevant things and people are not only perceived positively, but as superior to other alternatives. Attaining and maintaining positive self-esteem is accomplished by such views linking positive causes for action and positive traits to the self, relationship partners, and in-group members (all perceived to be better than others).

> **Better-than-average effect:** When people see themselves as better than others across most domains in a way that defies logic. Not all people can be above average in all qualities; some have to be average or below average. Despite this relentless fact of life, most people exaggerate their personal value across many dimensions.

Even people with *actual low ability* on a task will overestimate their ability, a bias that is known as the **Dunning–Kruger effect**. The bias is not for people of low ability to claim having more expertise than legitimate experts but for people of low ability to claim higher ability than they actually possess; people of low ability are unable to objectively assess their competence. Unfortunately, people who are incompetent often lack the skills needed to diagnose that incompetence (Dunning, 2011; Dunning & Helzer, 2014) and fail to learn when provided with feedback that they lack the very ability they presume to possess and that they would need to actually improve (e.g., Ehrlinger, Johnson, Banner, Dunning, & Kruger, 2008).

> **Dunning–Kruger effect:** A bias where people of low ability have an illusion of superiority and are unable to objectively assess their competence, leading them to overestimate their ability. Such people do not claim to have more expertise than legitimate experts, but do claim to have higher ability than they actually possess. Ironically, blindness to inefficacy instills a sense of superiority.

Another way in which positive illusions manifest as bias is to see anything we agree with as being popular or shared by the consensus. There is a "tendency to see one's own behavioral choices as relatively common and appropriate for the existing circumstances, while viewing alternative responses as uncommon, deviant, and inappropriate" (Ross, 1977,

p. 188). If people believe their interpretation of the world is the appropriate and correct view, this should lead to the false assumption that most people see things as they do. After all, other people receive the same information as you, and thus should respond to that information in the same way you would, given that your interpretation is the best! The **false consensus effect** is the name Ross, Greene, et al. (1977) gave to the belief that others will see

> **False consensus effect:** The belief that most others will see events and people identically to how you see them. This tendency to have a self-centered bias in consensus estimates leads people to fail to recognize that others may construe things differently than they do.

events and people identically to you—the tendency to have a self-centered bias in consensus estimates and fail to recognize the likelihood that others construe things differently. In an experiment illustrating this effect, Ross et al. asked undergraduates if they would be willing to walk around campus wearing a sign that said "REPENT." They then asked them what percentage of their classmates would be willing to act the same. For the students who said they would wear the embarrassing sign, they believed that 64% of other students would do the same. For the students who refused, it was estimated that 77% of other students would also refuse to wear the embarrassing sign. Obviously, it is impossible for more than 50% of the people to wear the sign and more than 50% of the people to refuse to wear the sign. Participants are revealing that they believe that most other people think and act like them. The cause of this miscalculation in estimates is our belief in our correctness. If true, then the effect should be less pronounced when people believe their choices reflect idiosyncratic oddities of their own personality. Gilovich, Jennings, and Jennings (1983) found this to be true; When people listed a dispositional explanation (an explanation linked to their own personality or disposition) for a choice they had made, there was no evidence for false consensus (to assume others would make the same choice). When they recognize explicitly that their view is a unique one, they no longer exhibit the bias that others will see the world as they do.

Another strategy for defending self-esteem is to develop a chronic tendency to prepare for and expect the worst. If one expects bad things to happen, one can prepare a ready-made excuse for failure that one can use as a rationalization should failure later appear. People can build walls of negative expectations that can buffer them from the harshness of negative feedback. Two such strategies that have been explored by social psychologists are reviewed next. The first is called **defensive pessimism**. Have you ever met a person (maybe

> **Defensive pessimism:** Rather than maintaining a positive sense of self and seeking reassurance from others to ward off negative thoughts of potential failure, this strategy regulates failure by obsessing about it. Defensive pessimism embraces impending failure fully, mentally playing out worst-case scenarios, thus motivating people to overprepare and, in so doing, avoid failure.

you are such a person) who worries that they have failed after every exam? They complain before any major event that it will go poorly, proclaiming "I will not succeed, I am doomed." What usually frustrates others about such people is that they are not doomed. In fact, more often than not they do better than most people. Their fears were unwarranted. But were these fears useless? Perhaps the fear motivated them to work extra hard to deal with the eventual task, thus making them well prepared for it and less likely to fail. Many of our life tasks (goals pursued over a long period of time that are central to our motivational system), such as doing well academically, are often confronted with difficulties, frustrations, anxieties, and self-doubts. The individual's style of appraising these hindrances leads to goals they pursue to overcome these obstacles (Cantor & Fleeson, 1991, 1994; Norem & Cantor, 1986). Defensive pessimists prepare for the possibility of failure by obsessing about the failure itself. Rather than trying to maintain a positive sense of self and ward off the negativity of possible failure by seeking reassurance, they embrace the idea of impending failure fully, mentally playing through worst-case scenarios, motivating them to overprepare and, in so doing, avoid failure. To protect from the sting of eventual failure they espouse pessimism, but this may ironically do more than soften the blow of failure; it may prevent it.

Sometimes people do more than imagine the worst-case scenario to defend the self. To defend the self, at times people actually put themselves in bad situations—they create conditions where they likely will fail. By creating real obstacles to success, they create a situational constraint that can serve as the reason for failure—that is, to the extent it is easy to form an external attribution for a negative outcome, the easier it will be to not have self-esteem placed at risk. Imagine the athlete who gets drunk the night before a big game, or the employee who avoids preparation to instead "help" a troubled friend before every big presentation, or a student who stays up too late studying so that exhaustion impedes test performance. These people have created external causes for failure, thus protecting themselves from being held personally responsible for that failure if it were to come. From the drunk athlete to the exhausted student, the creation of the excuse actually increases the chances that the excuse will be needed by making the person more likely to fail. **Self-handicapping** is said to occur when people actively try to "arrange the circumstances of their behavior so as to protect their conceptions of themselves as competent, intelligent persons" (Jones & Berglas, 1978, p. 200) and in so doing, ironically, do things that increase their chance of failure just so they can have a good excuse to account for that failure. Berglas and Jones (1978) provided evidence for the self-handicapping strategy. Research participants were asked to provide answers for extremely difficult questions that they most likely had to guess at. However, they then get false feedback that informs them they excelled on the test. After being given feedback that must have seemed miraculous to them, participants are again asked to answer similar types of questions. This creates a conundrum. How often can you expect to be lucky and get these difficult questions correct? Having created a context where the individual must be contemplating failure, the research team then introduced a manipulation to allow them to detect what types of strategies people adopt to deal with their fears. Do they attempt to place themselves in the best possible mental state to make their chances for success optimal, or do they create impediments that allow them to rationalize away any subsequent failure? To examine this, participants are next informed that the researchers are interested in studying the impact of drugs on intellectual performance. Participants are offered a choice between two harmless drugs: one that supposedly facilitates intellectual performance, the other supposedly interferes with it. The results revealed that participants chose the self-handicapping strategy; they prefer to take a drug that clearly diminishes the possibility for success, thus providing an escape route for self-esteem in the (likely) event that failure should strike.

> **Self-handicapping:** A strategy where people actively protect their self-concept by, ironically, doing things that increase chances of failing just so they have a rationalization to account for that failure. They are acting in ways that diminish the possibility of success, thus providing a shelter for self-esteem in the (now more likely) event that failure strikes.

Another example of what Taylor and Brown (1988) called unrealistically positive views of the self is observed in a bias relating to how one evaluates the future. Imagine how you would feel if you got the job of your dreams, found the perfect person to date or marry, had a number one single on the pop charts, or received a Nobel prize (all of these positive events have happened to people I know). Positive events such as these would make you extremely happy and produce a life of joy, right? Just as would winning a lottery for millions of dollars? Yet lottery winners do not report greater happiness, and people with number one songs often find themselves with tales of loss, depression, and substance abuse. As Wortman and Silver (1989) reported, typical events do not have a lasting impact on well-being, and unusual events (like winning the lottery or losing a friend to cancer) have less of an effect on long-term well-being than people expect. As we have already discussed, people have a tendency to maintain positive self-esteem, and this level of self-esteem, while temporarily impacted by the events in our day-to-day life, is relatively unchanged in the long haul. When predicting our futures, or at least engaging in **affective forecasting** (forecasting or predicting future affective/emotional states), we are inaccurate at judging the impact of both positive and negative events (Kahneman & Snell, 1992).

Affective forecasting: Predicting future affective/emotional states. An estimate of how one is going to feel about a specific event or person at some point in the future.

Focusing on positive events, there is a tendency for people to believe such events that will occur in their future will provide them with far greater lasting joy than they actually do. There is what is known as a **durability bias** in predicting the power of positive events, with durability meant to refer to the fact that we believe the positive consequences of such events for our emotional well-being are far more durable and long-lasting than reality bares them out to be. While we may be correct in predicting that some event will be positive, our shortcoming is evidenced by our inability to adequately gauge the duration, power, and impact of such events (Gilbert, Pinel, Wilson, Blumberg, & Wheatley, 1998). Gilbert et al. discuss a variety of reasons for this overly positive view of the impact of positive events. A first reason for the bias is described by what Schkade and Kahneman (1998) call the **focusing illusion**, whereby people making estimates about their future happiness after an event overly focus on the event in question and disregard a myriad of other future events that will also occur. When we imagine getting a number one song on the charts we might not focus on the ensuing pressure from the record company and fans, a relentless touring schedule that taxes one's physical and mental abilities, a prying press that destroys one's privacy, a disrupted home life, and failed romantic relationships.

Durability bias: An error people display in gauging how long-lasting the consequences of emotionally charged events will be on their future emotional well-being. Durability bias occurs when one believes that the positive and negative effects that impact their emotional state will be far more durable than they actually are.

Focusing illusion: When estimates about future happiness are overly focused on a salient current event and disregard the myriad of other future events yet to occur. By focusing too narrowly on a subset of factors that shape future happiness, the importance of the emotional state related to the current event is exaggerated.

A second reason is attributed to what Gilbert et al. (1998) refer to as **immune neglect**. Although people use positive illusions to ward off negative feelings, they do not realize they do so. They make an analogy between the positivity bias that promotes well-being in mental life and the immune system that promotes well-being in the physical health of the body. Just as the immune system wards off disease, the mental immune system promotes mental health through warding off negative self-views. However, if the mental immune system is to work, they argue it must work silently and somewhat outside of awareness. If we knew we were engaging in positive illusions—selectively ignoring negative information, rationalizing away our own inconsistencies, attributing our own positive and negative actions and outcomes in grossly divergent ways—the power of the positive illusion would be gone. For positive illusions to be successful as a psychological immune system, one must be able to neglect the fact that such an immune system is at work and is propping up psychological well-being. While we have a bias against seeing negative events in our future, we are also unable to recognize that bias in ourselves. The positive illusion here is the downplaying of negative events, and the failure to recognize our distorted sense of how likely and durable negative outcomes will be. For as

Immune neglect: The inability to see the positive illusions that ward off negative feelings. Just as the immune system wards off disease, the mental immune system promotes health through warding off negative self-views. However, a successful psychological immune system requires neglecting the fact that we engage in illusions to prop up psychological well-being.

sure as the sun will rise, there will inevitably be negative events we encounter in our future. We just remain immune to projecting them as likely occurrences, remaining blissfully unaware of our positive illusions.

Gilbert et al. (1998) examined durability bias in affective forecasting by asking assistant professors to forecast their affect if they were to be denied tenure. They then compared these predictions against how people actually feel after being denied tenure (by tracking down former assistant professors who had been denied tenure from the same university as the people doing the forecasting). Forecasters predicted they would be happier in the 5-year period following getting tenure than in the same 5-year period following being denied tenure. In actuality, people who had attained tenure were no happier in this 5-year period (or at least did not report being any happier) than people who had been denied tenure. Another experiment by Gilbert et al. highlighted the role of immune neglect in these biases to affective forecasting. Some participants made forecasts about their future affect by imagining how they would feel upon receiving negative feedback. Other participants did not imagine how they would feel, but made ratings immediately after actually going through a mock interview and being given negative feedback. Additionally, the experiment manipulated how easy or hard it was for positive illusions to be used to rationalize the event. Some participants were told the negative feedback about them was being provided by one person who was not highly qualified. Other participants were told the negative feedback about them was being provided by a skilled team. In support of the notion that immune neglect is at work in biasing estimates of future affect, people who forecast their affective reactions believed they would feel equally bad regardless of whether a rejection was caused by an individual or a skilled team, and that this negative affect would persist. Yet people who actually experienced rejection felt better as time progressed; it did not persist. This was especially true when an individual provided the negative feedback, because the person receiving the feedback had *positive illusions to unknowingly ward off the negativity by attributing it to the bias of the individual*. They blame negative feedback on a flawed evaluator. When imaging responses, people do not imagine using such a positive illusion. Instead they predict they will be equally devastated by negative feedback, irrespective of how (and by whom) it is delivered. They neglect the bias that ultimately will protect their self-esteem.

Yet another way positive illusions manifest is in the type of explanations we make, with a **self-serving bias** in attribution style that boosts and protects self-esteem. Over the last 50 years, research on causal attribution has shown that the correspondence bias, while pervasive, is not uniformly applied. The correspondence bias was described as a tendency to see traits as responsible for behaviors and outcomes that we observe. However, the overreliance on traits depends on motivation. When self-esteem is implicated, we use traits as explanations in a far more strategic way. If it is the self, or members of groups to which one belongs, then traits as explanations are reserved for positive outcomes. Negative outcomes are attributed to other causes. We not only have a tendency to see

> **Self-serving bias:** An attributional style which protects self-esteem by attributing causation to successful versus unsuccessful outcomes differently, dependent on whether it is the self or another who enacts the behavior. When judging the self, good outcomes are seen as internally caused, while bad outcomes are seen as externally caused.

ourselves positively but to avoid seeing ourselves negatively, and to rationalize away negative behavior and outcomes. As Hastorf, Schneider, and Polefka (1970) state, "we attribute success to our own dispositions and failure to external forces" (p. 73). This is the self-serving bias: If good at something, we see it as important; if bad, we see it as irrelevant. If there is a positive outcome we see traits as responsible, if negative it is bad luck.

Two examples of this self-serving bias were reviewed in Chapter 1 (Miller, 1976; Sicoly & Ross, 1977). An excellent early review of relevant research (and criticisms of that research) is provided by Bradley (1978). Here we review one more example. Stevens and Jones (1976) reasoned that if attribution can be used to protect self-esteem, then the self-protective attribution pattern should be most evident when self-esteem is threatened. Research participants had self-esteem threatened by giving them feedback that they consistently failed at a simple task. In addition to this false feedback, they also were told how other participants supposedly had performed. Some people were told 84% of others did the same as them, while others were told that only 16% had performed the same as them (most people consistently succeeded). The most threatening feedback is where one fails on the task and most other people succeed on the task. Explanations for the feedback (and defensiveness in explanations) were shown to vary as a function of the threat. Participants explained success on the task as due to ability, but failure to bad luck. When the feedback was most threatening, this pattern was most extreme—people assign their failure in the face of others' success to external factors, not their personal qualities.

Even when judging others, we are inclined to attribute the causes of unsuccessful versus successful outcomes differently dependent on who is enacting the behavior, and our motives relating to that person. If their behaviors are relevant to us, then their positive behaviors and outcomes are described by traits, while negative behaviors and outcomes are not! For example, ingroup members are perceived as superior to outgroup others (Tajfel & Turner, 1986) and relationship partners (e.g., spouses, friends, teammates) are perceived to be better than others (e.g., Aron, Aron, Tudor, & Nelson, 1991; Gagné & Lydon, 2004; Murray & Holmes, 1993). And when such relevant others engage in negative behavior, this can be just as threatening as receiving negative feedback about the self. Importantly, self-esteem is tied to the various groups or collectives with which we share an identity. The social identities we possess contribute to self-esteem, and the social groups themselves have esteem associated with them—**collective self-esteem**—that reflects on us as a member of that

Collective self-esteem: Self-esteem that is derived from the various groups or collectives with which we identify.

social group (e.g., Crocker & Luhtanen 1990; Crocker, Thompson, McGraw, & Ingerman, 1987). The self-serving style of making attributions that exists for the self is extended to such important others.

In one experiment it was shown that people with high levels of self-esteem become defensive in the type of attributions they form if an important group is threatened, thus undermining collective esteem. Crocker et al. (1987) examined individuals who belonged to either high-status or low-status sororities. The logic was that belonging to a low-status sorority group would cause negative social comparisons and low collective esteem, and this should trigger a defensive attribution pattern. Members of low-status sororities should be more likely to try to bolster their group's image and denigrate other groups, whereas members of high-status groups should not. They found evidence of this defensive attribution in people with high self-esteem who were in low-status groups. If a participant had both high self-esteem and membership in a high-status group, there was no threat and no reason to use a self-serving attribution style to bolster one's identity. If they had high self-esteem and belonged to a low-status group, then such bolstering occurred. (People with low self-esteem did not react this way. They bolstered self-esteem, and evaluated their sorority more favorably, regardless of the status of their sorority.)

The motivation to see the self in a positive light can cause one to attribute the behavior of significant others to dispositional causes when those behaviors are positive, and to external causes when they are negative. For people we dislike, the attribution pattern is reversed; members of outgroups suffer from a bias to explain away their positive behavior, and to blame their stable traits for negative behavior. Positive outcomes are attributed to the situation (it is seen as a fluke), whereas negative outcomes are easily attributed to them (e.g.,

Pettigrew, 1979; Shepperd et al., 2008; Taylor & Jaggi, 1974). Such an attributional style ensures that one's own group is not threatened by failures or shortcomings within the ranks, or by merit and virtue within the ranks of other groups. Heider (1958) referred to this point in saying, "attribution depends on the value of the other person in the life-space. If we are inclined to disparage him we shall attribute his failures to his own person, his successes to his good luck or unfair practices. When Nietzsche says 'Success is the greatest liar,' he refers to this error" (p. 361).

Pettigrew (1979) dubbed this group-level version of the self-serving bias the **ultimate attribution error**. Attributions formed toward a person from a group we do not belong to—an "outgroup"—may be negative and dispositional, even when the same negative behaviors performed by a member of our own "ingroup" would be seen as externally caused. In Chapter 11 we provide a detailed illustration of this point, where Taylor and Jaggi (1974) show that people account for negative acts done by one's own group and positive acts done by members of a disliked outgroup by using situational attributions to explain away the behavior. Similarly, people use dispositional attributions to account for positive behaviors performed by their own group and negative behaviors performed by members of other groups.

Ultimate attribution error: The term's title is a reference to the fundamental attribution, but rather than describing a general preference for describing people by using traits, it is a preference for using traits strategically to keep stereotypic beliefs in place. It is a bias toward using traits to describe disliked outgroups engaging in negative behavior and ingroups engaging in positive behavior. The preference for using traits evaporates if a disliked group engages in positive behavior, or if a preferred group engages in negative behavior.

If defensive attribution, in which one is motivated to enhance esteem, is actually what causes such differential responding, then a pattern of outgroup denigrating and ingroup enhancing attributions should be heightened under conditions that facilitate and enhance the motive to bolster self-esteem. To test this, Dunning, Leuenberger, and Sherman (1995) manipulated the extent to which esteem was threatened. Their research participants either succeed or fail at a task just prior to making evaluations of others. In some cases, the other people who were being evaluated were similar to the research participant, thus making evaluations of these "others" relevant to one's own esteem. In other cases, the people being evaluated were dissimilar to the participant. In this sense the evaluations being formed are similar to the ingroup and outgroup evaluations in Taylor and Jaggi's (1974) experiment. What Dunning et al. found was that when self-esteem was threatened, participants restored their positive sense of self through the types of attributions made; they made more positive evaluations of the similar others than of the dissimilar others, but only after failure (when esteem motives are high), not after a success.

Ingroup Favoritism Arising from Self-Esteem Needs

Chapter 1 introduced a fundamental type of prejudice: favoritism shown to people with whom we share an identity. It was stated that even trivial groups to which we have just been assigned, where the identity is new and virtually meaningless, are favored. Why would this be the case? Why is prejudice so easily activated in such minimal circumstances? First, consider the more global point made in Chapter 1 that thinking exists to provide meaning, and such meaning can help us prepare to act. Tajfel and Wilkes (1963) argued that when groups are encountered, deriving meaning is often promoted by being able to differentiate among the groups, to compare them against one another. They suggest that whenever grouping of almost any kind is made, people perceptually differentiate them and exaggerate the differences among the groups.[6] Such differentiation among groups exists even when self-esteem is not involved, and the groups are not even social groups. Perhaps to understand prejudice, we first need to understand this more basic need to differentiate things that are of a "same kind." To do so, Tajfel and Wilkes asked perceivers to make judgments not of people but of lines! Something as clear-cut as a line should not be judged differently simply because it has been labeled as being in one group versus another. Yet biased perception emerged from such groupings.

In their experiment, Tajfel and Wilkes (1963) presented a series of eight lines to research participants, with the lines grouped into two sets of four. Participants were asked to judge the difference in length between two consecutive lines. For half of the people the lines were grouped according to membership in a category that had meaning. The first four in the series were labeled as part of Group A, and the meaning attached to them was that lines from Group A were short. The last four lines in the series of eight lines were labeled as part of Group B, and the meaning attached to them was that lines from Group B were long. The other half of the participants saw the same eight lines, in the exact same order, but membership in Group A versus Group B now did not coincide with line length. Each group had long and short lines (see Figure 9.4).

Remarkably, if the lines were labeled as being part of a group that had meaning, the difference between the longest line in Group A (line 4) and the shortest line in Group B (line 5) was seen as greater than when these same lines were being judged without this frame of reference. People exaggerated the difference between lines from two different groups, perceiving these groups to be more different than they actually are. Categorization as a member of Group A led line 4 to be seen as more different from a neighboring line in Group B if a "stereotype" for the groups exists. Without a group "stereotype," the lines seemed similar. This is seen as due to a human tendency to make meaning—to latch on to what differentiates the groups and exaggerate that difference.

What happens if in addition to this drive for meaning there is a drive for self-esteem? If the groups in question are socially defined groups, and are groups to which we are linked, will the same tendency to differentiate one group from the other exist? And will that differentiation be an attempt to see positivity in one's own group? Tajfel and colleagues extended

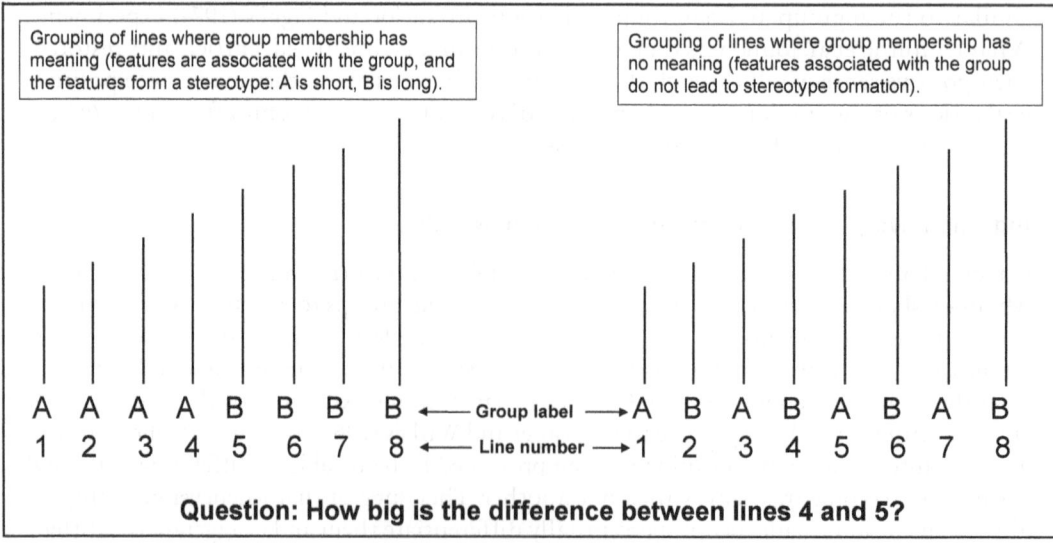

FIGURE 9.4. Mere categorization to a trivial, stereotyped group causes distortion.

this examination of seeing differences among groups to perceptions of groups of *people as opposed to lines*, showing that merely labeling a group as "us" versus "them" created **ingroup favoritism**. Such favoritism is illustrated through better evaluations of, and superior treatment of, "ingroup" members (e.g., Tajfel & Turner, 1979). While the prejudice to favor one's own group is perhaps strongest when the group in question is tied to an important identity, prejudice emerges to see the groups as different even if the group distinctions are trivial, as suggested above with judgments of lines.

> **Ingroup favoritism:** A preference shown to members of one's own group, regardless of whether one is aware of conferring such privilege on the group or not. Such favoritism is consistently illustrated through better evaluations of and superior treatment of "ingroup" members.

To illustrate just how fundamental the tendency is to favor "our own" over "others," initial illustrations attempted to create groups that existed in a vacuum, void of any real-world meaning. Even in a vacuum, so to speak, where all that is present is categorization based on meaningless criteria, our cognitive processing reveals a preference for people who are seen as "similar" to the perceiver—who share a meaningless identity. In this type of research the experimenters create a *minimal group* in which people are randomly assigned to meaningless groups based on a trivial feature of their personality they happen to share with others (such as if they prefer the paintings of Klee to Kandinsky, or overestimate versus underestimate the number of dots in an array). Tajfel et al. (1971) provided an early demonstration of the now highly replicated phenomenon that participants favor and value a minimally defined group to which they belong over other minimally defined groups to which they do not belong (e.g., Diehl, 1990; Otten, 2016). In this research the participants are first assigned to a group based on a supposed preference for one painting over another (asked for their preferences among a work by Klee vs. Kandinsky). Fellow ingroup members have never actually met. Participants are next asked to allocate points to ingroup members or outgroup members by choosing one payout option from among 13 provided to them. The participant can no way personally benefit from these payments—it will only benefit the other group members. They repeat this task numerous times using a different set of 13 payment options each time (see Figure 9.5).

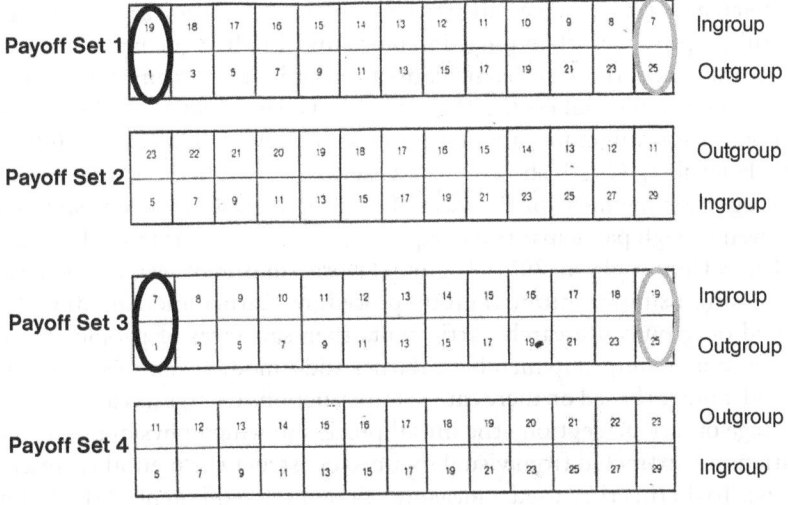

FIGURE 9.5. Sample payoff matrices in a minimal group experiment.

Remarkably, even though participants do not personally benefit, do not know their group members, never meet them, and have group membership based on the most minimal of features, they favor the ingroup. In fact, they often do so in a way where they attempt to maximize the differences between their own group and others. If responsible for the distribution of limited resources, participants do so in a way that creates a larger differ- ence between their own group and others, even at the expense of greater reward for their ingroup. What seems to matter is a superior comparison against others, not doing as well as one's group possibly can. In practical terms, people tend to choose having $10 distributed to their group if it meant another group getting nothing (a difference of $10 between the groups) rather than choosing getting $20 for their own group if it meant the other group got $15. The payoff matrices depicted in Figure 9.5 allow us to determine what strategies people are using. For example, in payoff set 1, the participants could choose to get the most possible reward for everyone (dishing out $32 total) by choosing the option circled in grey on the far right. Since these are all strangers, why not choose the option that pays the most possible money? But participants do not. They choose the option circled in black on the far left, which maximizes both the amount given to the ingroup ($19) and the differ- ence between the amount given to the ingroup versus the outgroup ($18). Which of these is most important: getting the most for the group, or maximizing the difference between the groups? Payoff set 3 allows us to test this. The option circled in grey on the far right offers the most ($19) to the ingroup (but offers even more—$25—to the outgroup). Yet participants prefer the option circled in black on the left, where the ingroup gets $7, the least out of all the options (but the amount they profit relative to the outgroup is greatest). Across dozens of such matrices one can examine the choices made. Results show people privilege their own group, and do so with a bias to maximize disparities among groups. Tajfel et al. (1971) state that

> when the subjects have a choice between acting in terms of maximum utilitarian advantage to all combined with maximum utilitarian advantage to members of their own group as against having their own group win on points at the sacrifice of both of these advantages, it is the win- ning that seems more important to them. (p. 172)

The preferences that emerge during the mere act of categorization into groups also extend to subtle processes of implicit inference and implicit memory. For example, the spontaneous inferences research participants form of ingroup members are more positive than those of outgroup members (e.g., Otten & Moskowitz, 2000) and they also form more negative spontaneous inferences about outgroups (e.g., Wigboldus et al., 2003). Bernstein, Young, and Hugenberg (2007) showed that assigning research participants to a group led to better recognition memory for the faces of ingroup members (as compared to outgroup members), even though participants had equal exposure to both types of faces (see also Van Bavel, Packer, & Cunningham, 2011). Ingroup favoritism is even seen at the lowest levels of perception. Using a similar minimal group procedure, Ratner and Amodio (2013) created ingroups and outgroups. Research participants then saw faces of people who were either labeled as ingroup or outgroup members. Ratner and Amodio examined "whether ingroup processing advantages based on mere category distinctions emerge as early as the structural encoding stage of face perception—the initial process in which physiognomic features and configurations are extracted from visual input to construct the mental representation of a face" (p. 299). To do this they used a measure of event-related potential (ERP) known to be associated with facial encoding processes. To be precise, they measured the N170 compo- nent of the ERP, "the earliest ERP component known to reflect the perceptual processing of a face" (p. 299). The amplitude of the N170 component served as the unit of measurement, with larger amplitudes signifying the superior structural encoding of faces. They found that the N170 amplitude was larger when the participants saw faces of a minimally defined ingroup member as compared to outgroup faces. This reveals a preference for processing the faces of people who are simply categorized as an ingroup member. Why do people show positive prejudice to an ingroup?

The research on ingroup favoritism suggests that we preference the groups to which we belong partly because this reflects positively on us. That self-esteem enhancement is not only attained through the way in which we think about the self but also determined by how we evaluate close others. The self is not an island, but a complex array of *social identities* that link the individual to various social groups (what Brewer, 1991, called the social self). To maintain a positive sense of self requires that people not only be biased in how they evaluate self-relevant information but to maintain positive views of the groups to which they are linked. Evaluations of others are biased because they are linked to us through social/group bonds. For example, Rubin, Hewstone, and Voci (2001) showed this bias to see an ingroup positively. Research participants learned about positive and negative qualities of ingroup members. They selectively generalized these behaviors to the group more globally. When the behaviors were positive the participants saw the behaviors as true of most group members—the group was seen as homogeneous when contemplating their positive traits. They found a bias to see the group as heterogeneous when it came to contemplating negative traits—they saw negative qualities as variable and not true of most group members.

The basic nature of these tendencies is made clear by the fact that the bias emerges in minimal groups. However, such favoritism toward an ingroup is even more prevalent when the groups in question are tied to identities of value and interest. The greater the value of the group, the greater its favorable outcomes and differentiation from others can reflect positively on the group. For example, when one of the social groups we identify with has succeeded at something, we take extra steps to highlight the fact that we are members of those groups. The behavior and status of the group can be used to bolster the self by one being able to **bask in reflective glory** (BIRG) of the achievements made by others with whom one identifies. In support of this idea, Cialdini et al. (1976) found that university students altered the manner in which they dressed the day following a victory by their football team. Fans bolster a positive sense of self by wearing the jerseys and hats of their favorite teams after a victory; this links the self to the social group and allows for the positivity associated with the achievement to extend from the group to the self.

> **Bask in reflective glory (BIRG):** When the positive behavior and status of a group with which one identifies is used to bolster the self by allowing one to associate oneself with the group's achievements.

When group identity is also tied to real-world advantages in domains that matter, identification with a group can lead to not only preference for the ingroup but denigrating groups to which we do not belong (see DiTomaso, 2015, for a review). There is a dark side to social identity in that positive esteem is not only attained by the achievements of one's own group, it is also attained through social comparison that tells us a disliked outgroup has poor outcomes (as we saw earlier in the research of Fein & Spencer, 1997). This can create a drive to derogate others in an attempt to produce comparisons in which our group compares favorably. There is now a large body of work that suggests that one cause of prejudice is the simple act of trying to promote positive group identity through such derogation of other groups. Rather than needing a history of dislike between groups, conflict over scarce resources, or ideological differences that lead to disdain, desires for positive social identity can create such ill will through social comparison processes aimed at trying to enhance the esteem of one's own group (see Ellemers & Haslam, 2012; Van Bavel & Packer, 2021, for reviews). One can even seek out such social comparison through the use of social media, which is perhaps why sites like Buzzfeed create headlines appealing to identity groups and social comparison (such as "9 Reasons to Hate the Woke Democrats"). These identity appeals generate clicks. We discuss this further in Chapter 11, and exit this topic here with this quote from Ellemers and Haslam:

"People's responses are thus understood in terms of subjective beliefs about different groups and the relations between them, rather than material interdependencies and instrumental concerns, objective individual and group characteristics, or individual difference variables" (p. 379).

Self-Esteem or Control?

Gilovich, Medvec, and Savitsky (2000) describe a bias they call the **spotlight effect**. This is a bias where people overestimate the extent to which they are the focus of attention and perceivers are noting things about them. Thus, if one is having a "bad hair" day, one is convinced it is the first thing others will notice. Gilovich et al. illustrated this bias by having research participants sit in a room with five other people while wearing what was at the time considered to be an embarrassing concert T-shirt. The student who wore the shirt then predicted how many of the other students in the room could recall and identify what was on the shirt. The students who wore the T-shirt predicted that nearly half of the others would know who was on the shirt. In reality, less than a quarter of the people recalled who was on the shirt. This belief in a metaphorical spotlight on the self perhaps is a bias of self-esteem—one thinks one is important enough to be the focus of attention. However, it is possible that this bias is less about self-esteem and more about motivations relating to *control and predictability*. Control is invoked in this bias because beliefs about how others see you are essential for making predictions about how they will react to you and how an ensuing interaction with them will unfold. As perceivers, we need to feel as if we can predict what others are like, and likely to do, and this hinges on a belief that we can see them accurately, and that they see us accurately. Perhaps it is not ego, but epistemic goals at work.

> **Spotlight effect:** A bias where people overestimate the extent to which they are the focus of attention and perceivers are noting things about them.

This control need should not only impact a belief that people can see our physical characteristics (our embarrassing shirt, our bad hair) but our psychological characteristics as well. Vorauer (2001) labeled this tendency to exaggerate the extent to which our internal states are easily seen by others as **transparency illusion**. This is a belief that our internal states, wants, desires, and goals are obvious to others. If you are feeling sad, yet have not told others, you will assume your heart is on your sleeve and your true self has bubbled to the surface, even though no discernible cues may actually be provided for others. Vorauer and Claude (1998) examined the transparency illusion by focusing on people involved in a negotiation, because in a negotiation, others must be able to read your objectives and intentions. Your ability to communicate these internal states will be a dominant determinant of whether the negotiation is successful. If you incorrectly assume these states are clear to others, and the transparency of your position is greatly exaggerated in your mind, the negotiation will be doomed. For example, you might think your adversary in the negotiation is being insensitive to your wishes and needs, when the problem actually is that you have not

> **Transparency illusion:** A tendency to exaggerate the extent to which our internal states are easily seen. Believing one's internal states, wants, desires, and goals are obvious to others. If you feel sad, yet have not said so, you assume it is observable by others, even though no discernible cues were provided for others.

adequately told them what you need. Thus, your hostile reaction to your adversary is actually a result of your own miscommunication, borne of transparency overestimation.

Gilovich, Savitsky, and Medvec (1998) explored the transparency illusion by looking at liars, not negotiators. How well are people able to predict whether their lies are transparent to others? People exaggerate their transparency here as well. For example, when participants were asked to lie to others when answering questions (e.g., "What is your favorite type of music?"), their estimates of how well others could detect the fact that they were lying was greatly exaggerated. Observers are not as good at detecting lies as we think they are. This is also true for lies of omission. If we attempt to conceal our emotions from others, failing to tell them how we truly feel, we fear our true emotions will nonetheless become apparent. Savitsky and Gilovich (1998) found that people who are nervous when speaking in public exaggerate how nervous others think they are. Despite trying to conceal our anxiety we still believe this anxiety leaks out and reveals our hidden insecurity. But this is an illusion; concealment of an emotional state typically works far better than our transparency illusion allows us to believe. While it is true that people are good at detecting nonverbal cues, we are not always sending the signals we feel we are.

Since this bias reflects your beliefs about other people's beliefs and impressions about you, it is a case of **metaperception**. And since it reflects a concern with what you believe others believe, the more self-conscious you are, the greater the bias (e.g., Vorauer & Ross, 1999). If we overestimate the extent to which others can see our internal states, the more accessible those internal states are to us, and the more we will think others can see them. Self-awareness is known to heighten the accessibility of self-relevant information (e.g., Carver & Scheier, 1978; Fenigstein, Scheier, & Buss, 1975). This has been shown in a variety of ways. Having people perform a task while in front of a mirror, or when a camera is pointed at them, can heighten self-awareness and lead to the increased accessibility of one's self-knowledge (Duval & Wicklund, 1972). Vorauer and Ross utilized these facts to illustrate that increased self-awareness heightens self-relevant thoughts, and in so doing promotes the transparency illusion.

> **Metaperception:** Beliefs about other people's beliefs and impressions about you.

CONCLUSIONS

Scientists, even naïve ones, should consider the facts unfiltered by desires. Yet despite following rules like scientists, our social cognition is also biased by what we want to see. People are motivated processors of information (e.g., Chaiken et al., 1989; Kruglanski, 1990) who flexibly interpret information in line with goals. These goals must be pursued within the limitations set by the capabilities of the processing system, creating a necessary compromise among desires to think deeply and structural barriers to doing so. Through habit we develop ways to implicitly pursue goals, and when such efficiency is lacking, we have the ability to dedicate the available processing resources to those items that matter. This notion of people as motivated tacticians has replaced the cognitive miser as the dominant metaphor for describing social-cognitive processing (e.g., Fiske & Taylor, 1991). It is not because we are lazy that we come to rely on stereotypes and heuristics. Many of the biases we see in how people judge, evaluate, and decide arise from some core set of motives: a desire to avoid threat, a need to enhance self-esteem, motives to be consistent, and motives to produce meaning efficiently. A shift in goals will shift the type of bias that is observed.

The goals we pursue can be expressed through conscious and effortful reasoning processes, but they can also operate implicitly to shape perception, attention, categorization, and inference all outside of awareness. Processes that feel beyond our control because of their implicit nature, such as the triggering of stereotypes, or the preference to use traits in explaining behavior, are in actuality choices made during goal pursuit. The goal is just implicit, and the choices occur outside awareness. Stereotyping is not inevitable; an implicit goal to produce meaning efficiently may promote stereotyping, but by changing the motivation that the individual is pursuing at the implicit level we can control stereotyping. Cognitive processing, even when implicit, is in a sense a tool we use to help us achieve the ends specified by the goal we have set in that context.

Long ago, Kurt Lewin described how our goals can direct our implicit cognition. He did this with an anecdote—when one has an important letter in one's pocket that needs to be mailed, postal boxes suddenly appear in the environment where they had never been noticed before. A street one walks along every day may contain mailboxes every four blocks, but one had never noticed them—not even in a year of walking that street every day. However, when one suddenly has a new goal that requires a mailbox, without consciously looking for them, the mailboxes suddenly appear. The shift in goals changes the way attentional filters are operating. Never one to rely simply on anecdotes, Lewin and his students set about performing a set of experiments that were foundational to the new field of social psychology that showed the power of goals to shape cognition. We review some of these experiments later in the book. For now we simply underscore the point that cognition is often in the service of, and biased by, the goals of the perceiver. Whether it be inhibiting taboo words, suppressing stereotypes, or attention being captured by stimuli that have affordance for the individual, our goals bias how we think.

The chapter ended with a discussion of several lines of research that identify components of a self-system that contribute to how one manages the needs for positive esteem, control, and belonging simultaneously. Brewer (1991) sees the individual as in a constant state of juggling the need to assimilate with and join similar others from whom one can attain a sense of belonging, with attempting to maintain some sense of positive distinctiveness and uniqueness. Of course, we can at times use groups to establish both a sense of belonging and a personal sense of distinctiveness if the group is itself a marker of distinctiveness. In the film *The Social Network* it was the distinctiveness (and exclusivity) of joining a Harvard University Facebook account that spawned the initial idea for that social network. A "friend" request was seen as a desire to enter an exclusive set that makes you both belonging to something large but also distinct. Thus, social identities can at times allow both of these goals to be accomplished through membership in groups. Group settings shift the sense of self from a focus purely on self-esteem and a concern with "I" to group-level concerns, even willing to suffer personal costs for the success of the group (e.g., Brewer & Gardner, 1996; Brewer & Kramer, 1986). When we value a group identity, belonging needs and the distinctiveness of the identity we receive from that group membership can overpower self-esteem needs. For example, Packer (2008) discusses how people will take on the potential humiliation and ostracism of dissenting from a group if they believe their act of dissent will enhance the group. Self-esteem is an important element of identity, but it is not the sole motivator of how we act or how we show bias. To understand bias, we often need to understand the motivations that exist for the person in that specific context.

NOTES

1. Even subliminal faces capture attention on this task, but only if they appear on the left side of the visual field. This suggests the brain's right hemisphere is responsible for detecting

threat (consistent with research suggesting that the right hemisphere exerts dominance when perceiving emotional faces, and emotional processing more generally).

2. It should be noted that in research on implicit inferences, the negative acts that promote implicit trait inferences are also extreme, and it could be this extremity that causes them to be diagnostic rather than negativity. Other research on implicit inferences that uses behaviors that are less extreme does not show a negativity bias (e.g., Olcaysoy Okten & Moskowitz, 2020a; Olcaysoy Okten et al., 2019; Todorov, Gobbini, Evans, & Haxby, 2007; Willis & Todorov, 2006). That research highlights the fact that there are times when positive behavior offers more of an affordance to a perceiver than negative behavior. For example, if judging ability, positive ability on a difficult task is more diagnostic than failure (e.g., Skowronski & Carlston, 1987).

3. Another example is provided by Hudson and Ghani (2021), who find that the traits people assumed gay men and lesbian women typically have—descriptive stereotypes such as gender inversion—diverge from the traits people believe gay men and lesbian women *should* have.

4. In many ways the theory of symbolic self-completion and the theory of cognitive dissonance are similar ideas that are simply being applied in two domains: one to attitude change and one to goal pursuit. This similarity is likely due to the fact that the theorists who developed each theory were students of Kurt Lewin, whose research on "tension states" arising from "discrepancies" is at the heart of each approach.

5. Using a personal anecdote, in 2017 I started chairing an award committee that honors a career of distinguished contribution to the field of social cognition. In my 6 years leading this committee we have given out nine awards. At a conference in February 2023 this award was used as an exemplar of how award winners in the field of social psychology *generally lack diversity*. The speaker put up the faces of all of the winners for the award, starting in 1998, to make the point that, as in the field generally, award winners lack diversity. They showed that since 1998 only two non-White people had won the award, and most winners were men. As the current chair of the committee to decide on the winner, it was easy to feel as if my acts had contributed to others feeling victimized by racism and sexism. I felt bad. Does pointing to my belief that I work hard, or my wife's belief that I am a good parent, ease the dissonance or incompleteness? It did not. Only stepping up efforts to do better toward pursuing my egalitarian goals, or pointing to symbols that show I am on the path to achieving those goals, counteract the incompleteness. For example, out of the nine awards we have distributed in my time as chair, the majority were to women, and two were to people who do not identify as White (and of the winners who were White, many were scholars not from North America, another group largely neglected in the past). These facts serve as symbols I can point to that help to address the incompleteness caused by the facts shared by the conference speaker.

6. As an anecdote, when my son Ben was 1 year old I described to a friend that Ben had just been ill and had vomited for the first time. The friend looked at her young girl sitting next to her and proclaimed, "She is not the vomiting type." As if vomiting when struck by a virus was an attribute one could (or could not) choose to possess. This friend's natural tendency was to group her and her child, and to then differentiate their group from the negative attributes of another group (in this case, me and my child!). In this case, this type of reflexive differentiation among groups likely enhanced my friend's self-esteem, as well as differentiating them from us.

CHAPTER 10

Beyond the Information Given
RESPONDING GUIDED BY PRIMING

Pretend that you are a manager for a company interviewing a prospective employee. They describe to you how they had made a great deal of money for their prior organization by investing a large amount of the company's resources in a new technology, which happened to succeed wildly. This behavior is ambiguous—it can be seen as reckless (risking a huge amount of resources on an unproven venture) or it can be seen as bold and adventurous. Your company avoids recklessness by policy, but has values that support boldness. How will this prospective employee be interpreted, with their opportunity for employment hanging in the balance? It may be the case that simply thinking about recklessness earlier in the day, in a totally different domain (such as reading an article about an underwater expedition that neglected regulations and led to the craft imploding and killing all on board), might cause you to see the interviewee as reckless. Or perhaps their gender might trigger a stereotype that leads you to think of recklessness without realizing it, and you then attribute that recklessness to their behavior.

Imagine you observe two men talking to each other when one suddenly shoves the other one. How would you interpret this act? You might think the two men are friends, and that one of them said something funny or obnoxious, and the shove was a playful act acknowledging the sarcasm. Alternatively, you could see the shove as an act of hostility or threat, with one man acting violently toward the other. We would like to think that decisions about how to interpret such acts are made by a careful consideration of the context, without rushing to judgment. However, decisions such as these are made all too often without much thought, but based on whatever comes to mind most easily in the moment. For example, Duncan (1976) showed that in the situation just described, people judge the shove based on a stereotype that they may not even realize they possess, let alone use. White research participants observed such an ambiguous shove and were asked to describe why it happened. Some participants observed an interaction where a White person shoved a Black person; others an interaction where a Black person shoved a White person. The results are striking. When a Black person shoves a White person, the participants label this act as violent 75% of the time. However, when a White person shoves a Black person, it is seen as violent only 17% of the time. If not violent, what then? The act is labeled as playful 42% of the time (as opposed to the act being labeled as playful only 6% of the time when a Black person shoves a White person). A similar pattern was found when examining whether the cause for the behavior is seen as internal to the person, or something in the situation. When Black men do the shoving, personal causes are high and situational causes are low; White men doing the shoving are seen with a pattern of low personal and high situational causation.

Race, ethnicity, age, gender, and other categories may have stereotypes associated with them. As described in Chapter 2, these qualities can be activated when the category is triggered. This spreading activation makes those particular thoughts ready to be used, whether the person intends to use them or not, or is even aware of their activation. Stereotypes being triggered are just one way some subset of information becomes "perceptually ready." We might observe a behavior and it could trigger associated thoughts; we might read a description of a person; and we may have been told a story about someone we know by a mutual acquaintance. In each of these cases some qualities—traits, goals, attitudes—are triggered, perhaps without us realizing it or thinking much about it. And just because they are triggered, we may be more likely to use them when interpreting the events and people we encounter shortly afterward. In Chapter 8 we defined *accessibility* as when a particular construct has a heightened state of potential use, one that makes it more easily retrieved from memory and gives it an advantage in meaning making. When a concept is not lying dormant in long-term memory but has a state of accessibility, this increased activation arises from two potential reasons: (1) the perceiver has either been recently or frequently thinking about the construct, or (2) the perceiver has a long-standing tendency to retrieve that construct from memory. The former type of accessibility is known as **temporary accessibility**, in which what is accessible in your mind is determined by what you have been recently exposed to in your environment. The environment might trigger a particular thought, or you might actually see an example in the environment (whether you are aware of having seen it or not) that leads to that construct being retrieved from memory. This triggering of a concept in the moment, temporarily pulling a concept from long-term memory, is known as **priming**, and the stimulus that causes the concept to be triggered is known as the **prime**. The effect that accessible information has on judgment is called a **priming effect**. In the example above, the stimulus that serves as the prime is the race of the person observed shoving someone, and the priming that occurs is the triggering of the associated stereotype. The priming effect is judging the person as more violent and threatening because the stereotype of Black men was primed.

In contrast to this incidental and momentary triggering of a construct from memory, **chronic accessibility** is when habit and repetition cause a unique set of constructs to be typically encountered, leading these constructs to have a permanent state of readiness for use. Kelly (1955) argued that people have routine and habitual experiences in life that make specific sets of social situations frequent and that

Temporary accessibility: When what is accessible in the mind is determined by what one has recently been exposed to in the environment, the accessibility of which will fade as time passes from the moment of exposure.

Priming: The retrieval of a particular thought from memory, either from seeing an example or a related construct. This makes that construct accessible, whether one is aware of this process or not. Priming is when exposure to a construct leads to retrieval of that construct from memory.

Prime: The stimulus that causes the priming of a concept.

Priming effect: The effect that accessible information has on the judgment of some new information, or on any cognitive process relating to a new stimulus.

Chronic accessibility: When what is accessible in the mind is determined by habit and repetition, causing a unique set of constructs to be typically encountered and leading these constructs to have a permanent state of readiness for use.

result in the repetition of specific types of social behavior. People are repeatedly in situations that call for kindness or helpfulness or intelligence, and so on, dependent on the types of daily routines they repeatedly enact, or traits that lead them to consistently pursue these types of behaviors. This personal history creates a permanent screen or filter through which the person's world is experienced. According to Kelly, constructs that are chronically accessible serve as a "scanning pattern which a person continually projects upon his world. As he sweeps back and forth across his perceptual field he picks up blips of meaning" (p. 145). A student who spends an inordinate amount of time with friends who focus on scholarship and making the most of educational opportunities will have constructs related to intelligence and hard work chronically ready to be used to interpret other people. Another student, who is immersed in a group of friends consumed by social events, drinking, and people's physical appearance will have constructs related to socializing and fashion chronically ready to be used to interpret other people. These values are frequently encountered and endorsed and come to have a sort of favored status over other concepts that are less frequently encountered and endorsed. This relative state of readiness to view the world through the lens of these concepts makes them especially likely to use the concepts when encountering a person (or people) to whom those concepts might be relevant. Upon hearing a prominent lecturer, the first type of person may be inspired to think about their positions on issues while the latter person may have only remarks about the color of the lecturer's shirt, or the style of their haircut, to offer (not because they disliked the talk—which they may have—but because they have a *perceptual readiness* to see the world a specific way). In Chapter 5 we described political orientation as able to create such a chronic lens through which the world is viewed: a preparedness to see the world one way.

Most people find the idea that their judgment and decision making can be determined by whatever happens to be accessible, without them even realizing it is accessible, difficult to embrace. Being biased by motives and self-interest (as was described in Chapter 9 and the discussion of motivated reasoning) may be an unfair way to judge, but at least it seems easy to grasp as to why we do it. Accessibility effects seem far less justifiable, more like magic than science, and people have an inherent distrust that we actually are so capriciously influenced, in a way that does not even serve our self-interest. Given that an entire chapter is dedicated to these effects here, you might infer that the phenomenon is seen here as real, and complex; it is moderated by many variables that determine *if* accessible constructs have an influence and *how* accessible constructs have an influence. As you may intuit, your judgment of how well you performed on an incredibly easy exam or puzzle is unlikely to be influenced by what is accessible. It is also unlikely that your assessment of something that is universally disliked—such as a cockroach—is biased by accessibility. Your judgment of something important—such as the personality of your cousin's new spouse—is unlikely to be shaped by an article you read just prior to meeting them. The effects of information being primed or accessible do not always emerge, but require *certain conditions*. Additionally, the direction of the influence, *how* you are influenced, will also differ dependent on conditions. This does not make the phenomenon less important or less real, it merely means we need to understand the factors that shape when and how this influence is exerted.

Before turning to examine some of those factors, we briefly illustrate accessibility. Despite any skepticism that accessibility exerts an influence, the phenomenon is easy to illustrate. If I ask you to name a nut that comes in a shell, and then ask you to think of an animal, most people generate a peanut for the nut and an elephant as the animal of choice. The peanut, for most readers of this book, is the most accessible shelled nut. And as we reviewed in Chapters 2 and 4 when discussing associations among related constructs,

Meyer and Schvandeveldt (1971) showed that when a construct such as "doctor" is retrieved from memory, associated constructs such as "nurse" are made accessible as well. Peanuts are associated with elephants, but not so directly that asking you to think of a peanut would have made you consciously aware that "elephant" had also been made accessible. When later asked to decide which from among hundreds of animals to select, you chose the most accessible one: the elephant. Consider another example: Complete this fragment of a six-letter word by filling in the missing three letters (the three blanks at the start of the word) to form an English word: "___ect."

There are many possible answers: "reject," "inject," "effect," "detect," "affect," "select," and so on. Yet most people answer this question with the word "insect." Why? Because in the third sentence of the prior paragraph the word "cockroach" was used. Although there was no mention of "insect" directly, "cockroach" likely made you unconsciously retrieve "insect" from memory via spreading activation, making it temporarily primed. This influenced your word completion; even though your answer to the problem, to you, felt unbiased. In fact, I just realized I used the word "capriciously" two paragraphs ago, a word I rarely use, and just now noticed it was used in a news story I read earlier today. Another illustration of priming is one we all identify with. We have all found ourselves at times whistling, humming, or singing a song, only to wonder whether it was actually playing in the shop or grocery store we just left. How can you not even be sure you heard a tune, yet find yourself singing it nonetheless? It is because the song has been made accessible without you realizing it and has influenced your own responses despite you being unaware of its influence (or the fact that you even encountered the song).

As a final example, most likely you would describe the last symbol in the following string as a letter: *A a, C c, L l*. However, here is the exact same stimulus presented in a different string: 4, 3, 2, 1. How would you describe it now? The exact same stimulus gets interpreted differently because *it fits equally well into two, nonoverlapping categories*. The way in which it is judged is determined by what we are ready to see and what concepts have been made accessible (numbers or letters). Many of the behaviors we observe in the self and in others are similar in this regard: They can be placed into more than one non-overlapping category. The person who helps another person can be seen as kind, ingratiating, or even manipulative. The Senator who opposes kneeling during the "National Anthem" can be seen as patriotic, racist, or sycophantic. The interviewee who invested large resources in a new technology can be seen as bold or reckless. The President who invades a foreign country can be seen as a forward thinker, or cynical, a liberator, aggressive, or manipulative. A shove can be playful or violent. Many of the social behaviors we observe are open to such multiple interpretations; they are able to be categorized in alternative ways with equal likelihood, often with these potential interpretations being quite distinct and leading to drastically different implications (Kanouse & Hanson, 1972). The interpretation that is chosen can be determined simply by whatever concept happens to be accessible.

CHRONIC ACCESSIBILITY

At the start of the chapter we described two reasons that constructs could be perceptually ready: temporary accessibility and chronic accessibility. Let us start by examining evidence for priming effects that arise from chronic accessibility. People who have routines that frequently place them in contact with the same stimuli will have that concept in a permanent state of perceptual readiness. For example, motives and values can create a stable way of interacting with the world that produce such a state. With chronic accessibility, there is no prime causing the construct to be activated and retrieved. How then do some constructs have a readiness over others? As just stated, these certain constructs may have a permanent state of heightened activation, with accessibility always maintained at higher default levels than other constructs. "To the extent that people's social experiences vary in respect to which constructs are frequently activated (e.g., long-term differences in socialization experiences, goals), one would expect there to be individual differences in construct accessibility" (Higgins, King, & Mavin, 1982, p. 36). Eitam and Higgins (2010) propose an alternative way of thinking about chronic accessibility. They propose it is a matter of *motivational relevance*. Constructs that are important to the self are more relevant to the person, and this relevance is a permanent aspect of the representation, like a tag that identifies it as important. If a construct has such a tag of relevance that makes it more relevant than other constructs in memory, then it has an advantage when related behavior is observed. For example, if generosity is highly relevant to a person, it may not be that generosity is permanently in a state of accessibility, but is tagged as highly relevant and makes one better able to detect situations and people that invoke generosity. Higgins and Eitam propose that when behavior is observed we do a fast determination of its personal relevance. Constructs that are tagged as motivationally relevant will be faster and easier to be seen as relevant to that behavior. At the moment a behavior is observed, if a relevance assessment identifies that generosity is relevant, generosity then becomes accessible and jumps out to meet the behavior and capture its meaning. Thus, it is not that constructs have a permanent state of being primed, it is that when a stimulus appears, the relevant constructs will be more easily activated at that moment and thus be ready to provide an interpretation. *Chronic relevance* is perhaps a better term than *chronic accessibility* from this view, with relevance then causing accessibility in the moment.

Regardless of which view is correct, the impact is the same. Chronically accessible concepts free people from needing to consciously scan the environment for things that matter. Chronic concepts can pick and select such information from the environment without us needing to ask them to do the job (e.g., Erdelyi, 1974; Kelly, 1955). They have permanent relevance that is automatically assessed for its applicability to new stimuli (e.g., Eitam & Higgins, 2010).

Chronically Accessible Knowledge and Judgment

Higgins et al. (1982) sought to illustrate that chronic accessibility would impact impression formation. The same information should be interpreted differently by different individuals as a function of their chronically accessible constructs. However, such influences are unlikely to become aware to the individual (since they represent a permanent aspect of how they see the world). To explore these issues, Higgins et al. first assessed what concepts were chronically accessible to their research participants. They asked people to list up to 10 traits that described a type of person that they (1) liked, (2) disliked, (3) sought out, (4) avoided, and (5) frequently encountered. These questions were used to ascertain the types of traits each individual had chronically accessible. From these traits an essay was constructed (tailored to each participant) that described a person who performed behaviors that implied traits. Half of the behaviors in the essay implied traits consistent with the participant's chronically accessible concepts, and half implied traits not chronically accessible to the participant. The task was to read the essay, form an impression of the person, and reproduce the essay from memory. They did not know that these tasks had any link to the earlier task where they listed traits of people they liked, sought out, and so on. The findings suggested that chronic accessibility determined the impressions formed and the behaviors that were remembered: "the effects of construct individuality on impressions and reproductions were found a week after subjects' accessible trait constructs were elicited . . . an individual's accessible constructs remain fairly consistent over time" (p. 42).

Bargh (1982) illustrated that chronically accessible knowledge has an impact on not only the types of impressions people form but on the lower-level cognitive processes of attention and perception: what information in the environment automatically captures attention. Bargh identified people who had the trait "independence" chronically accessible, and participants who did not. It was predicted that participants with chronic accessibility would detect and attend to words relevant to their chronically accessible knowledge more easily, and that such words would draw attention if attention was focused elsewhere. To test the hypothesis, Bargh used a *dichotic listening task*, reviewed in Chapter 4 (e.g., Kahneman, 1973). In this task people wear headphones and have separate streams of information presented to each ear. They are told to ignore information presented in one ear and attend to information in the other (repeating the information in the attended ear out loud, a task known as shadowing). Bargh manipulated the type of information presented in each ear. Half the participants heard adjectives relevant to the chronically accessible concept "independence," as well as adjectives irrelevant to independence in the ear they were to ignore. The other half of the participants also heard both adjectives relevant to and irrelevant to independence, but they heard them in the ear to which they were attending—these words were being shadowed, not ignored. In the other ear, all participants heard nouns irrelevant to independence.

Is attention automatically drawn to chronically accessible constructs? To see whether attention was being uncontrollably drawn to the ear that had such information, people were asked to perform a task simultaneous to the dichotic listening task: turning off a light whenever it came on. The light was rigged so it sometimes came on precisely at the moment when relevant information was being presented. If people are automatically drawn to that chronically accessible information, it should impact on both the shadowing task and the task of turning off the light. If attention to the shadowing task is distracted and interfered with, one has fewer attentional resources to dedicate to turning off the light, and response time will be slowed. If attention to the shadowing task is facilitated, one has greater attentional resources to dedicate to other tasks and responses to the light will be faster. Thus, we can learn whether chronic accessibility impacts attention to the shadowing task by measuring if response time to the light is slowed versus quickened when a chronically accessible word is presented in the ignored ear versus the ear where one is focused (and such effects should not occur for people without chronic accessibility).

When chronically accessible information was presented in the ear people were attending to as part of the shadowing task, performance on both the shadowing task and the speed with which participants turned off the light was facilitated; it automatically directed attention. When chronically accessible words were presented to the ear people were ignoring, response times to the light task were longer, indicating that people were not ignoring the words; attention was automatically drawn to them. This same pattern was found for response times to the shadowing task: "automatic processing of the self-relevant information facilitated the shadowing task when part of the attended channel, and inhibited performance when on the rejected channel" (Bargh, 1982, p. 433). A conceptual replication of this finding of chronicity guiding attention was reviewed in Chapter 3, where Bargh and Pratto (1986) used a Stroop-like paradigm.

Depression as Chronic Accessibility of Negative Beliefs

Chronic perceptual and explanatory styles have become increasingly popular in explaining the effects of depression. Beck (1976) proposed a cognitive model of depression in which a **depressive schema** develops, one in which the depressed individual has developed a chronic style of perseverating on negative beliefs and explanations for events that comes to lead to increased negative affect and feelings of helplessness. The depressive self-schema is so pervasive in the individual with depression that it pervades all levels of psychological functioning; it guides the types of beliefs one holds, the types of explanations one generates for positive and negative outcomes, and the types of interpretations one forms for the behavior of others. The more accessible the schema becomes, the greater the range of events seen in the light of this schema, and an ever-widening range of behaviors are seen as validating and supporting the negative self-views that have come to characterize the self-concept.

> **Depressive schema:** A chronic style of perseverating on negative beliefs and explanations for events that eventually leads to negative affect, depressed mood, and feelings of helplessness.

Beck (1976) argued that this depressive schema spins its negative web over perception and interpretation without individuals' awareness; one concludes that the world is a negative and threatening place where failure predominates. We would not want to label the process as wholly automatic, since cognitive theories of depression also posit that people have the ability to control such thoughts. But, nonetheless, this is a pervasive and silent process of seeing the world through the lens of a negative self-concept that constitutes a chronic belief system. Seligman (1975, 1990) and his colleagues took Beck's cognitive formulation of depression and investigated how these schemas impact on the types of attributions depressed people arrive at for negative events. The Seligman group developed the idea that chronic accessibility manifests as **explanatory styles**—chronic tendencies to overrely on specific types of information that one is prepared to use when forming attributions (e.g., Anderson, Horowitz, & French, 1983). What sorts of "styles" develop?

> **Explanatory styles:** A chronic tendency to overrely on specific types of information that one is prepared to use when forming attributions. Seligman (1990) identified two broad styles of explaining behavior—the optimistic and the pessimistic.

Seligman (1990) identified two broad styles: the optimistic and pessimistic style of explaining behavior. These styles determine not only how one makes attributions for the behavior of others but guide the attributions one makes for one's own behavior and one's own consequences. The optimistic style is one in which positive events are seen as something stable and dispositional and global. It is a chronic way of seeing the world in which good events are seen as caused by you, pervading everything you do, and doing so across situations and over time. The pessimistic style is the opposite. It is the tendency to see negative events as something stable, dispositional, and global. You see bad things as caused by you, pervading everything you do, and stable across time and situations. Seligman's concern was with how these attributional or explanatory styles impact mental and physical health, arriving at the conclusion that explanatory style has long-term effects for well-being across a wide variety of domains. Most centrally, Seligman (along with Albert Ellis and Aaron T. Beck) suggested depression is caused by one's explanatory style.

Seligman (1990) has marshaled two general types of evidence to support the idea that chronic attribution styles lead to depression. The first is correlational in nature and involves measuring (1) the degree to which a person is depressed, and (2) what type of attributional style people have. Such research has consistently revealed that depression and the pessimistic attribution style are correlated. People who attribute negative events to internal, stable, and pervasive causes are more likely to be depressed. Of course, it could well be that it is not this attribution style that causes depression, but depression causes one to adopt this attributional style. If we want to establish that people's styles are what determine their mental health we need to examine one's styles ahead of time and see how well people protect themselves from depression when life eventually beats down one's door. Such evidence has also been gathered, and reveals that people with pessimistic styles are more prone to depression following failure and negative life events than people with an optimistic style. A compelling example comes from the Princeton–Penn longitudinal study, an experiment that followed children for 5 years, starting in the third grade, to examine how their attributional styles related to the development of depression as the children aged. Children with pessimistic styles were more likely to develop depression and in turn do poorly in school. A style of seeing negative events in a pervasive, personal, and persistent (permanent) way leads to depression (Nolen-Hoeksema, Girgus, & Seligman, 1992).

The implications of these findings range from the pragmatic to the therapeutic. For example, if depression is caused by pervasive, automatic thoughts that assign negative events to the permanent and global nature of the self, treatment for depression would involve (1) training people to identify these thoughts, (2) trying to marshal contrary evidence to the conclusions suggested by such thoughts, (3) teaching people new styles of explaining negative events that can replace the automatic ones currently springing to mind, and (4) developing automatic strategies for recognizing when pessimistic explanations are likely to be made and developing new automatic associations that move one toward more self-affirming explanations.

Bargh and Tota (1988) suggest Beck's (1976) notion of the depressive self-schema is tied to the automatic triggering of negative thoughts linked to the self-concept. People who are depressed and those who are not depressed differ in the constructs that are chronically accessible. People who are depressed are said to be people who have chronic accessibility for negative information, and, it is this increased accessibility that gives rise to differences in explanatory style and depressed affect. Spielman and Bargh (1990) argued that "once [an] event is recognized as a negative one, other negative events may also become accessible in memory, thus leading to the globality, or over-generalization, that is characteristic of depression" (p. 119). There is a triggering of negative beliefs, concepts, and traits, and this spreads through the associative network providing a web of negativity for interpreting the meaning of self-relevant events. Information that is chronically accessible was earlier shown to impact social judgments more broadly, including the perception of other people, and not only self-judgments. In contrast, Bargh and Tota (1988) claim "depressed individuals appear to differ from non-depressed individuals mainly in the content of their self-referential thought and not so much in the content of their more general social-perceptual constructs. The greater accessibility of negative concepts in depression seems to be conditional on the activation of the self-concept" (p. 926). Thus, a person who is depressed should have negative thoughts automatically triggered if the self is relevant to a context, but not if judging others.

Chronically Accessible Needs, Goals, and Values

Throughout this book we have reviewed the work of Jerome Bruner and his colleagues that was referred to as a "New Look" in perception research that emerged in the 1940s. What was new about this approach to perception was that it argued that perception was more than a transcription of the environment by the senses, and instead involved subjective twists of the data that were bombarding the perceptual system. These subjective twists were said to arise from the needs and states of perceptual readiness of the person doing the perceiving. People's needs, values, and goals that are habitually pursued were described as making people chronically ready to detect and perceive related stimuli from the environment. The chronic accessibility of certain concepts was attained because of the relevance of these concepts to the person's needs and values, and that heightened accessibility guided perceptual processing to detect stimuli relevant to these needs and values (e.g., Bruner & Goodman, 1947; McGinnies, 1949; Postman et al., 1948).

Bargh (1990) connected research on automatic processing and priming from the last quarter of the 20th century to the New Look research from 50 years earlier. That connection was made by Bargh proposing that much of human interpersonal behavior was directed by what he called "auto-motives." **Auto-motives** were defined as chronically accessible goals, motives, and needs that had the power to exert an influence on attention, judgment, and behavior across a wide array of interpersonal situations. The pursuit of these goals is initiated by cues in the environment—it is primed; the feeling of conscious willing is not needed to trigger goal pursuit, all that is needed are cues embedded in the context that signal this context affords one the opportunity to pursue an accessible goal. "Chronic goals and intents, and the procedures and plans associated with them, may become directly and automatically linked in memory with representations of environmental features to which they are frequently and consistently associated" (p. 100). Thus, chronic goals lie in wait, and when appropriate contexts appear, these contexts trigger a goal, and also trigger pursuit of the goal. A goal's chronic state of accessibility allows it to function outside awareness once an appropriate context is entered. In my own research I have moved away from calling this phenomenon an "auto-motive" because our research shows that these effects are not fully automatic. For example, one might have a goal to stereotype a particular group of people that is chronically accessible, but this does not mean that whenever such a person is encountered that the goal to stereotype will be triggered. One might have other accessible goals that compete with stereotyping, and these might be primed instead (we review a detailed example of this below). Using another example, one might have a chronic goal to eat certain types of delicious and fattening foods (such as cake and pie), but this does not mean that this goal will be triggered if one sees a cake. One can adopt health-related goals that are instead triggered when one sees fattening foods. In each case, goals are being primed outside awareness and without the experience of conscious intent, which is the point of our discussion here. The subtler point—that goal priming is not truly automatic because it is controllable—has led us to call this phenomenon **implicit volition** (e.g., Moskowitz, 2014), so as not to suggest it is inevitable and "automatic." We are not automatons (but we are easily and invisibly swayed).

> **Auto-motives (implicit volition):** Accessible goals, motives, and needs that have the power to exert an influence on cognition and behavior. Goal pursuit is initiated by cues in the environment without the feeling of conscious willing. All that is needed are contextual cues signaling that one is afforded an opportunity to pursue an accessible goal.

A large literature has been building to provide evidence of the impact of chronically accessible goals on how we perceive and judge others. Once a goal, need, motive, or value is primed, it shapes the way we interpret the behavior we see, the types of attributions we form for the people performing those behaviors, and the opinions we are ready to express. Among the chronic motives that influence how we judge other people are motivation to respond without prejudice (Plant & Devine, 1998), system justification (Jost, 2020), need for structure (Thompson, Naccarato, Moskowitz, & Parker, 2001), social dominance orientation (Pratto, Sidanius, Stallworth, & Malle, 1994), control motivation (Pittman & D'Agostino, 1989; Pittman & Pittman, 1980), bias awareness (Perry et al., 2015), locus of control (Lefcourt, 1976; Rotter, 1966), need for cognition (Cacioppo & Petty, 1982), need to evaluate (Jarvis & Petty, 1996), fairness (Moskowitz, 2010), and uncertainty orientation (Sorrentino & Short, 1986). Due to space constraints, we review only two examples.

Moskowitz et al. (2000) were interested in establishing that when one has a chronic goal, this goal will be triggered by an appropriate cue in the environment. Given the presence of such cues, two things would happen: First, the goal will be made accessible and direct attention to those stimuli that are compatible with the goal (that present an opportunity to pursue the goal). Second, the goal's activation will disrupt incompatible processing from occurring, a process known as **goal shielding**. Their focus was on fairness goals, or what they called chronic egalitarianism. Does the presence of cues in the environment that signal that an opportunity to be egalitarian is present lead to the increased accessibility of chronic egalitarian goals and the subsequent ability for those goals to direct what one attends to? Will shielding of the goal occur when the cue is detected by disrupting incompatible processing (in this case, by inhibiting stereotypes)? To be more specific, the interpersonal cue that was used was whether the face of a member of a minority group that has historically been treated in a nonegalitarian way was present. Members of an historically disparaged minority group represent an opportunity to act in an egalitarian way, being that they are often the targets of injustice. The measure of whether chronic egalitarian goals were triggered by such faces and then impact attention was whether people were able to detect stimuli relevant to egalitarian goals in their environment more quickly than other types of stimuli following exposure to these cues. Thus, for a White person with chronic egalitarian goals, the presence of a Black man should trigger those egalitarian goals, whereas the same man, encountered by a person without chronic goals, would not. Moskowitz et al. identified people who were chronic egalitarians and people who were not (nonchronics very well may value fairness, just not enough for it to be a dominant life goal). These two groups of participants were asked to engage in a perception task where they had to identify words that flash on a computer monitor. Some words are relevant to the goal of egalitarianism ("equity," "tolerance," "fairness," etc.), some are not ("humility," "courteous," "responsible," etc.). Additionally, each word is preceded by a face, a yearbook picture of either a White man or a Black man. It was predicted that seeing faces of Black men would trigger egalitarian goals in chronic egalitarians but not in nonchronics. Pictures of White men would afford no opportunity to think or act in an egalitarian way and would not trigger egalitarian goals. The triggering of the goals would be evidenced in the speed of responding to the words. This is what was found. People labeled as having chronic egalitarian goals had these goals triggered by the mere presence of a goal-relevant stimulus (a Black man). These goals, once triggered, impact attention and perception. Such individuals were faster to perceive words relevant to the goal of egalitarianism in their environment, but showed no increased speed to perceiving words irrelevant to the goal. In a second experiment they similarly showed that chronic egalitarians did not stereotype after encountering the face of a Black man, a form of goal shielding; rather than stereotype, their first response is to be fair.

> **Goal shielding:** When the activation of a goal disrupts incompatible processing (cognition and behavior that would interfere with the successful completion of the goal) from occurring.

In a second example of implicit volition, Fitzsimons and Bargh (2003) proposed that most important interpersonal relationships that we have with other people can be characterized by a set of chronic goals—whether it be the goal to make our mother proud or the goal to be supportive and helpful to our friends. Because these goals are chronically associated with these specific relationship partners, the presence of these people trigger these goals and impact our behavior, regardless of whether we are consciously aware of the goal being triggered. When with friends we nonconsciously start acting helpful, when with our mother we begin to act in situation-appropriate ways that might make her proud. In fact, we do not even need these relationship partners to be physically present to trigger these goals automatically and to start behaving in ways consistent with these goals. Any cues in the environment that might remind us of our mother would trigger the chronic goals we have associated with our mother and lead to behavior consistent with that goal. Thus, cues in the context that are associated with any of a number of our specific relationships can trigger whatever goals are associated with those relationships and lead to behavior that is aimed at delivering that specific goal.

Fitzsimons and Bargh (2003) provide several illustrations of how the chronic goals associated with specific relationship partners can be primed by the cues in one's current environment and impact on how one acts. In one experiment they relied on the fact that people seem to have chronic helping goals associated with close friendships. Therefore, they had people simply think about their friends and then measured whether such people were subsequently more likely to help others (thus indicating that thinking about the friend primed the goal to help, and this impacted on how they chose to act). As predicted, people who thought about a friend actually chose to help a stranger to a greater degree than when they had previously been asked to think about a coworker. Another experiment illustrated the powerful motivating influence of one's mother. Research participants were first classified as being people who either possessed the chronic goal of making their mother proud or people who did not have this chronic goal associated with their relationship with their mother. Participants then had thoughts about their mother triggered (or not) by asking half of them to describe their mother's appearance. Following this they worked on a task aimed at detecting whether there were behavioral differences between the groups. The task involved generating as many words as possible from a series of scrambled letters. Participants asked to think about their mothers showed a difference in how well they performed on the task as a function of their relationship with their mothers. Those who had the goal of "making mom proud" had these chronic goals triggered, whereas people who did not have this goal associated with their mother did not. Once this goal was primed, these participants outperformed all the other people in the experiment on the word-scramble task. They implicitly made their mothers proud by trying harder and doing better.

FIVE "A's" OF PRIMING EFFECTS: ACCESSIBILITY STRENGTH, AMBIGUITY, APPLICABILITY, ASSERTIBILITY, AND AWARENESS

Hopefully these examples of priming effects from chronic accessibility have helped to remove skepticism that people are influenced by what is accessible. Next, let us explore similar types of effects that arise from temporary accessibility, and the factors that determine if/when such an influence will occur from a force that you do not recognize as even being present. To do so, we first look at a sample experiment that illustrates temporary accessibility effects and analyze it according to these factors. It is the very first experiment to demonstrate social priming effects.

Higgins et al. (1977) introduced a classic procedure now used in many studies that illustrate the influence of temporarily accessible constructs. It was reviewed briefly in Chapter 4. The procedure is divided into two parts: the priming task and the judgment task (see Figure 10.1). In their priming task, people were incidentally exposed to information—in this case, traits—in order to make those traits (and their associated concepts) accessible. These traits were shown to research participants as part of a so-called perception task.

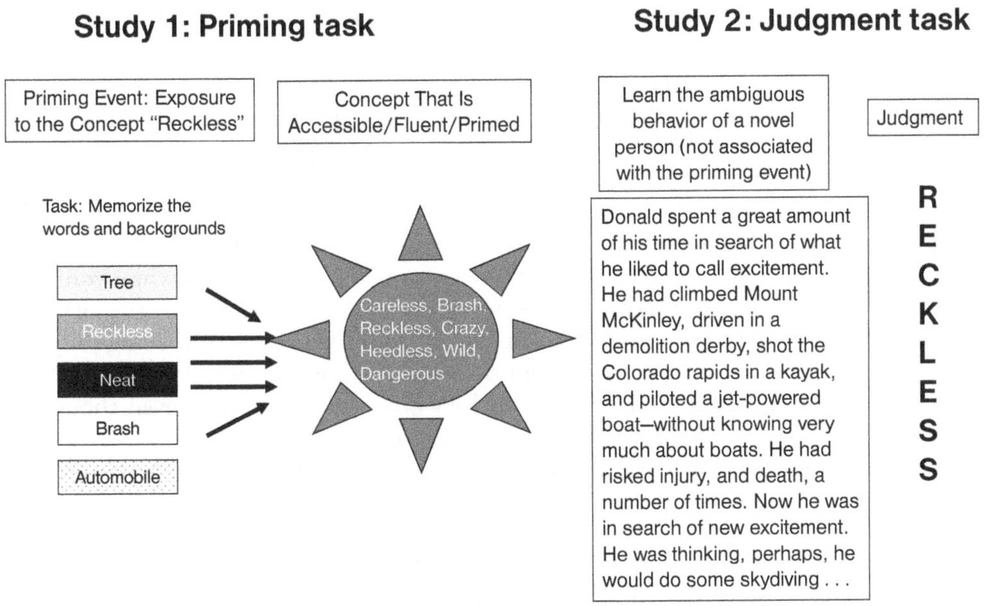

Study 1: Priming task

| Priming Event: Exposure to the Concept "Reckless" | | Concept That Is Accessible/Fluent/Primed |

Task: Memorize the words and backgrounds

| Tree |
| Reckless |
| Neat |
| Brash |
| Automobile |

Careless, Brash, Reckless, Crazy, Heedless, Wild, Dangerous

Study 2: Judgment task

| Learn the ambiguous behavior of a novel person (not associated with the priming event) | | Judgment |

Donald spent a great amount of his time in search of what he liked to call excitement. He had climbed Mount McKinley, driven in a demolition derby, shot the Colorado rapids in a kayak, and piloted a jet-powered boat—without knowing very much about boats. He had risked injury, and death, a number of times. Now he was in search of new excitement. He was thinking, perhaps, he would do some skydiving . . .

R
E
C
K
L
E
S
S

FIGURE 10.1. The "two-study" paradigm for examining priming effects.

Participants were shown a series of slides that contained words printed on a colored background, and they were asked to name the color of the background. However, prior to each slide they also received a "memory" word that they were to repeat 8–10 seconds later, after they had noted the color of the slide. These memory words were carefully selected so that four of them were used to prime four separate traits. One group of participants, for example, saw the traits reckless, conceited, aloof, and stubborn. A second group of participants saw the traits adventurous, confident, independent, and persistent. The perception task was actually being used, unbeknownst to participants, to prime these traits. However, there is nothing special about using a perception task to "prime" people. Any task that can bring a piece of information out of long-term memory in an incidental way, without the participant knowing it can influence them, can successfully serve as the priming task. The primes (the traits shown) in each set were specifically chosen to be foils for one another—they represent two ways a behavior that will soon be presented can be interpreted. The behavior will fit equally well into two nonoverlapping categories, and those categories are now primed: reckless versus adventurous, confident versus conceited, and so on.

Once this priming task is completed, participants are then asked to perform an ostensibly separate "reading comprehension" task. In this task, the participants learn about a person described as having performed a series of behaviors. The behaviors are always *ambiguous* in that each could be characterized in at least two, nonoverlapping ways (e.g., driving a jet-powered boat without knowing much about such devices could be characterized as reckless or as adventurous behavior). Importantly, the concepts primed in the first task are relevant to one of these possible nonoverlapping impressions that might be reached regarding the behavior—that is, the ambiguous behavior was relevant to the trait dimensions previously primed. This allows researchers to examine whether having the concept primed in the first task impacts how the behavior is seen in the second task. Does having "adventurous" primed, versus "reckless" being primed, make people see that particular behavior (driving a boat) as more adventurous? There are four ambiguous behaviors, each relevant to one of the four primed traits.

Finally, after having been primed and having read about the four ambiguous behaviors of the person, the participants then made judgments (formed impressions) of that person. What the research showed was that having been exposed to traits (e.g., reckless) in "Task 1" impacted which of the two, nonoverlapping ways the ambiguous behavior was interpreted. If you had been exposed to the words "reckless," "conceited," "aloof," and "stubborn" in the first task, you would see a person (whose behavior has nothing to do with the perception task just performed) as more reckless than adventurous, more conceited than confident, and so on. Of course, if you had been incidentally exposed to the words "adventurous," "confident," and "persistent" in the first task, you would see the person being judged as more adventurous than reckless, more confident than conceited, and so on. Trivial exposure to these concepts in Task 1 determined how a person was judged, even though the person had nothing to do with why those traits were accessible.

Higgins et al. (1977) illustrated that the judgments made by perceivers matched the accessible constructs, without the participants realizing such an influence exists. However, they also introduced some limitations and qualifiers to this influence that are quite important. The first qualifier is that a priming effect depends on the accessibility strength. An extremely weak level of construct accessibility might not have an effect.

Accessibility Strength

Bruner (1957) noted that as accessibility increases, less stimulus input is needed for that category to be used, and a wider range of stimuli will be captured by the accessible category. And as the **strength of accessibility** increases, the likelihood of an influence on judgment increases. Thus, when the degree to which one is primed with "hostile" increases, (1) a wider range of behaviors might be seen as relevant to hostility, and (2) fewer indicators of hostility might be needed to label the behavior as hostile. As the strength of accessibility increases, the person who is primed becomes even more "ready" to see hostility, needing less input to see it.

> **Strength of accessibility:** The level of accessibility of constructs can vary dependent on factors such as how recently or frequently the prime was seen. As accessibility increases, less stimulus input is needed for that category to be used, and a wider range of stimuli will be captured by the accessible category.

To illustrate this, Bargh and Pietromonaco (1982) manipulated how strongly the primed concept was activated. In a "first study" they presented participants with 100 words. Either 20 or 80% of the words presented were related to the trait "hostile" (e.g., "hostile," "unkind," punch," "hate," "hurt," "rude," "stab"), thus manipulating the strength of the priming and creating two groups: strongly (80%) versus weakly (20%) primed. Given the prediction that strength of accessibility should impact judgment, they expected to see people in the 80% condition judge a person they later encountered to be more hostile than people in the 20% condition or a third group of people in a 0% condition (who were never incidentally exposed to hostility in Task 1). Are people primed to see the world in terms of the construct of "hostility"? The results showed that the behavior seen in "Task 2" was judged more hostile in the 80 than 20% condition. The more frequently one is exposed to a construct, the stronger the accessibility (and its effects).

Srull and Wyer (1979) had provided similar evidence. They made concepts accessible by having participants read sets of four words that did not form a grammatically correct sentence. The task was to take three of the four words from a given set and use them to form a sentence. The priming occurred by the concepts implied by the sentences. For example, one set included the words "the hug boy kiss," and any use of three words to form a correct sentence (e.g., "hug the boy") must imply the concept of "kindness." The experiment then manipulated how frequently participants were primed. Some were primed by seeing 30 items, 20% of which were related to the concept "kind." Other participants read 30 items, 80% of which were related to kindness. Further, some participants read 60 items, with either 20 or 80% of the items related to kindness. Obviously, the person who sees 60 items, 80% of which are related to kindness, has encountered the concept of kindness more frequently than the person who saw 30 items, 20% of which were related to kindness. What impact does frequency of priming have on the strength of the activation? To test this, participants next read about a person whose behavior was ambiguous with regard to the primed quality (kindness). They rated this person along a variety of trait dimensions. Accessibility effects were greatest the more frequently a concept had been activated (such as 60 sentences that had 80% of the items related to the prime). Such research illustrates that the likelihood that one construct will win the metaphorical "race" to "capture" a stimulus against other competing constructs is linked to the construct's strength of activation. Weakly primed constructs may have no influence. The stronger the accessibility, the more likely it exerts an effect (so that if one has recently been exposed to a concept, such as hostile, it will capture the stimulus and be used to judge the person, as opposed to other potential constructs that could also fit, such as playful, but are not accessible).

Priming effects, when they are instances of temporary accessibility, will fade as the strength of the priming fades. Some have used a metaphor of an *energy cell or battery charge* to describe these temporary effects—when a construct is primed it will be strongly charged, but the charge can dissipate, and with that dissipation comes a faded influence. Higgins (1996a) describes "priming effects in terms of the heightening and the dissipation of excitation (or energy levels) from stimulation and decay" (p. 147). Using this metaphor, Higgins, Bargh, and Lombardi (1985) proposed that with priming, a concept "accumulates charge" until its level of activation reaches a threshold where it is accessible enough to exert an influence. Once the activation level passes that threshold it continues to accumulate charge, becoming not only activated but strongly activated, and more likely to exert an effect on judgment.

Not only is the impact on judgment greater when accessibility strength is greater, so too is the duration of the construct's accessibility (e.g., Bargh, Lombardi, & Higgins, 1988). If accessibility is like a charged energy cell, then a stronger charge should be a longer-lasting charge. Stronger accessibility, or a larger degree of excitation, has a longer-lasting influence than a more weakly primed construct. But just how long in real time do priming effects typically last? Srull and Wyer (1979) offer an initial answer to the question by manipulating how much time had elapsed since encountering the priming event (how recently the concept was activated). In addition to manipulating how frequently the prime had been encountered (80% of 60 puzzles vs. 20% of 30 puzzles), they also manipulated the delay to when the second "unrelated" task was performed. To measure how long the accessibility lasted, some participants were asked to make a judgment of a person whose behavior was known to be ambiguous with regard to kindness immediately after performing the first (priming) task. The time interval for making this judgment was varied, with other participants making the judgment after waiting 1 hour from the first task, and yet others being asked to wait 1 day (24 hours). They found that the length of time that accessibility was able to impact judgment depended on the strength of the prime. Weakly primed constructs (primed by 20% of 30 puzzles) were only able to impact judgment immediately. The priming effect lasted only a matter of minutes. However, more strongly primed constructs (primed by 80% of 60 puzzles) did not see the influence fade even an hour later. Srull and Wyer concluded that frequent priming led to effects that persisted through an hour, and beyond: "they are some-times detectable even after 24 hours" (p. 1670).

In summary, accessibility is stronger the more recently one has been exposed to a con-struct. Influence is greater from having been exposed to the concept of hostility 5 minutes ago as compared to 1 hour ago. However, extending this finding, both Higgins et al. (1985) and Srull and Wyer (1979, 1980) show that the strength and duration of the accessibility are not only connected with what concept has recently been encountered but the frequency with which one encounters that concept. The more frequently one encounters (or contem-plates) the primed concept (such as when 80% vs. 20% of the stimuli prime the same con-cept), the stronger the accessibility, and the longer the duration of its heightened accessibil-ity. Whereas a recent prime fades quite quickly, the frequently primed concept has strong initial effects and persistent effects that survived an hour, and at times, a day. And, recent and frequent priming work in concert with each other so that it is not the accessibility *at the time priming stops* but the accessibility *at the time the judgment is made* that matters—that is, a recent prime might be more powerful immediately after having been primed—however, a frequent prime might surpass the recent prime in strength of accessibility as time passes. Imagine observing one person shove another person, as you were asked to do at the start of this chapter. If I primed you with "playful" frequently, but with "violent" recently, then you might interpret an ambiguous shove as violent if the judgment happened right away. But if the judgment is made 30 minutes after the priming has stopped, the frequent priming of "playful" would be stronger and have a larger influence. The decay rate for a frequently primed construct might be slower than the decay rate of the recently primed construct.

This is precisely what Higgins et al. (1985) demonstrated experimentally. They primed participants with one concept repeatedly ("independent"), but the same participants were primed with another concept more recently ("aloof"). Therefore, two constructs were primed, each being potentially useful for describing a behavior they then had to judge: a person act-ing in a standoffish manner. Is the person seen as independent or aloof? The answer was that it *depends on the length of the delay between when a construct was primed and when the judg-ment was made*. When the delay was brief (15 seconds), the recently primed concept was more accessible and guided judgment. When the delay was of a longer duration (2 minutes), the frequently primed concept was now more accessible and guided judgment. The excitation level of a construct decreases over time since the last encounter with the priming stimulus, but *the decay function is not uniform* because the level of excitation is not merely tied to how long since the priming event has been encountered but how often it has been encountered. Frequency and recency of activation each impact the duration of accessibility effects, some-times in ways that are compatible, but potentially in ways that are incompatible.

Bargh, Bond, Lombardi, and Tota (1986) pointed out that temporary and chronic sources of accessibility can be present at the same time. The two separate influences can be antagonistic to each other (such as when one's chronically accessible construct is kind-ness, and one's temporarily accessible construct is manipulativeness), or they can facilitate each other. Bargh et al. posit that when two constructs facilitate each other, the effects are additive such that a chronically accessible construct can have its level of excitation (or the strength of its accessibility) heightened by an encounter with a stimulus that makes the same concept temporarily accessible. Thus, the degree of accessibility, or the "charge" associated with a concept, is not determined solely by what has recently been encountered but by what is chronically accessible, and the interaction of the two sources of accessibility.

While accessibility strength makes an influence on judgment more likely, this occurs within the confines of the fact that the behavior being judged must first be identified as having features that at least make the item relevant to the category. The wide range of stimuli/behavior that may be captured by an accessible construct is not so wide that it extends to all behavior. *The behavior must be applicable to the prime.* Behaviors indicating tiredness, shyness, or conscientiousness are not seen as hostile, no matter how strongly hostility is primed. Additionally, the behavior must be ambiguous enough to be influenced by the prime. A clearly hostile person will not be seen as more hostile (nor will a clearly passive person). We turn to exploring these two factors next.

Ambiguity

A central qualifier to finding a priming effect is that an accessible construct will have an influence on judgment only when the person being judged behaves in a manner that is open to interpretation—that is, the person's behavior must be either equally relevant to at least two, alternative, nonoverlapping constructs, or be vague. "In an ostensibly unrelated second task, subjects read a behavioral description of a stimulus person that was ambiguous regarding hostility, and then rated the stimulus person on several trait dimensions" (Bargh & Pietromonaco, 1982, p. 437). If a priming effect is to occur, why is **ambiguity** an essential characteristic of the behavior of the person being judged? When we observe a person act in a highly diagnostic, unwaveringly clear fashion, there is little room left for a perceiver's implicit biases to have an impact. If someone is acting in an unambiguously kind way, priming them with hostility will not lead you to the judgment of "hostility." If someone acts in a clearly counterstereotypic way, an accessible stereotype will not be used in one's impression (e.g., Locksley, Borgida, Brekke, & Hepburn, 1980; see Chapters 5 and 8).

> **Ambiguity:** Behavior or contexts that are not unwaveringly clear but open to interpretation. That is, it must be either equally relevant to at least two, alternative, nonoverlapping interpretations, or be vague.

Thus, accessibility effects are dependent on the stimulus information being ambiguous. When we are forming impressions of people whose traits are so evident in their behavior that their behavior impels one and only one interpretation, then accessibility of a construct will not matter much at all. But if the acts observed remotely lend themselves to subjective twists and spin, as is the case with much social behavior, then perceivers will interpret the actions in line with what is suggested by their accessible concepts. This is why experiments on priming effects must pretest the behaviors they ask people to judge, to make certain the behaviors are equally descriptive of at least two different traits: such as reckless versus adventurous, or persistent versus stubborn. If the behavior is not ambiguous, one should not expect to replicate a priming effect; the effect is not magic and does not just appear when primed. It is an influence that emerges when conditions allow for it, and ambiguity of behavior is one such condition.

Applicability

The **applicability** of a primed concept to a stimulus/target/person that is being judged is a question of how relevant the accessible information is relative to the information one is attempting to understand. Herr (1986) has said:

> **Applicability:** The relevance of accessible information to the information one is attempting to understand. If they are potentially in the same semantic domain then the behavior is relevant to the primed construct; there is applicability.

> Priming a category increases the likelihood that it will be applied to new incoming information, so long as the category

is applicable to the stimulus. The stimulus will then be categorized as an instance of that category . . . [the primed category] is accessed first for encoding that new information, provided
that the category is relevant and applicable. (p. 1107)

We review here two distinct ways a primed construct may be applicable to one's subsequent response. One way is in semantic meaning. Does the primed concept offer a way
to interpret the new information based on a shared meaning? For example, the concept of
"reckless" may have been primed, but it will have no influence if the behavior being judged
is unrelated to recklessness in any way—for example, if one is performing a behavior that
is ambiguously intelligent versus lucky (or any behavior that does not share semantic overlap with "reckless"). As perceivers, we do not attempt to foist whatever concepts that have
been brought to mind upon every person we encounter. When notions of intelligence are
brought to mind, increasing the accessibility of this concept, and we then are introduced
to our cousin's spouse, Perri, who acts in a manner that fits equally well to several alternative, nonoverlapping categories, how is the spouse judged? The answer is that accessible
information exerts an impact on our judgment only if the person we are judging is behaving
in a fashion that is relevant/applicable. If Perri's behavior is unrelated to intelligence (the
behavior is applicable to the qualities tired or bored), the prime "intelligent" should have
no impact. If a concept is "perceptually ready," this should not be interpreted to mean it is
a perceptual "given."

Higgins et al. (1977) thought this point central to understanding accessibility effects.
To illustrate the role of applicability in determining when accessible information is used,
they manipulated whether the behavior that was observed was applicable to the accessible
category. We already discussed the behavior being judged in their experiment: A person
acted in a way that could be seen as reckless or adventurous, in a way that could be seen as
confident or conceited, in a fashion that was independent or aloof, and in a manner that
could be seen as persistent or as stubborn. And we already discussed how the interpretation a perceiver arrived at was determined by what was accessible, so the behavior was seen
as similar to the accessible information. What we did not mention was that in addition
to the experiment "priming" either the positive or negative versions of the possible interpretations for the behavior (e.g., confident vs. conceited), it also manipulated whether the
concepts being primed were applicable to the behavior being judged. Therefore, some participants were exposed to trait words in the initial "perception" task that were relevant to
the behavior that would soon be judged, and some saw trait words that were not applicable.
This resulted in four types of primes: positive and applicable (adventurous, confident, independent, and persistent), negative and applicable (reckless, conceited, aloof, and stubborn),
positive and nonapplicable (neat, satirical, and grateful), and negative and nonapplicable
(disrespectful, listless, clumsy, and shy).

They found that, as was noted already, applicable primes shaded the type of judgment
made regarding the behavior. This difference in judgments *did not* emerge when nonapplicable concepts were primed. What these results suggest is that people do not "see" the concepts that are accessible to them in all places they look, they only see them in the relevant
places. But, if the person being observed behaves in a way that is perhaps even remotely
relevant, given that we are perceptually ready to see that behavior, our accessible category
may exert an influence. The results also mean that accessibility effects are truly linked to
the specific constructs that are primed. It is not the case that the effects of Higgins et al.
(1977) are due to people simply being ready to see others positively when primed with positive concepts. The behavior must be relevant and applicable to the accessible concepts not
in their affective tone but in the meaning they suggest. People primed with shyness do not

see a person as shy if their behavior does not fit it, nor do they come to see the person as negative or positive in a general sense.

Just how wide can the gap between the behavior and the concept be in order for it to still be seen as relevant and applicable? When behavior is clearly not shy or intelligent, it will not be seen as such even if shyness or intelligence is strongly primed. While it may be the case that the range of stimuli/behavior that may be captured by a prime does not extend to all behavior, it is also the case that the stronger the accessibility, the wider the range of behaviors and stimuli that will be captured and be deemed as relevant. Higgins and Brendl (1995) examined this component of the notion of applicability—namely, that "applicability" is a relative term, and what is deemed as applicable can vary along with the strength of the accessible concept. Thus, on the one hand, applicability is, in some sense, an absolute thing—generous behavior is unlikely to be seen as applicable to the concept of shy. On the other hand, there are perhaps a host of behaviors that might be seen as relevant to the concept of shyness, dependent upon just how ready one is to see that trait in others. The judgment of applicability is not solely based on the features of the stimulus but on the strength of the excitation of the accessible construct.

Higgins and Brendl (1995) examined this by manipulating the behavioral information. For some participants the behavior was vaguely related to the trait of conceited. For other participants the behavior was not vague; it was either clearly applicable to the trait "conceited" or clearly applicable to the trait "confident." The participants who read about these behaviors and judged the person performing them were first primed so that they had varying degrees of accessibility of the trait conceited or confident. The most important finding emerging from this research was that when the behavior being judged was, as they labeled it, "extremely vague," the strength of activation compensated for the weakness of the stimulus. The more accessible a construct (conceited), the more likely a vague behavior was seen as similar to the primed construct (the person was more likely to be judged as having acted in a conceited way). Higgins and Brendl conclude that applicability determines the influence, but applicability is somewhat subjective.

A second way a prime can be applicable, aside from its semantic similarity to the behavior, is regarding its **motivational relevance**. One must have the goal to make a judgment, or have a goal to use the primed construct. For example, in cognitive psychology studies it is known that if a perceiver is responding to a target with the goal of counting the number of syllables, identifying how many vowels are present, or with circling each instance of a particular letter, rather than reading the material to find meaning, then priming effects do not occur (e.g., Friedrich, Henik, & Tzelgov, 1991; Parkin, 1979). Without the goal of inferring meaning, the prime is no longer relevant to, or applicable with, the task at hand. Even if the prime and the behavior being judged have semantic relevance to each other, using the prime might not be deemed relevant if the prime is not motivationally relevant. For example, a person might be primed with the concept "egalitarian," yet be a person for whom that construct is not personally relevant. Such a person could be primed with egalitarian, yet may fail to see how that construct is applicable to any judgment they make. Its lack of relevance to them (motivationally) would disrupt any priming effect.

> **Motivational relevance:** It is possible for a construct to be accessible but for there to be no motivation to make a judgment. Motivational relevance is when there is a match between a primed construct and one's goals relating to using that construct.

That is an extreme example, where a construct lacks any motivational relevance to a person, ever. But motivational relevance can be easily manipulated from moment to moment. For example, Holland, Hendriks, and Aarts (2005) manipulated not merely if the semantic meaning of "clean" was primed but if the research participant additionally had the *goal* to clean, giving that construct motivational relevance. To prime the goal of "clean," they exposed half of their research participants to the odor of a popular cleaning product. However, they did this very subtly, so that the odor could barely be detected. They placed some participants in a room that contained the faint odor of cleaning fluid, while others waited in a room without the odor. To detect whether they then engaged in motivationally relevant behavior, they gave all the participants a messy cookie to eat, one that crumbled to pieces on the table quite easily. They showed that being in a room with a slight, hard-to-detect odor of cleaning fluid makes people more likely to clean the table after eating the cookie. They engage in the relevant goal.

Perhaps the clearest way to illustrate the importance of motivational relevance for a priming effect to occur is to illustrate that when the person has a goal that is relevant to a prime, they respond in ways determined by the prime. However, if the goal is terminated, so that one is no longer experiencing the motivation associated with it, the prime no longer has an effect—that is, the semantic meaning of the construct is primed, but it has no motivational relevance, and hence exerts no effect on how we respond. Let us return to the example above. If participants were all primed with the goal of being egalitarian, they should all be ready to respond in prime-relevant ways if a goal-relevant person is encountered. For example, as reviewed above, Moskowitz et al. (2000) showed that a White person who is primed with egalitarianism should be "ready" to direct attention (without realizing it) to people who afford one an opportunity to be egalitarian (such as a Black man), but show no such priming effect to people who are not motivationally relevant (such as a White man). However, if egalitarianism is no longer motivationally relevant, the priming effect should disappear. Martin and Tesser (2009) illustrate that *success at a goal lowers its accessibility*—one no longer needs to strive to attain a state that has already been attained. If one has a goal to study for an exam, an amazing study session will lower one's motivation to continue studying. If one has a goal to achieve, a salient achievement would lower the striving to achieve (and might increase the goal to celebrate). Following the logic that a goal persists in being relevant until it is attained, then if one feels success at being egalitarian in the moment, the goal would lose its motivational relevance to one's behavior (even though the semantic meaning of "egalitarian" would still be accessible). In our research (e.g., Moskowitz et al., 2011; Moskowitz & Stone, 2012), White research participants were primed with a goal to be egalitarian. This led to a priming effect. When encountering Black men, they responded in a more egalitarian way, with reduced stereotyping. However, they no longer showed a priming effect if they were primed with having an egalitarian goal by affirming that goal. Thoughts about achieving an egalitarian goal, though increasing its semantic accessibility, minimized its motivational relevance.

Another illustration that the motivational relevance of a prime determines whether there is an effect of the prime was provided by Strahan, Spencer, and Zanna (2002). Half of their research participants were subliminally primed with "thirst." However, prior to the priming, a goal relating to thirst was created in all of the participants by asking them not to eat or drink for 3 hours before the experiment. All participants arrived in the motivationally relevant state of being thirsty. However, when they arrived at the lab they were allowed to eat, and then half of them were asked to cleanse the palate by drinking water. Now there were two groups created: one that had the motivational state removed (no longer thirsty), and one that still had the state of being thirsty. This is when the priming task occurred. The issue at hand is, does being primed with "thirst" lead to a priming effect, or does it only do so when the prime is motivationally relevant (for the people who are still thirsty)? To answer this, participants were allowed to have a drink after the priming task was done, and the researchers measured beverage consumption. They found that priming effects on beverage consumption occurred only if the goal was active. People had more to drink if primed with thirst than if primed with control words, but only if they were thirsty when primed. A prime needs to be motivationally relevant to have an effect (see also Bargh, Gollwitzer, Lee-Chai, Barndollar, & Troetschel, 2001).

Assertibility

Oftentimes we feel we simply are not allowed to assert a particular opinion. A sense that our expectations, stereotypes, and accessible constructs should not be asserted (whether due to conformity pressures, political correctness, or our own sense of values informing us that to do so is unjust) can limit the degree to which priming effects occur. As was noted in the discussion of ambiguity, one factor that determines what we assert about a person whose behavior we have observed is the quality of the stimulus information. Information about another person's behavior may stray too far from being ambiguous to allow accessible constructs to have an impact on our impressions. We examined the case where the information strays from ambiguity in the direction of *increased clarity* (diagnostic information suggests one clear interpretation). However, there is another direction information may travel away from being ambiguous, and that is when information is just plain *uninformative*. Ambiguous information is information that has multiple possible alternative interpretations, but at least it has possible interpretations. Uninformative information does not suggest any particular interpretation. If the behavior of a person we observe is uninformative, then we may see a constraint on the willingness to assert an impression that is consistent with an accessible construct. Stimuli that are uninformative leave an accessible construct no room to have an impact, because it lacks **assertibility**; perceivers do not feel **licensed** to express any impression (e.g., Monin & Miller, 2001). By saying a perceiver lacks the feeling they have license, it is meant that people are unwilling to assert an impression due to having insufficient information. Thus, the prime will not have any influence on judgment if a person is reluctant to judge; the stimulus information must provide an opportunity for one to formulate what could be considered a valid and justifiable impression. With ambiguous behavior one can twist it to see evidence. With uninformative stimuli one is reluctant to say anything.

> **Assertibility (feeling licensed):** When a perceiver feels that they are allowed to express a particular opinion. There are many instances in which a perceiver has a sense that their accessible constructs should not be expressed. Assertibility refers to instances where they feel doing so is warranted and expressing judgment is not constrained.

A stimulus being uninformative is not the only factor that determines whether a feeling of assertibility exists. Another factor is whether the perceiver believes a social constraint exists that does not allow one to express a particular judgment. Many thoughts may cross our mind that we know are not appropriate, allowable, or acceptable to utter or to use in our judgments of others; they are not socially sanctioned thoughts. Thus, even if a behavior is ambiguous and relevant to one of our accessible thoughts, we may still prevent ourselves from using such thoughts because of the social constraint. In essence, we need a license to speak our mind, and some situations clearly revoke that license. A classic demonstration of this lack of assertibility (a removal of one's license to judge) was provided by Darley and Gross (1983), which we reviewed in Chapter 5. Darley and Gross primed research participants with the stereotype of either rich or poor people. They then judged the intelligence of a girl in a classroom. However, they found that participants do not always show a priming effect and use this stereotype. They must feel licensed to use a stereotype, and if they do not feel as if it is allowable to do so, they do not. Their research participants refrained from using their stereotypes until the stereotype could be tested against some evidence. If participants saw a video of a girl's school performance, they then felt licensed to make a stereotypic judgment. After viewing a video of her ambiguous test performance, they stereotyped her. If told she is in fourth grade, and primed with "poverty," then they rate her abilities as being below the fourth-grade level. However, if asked for a judgment without having any behavioral evidence on which to base their evaluation, they do not show a priming effect. If told the girl is in fourth grade, but get no other information (no video of her test performance), then they rate her abilities as being at a fourth-grade level. This suggests a somewhat happy conclusion: People only judge other people according to a stereotype if they feel there is evidence on which to base a judgment (what Yzerbyt et al., 1994, called a feeling that the target is worthy of being judged). The somewhat unhappy conclusion that we must use to qualify that statement is that the amount of evidence it takes for a perceiver to decide the stereotype is correct is quite small, and can factually be ambiguous in its support. In the Darley and Gross experiment, the girl was judged in a stereotypic way when all that was provided was vague and mixed feedback about her ability.

To illustrate the notion of assertibility, and its impact on impression formation, we describe another experiment, one by Monin and Miller (2001). They argue that for accessible information to influence one's social judgments, one must feel that it is warranted to use such information, that one has "license" to do so. Concerns over licensing can initially constrain the impact accessible constructs have on judgment. However, once one's license is returned to the individual (a feeling that the use of accessible constructs is warranted), their accessible constructs now drive their impressions. The logic of their research hinges on the belief that people sometimes become so comfortable in the public perception that they are fair and just, they soon feel as if they no longer need to guard against what they say and do. The public perception of them is so strong that one need not be concerned about damaging it. Thus, once one becomes convinced others see them as fair, or one becomes secure in one's own sense of self as fair, one now feels no obligation to censor one's biases and stereotypes from impacting on judgments. Whereas concerns about what one may or may not assert—what is socially licensed and allowable—may initially constrain accessibility effects; these constraints eventually become lifted if one feels sufficient credentials as a fair person have been established that will not be damaged by what one says. Once this social constraint is lifted, one is licensed to react according to whatever is perceptually ready.

Monin and Miller (2001) illustrated that people make judgments that are consistent with accessible concepts only after they have first established credentials that would seemingly allow them to get away with a behavior, secure in the knowledge that they have a license to judge others. In their research the accessible concepts being examined were stereotypes, and the logic was that social norms prohibit using stereotypes to judge someone in a stereotypical way. However, if a person had the opportunity to illustrate that they were nonprejudiced, to establish credentials as a fair person, such a person would now, ironically, feel free to stereotype others! Their credentials as a fair person make them feel immune to the social constraints, because their public image as being a nonprejudiced person protects them from being seen as biased if they said something politically incorrect. For example, participants were asked to make a choice between candidates for a job. The job was stereotypically male, and the job candidates included both men and women. The accessibility of the stereotype should lead people to see the male candidate as fitting the job better. However, using stereotypes to make a hiring decision is not licensed by society. In the absence of any information that one can use to justify their decision, relying on the stereotype alone would be a blatantly bad thing to do. Thus, in the absence of either diagnostic information about the candidates or ambiguous information about them, participants should be unable to assert any preference, regardless of whether the stereotype is accessible. However, this constraint should disappear if participants feel they have the license to stereotype. This is precisely what was found: priming effects were more likely to occur after participants first had the opportunity to establish their credentials as a nonsexist person. These credentials were established by allowing some of the participants to express their disagreement with blatantly sexist statements. This disagreement, ironically, licenses them to go ahead and use the sexist constructs that were accessible. Without the buildup of credentials, people do not feel allowed to assert a judgment that aligns their judgment (Who is the best candidate for the job?) with the accessible stereotype.

Social pressure is another force that determines what we feel licensed to assert. What you are willing to assert in private is often different from what you assert in public because social forces censor people. Thus, social forces may inhibit one's sense of feeling licensed to say what one thinks. It can even alter the very type of judgment that is formed. One such social pressure comes from needing to justify one's decisions and impressions to others. Being held publicly *accountable* for one's judgments motivates people to be more accurate in how they evaluate information and more deliberate in considering what types of factors should influence one's judgment. Accountability leads people to think through issues in a careful and thorough fashion in order to form a position that is defensible (Tetlock, 1985). It motivates people to contemplate the arguments on both sides of an issue to prepare for the criticisms of others and have a well-articulated and carefully constructed point of view.

Thompson et al. (1994) predicted that priming effects would be eliminated when people were accountable. Rather than relying on what is most accessible to shape judgment, a person concerned with justifying judgments will draw conclusions from a precise evaluation of the data, rather than a quick and effortless application of whatever interpretation is perceptually ready. Accountability alters what people feel licensed to assert, and this sense of what one is licensed to assert determines whether accessible constructs are used in forming an impression. Thompson et al. primed people with concepts such as "reckless" or "adventurous" and "persistent" or "stubborn," and then looked to see whether people assimilated their judgment of an ambiguous target to fit with the accessible information. Half the participants were accountable to others for the judgments being formed, half were not. As predicted, when not accountable, priming effect emerged; when accountable, judging the targets as similar to the accessible traits did not occur. When people were accountable, they no longer asserted that the target resembled whatever perceptually ready information was accessible.

Awareness

When discussing priming effects there are generally three distinct things of which one does or does not become aware. The first is **awareness of the prime** itself. If notions of warmth are primed by holding a hot coffee cup (as with Williams & Bargh's, [2008] research reviewed in Chapter 2), one is aware that the cup (the prime) is hot, and in the moment likely consciously registered a thought about it being hot. Yet that thought likely recedes from consciousness quickly. If the construct "reckless" is primed by being asked to memorize the word during a color perception task, one is aware of it while attempting to memorize it, though it too likely recedes from consciousness quickly once that task has ended. If a song is primed from having heard it in the grocery store, one was certainly aware the song was playing when in the store, even if one has no explicit memory of having heard it a mere 5 minutes later when driving home. Many tasks that incidentally prime a construct still require conscious processing of the prime, and one is aware of having

> **Awareness of the prime:** The issue of whether one is aware that a prime was even present. Can one consciously detect the exposure to the information that made a given construct accessible?

been exposed to the prime. However, it is also possible to not be aware that one has been exposed to a prime. Bargh and Pietromonaco (1982) used **subliminal priming** by flashing the prime word ("hostile," in their case) at speeds too fast for conscious recognition. Participants were primed with "hostile" despite not being aware they ever even saw the word. Moskowitz and Roman (1992) explored a more natural way people might be primed without awareness. Their participants self-generated primes outside of consciousness. To do so they simply had participants read sentences that implied a trait, but that did not mention the trait—that is, their participants formed spontaneous trait inferences outside of awareness. Without knowing they had inferred a trait, such as "cautious," the participants had primed the construct "cautious" with their implicit inference.

> **Subliminal priming:** Making a construct accessible through the prime being exposed to the perceiver at speeds too fast for conscious recognition.

> **Awareness of the state of accessibility:** Unlike awareness of the prime, which was concerned with whether the exposure to the prime was consciously detected, the concern here is with awareness of the mental representation attaining heightened accessibility. One might be aware of having seen a prime, yet not aware that it created increased accessibility.

> **Awareness of the influence of the heightened accessibility on responding:** Once a prime creates a heightened state of accessibility, that accessibility may influence the person (altering their judgment, decision making, or behavior). When one is unaware of this influence, it creates a silent form of bias, an implicit bias.

Secondly, one may lack **awareness of the state of accessibility**. This is a distinction between awareness of the prime versus awareness of the priming. One might be aware of having seen a prime (such as the hot coffee cup), yet not be aware that it created an increase in accessibility of the construct "warm." Often people have no awareness of accessibility, but as discussed in Chapter 8 when reviewing feelings of familiarity, people do at times develop a sense that information is accessible.

The third thing that one may, or may not, be aware of is **awareness of the priming effect—the influence of the heightened accessibility on responding**. Once a prime creates a heightened state of accessibility, that accessibility can influence the person (altering either their judgment, decision making, or behavior). When one is not aware of this influence, it creates a silent form of bias, an implicit bias. Throughout this chapter we have described experiments that use a "two-study" format in order to promote participants being unaware that the prime could influence them. If people believe that they are performing two totally unrelated tasks, there would be no reason to suspect one task would influence the other. Consider an experiment by Dijksterhuis and Van Knippenberg (1998), who primed research participants in the Netherlands with stereotypes of groups known to be associated with either intelligent behavior or moronic behavior, and then looked at whether the priming caused the participants (in a second, unrelated task) to act either more, or less, intelligently. In a "first study" participants were asked to think about either professors or about soccer hooligans. This was meant to prime the construct of intelligence (when thinking about professors) versus stupid and careless (soccer hooligans). Participants were then asked to perform a "second study" that on the surface did not possibly seem related to the first study. They were asked to take a test and to try to get the best score possible. The results showed a priming effect: the people for whom college professors (the intelligent group) were accessible subsequently performed better on the test, while people asked to think about soccer hooligans performed worse. Something seemingly unmovable, like intellectual ability measured by performance on a test, was shaped by the primes people were exposed to prior to test taking. People act smarter when primed with stereotypes of smart people. The separation of the two tasks suggested that participants were not aware of this influence. A lack of awareness of an influence is especially likely if the two tasks are not only separated but look nothing like each other, such as judging the behavior of a person (Task 2, the judgment task) and trying to form sentences from words, or trying to memorize words (Task 1, the priming task).

Consider an experiment by Bargh et al. (1996) that was reviewed in Chapter 2. In a first task they exposed research participants to words associated with the stereotype of older adults (such as Florida and forgetful), notably leaving out the quality "slow" that they assumed would also be primed through spreading activation due to its association with the other primes. The second task looked in no way similar to the first, or even like a task at all. Participants were simply told the experiment was done and could walk down the hallway to the elevator. The dependent measure of interest was how slowly the participants walked while exiting, with "exiting" being the second task. They found that participants who had the older adults stereotype accessible walked more slowly. The dissimilarity of the two tasks suggested that participants were not aware of this influence.

How might a researcher *know for certain* that the participants in their experiment are not aware of the influence of the prime? One guaranteed way to do so (though not the only way) is to follow the procedure of Bargh and Pietromonaco (1982). They presented the prime subliminally. If one is never aware of having seen a word, it would be impossible for one to be aware of any impact that word might have on one's later judgments and impressions. This should not be taken to mean a concept must be subliminal for it to exert an influence on our judgment. Rather, all that is needed is for us to remain naïve as to the influence being exerted—whether we are aware or not that there is an impact on our later thoughts and actions (Bargh, 1992). What happens if one *is* made aware that an influence exists on one's responding? Of course, if made aware of the influence of the heightened accessibility on responding, one could correct for this influence and produce an unbiased response, free of the priming effect. However, attempts to correct a priming effect could result in bias. In Chapter 8 this was discussed as arising from a correction process, where a perceiver is aware of a potential influence on their judgment, and this force is one they do not want as an influence, so they attempt to remove its influence. However, in doing so, responding may be altered in a way that creates a new bias (one that conforms to whatever theory of influence was guiding the correction process). We turn to these issues next.

This chapter began by asserting that the nature of priming effects is complex, and will change dependent on a set of factors. We just reviewed five such factors that shape the nature of the effect (and if a replication will succeed). None of the factors reviewed thus far touched on the nature of the prime itself. We saw examples of a cup of coffee as a prime (warm), a trait as a prime (cautious, confident, independent), and a stereotype as a prime (professor, hooligan, old person). However, these were all examples of schemas being made accessible—abstract representations of broad categories. In Chapter 2 we saw that mental representations are not always broad and abstract. At times they can be *exemplars* that are narrow and specific. These factors (prime type) are also important for determining the nature of priming effects.

ASSIMILATION EFFECTS AND CONTRAST EFFECTS

There are two types of effects of an accessible construct that are typically discussed: two types of priming effects. One effect is that the behavior that is being judged, or the target stimulus to which one is responding, is seen as *similar to* the primed construct. This drawing of one's response toward an accessible construct is known as *assimilation*. Thus far, all of the examples of priming effects that have been reviewed in this chapter have been assimilation effects, whether the response was a judgment that makes a target seem similar to a primed construct, or a decision or behavior that is consistent with the primed construct. However, in several other chapters of this book we have also reviewed *contrast effects*, and these too can emerge when a construct has heightened accessibility (is primed). Contrast effects occur when the behavior that is being judged, or the target stimulus to which one is responding, is seen as *dissimilar to* the prime. The impact of a primed construct (such as "cautious") is to make the target of judgment seem less like it, to push judgment in the direction opposite of the prime ("reckless"). In this section we explore how type of prime helps to shape whether assimilation or contrast emerges.

Primes as Filters versus Standards of Comparison

Throughout this book we have seen two distinct ways in which people make meaning. People can use existing information as a filter through which new information passes, twisting the way that information is interpreted. This often produces a confirmation bias. People can also use existing information as a standard against which new information is compared, with similarity leading to assimilation and dissimilarity leading to contrast. For example, with the Ebbinghaus illusion the dissimilarity in size between an inner circle and the outer circles orbiting it led to a contrast in the perception of the inner circle's size. These same issues determine the nature of priming effects, with assimilation or contrast dependent on whether the prime is used as a filter or a comparison standard. Although not an absolute, exemplars often are used as standards of comparison and schemas/stereotypes are often used as filters. Why is this the case?

Exemplars as primes (e.g., Hitler, Martin Luther King Jr., Shark, Grandpa Simpson) differ from traits or stereotypes as primes (e.g., evil, activist, ferocious, older adults) in terms of how distinctive they are, how abstract/narrow they are, and in how exclusive they are (there are many ways to be evil but only one way to be Hitler). Stapel and Koomen (2001) asserted that the narrower, more exclusive, and more distinctive a primed category, the more likely it is that it will be used as a comparison standard. This is why extreme exemplars, such as Hitler, are likely to be used as comparison standards: they possess all of these features. Traits—such as "evil"—possess none of these features. Traits are abstract concepts and as such are less likely to be used as comparison standards and more likely to serve as filters. As stated above, these are not absolutes—exemplars can serve as filters, and traits can serve as comparison standards (especially if the trait was made less abstract and more distinctive). For example, if you learned "Bob is smart" and a picture of Bob was also provided, the picture would promote seeing the trait less abstractly, and could more easily trigger standard-of-comparison processes. Thus, the main point to be made here is not that traits and stereotypes are always associated with a filtering process or exemplars always lead to using comparison processes. It is that *whether assimilation or contrast will occur depends on the type of processing* being used—whether comparison or filtering processes are engaged. Comparison may be easier to instigate with exemplars, but it is possible for traits to do so. Filtering processes may be easier to instigate with more abstract constructs serving as primes, but it is possible for exemplars to do so.

The question we turn to next is that of how comparison processes and filtering processes determine whether assimilation or contrast effects will be found. A standard-of-comparison process is one in which new and applicable stimuli are evaluated against a primed concept (e.g., Herr, 1986; Herr et al., 1983). For example, if one is primed with an exemplar that in one's culture represents extreme hostility (in the United States such examples include Adolf Hitler, Charles Manson, Osama Bin Laden), then if judging a subsequently encountered person behaving in an ambiguous way that is relevant to hostility, their behavior will be compared against the accessible exemplar. Compared to Hitler, a person behaving in a way that is ambiguously aggressive or hostile does not seem hostile at all. Rather than the perception of the person being drawn toward the accessible construct, it is pushed away. A contrast effect emerges because the ambiguous behavior pales in comparison to the narrow and specific case of evil. For instance, Herr (1986) found that increasing accessibility of the construct "hostility" through exposing participants to hostile exemplars as primes led to subsequent impressions that a target person was *less* hostile (as compared to a control group). Similarly, Herr et al. found that accessible exemplars led to contrast effects by using nonhuman stimuli (exemplars of animals) as primes. The construct "hostile" was made accessible by exposing participants to ferocious (e.g., grizzly bear, shark) and nonferocious (e.g., dove, kitten) animal exemplars. They then judge the ferocity of a new, ambiguous animal. Accessible exemplars led to contrast. If the concept of "shark" was accessible, the ambiguous animal was seen as not very fierce; if "kitten" was accessible, the animal was judged as fierce.

Dijksterhuis et al. (1998) provide another example illustrating that priming people with an exemplar triggers a contrast effect. Rather than showing a contrast in judgment, they showed a contrast in behavior. They argued that if the prime is an exemplar, one should *act* in the manner opposite to what the prime implied. In one experiment, Dutch research participants were primed with an exemplar of older adults by having the participants think about the Dutch Queen Mother. It was found that participants walked faster following this prime—a contrast effect.

Standard-of-comparison processes do not always produce contrast effects. As described in Chapter 8, this depends on whether the new information falls within a latitude of acceptance or a latitude of rejection. When the new behavior, such as ambiguously hostile behavior, is clearly dissimilar to the comparison standard, such as Hitler, then contrast occurs. In the language of social judgment theory, the extreme prime is more likely to set a judgment standard in which the moderate behavior of others will fall into the latitude of rejection. However, if the new behavior is similar to the comparison standard, then assimilation will occur. For example, when a less extreme exemplar of hostility (such as Larry David rather than Hitler) is used, then the new behavior to be judged (if ambiguously hostile) will fall in the latitude of acceptance. The new behavior will seem similar to the standard, sharing many features, and evaluation will be drawn toward the prime. The behavior will be assimilated into the standard. Herr (1986) found that whereas extremely hostile exemplars led to contrast effects, moderately hostile primes serving as standards of comparison, such as "Alice Cooper" and "Joe Frazier" (well-known people from the 1970s—a rock star and a boxer, respectively), led to an assimilation effect. A person who behaved in an ambiguously hostile way was assigned judgments of greater hostility when primed with these standards of comparison. In sum, contrast increases as the primes that serve as the standards of comparison increase in extremity; more extreme exemplars share fewer features with a target, seem more dissimilar, and serve as more distant judgmental anchors against which the new behavior pales (it falls within the latitude of rejection).

A filtering process is one in which a primed concept is used to provide a framework through which new and applicable stimuli are interpreted (e.g., Bargh & Pietromonaco, 1982; Higgins et al., 1977; Srull & Wyer, 1979). Rather than evaluating the new behavior against the prime, the new behavior is interpreted through the filter of the prime. For example, if one is primed with a trait that represents an abstract construct (such as hostility), subsequent people who are behaving in an ambiguous way that is relevant to hostility will have that behavior interpreted as similar to the accessible construct. Due to the readiness to see hostility, the perception of the person is drawn toward the accessible construct, applying that readiness to the behavior rather than attributing it to its correct source, an unseen and undetected prime (e.g., Higgins, 1996a). As explained in Chapters 4 and 8, they will misattribute the accessibility of "hostility" from the prime (which they do not recognize) to the behavior (which they do recognize and are asked to judge). Many examples of such a filtering process have been reviewed in this chapter (e.g., Bargh et al., 1996; Bargh & Pietro-monaco, 1982; Dijksterhuis & Van Knippenberg, 1998; Higgins et al., 1977, 1985; Higgins & Brendl, 1995; Srull & Wyer, 1979, 1980; Thompson et al., 1994). Other examples have been seen throughout the book (e.g., Banaji et al., 1993; Devine, 1989; Martin, 1986; Moskowitz & Roman, 1992; Schwarz, Bless, et al., 1991).

Filtering processes do not always produce assimilation effects. As discussed in Chapter 8, such processes can produce a contrast effect due to correction attempts. When people perceive a primed construct to be a biasing influence on their judgment—they become aware of being influenced—they will attempt to remove this potential source of bias from their judgment (e.g., Martin, 1986; Martin et al., 1990; Moskowitz & Roman, 1992; Moskowitz & Skurnik, 1999; Strack et al., 1993). Contrast arises from people having difficulty determining whether their judgment was shaped by the behavior of the target (what seems a reason-able basis for judgment) or the primed construct (what seems a biased basis for judgment). When one attempts to correct for the prime's unwanted influence, and exclude information related to the prime from one's judgment, one may extract part of one's genuine reaction to the target. Certainly, it is possible that when adjusting judgment for a potential biasing influence one can be accurate and correctly partial out *only* those contributions to judg-ment uniquely contributed by the biasing force. However, people "may not make a perfect discrimination between their reaction to the priming task and their reaction to the target" (Martin et al., 1990, p. 28). In such instances they remove too much of the primed construct and end up seeing the person more unlike the prime—a contrast effect.

For example, if the trait "reckless" is primed, this trait now has increased accessibility. If one then encounters an ambiguously reckless versus bold person, one's genuine reac-tion to that person's behavior—in the absence of the prime—would contain both elements of recklessness and boldness. However, if the prime is being used to help one interpret a stimulus, then one's reaction now includes the genuine reaction that is equal parts reck-lessness and boldness, as well as extra notions of recklessness that are contributed by the prime. Thus, the perceiver judges the person to be reckless. Finally, if one becomes aware of the fact that the prime was altering their genuine reaction, and wants to remove that bias-ing influence from one's judgment, a process occurs where one must adjust or correct that judgment and eliminate this unwanted influence. But since the two sources of influence (one's real reaction to the person untainted by the prime, and the elements contributed by the accessible construct) have been merged, separating them is difficult and imprecise. In the process of adjusting judgment for the unwanted influence (removing reckless), one may overadjust. By overadjust we mean one removes part of one's real reaction to the person, untainted by the prime. The result is that one's reaction to the person is left with too little of the concept "reckless" and the concept "bold" is now overrepresented. This is a contrast effect. Rather than judgment being drawn toward the prime, a judgment is produced that has fewer elements of the prime. This is depicted in Figure 10.2, where a reckless prime leads to the impression of the person as bold.

Several examples illustrating such a correction process leading to contrast were already reviewed in Chapter 8. For example, Moskowitz and Roman (1992) had some research par-ticipants form implicit first impressions, while others formed explicit first impressions, from behaviors they read. The questions of interest were whether these first impressions

A. **Priming occurs: Elements associated with a reckless prime, in grey font, become accessible.**

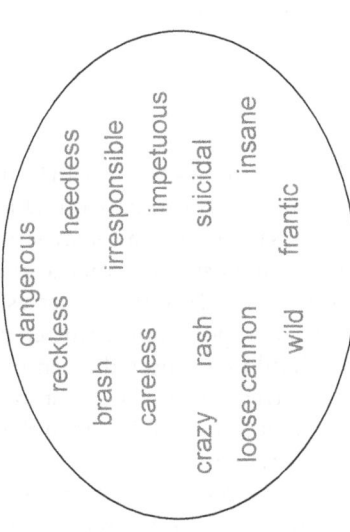

dangerous
reckless   heedless
brash   irresponsible
careless   impetuous
crazy   rash   suicidal
loose cannon   insane
wild   frantic

B. **Ambiguous behavior is observed: Elements that suggest "bold" as a trait are italicized; elements that suggest "reckless" as a trait are in grey font).**

bold   reckless
adventurous   dangerous
gutsy   brave   careless
dauntless   crazy   rash
fearless   loose cannon
daredevil   wild
courageous   frantic   brash
daring

C. **Assimilation effect: The behavior is drawn toward the prime so that the prime dominates judgment. Influence of the prime is indicated by bold words, including words in the intersection of the two ovals that were present in the ambiguous behavior.**

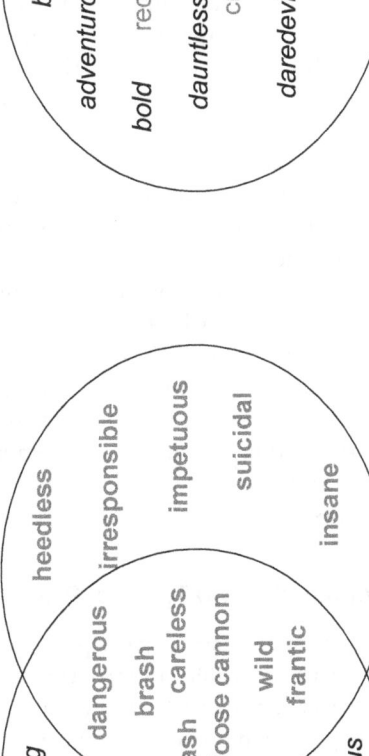

heedless
daring
brave   dangerous   irresponsible
adventurous   brash   impetuous
reckless   rash   careless
gutsy   bold   loose cannon   suicidal
dauntless   wild
fearless   frantic
crazy   insane
daredevil
courageous

D. **Awareness of an influence leads to correction: The prime's influence is removed along with some of one's genuine reaction. The final impression includes only two reckless items originally associated with the behavior, creating contrast. The person is seen as bold.**

brave
adventurous   daring
bold   reckless   gutsy
dauntless   fearless
crazy
daredevil   courageous

FIGURE 10.2. Correction process leading to a contrast effect.

prime a trait, and does that trait then lead to assimilation or contrast in a later judgment? They found that people who formed an explicit impression were aware that the trait they had inferred about the person could exert a bias on their later judgment. This concern motivated them to correct the later judgment so it was not biased by the primed trait. But in removing this influence a contrast effect was produced so the later judgment was shown to be the opposite of the primed trait. However, people who formed implicit first impressions were not aware of its potential to bias the second judgment. This lack of awareness of the first impression made the second judgment consistent with the first (implicit) impression. There was assimilation. Todorov (2023) made a similar argument regarding trait inferences drawn from faces rather than from behaviors. People likely lack awareness that facial information triggers a trait and biases their judgment. When explicitly asked to evaluate a face, participants respond much like those who Moskowitz and Roman explicitly asked to form an impression. They recognize an opportunity for bias and correct it. However, when not prompted to form an impression of a person's face, then people act similar to Moskowitz and Roman's participants who formed spontaneous impressions from behavior. It does not consciously occur to them that they were forming trait inferences or evaluating others.

Further evidence that awareness of the prime leads to an attempt to correct for it is provided by research findings that use enhanced memory for the prime words at the end of the experiment as a proxy for awareness. The argument is that if memory for the prime is strong when making the judgment, then the primes are present in consciousness, and this increased awareness makes one more prone to seeing the prime as an influence that needs to be removed. Such research illustrates that when there is a heightened memory for the primes, there is also a heightened amount of contrast in the judgments the participants formed (e.g., Lombardi et al., 1987; Newman & Uleman, 1990). For example, Strack et al. (1993) primed people with traits and asked half of the participants to remember the primed traits just prior to reading about a target. Thus, half of the people had superior memory for the primes, and this heightened awareness could trigger correction processes. They found that participants who had poor memory for the primes showed assimilation, whereas participants in the condition with high memory for the prime words showed contrast in their judgments.

Comparing the Two Types of Processes

We have been discussing two separate ways in which one's judgment of a person can be influenced by an accessible construct: filtering (or interpretation) versus comparison. One difference between the two types of processes concerns the types of accessible constructs that often trigger each process. Comparison processes were triggered most easily when accessible constructs were created by people being exposed to exemplars, while filtering processes were triggered most easily by people being exposed to traits or stereotypes. Another difference is that the two processes suggest that different judgments should be expected when primes are extreme versus moderate. With comparison processes, extreme exemplars as standards lead to contrast effects, whereas more moderate exemplars as standards fall within the latitude of acceptance and lead to assimilation. However, with filtering processes, it is moderate primes that lead to contrast effects. These primes can be recognized as a potential source of bias, so people try to correct for this "contamination" to their judgment. Extreme traits lead to *less* contrast because one would be less likely to see something so extreme as a source of bias; it instead seems so different from the target behavior as to be irrelevant. These differences were tested directly in a study by Moskowitz and Skurnik (1999).

Moskowitz and Skurnik (1999) proposed that features of the prime—not simply whether the prime is an exemplar or a trait, but its *extremity*—determine the type of priming effect. They reasoned that when a concept is triggered by a *moderate trait* prime (e.g., troublesome, hostile) one is more likely to get contrast in judgment than when triggered by an *extreme trait* prime (e.g., murderous, malevolent). Moderate primes, more so than extreme primes, are seen as sharing relatively more features with ambiguous target behaviors. A moderately hostile prime, such as "troublesome," is perceived as a more appropriate characterization of ambiguously hostile behavior (such as arguing with a store clerk) than an extremely hostile prime, such as "malevolent." The consequence is that once one becomes aware of a prime's increased accessibility, moderate primes are more likely to be seen as having potentially contaminated one's reaction to the target and less likely to be seen as irrelevant to the target's ambiguous behaviors—extreme traits will not. Malevolence hardly seems applicable to the behavior observed, so becoming aware of the possibility for its influence does not make one likely to conclude that it did actually have an influence. The more likely the prime is seen as having contaminated one's reaction, the more one will adjust one's initial reaction to the target to correct for the prime's influence, and the more likely one will have removed part of one's genuine reaction. However, the opposite pattern is predicted to emerge with exemplar primes: increased extremity produces a greater likelihood of contrast than moderate exemplars. The reasoning was explained above. The more extreme the prime being used as a standard in comparison, the greater the perceived dissimilarity between the standard and the ambiguous behavior, the greater the contrast. Relative to Hitler, this person isn't hostile, and the more Hitleresque the exemplar, the greater the contrast.

To illustrate these processing differences, Moskowitz and Skurnik (1999) manipulated prime type (exemplar, trait) and prime extremity (moderate, extreme). They primed concepts by exposing research participants to either extreme traits (e.g., malicious, malevolent), moderate traits (e.g., unfair, troublesome), extreme exemplars (e.g., Mike Tyson, Dracula), or moderate exemplars (e.g., Bart Simpson, Kurt Cobain) that were pretested to be relevant to the concept "hostility." They then had participants read about a person acting in an ambiguously hostile manner. They found that extreme exemplars were more likely to produce contrast effects than moderate exemplars. Yet a different pattern of findings emerged for trait primes. When traits were used as primes, greater contrast was seen with moderate rather than extreme primes. Moskowitz and Skurnik concluded that these findings tease apart the different processes that produce contrast. Extreme but not moderate exemplars yielding contrast suggest a standard-of-comparison process was being used in which the more extreme the standard relative to the judgment target, the more distinct it is, and the more likely contrast is produced. Moderate but not extreme traits yielding contrast suggest that a correction process was used in which the more extreme the prime, the less the prime target feature overlap, and the less likely one will suspect an influence of the prime for which one needs to correct.

These findings are complex. A priming effect can be one of assimilation or contrast. The effect can occur through standard-of-comparison processes or through a totally separate process impacting how information is interpreted through a "filter." The prime being a trait versus an exemplar matters for the nature of the effect, as does the extremity of the prime. If one is aware of the prime's influence, the effect might reverse. If the behavior is not ambiguous or applicable to the prime, there might be no effect at all. If norms or feeling a lack of license exist, the effect would also dissipate. If accessibility strength is strong, effects are more likely.

STEREOTYPING AS A PRIMING EFFECT

One of the most important types of constructs that can be primed, and then shape how people are seen and judged, is a stereotype. This type of stereotyping need not involve any pernicious intent, and can arise simply in the manner described throughout this chapter: A cue (such as skin tone) triggers a category, and the traits that are associated with that category then shape how ambiguous behavior is then seen. The stereotyped person is then judged and treated in an unfair manner, one guided by the existing stereotype and not their own qualities. Without intending to be biased, a perceiver could then unintentionally reinforce a stereotypic impression through the perceiver coming to believe they see new evidence in support of that impression. This is a type of confirmation bias, one where the thing being confirmed (a stereotype) is not recognized by the perceiver as primed, and the influence it has on how another person is judged is never detected. We have already reviewed several examples of this kind of implicit stereotyping when we described "misattribution procedures" in Chapters 4, 6, and 8. Of course, a discussion of this form of stereotyping is included in this chapter because the argument is simply that in some cases, stereotyping is nothing more than a priming effect. As depicted in Figure 10.1, a stimulus may trigger a concept (in this case, a stereotype), and the behavior of the person judged, even if ambiguous, will come to be seen in a way that confirms the primed stereotype. Once one has consciously believed to have seen confirming evidence, the person has been judged unfairly, and the stereotypic association of the category and the trait is strengthened.

Devine (1989) was the first to describe a form of stereotyping that is no different from priming more generally, and offered a model that explained why stereotyping not only persists but can potentially be strengthened, even among people with propositional learning that rejects the stereotype. Devine identified two distinct processing stages in this type of stereotyping. The first stage is the activation of the stereotype, the second is the application of the stereotype in perception, attention, judgment, behavior, and so on. This has come to be known as a **dissociation model of stereotyping** because it specifies two dissociable stages that operate under different guiding cognitive processes. The first stage is described

Dissociation model of stereotyping: A model specifying two dissociable stages to stereotyping. The first is a set of implicit processes where a person is categorized into a group and associated stereotypes get triggered through spreading activation. The second involves the application of the activated stereotype to whatever task in which one is currently engaged.

Stereotype activation: Within a half-second of seeing a person, and without realizing it, perceivers detect features, assign the person to a category, and retrieve from memory the category's associated attributes. Stereotypic knowledge is then ready to be used to identify and understand subsequent people (particularly people relevant to the category).

as a set of *implicit and effortless* processes in which a person is categorized into a group and the related stereotypes and affect that are associated with that group get triggered through priming and spreading activation. The second stage involves the application of these accessible traits to the task in which one is currently engaged, which is usually described as a more effortful process (e.g., judging a person, evaluating performance, deciding how to act). These responses can be influenced without one realizing it by the implicit priming. Thus, one comes to judge a person in a way that confirms the stereotype, providing new evidence to support that stereotype (even though the evidence did not actually support the stereotype, it was merely perceived that way). According to the logic of the dissociation model, bias is not inevitable, because one could disrupt this priming effect if motivated to do so at the second stage (see Figure 10.3).

Dovidio et al. (1986) performed the first experiment illustrating the first stage of this process, where **stereotype activation** occurs. Research participants responded to pairs

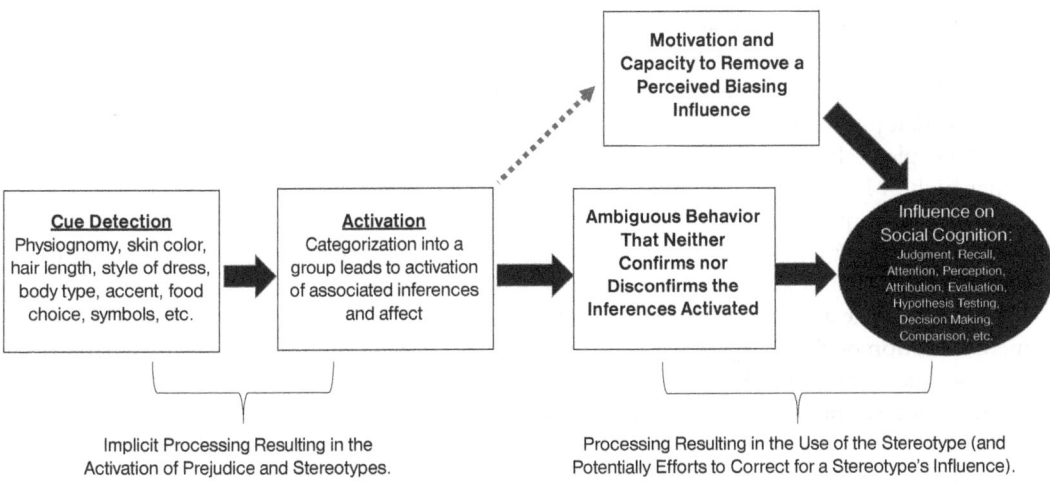

FIGURE 10.3. A dissociation model of stereotyping.

of words on a monitor. For some of these pairs, a social group (such as "Black") was the first word presented in the pair, and the second word was a trait. Participants were asked to press a button marked "yes" if the second word in a given pair could potentially be conceived of as a trait possessed by a member of the group just seen. Thus, one might see the pairing of "White–Ambitious" or "Black–Athletic." On the critical trials the correct answer is always "yes," since any trait could describe any group of people. Speed of responding "yes" was the measure of stereotype activation. People were faster to respond "yes" when pairings were stereotypical, providing evidence that the group had activated the stereotype. This triggering of a stereotype should be reciprocal. Thoughts of the group will trigger the associated items in the stereotype, and thoughts of some of the associated items in the stereotype should trigger the group. As Eberhardt, Goff, Purdie, and Davies (2004) put it, "we argue that just as Black faces and Black bodies can trigger thoughts of crime, thinking of crime can trigger thoughts of Black people" (p. 876). To illustrate this, Eberhardt et al. showed not only that activating the category "Black man" (vs. "White man") primes thoughts of crime but that exposing White participants to crime-relevant objects (such as a gun) primed thoughts of Black men. They suggest that this bidirectionality in the triggering of both the stereotype and the group contributes to why stereotypes are so durable. With two associative routes, the association can be activated outside awareness (and used more often).

Devine (1989) was the first to illustrate both stages in Figure 10.3 in an experiment—the stereotype is activated, and as with other priming effects, it is then used to guide judgment. White research participants were subliminally shown characteristics stereotypically associated with the group "Black" (e.g., poor, lazy, athletic). Because this category was triggered outside awareness, there were two consequences posited: (1) due to spreading activation, the entire stereotype would be triggered, including an aspect of the stereotype that was deliberately not shown: "hostile/aggressive"; and (2) judgments would reflect this stereotype regardless of the participants' explicit beliefs about the group stereotype. That because these two processes are dissociated, even people who express low prejudiced beliefs would have their explicit judgments made in Stage 2 influenced by the stereotype activated in

Stage 1 *if they were unaware of its influence*. If they were to become aware of this influence, the argument was that the first process would still occur (the stereotype is activated), but a second and separate process would overwrite it so that no influence would be exerted on one's explicit judgment.

To explore these predictions, Devine (1989) recruited research participants who were either high or low in prejudice beliefs. Participants were shown either a list that contained 80 words relevant to the stereotype of African Americans and 20 neutral words (to activate the stereotype), or a list with 80 neutral words and 20 stereotypic ones (to not activate the stereotype, or at least activate it very weakly). To make certain that the stereotype was being triggered outside awareness, the words were presented by flashing them subliminally. The mere detection of the stereotypic words outside of awareness should activate the entire stereotype, such that "hostility" was also activated, even though never shown as part of the stimuli. In a supposed second task, participants read about a person whose behavior was pretested to be ambiguous on the quality of "hostility," and then formed an impression of the person. The prediction was that while low-prejudiced people may be able to prevent themselves from using a stereotype if they were aware of its existence, they will not be able to stop the stereotype from being activated. These are distinct processes. And if the person is not aware of the stereotype's activation, a person would not be able to control the use of that stereotype when judging and acting. They would, without realizing it, confirm the stereotype and see evidence that supports it. This is precisely what is found. Those without a stereotype primed accurately saw the behavior as ambiguous with regard to its hostility. Those with a stereotype that was implicitly primed made judgments that labeled the person as hostile. Remarkably, the study shows that even low-prejudice people end up judging a person in a stereotype-confirming way, without having any idea that either the stereotype has been activated or that their judgment is influenced in any way. They saw evidence that was not there not because of ill will, but because of priming.

This experiment was groundbreaking in its ability to establish the implicit nature of stereotype activation, and its dissociation from the use of the stereotype. For the first time it was illustrated that not only are stereotypes brought to mind easily and efficiently, but it happens fully without awareness and even among people who do not intend to stereotype and who explicitly reject stereotypes (low-prejudice people). The findings show that (1) a stereotype is *easily* activated, including elements of the stereotype not seen; (2) its state of activation makes one ready to use that stereotype in an *efficient* way; (3) these processes are not consciously *intended*; 4) that they occur *without people being aware*; and (5) separate explicit processes allow people to control and correct these influences if a person is aware they exist. This paints a sobering picture despite the possibility for control. Stereotype use is pervasive, especially because people do not realize their stereotypes are triggered or impacting them. For this reason, the stereotype exerts an invisible influence on judgment; people see evidence that reinforces a stereotype even when no evidence exists. A variety of types of evidence support this idea that if a stereotype is primed, we see evidence to support our stereotypes, thus reinforcing it. In an example reviewed in Chapter 4, Banaji et al. (1993) showed that men with a stereotype of women primed in a first task, later judged a woman in a more stereotypic way. They read about a woman's behavior and made judgments about her. The key was that the behaviors described a person who acted in a manner mostly irrelevant to gender stereotypes, but a small subset of behaviors were weakly related to the stereotype. The judgments clearly showed that the stereotype was activated implicitly, and in a separate explicit process a judgment was made that the woman's behavior provided evidence of the stereotype.

Here are a few more examples that extend the illustrations of this phenomenon beyond judgment of an ambiguous behavior. Implicit stereotypes also distort the perception of faces, skin tone, and body shape so that they are seen (and remembered) as more stereotypic. For example, Macrae and Martin (2007) showed that gender could be triggered using hairstyle, and this was sufficient to also trigger the stereotype of the group (e.g., long hair activated "woman" and its associated stereotype). More importantly, the triggered stereotype then altered the perception of a person's gender. A woman with short hair was more likely to be perceived as a man, and a man with long hair was more likely to be perceived as a woman. This suggests that stereotypes can be triggered by specific features of a person, and once that stereotype is activated, it can lead to errors in how that person is perceived. Additional support for such an effect was provided in research by Livingston and Brewer (2002). They showed that Black men with Afrocentric facial features elicited more stereotypic reactions in White research participants than Black men with fewer facial features that were prototypical of the category. Thus, people come to see the man more negatively simply because his facial features are able to strongly prime an implicit stereotype.

Further supporting the idea that it is the facial features that trigger the stereotype, which then alters the reaction, Blair and colleagues (Blair, Chapleau, & Judd, 2005; Blair, Judd, & Chapleau, 2004; Blair, Judd, Sadler, & Jenkins, 2002) showed the same type of effect when faces of White men were given Afrocentric facial features. When an image of a White person's face was morphed to have facial features that are associated with Black men, the stereotype of Black men was primed and the White target was judged more negatively. In a final example, Eberhardt et al. (2003) created racially ambiguous faces by morphing two faces: 50% White man's face and 50% Black man's face. The image was accompanied by a label that either specified it as White or Black, thus priming one racial category. They then tested to see how face perception was distorted by priming of the stereotype. Participants were asked to draw the person's face as best as they could, providing a measure of what the person perceived; stereotypicality of drawings were later rated by judges. The results showed that what is perceived is more stereotypic than what was presented. An ambiguous face was seen to have the facial features and skin tone consistent with the prime. Faces labeled "Black" were seen as having darker skin and broader noses than the same faces labeled "White." In a second study using a memory measure a similar finding emerged. The primed stereotype distorted memory of the ambiguous face of a person from another race in a way consistent with the stereotype.

Such a dissociation model does not suggest people are doomed to *use* stereotypes once activated. They can utilize conscious control to suppress any influence that a triggered stereotype might exert.[1] Devine (1989) argues that people differ in how they effortfully exert control when explicitly processing. These processes involve conscious choices. An individual may choose to exert conscious control over a first impression and decide to engage in the effort of attempting to make sure the response selected is free from bias. This is often thought of as first requiring one to become aware of bias (such as acknowledging that a stereotype may have been activated and could exert an unwanted influence), to then have the motivation to be unbiased and to engage in strategies to mitigate bias, and to have the capacity to do so. However, a point often neglected (despite my having stressed it for over 30 years) is that people are also not doomed to have stereotypes *activated*. The implicit processes of the first stage can also be controlled. There are two dissociable stages, and two discrete forms of control that can be exerted at each stage. We return to this idea of how to update and change an implicit stereotype, even controlling the priming of the stereotype (despite it being an implicit process), in Chapters 12 and 13.

CONCLUSIONS

The influence of accessible information on cognition was eloquently stated by James (1890/1950):

> The object we wish to capture with our attention may be very weak, a small noise in the midst of a crowd, and the way not to miss it is to prepare for it by either rehearsing it mentally or actually coming into contact with an exemplar. In doing so, this preparation partly consists of the creation of an imaginary duplicate of the object in the mind, which shall stand ready to receive the outward impression. . . . When watching for the distant clock to strike, our mind is so filled with its image that at every moment we think we hear the longed for or dreaded sound. So of an awaited footstep. Every stir in the wood is for the hunter his game; for the fugitive his pursuers . . . the image in the mind is the attention. (p. 442)

While the examples in the quote above imply consciousness of the "readiness" to respond, we have reviewed in this chapter how such readiness can occur outside of conscious awareness. Just as we prepare to paint by priming the wall to make the final action more fluid and smooth, or prime the mower to make it ready to start, we prime our judgment and action with "an imaginary duplicate of the object in the mind," with an accessible mental representation.

If a stimulus is ambiguous, or when a stimulus is somehow impoverished (such as when it is dark, far away, blurry, or otherwise hard to see), people have categories accessible that they are perceptually ready to use to help in perceiving and making sense of the stimulus. Accessibility effects were first experimentally studied (under a different name) in the 1940s with a focus on primed goals and values (see Bruner, 1957; Erdelyi, 1974, for reviews). Priming, however, can exist for semantic knowledge as well, with the following effects (Bruner, 1957):

> The greater the accessibility of a category, (a) the less the input necessary for a categorization to occur in terms of this category, (b) the wider the range of characteristics that will be "accepted" as fitting the category in question, (c) the more likely that categories that provide a better or equally good fit for the input will be masked. To put it in more ordinary language: apples will be more easily and swiftly recognized, a wider range of things will be identified or misidentified as apples, and in consequence the correct or best fitting identity of these other inputs will be masked. This is what is intended by accessibility. (pp. 129–130)

Bruner (1957) thus identified three general effects of accessibility on perception of a stimulus. First, the greater the accessibility, the less the input necessary for a categorization to occur; you will be able to categorize a person or identify an object based on fewer features. Readiness leads the accessible item to be seen when there is degraded stimuli, when there is little evidence, and when there is ambiguity. If we have been raised on an apple orchard, we are quicker and better able to identify a tree in the distance as an apple tree. If the trait "hostility" is chronically accessible, the more quickly we will label a behavior as hostile, even if the behavior is ambiguous. Second, a wide range of characteristics will be accepted as fitting the category; we are ready to accept something that resembles the accessible item as an instance of it (this leads to misidentifying ambiguous stimuli due to too broadly applying the construct). For example, a broader range of behavior is subsequently interpreted as being a hostile act if the trait hostility is accessible. Third, competing explanations that provide an equally good fit for the input will be masked. Once we are ready to categorize something as an apple tree, alternative categories (e.g., pear tree) are more difficult to see if they are in fact the reality.

Accessible categories allow perceivers to "go beyond the information given" (Bruner, 1957) and to construct a reality more full than what the actual stimulus may have suggested by itself. Accessible information not only colors what we see but fills in the gaps and extends what we see to features not even present. It shapes our judgments, often assimilating new information to match the accessible construct, but also leading to contrast effects where we see the information as being dissimilar to what we were ready to see. If we had just seen the movie *Call of the Wild,* an animal we later see in the distance and which is obscured by the woods is more likely to be seen as a wolf. These effects extend to behavior, as well as attention, categorization, and judgment. However, this does not mean our behavior is pushed around like we are puppets by implicit primes.

Consider the case of subliminal priming. There has long been discussion of whether this can be an effective marketing tool to change attitudes and behavior. In the 1960s a famous experiment was unleashed on the consuming public. A researcher had infiltrated a movie theater to investigate the effects of subliminal advertisements on what sort of products people purchased at the candy/popcorn stand. It was reported that the words "drink Coke" being subliminally flashed in a movie theater led to sales of Coca-Cola going up by 18%. Why would people leave their seats to buy Coke following this subliminal message? It turns out, the real answer is "they would not." The famous experiment was in fact a fraud—the data reported were fabricated.

Strahan et al. (2002) suggest that this does not mean that behavior is never influenced by a subliminal prime. However, for subliminal priming to alter how you behave you must first have the goal to behave. The prime could then influence behavior if the concepts primed are consistent with the actions needed to attain the goal. One would not get up and drink Coke if one was not thirsty, simply because of a prime. However, if you were already thirsty and contemplating a trip to the concession stand, a subliminal prime could impact how you act (what beverage you select). If you are motivated to judge or evaluate a person, a prime could impact what you think you see (if the behavior is ambiguous and applicable to the prime).

Consider the following events reported by the Associated Press on September 13, 2000 ("Bush Dismisses 'Rat' Allegation"), during the Presidential election between George Bush and Al Gore:

> A GOP commercial that subtly flashes the word "RATS" across the screen is coming off the air amid allegations the Republicans were trying to send a subliminal message about Al Gore. George W. Bush called the notion "bizarre and weird," and his campaign made light of it all. The GOP admaker said he was just trying to make the spot visually interesting. But Gore's campaign and experts in political advertising said the word choice—as an announcer was denouncing Gore's Medicare plan—could hardly have been an accident. . . . Bush noted that the word appears only fleetingly—for a tiny fraction of a second. Played at full speed, it's barely noticeable, particularly if the viewer isn't looking for the word. "One frame out of 900 hardly in my judgment makes a conspiracy" [said Bush].

As images flashed on the screen during the advertisement, the word "bureaucrats" (included among the images) did something odd only very few people could see with the naked eye (and thus was subliminal to most people). The letters *R, A, T,* and *S* jumped out, very quickly, from the word "bureaucrats" so *RATS* was exposed to viewers just as a summary of Gore's views on Medicare were summarized on the screen. Democrats claimed Bush used subliminal messages, in this case priming the concept "rat," to try to make people form negative impressions of Gore. Bush declared this was not a case of "subliminable" advertising. He pressed Americans to see that the flashing of the word "rats" was an honest mistake that could have no effect on a voter's evaluations. Our focus in this chapter is not on the fact that a man running for President could not pronounce the word "subliminal," or that letters do not mistakenly appear to leap off of film, but must be artfully made to do so by a professional. Rather, our focus is on whether subliminal information, or information primed in any way that makes its influence outside our awareness, has any impact on judgment or behavior. Can concepts be made accessible (even by subliminal flashes)? Do they impact us?

George W. Bush was incorrect in assuming subliminal concepts can have no impact. We should not necessarily ignore a small number of "frames" embedded within thousands on film, nor should we ignore the power of that which we do not see. But the issue we must be concerned with is when, how, and why such forces, that feel as if they should be random and meaningless, have an impact (and thus, allow us to know whether subliminal words in a political commercial could have an influence). An irrelevant or unambiguous target would not be influenced by such a prime. However, if a person did not have a firm opinion of Al Gore (Gore was ambiguous), and if Gore's policy on the behavior in question (the advertisement was discussing his health care policy) was ambiguously sleazy/opportunistic (it is relevant to the prime), then priming people with the word "RATS," and then presenting people with an image of Al Gore and asking them to form an opinion of his health care policy and of him as a candidate, should cause those people without firm opinions (the undecided voters such campaign commercials are designed to influence) to be influenced by the prime when judging Gore. Based on our existing knowledge, we would have to conclude that this campaign trick may have worked for a limited number of perceivers if the influence was assimilation, and it may have backfired if the influence was to cause a contrast effect. Both chronic and temporary primes can influence what we see and think, regardless of whether it is shaping judgment of a target in an ad campaign, negatively influencing how a member of a stereotyped group is judged, forming a skewed impression of a job candidate, or simply assessing a new person one has met. This occurs without us seeing the influence, and thus leading us to feel as if the person being judged has displayed that quality, even if their action is ambiguous and only weakly relevant. These types of misattributions from the prime to the stimulus, a priming effect, can shape what we think we know, and in turn bias how we act.

NOTE

1. And the dotted line in Figure 10.3 represents the possibility that, at times, the category that is triggered might even initiate the motivation to be unbiased, a topic we return to in Chapter 12.

CHAPTER 11

Prejudice and Stereotyping

Prejudice and stereotypes are two distinct types of mental representations. Though often treated interchangeably by lay people, they represent different types of impressions about a target group (e.g., Amodio & Devine, 2006). As noted in Chapter 3, *prejudice* is an affective prejudgment of a group of people, usually a negative one. It is an association between *evaluations* of a group—positive or negative attitudes—with the group category. Once such associations among evaluation/affect and a specific social group develops, it remains possible that such associations are triggered outside conscious awareness (e.g., Bargh et al., 1992; Fazio et al., 1986). If triggered, these attitudes are typically applied to individual members of the group, without one being aware of the attitude accessibility or its influence on judgment (though one may, or may not, be aware that a judgment is being made). Allport (1954) defined prejudice as containing "two essential ingredients. There must be an attitude of favor or disfavor; and it must be related to an over-generalized (and therefore erroneous) belief" (p. 13). Few would argue that *erroneous*, predetermined feelings of dislike toward a group of people are good. However, it is also likely that few would argue that negative prejudice would be adaptive if *not erroneous* (such as a dislike for rapists, child molesters, serial killers, Nazis, treasonous insurrectionists, physically abusive people, murderous tyrants, etc.). Allport's definition introduces subjectivity: it suggests that a prejudgment is not prejudice if it is warranted—if the feeling is not based on erroneous beliefs. Such a definition allows one to excuse negative attitudes by arguing that "in that culture, at that time, the belief was not thought to be erroneous." Was enslavement of Hebrew people by Egyptian rulers in ancient times an example of prejudice? If prejudice is defined by the notion of there being sufficient warrant, one could argue that if Egyptians accepted group superiority as a fact, then the slavery in their culture was not prejudice. This is why the definition of prejudice offered above, and other modern definitions, only require a prejudgment about a group. Examinations of whether it is warranted or not is a separate matter.

The word "stereotype" comes from the early world of printing and photography to describe a procedure developed in 1798 for duplicating something in order to use it, not the original, in the printing process. Walter Lippmann introduced its modern use—to refer to a way of thinking—in his 1922 book *Public Opinion*. Lippmann described stereotypes simply as mental snapshots that reproduce the outside world in the mind of a person. Lippmann

called stereotypes pictures in our heads, with the term combining the 19th-century meanings of the photography term for the procedure by which images of the world are reproduced on film—a *daguerreotype*—with the printing term *stereotype*. Unlike prejudice, which is
how we *evaluate* a group, *stereotypes* are *semantic knowledge* we possess about a group. They are
information about the personal qualities, characteristics, physical features, typical behaviors, and value system that are associated with a social group. They are mental representations that describe (and prescribe the behavior of) a class of people. If triggered, these
associated pieces of semantic knowledge are typically applied to individual members of the
group, without one being aware of the stereotype's accessibility or its influence on judgment
(though one may, or may not, be aware that a judgment is being made). As with prejudice,
accuracy of a stereotype is not essential to the definition. A stereotype may start from a
kernel of truth, making it easy for a biased person to find some true fact to point to as justification for their stereotype (Prothro & Melikian, 1955). A biased person can argue for the
validity of the stereotype if they can identify a subset of elements or qualities that define
the stereotype that are true of the group. But a stereotype can be 100% false. And another
stereotype can start from a kernel of truth but develop further in a way that is mostly
false. And yet another can be mostly true. Its validity is a separate (but important) matter.
Stereotypes become a societal concern when riddled with falsities and overgeneralized to
individuals. Yet they persist because of the functions they serve (as described in Chapter 2)
and for the reasons first impressions persist (as described in Chapters 5 and 6). We repeat a
review of such reasons shortly.

In *dissociation model of stereotyping* presented in Chapter 10, bias arising from the accessibility of prejudice or stereotypes was described as happening through a set of dissociated
processes (as depicted in Figure 10.3). One set of processes involves the activation and heightened perceptual readiness of stereotypes and prejudice. A separate set of processes involves
the use of these accessible constructs to shape attention, our impressions of the group (and
individual group members), how one behaves, and a host of other types of responses. Many
examples of these dissociated processes producing bias have been offered throughout the
book. Although research on stereotyping and prejudice as a cognitive process began in the
1970s, in 1954 Gordon Allport had already proposed how stereotypes could emerge from
normal cognitive function. Allport stated:

> What I sense, what I perceive, and what I think become blended into one single act of cognition.
> When I meet a [Black man], his blackness is conveyed to me by sensation, but the fact that he is
> a man, also a member of a certain race, and that he accordingly may have other attributes of the
> group (which I think I know about) are all added by past experience. (p. 165)

Allport (1954) spoke of laws of association that bind together categories and attributes
to form stereotypes, such as the associations formed among group membership and traits.
He introduced the idea that as the category is triggered after perceptual experience detects
features that render it relevant, the associated attributes will be triggered as well. Allport
summarized this process well: "every event has certain marks that serve as a cue. . . . When
we see a red-breasted bird, we say to ourselves 'robin.' . . . A person with dark brown skin will
activate whatever concept of Negro is dominant in our mind" (p. 21). This is a prominent
theme of the literature on prejudice and stereotyping. Even if not conscious of it, activation
creates a state of perceptual readiness. And with a prejudiced attitude or a stereotype ready
to be used, it can exert a biasing influence on how subsequent social cognition unfolds,
especially if the stimuli next encountered are ambiguous and the impact of the stereotype is

one in which the perceiver is not aware. This processing model raises important questions—for example, the question of whether bias is inevitable versus controllable. Or the question of whether control over bias is effortful and requires conscious exertion versus being effortless and easily regulated with a shift in one's goals. Or the question of how controlling bias might differ if one is focused on regulating the processes that give rise to the *activation* of the mental representation versus the processes governing its subsequent *use*. Or the question of whether raising awareness of bias will result in a desire to mitigate that bias in the future or a desire to deny that the bias is problematic. Those questions, that concern the control of bias and the updating of stereotypes and prejudice, are addressed in Chapter 13. Here we turn to extending the investigation of stereotyping and prejudice beyond this one form in which the bias manifests as a priming effect. With that having been reviewed in Chapter 10, let us turn to other questions relating to prejudice and stereotyping. We first look at the impact that *prejudice* has on social cognition, and then turn to *stereotypes*.

WHY IS EXPLICIT PREJUDICE EASILY ACTIVATED?

The broad history of scholarship on prejudice, as well as how most laypeople have historically thought about prejudice, is on its explicit forms. Gordon Allport illustrated this old-fashioned form of prejudice in the opening sentences of his 1954 book, *The Nature of Prejudice*: "In Rhodesia a white truck driver passed a group of idle natives and muttered, 'They're lazy brutes.' A few hours later he saw natives heaving two-hundred pound sacks of grain onto a truck. . . . 'Savages,' he grumbled" (p. 3).

Writing in *The New York Times* nearly 70 years later (March 17, 2023), Pamela Paul (Paul, 2017) reveals little progress. She describes prejudiced reactions to a Black high school student who was walking in the corridor during the school's morning pledge of allegiance to the United States, such as one online comment suggesting that she "go back to her monkey cage in Africa if she doesn't like to recite the pledge to the country that's doing her and her retarded family a favor by letting them live among decent humans." This type of overt hate has historically been a target of concern for the social sciences. A concern with *implicit attitudes* and the triggering of negative attitudes outside awareness is a newer concern; it arose in the United States in the period after civil rights laws were passed in the 1960s. Norms concerning how we publicly talk about race and gender began to slowly change, even if attitudes did not. New norms required people to mask their bias, even from themselves, giving rise to a concern with implicit forms of bias. However, as shown by the examples above, prejudice is hardly only expressed in this implicit form. When Katz and Braly (1933) undertook their early exploration of bias in the United States, they merely had to ask people to openly tell them the qualities they explicitly associated with 10 groups (Black people, Turkish people, Jews, Germans, Chinese people, etc.). Current norms ask us to stifle such free expression of bias, but this does not mean explicit bias has been vanquished.

Despite the commonness of holding overtly prejudice beliefs certainly waning over the last century, there are many examples of people who still proudly endorse race, sexual orientation, religious, and gender superiority (e.g., Campbell & Brauer, 2021). And when the typical person contemplates the causes of prejudice, there is a tendency to see it as attributable (in large part) to this type of explicitly biased person. An image is conjured of a person who reacts to members of social groups that are not their own with emotions and attitudes such as hate, disregard, fear, anxiety, avoidance, pity, and envy. These biased people promote negative beliefs about outgroups, such as their laziness, clannishness, dangerousness, immorality, lack of intelligence, and incompetence. It is this prejudice personality type, these "others," to whom the typical person imagines the social ills that are attributed to prejudice should be linked. The moral conundrum of prejudice is placed squarely at the feet of these blatantly deplorable others, freeing one from imagining any personal culpability and feeling safe in one's own distinction from these "bad" people. Who are these "deplorables" assuaging collective guilt and personal culpability?

In Chapter 4 we reviewed projective tests used in the 1950s to reveal prejudiced individuals. We also saw how measures of authoritarianism and ethnocentrism could be used to assess explicit prejudice. In more recent years we have seen measures of racism (Henry & Sears, 2002; McConahay, 1986) and sexism (Glick & Fiske, 1996) that have emerged as ways to identify people who are high in prejudice. People who exhibit this old-fashioned type of prejudice will unashamedly express negative attitudes and beliefs about the social groups they openly dislike. For example, Monteith, Devine, and Zuwerink (1993) used a measure of prejudice to identify one group of heterosexual research participants who were high in prejudice and another group that were low in prejudice. They asked each group to honestly contemplate how they actually would act during four hypothetical encounters with homosexuals that were provided for them, using their own personal standards as a guide. They then asked the participants to again contemplate the same encounters with homosexuals, and this time to report how they *should* act in each situation if using what the culture suggests is appropriate as a standard (what we earlier called an ought standard in Chapter 8). How do people react when a discrepancy arises among how one should act and how one would act? As might be expected, low-prejudice people are bothered by not meeting societal standards: They feel guilt and shame. However, high-prejudice people hold no remorse or shame if responding in ways that violate what others say is appropriate. Their prejudice is explicit and proudly endorsed, knowing full well it is discrepant with what others say is appropriate. We next explore motivations that encourage such explicit prejudice.

System Justification

Some of the time a person's explicit prejudice might take the form of endorsing a hierarchical and stratified society that marks some groups of people as inferior to others, with their lower status as proof of their inadequacies. For example, earlier in this book we reviewed *system justification* as causing motivated reasoning to produce conclusions, bolstered by cherry-picked evidence, to support the status quo (e.g., Jost, 2020). System justification was defined as a motivation to defend the social systems that support the culture in which one lives. Without a belief in the value and reliability of the social, economic, and political systems that allow one's culture to function, the world would be seen as chaotic and riddled with uncertainty. To varying degrees, people are motivated to justify the systems that support their daily life.

A person with high levels of system justification uses prejudice to support why disparities exist among groups. If some groups are disadvantaged relative to others, it must be because the outcomes meted out are justified. To think otherwise would lead such people to have to question the foundation on which the entire system sustaining their existence is built. System justification, therefore, is one reason prejudiced attitudes are activated easily. People are motivated to maintain structural biases that keep the groups to which they belong (or aspire to belong to) in a favored status. This allows them to openly endorse the disparities such a system produces. Of course, it is not just prejudice to others that results from high system justification. If one's own group is itself disadvantaged and at the bottom of the hierarchy, one can come to accept this as well, rather than challenge the system. Overt prejudice toward a group (usually another, but at times one's own) can be activated from motives relating to system justification.

Social Dominance Orientation

Rather than needing to justify a particular structural system, people can also differ in their motivation to simply prefer hierarchies. Sidanius (1993; see also Pratto et al., 1994) identified what is called **social dominance orientation (SDO)**—a chronic motive to have the hierarchical nature between groups maintained, or "the extent to which one desires that one's in-group dominate and be superior to out-groups" (p. 742). SDO manifests through **hierarchy-legitimizing myths**. These are cultural beliefs and ideologies present in a society that "minimize conflict among groups by indicating how individuals and social institutions should allocate things of positive or negative social value, such as jobs, gold, blankets, government appointments, prison terms, and disease" (p. 741). SDO is sustained in some cultures through *paternalistic myths* that specify that the dominance of one group over another group serves society. This myth supports hegemony, which is then used to legitimize

> **Social Dominance Orientation (SDO):** A motivation for one's ingroup to be superior to outgroups and to dominate outgroups.
>
> **Hierarchy-legitimizing myths:** An element of the theory of SDO that specifies a set of cultural beliefs and ideologies present in society that indicate and justify how things of social value to individuals and social institutions should be allocated.

forms of social dominance (e.g., governing people who were perceived as incapable of governing themselves) such as colonialism, slavery, and patriarchy. Other cultures see SDO sustained through *sacred myths* that specify a divine order (such as a right of monarchs to rule, or a religiously defined mandate for one group to govern another). Yet other cultures have *meritocratic myths* that sustain the social order. For example, the differences found among liberals and conservatives in the United States in how they form moral inferences and reason about causality (personal vs. situational) is justified by each group's belief in meritocracy (e.g., Kugler, Jost, & Noorbaloochi, 2014).

There are two paths through which social dominance is said to be exerted. The first is by determining the attitudes of individual people toward things such as race relations and social policy—that is, the type of person who is high in SDO is likely to be high in prejudice. White people high in SDO were more likely to express anti-Black sentiment, and men high in SDO were more likely to express anti-female sentiment in surveys about these groups (relative to people low in SDO). As with system justification, such impressions help to rationalize the reasons for the lower standing of some groups in the societal hierarchy. Pratto et al. (1994) showed that SDO is correlated with endorsements of "racism, nationalism, ethnocentrism, militarism, law and order, and pro-establishment politics" (p. 757). Thus, one reason explicit prejudice is easily activated in some people is because they are motivated to support hierarchies.

SDO is not only exerted through individuals developing prejudiced attitudes but is also said to be exerted by impacting the social structures that determine the opportunities and penalties that face people from different social groups. A stratified system creates access to and control over resources to a dominant group (such as political power), which promotes affiliation, kinship, and nepotism among members of a dominant group. At the same time, such a stratified social structure discourages defiance from inferior groups. This can occur through beliefs that help perpetuate the myth that the structure is justifiable and just, or through systematic terror, violence, and aggression (Sidanius, 1993). A subordinate group might incur harsh punishments for questioning the social order and challenging the structures that help keep it in place.

Social Identity Theory

Throughout this book we have reviewed the powerful effects of the motivation to enhance self-esteem. We engage in self-enhancement processes to defend self-esteem and promote positive (and ward off negative) evaluations. The same type of defensiveness is used to enhance the esteem we derive from the groups with which we identify. From the earliest moments of life, we enter into social groups, often starting with families and religions, and evolving into ethnic and socioeconomic communities, school affiliations, fraternities, sports teams and work groups, and so on, all helping to satisfy the need to belong (e.g., Baumeister & Leary, 1995). These groups become linked to the self-concept, creating a complex, layered notion of the self that has the individual at its core, but a sphere of social influences that are essential to it as well (e.g., Brewer, 1991). If these groups are perceived as doing well through positive evaluations against other groups, then it reflects positively on us. This creates a positive sense of self through promoting a positive social identity (e.g., Brewer, 1991; Tajfel & Turner, 1986) and what Crocker and Luhtanen (1990) called high collective self-esteem (self-esteem that is derived from the various groups or collectives with which we identify). This fact is the essence of an influential theory of prejudice known as **social identity theory** (SIT; e.g., Tajfel & Turner, 1986). According to SIT, esteem enhancement impacts prejudiced evaluations of others in the following ways:

> **Social identity theory (SIT):** A theory stating that prejudice arises from goals to enhance and defend self-esteem derived from groups with which we identify. It argues that we engage in comparisons of the "ingroup" against other "outgroups" to promote positive (and ward off negative) ingroup evaluations. Both positive ingroup prejudice and negative outgroup prejudice accomplish this.

> 1) Individuals strive to maintain or enhance their self-esteem: they strive for a positive self-concept, 2) Social groups or categories and the membership in them are associated with positive or negative value connotations. Hence, social identity may be positive or negative according to the evaluations, 3) The evaluation of one's own group is determined with reference to specific other groups through social comparison. (p. 16)

Thus, the theory specifies a motivation to enhance self-esteem as essential to prejudice, and it specifies a process through which that positive esteem can be achieved: through the evaluation of one's own group against other groups by engaging in social comparison (comparisons of their own "ingroup" made against other "outgroups"). We use comparisons of our group against others to promote positive (and ward off negative) evaluations—to enhance the esteem we derive from the groups with which we identify. When these evaluations reveal our group as doing well it reflects positively on us. For example, if a social comparison reveals information that threatens the positive evaluation one has of one's group (such as a suggestion that one's group is relatively lacking in morality), a strong social identity will lead one to justify and defend the group. One can rationalize away the negative results of the social comparison (e.g., Branscombe, Ellemers, Spears, & Doosje, 1999; Ellemers & Van den Bos, 2012). According to the theory, people strategically use social comparison processes to enhance the positivity assigned to the group (see Figure 11.1). How can one enhance positive evaluation of one's group as a result of a comparison with other groups? As shown in Chapter 9, this can be achieved by both ingroup favoritism and outgroup derogation.

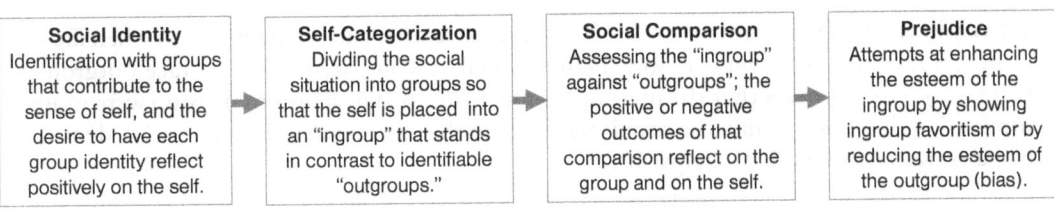

Social Identity	Self-Categorization	Social Comparison	Prejudice
Identification with groups that contribute to the sense of self, and the desire to have each group identity reflect positively on the self.	Dividing the social situation into groups so that the self is placed into an "ingroup" that stands in contrast to identifiable "outgroups."	Assessing the "ingroup" against "outgroups"; the positive or negative outcomes of that comparison reflect on the group and on the self.	Attempts at enhancing the esteem of the ingroup by showing ingroup favoritism or by reducing the esteem of the outgroup (bias).

FIGURE 11.1. Social identity theory.

One way to explore whether ingroup favoritism or outgroup dislike is useful to enhance esteem and create a positive identity is to manipulate identity threat. This type of identity threat can happen when a social comparison reflects negatively on an identity group, or when personal esteem is undermined and needs enhancing. In Chapter 9 we saw evidence from the research of Fein and Spencer (1997; Spencer et al., 1998) that a threat to the self leads to increased prejudice toward the outgroup. A generalized threat that had nothing to do with group identity (feedback about poor performance on an intelligence test) led to prejudice, which in turn bolstered self-esteem. A threat to a social identity has a similar effect. This can also occur when one's status in the group is threatened and one needs to reaffirm one's credentials as a group member to remove the threat of losing an identity. Branscombe et al. (1999) created the possibility that one might be rejected by an ingroup, making their research participants feel the threat to their sense of belonging to the group. This caused an increase in derogation of an outgroup—an attempt to use outgroup disdain as a way to reassert ingroup status and one's sense of belonging.

Rather than induce threat to the group, another way to explore whether social identity concerns are sustained through prejudice is to make a group membership momentarily important. Does ingroup favoritism emerge to a group when membership in it is made important in the moment? Ashburn-Nardo, Voils, and Monteith (2001) created minimal groups (as described in Chapter 9) to explore this. They found that participants showed ingroup favoritism to these minimal groups even on an implicit measure of attitudes (the Implicit Association Test [IAT]).[1] Does this favoritism to a minimal group created in the moment occur even at the expense of other group memberships that would otherwise be protected and enhanced? For example, identification with a racial group often leads to outgroup prejudice and ingroup favoritism. However, if a new group membership was created that cut across racial lines, would the new group be the group that is favored, and the racial division becomes momentarily meaningless? Van Bavel and Cunningham (2009) provided an illustration by pitting an existing group identity (race) against a minimal group identity made relevant in the experiment. They show that creating minimal groups that included both Black and White ingroup members led the research participants to show favoritism to the minimal ingroup and to stop exhibiting prejudice to people from a racial outgroup. To explore this, they manipulated whether the minimally defined groups contained only members of the same race as the participant versus the group including people of a different race. Racial prejudice was eliminated when the newly created ingroup included people of both races. Ingroup members of a different race were favored over same-race people who were part of the outgroup. Social identity goals to this momentarily important group seemed to trump long-standing racial bias. This was true of explicit racial prejudice and *implicit* prejudice, as measured using an IAT. The type of prejudice people show depends on the group they identify with in the moment—on the salient social identity specifying which people are "outgroup" members, and to be disliked. Van Bavel et al. (2008) even found greater activity in the amygdala (a structure in the brain associated with goal relevance) when faces of mixed-race ingroup members were being evaluated (compared to mixed-race outgroup members). This suggests that the ingroup members defined by a minimal group were more motivationally relevant than the people with whom the participants shared a racial identity (see also Kubota, Banaji, & Phelps, 2012).

Enhancing positive esteem is not the only key motivation SIT stipulates is associated with the comparison processes in which group members engage. Comparison not only allows one to evaluate the relative positivity of one's group, but its relative distinctiveness. Pursuing a **distinctiveness goal** when engaged in comparison to another group allows for the ingroup to be seen as unique, which also confers value on the group (e.g., Turner & Reynolds, 2001). Brewer (1991; Pickett & Brewer, 2001) argued that humans strive to belong to and assimilate with a group of others, but simultaneously they strive to be perceived as unique and distinctive. Group identities can accomplish each goal, giving one both a sense of belonging to something larger than the self and a sense of distinctiveness by the group's ability to be assessed as unique in comparison to other groups. Individuals strive for group identities that provide **optimal distinctiveness**, that balance the needs for belonging/inclusion and needs for differentiation so that both of these needs are not only met, but promote cooperative interdependence among group members and mutually beneficial goal achievement (Brewer, 1991). Highly inclusive, superordinate social groups, such as American or human, are less likely to be ones that create optimal distinctiveness. It is instead found in overlapping lower-level identities of smaller social categories such as religious groups and political affiliations. Hornsey and Jetten (2004) suggest that members of minority groups identify more strongly with their group than members of majority groups because a minority group more easily satisfies both a motivation to belong and a motivation to be distinct. Differentiation of one's group from another, or attempting to maximize or make optimal the group's distinctiveness, can create trust and cooperation among the ingroup members who are in pursuit of shared goals. Indeed, many goals cannot be achieved in isolation, without joining a group, and groups that are optimally distinct provide one with a depersonalized trust in others that makes achieving such goals most likely. It soothes one when feeling isolated and ostracized, but also provides a unique identity when feeling lost in the collective. However, it may also lead to active distrust and competition with an outgroup, particularly when conflict over resources exists among the groups.

In summary, there is motivation to create a sense of positivity and superiority for the group, to make a group as distinctive and separate from others as possible, and to engender a sense of positivity toward the self as a member of the distinctive and positive group. Brewer (1999) argued that mere categorization into ingroup and outgroup is enough to produce ingroup favoritism. It can create prejudice without a history of antagonism, without competition over scarce resources or power. This is not to say that real conflict over resources and power struggles are irrelevant to group conflict. They are obviously relevant and can create antagonism and intergroup conflict above and beyond mere favoritism for one's own group (e.g., Campbell, 1963; Sherif, 1967; Sidanius, 1993). But such competition is not necessary. The need for a positive and distinctive social identity can be enough to lead

Distinctiveness goal: Humans strive to belong to groups to enhance esteem and reduce uncertainty, but also to be perceived as unique and distinctive. Part of the sense of identity uniqueness we experience is derived from groups we belong to seeming unique and different (in a positive way) in comparison to another group.

Optimal distinctiveness: Balancing the needs for belonging/inclusion and for differentiation so that both of these needs are not only met, but promote cooperative interdependence among group members and mutually beneficial goal achievement. When group membership allows one to easily satisfy *both* a motivation to belong and a motivation to maximize or make optimal the group's distinctiveness.

to favoritism and privilege for an ingroup, which can, under the correct conditions, develop into disparagement and disdain of an outgroup. Of course, when social identity motives combine with resource competition and threat, an ingroup member should derogate the outgroup with even higher levels of prejudice and should favor the ingroup even more (e.g., Branscombe et al., 1999; Cikara, Botvinick, & Fiske, 2011).

Self-Categorization Theory

Since its introduction in the 1970s, SIT has evolved with research on **self-categorization theory**, which extends the theorizing to a more specific focus on the role of how being categorized into a group helps to remove uncertainty (e.g., Turner et al., 1987). It posits that in addition to yielding distinctiveness, belonging, and positivity, groups tell us how and what to think, which helps give meaning to people. Hogg (2000) argues that categorizing the self into a group of similar others provides such a reduction to uncertainty through specifying group norms that clearly define what is, and what is not, appropriate (as well as offering prescriptions about how one should behave). When we identify strongly with an ingroup we see all ingroup members as equally governed by norms, and in a manner interchangeable with one another with regard to the influence of group-level norms on behavior. When a person self-categorizes as a member of an ingroup they start to think and feel as a representative of the group, not autonomously. They undergo a shift in identity from "I" to "we," from "me" to "us." Hornsey (2008) describes this notion of **depersonalization** as a cornerstone of self-categorization theory. Depersonalization is the idea that categorizing the self into that group allows one to see the self and other members of the group as "interchangeable exemplars of the group prototype" (p. 208). They see themselves less as individuals, and surrender individual identity to the group prototype—"depersonalizing." This helps to reduce uncertainty by specifying for each person the group norms, values, goals, and beliefs to adopt.

> **Self-categorization theory:** A theory that extends SIT to include not only goals of esteem enhancement, but uncertainty reduction. It posits that being categorized into a group reduces uncertainty through specifying group norms that define what is, and is not, appropriate (as well as offering prescriptions about how one should behave).

> **Depersonalization:** When people see group members (including the self) as interchangeable exemplars of group prototypes. If self-categorizing as an ingroup member, one starts to think, act, and feel as a representative of the group. They surrender individual identity, with a shift in identity from "I" to "we" and from "me" to "us."

When a group is strongly defined, with clear boundaries and norms, their specified ways to think, feel, and act are especially useful at times of uncertainty. Therefore, especially during times where people are concerned about how to behave, and social life introduces high levels of uncertainty, affiliating with and depersonalizing the self into a group can provide a guide for how to be (Hogg & Blaylock, 2012). This is especially true for groups that have high entitativity and offer clear and distinctive boundaries to competing groups (e.g., Hogg, 2014; Jetten, Hogg, & Mullin, 2000). In almost every country, and during almost any historical period, one can point to increases in tribalism and a group mentality marked by polarization as the times become more uncertain and people feel heightened threat. For example, Sherman, Hogg, and Maitner (2009) found that a combination of the feeling of uncertainty and identifying with a group characterized by high entitativity (such as a political party) led to polarization and an increase in prototypical responses. It is not only the uncertainty of the times that lead people to embrace categorization into a group, but some people simply have a stronger desire to identify with a group. The more strongly one identifies with a group, the more one will depersonalize and comply with group norms (e.g., Barreto & Ellemers, 2003; Hogg & Reid, 2006; Jetten, Spears, & Manstead, 1996; Packer, 2008).

Shifting Norms and the Modern-Day Expression of Prejudice

To end this section on explicit prejudice, it is important to note that even if social norms make the expression of explicit prejudice less likely, this does not mean the existence of explicit prejudice is minimized. We saw examples of this in Chapter 2 when discussing the Bradley effect. To appear nonracist, a White person may say they will vote for a Black political candidate, yet know full well they would not. More subtle measures are needed to assess explicit prejudice as norms that label such prejudice as unacceptable develop. It is not simply that norms about what is acceptable to say have changed, making prejudice less likely to be expressed. It is also the case that stereotypes about groups, what we believe are the facts about a group, can change with time. The stereotypes expressed by Katz and Braly's (1933) research participants are different from the stereotypes that exist today. Yet, while beliefs about the qualities that describe a group (stereotypes) may change over time, negative affect associated with the group appears to be more stable; the traits comprising the stereotype change, but the negative affect associated with the group remains (Devine & Elliot, 1995). This can lead to a situation where one believes one does not hold stereotypes (and perhaps does not) but still has explicit negative feelings for the group. One would be left with explicit prejudice even if stereotypes were not strongly held.

Aversive racism, as discussed in Chapter 3, represents a more common form of a separation of negative feelings and positive beliefs. Rather than having explicit negative feelings, aversive racism is when the negative reaction is unrecognized by the person. The person can truly believe that their feelings toward the group in question are not at all negative due to their explicit rejection of the stereotype. However, the implicit association that links negative reactions to the group can be dissociated from these explicit responses. Both exist. One is undetected, but lack of detection does not mean it has no influence. Throughout this book there have been summaries of research on implicit prejudice that were meant to illustrate the extent to which prejudice can exist in a person outside of awareness. Our focus next is to explore the variety of ways that invisible prejudice can influence how we respond without our awareness of that influence.

IMPLICIT PREJUDICE: UNCONSCIOUSLY HELD NEGATIVE ATTITUDES ABOUT GROUPS

As reviewed in Chapter 3, attitudes are among the first things we assess when encountering a person; triggered within a half-second without the person's intention to evaluate, or without awareness of having evaluated. This activation of attitudes has a functional nature that helps an individual to avoid harm and seek help, to quickly decide who is friend and who is foe. However, despite its functional nature, the implicit activation of attitudes can often lead to bias (e.g., Banaji & Greenwald, 2013). When social groups are the attitude object, the evaluation associated with this group will be triggered, just as it would be for any attitude object. This means that feelings of dislike (or favoritism) can be activated without our intention and without our awareness. It also means we may not realize we have negative attitudes or that we are experiencing negative affect toward a group in a given moment, even when we are. We can prejudge a person positively or negatively in an implicit manner due to these natural cognitive events that, from their functional nature, become habit. While explicit prejudice is a serious problem, we should not allow it to mask the separate problem of subtle and implicit prejudice.

In addition to the fact that attitudes can become implicitly activated, Yoshida et al. (2012) argue that this is true of norms, as well. For example, if a man is repeatedly exposed to other men in their group who believe that gender bias is nonexistent, the goal of belonging to this group could lead our individual man to associate that men in his group dislike women, or at least feel that other men feel gender bias is unproblematic. Even if the man in question is himself extremely concerned with gender bias in his group more generally, he will be sensitive to those attitudes that have consensus in the groups to which he belongs. His knowledge of the shared evaluations among other men, or of the group norms, become associated with the group. As such, the norms that specify how others feel and what others say is appropriate can become important determinants of how we respond (e.g., Tankard & Paluck, 2017). It can lead to prejudice in a person who personally does not share the attitude, without that person realizing information processing was influenced by these implicit norms. As Yoshida et al. state:

> It may be the case that when people are exposed to a negative depiction or treatment of a group (as may occur after hearing a racist joke) even those who are low in both implicit and explicit prejudice may engage in discrimination. This influence of implicit normative evaluations would suggest that culture has a broader impact than simply its influence on individuals' attitudes and beliefs. Much as people develop the accent of those they often hear speaking, we argue that people develop implicit normative evaluations that reflect the way objects of evaluation (including social groups) are depicted and treated in their society. For example, if female engineers are regularly depicted and treated negatively, then people are likely to develop negative implicit normative evaluations about female engineers even if their explicit and implicit attitudes about female engineers are positive. (p. 705)

When attitudes and norms are implicitly activated, the resulting prejudice can have dire consequences. The groups toward whom such biases are held feel the disparate treatment just as acutely as they do when the bias originates from intended forms of disparate treatment. Let us turn to an example from the medical community. As reported in Chapter 3, research examining bias in doctors and nurses has shown that physicians were only 60% as likely to suggest a top-rated diagnostic test for Black "heart patients" as for White patients. This was true even when Black patients presented the same symptoms and gave identical information about themselves. Black patients are also known to be treated differently by doctors not only in terms of the medical treatments suggested, but the interpersonal style/treatment exhibited during patient–doctor interactions. They are less likely to receive empathy from their physician and are less likely to be included in the decision-making process, with results showing that they receive less information about their conditions than White patients. One experiment found that physicians described Black patients as more likely to abuse drugs, less intelligent, less likely to comply with medical recommendations, and less educated. These effects emerged even after controlling for patient age, gender, socioeconomic status (SES), and degree of illness. We could use similar data to tell the same tale of prejudice leading to disparity in education, bank loans, criminal justice, job hiring and promotion, targets of gun violence—in almost every domain of life.[2]

Intersectionality and Colorism

Such statistics are focused only on people who are being discriminated against due to membership in a single minority group. However, multiracial people create ambiguities for perceivers, and unique stereotypes, due to the intersection of two racial identities (e.g.,

Chen, 2019; Chen et al., 2018; Eberhardt et al., 2003). As Petsko and Bodenhausen (2020) review, the nature of prejudice (and stereotyping) is complicated by **intersectionality**. Intersectionality is defined as a person having more than one social category with which they are identified and evaluated so that multiple (perhaps interlocking) group stereotypes and evaluative responses could be brought to bear on evaluation (e.g., Cole, 2009; Dupree, 2022; Goff & Kahn, 2013; Petsko & Bodenhausen, 2019; Plaut, 2010; Purdie-Vaughns & Eibach, 2008; Sesko & Biernat, 2010; Sim, Almaraz, & Hugenberg, 2022). These multiple categories (such as race and status, race and gender, age and gender, etc.) can each have an impact separately, or could interact in interesting ways, such as when the bias against Black men in leadership positions reverses if the man is also perceived to be gay (Wilson, Remedios, & Rule, 2017), or when the bias to exhibit backlash against White women exerting dominance in the workplace is diminished for Black women exerting dominance (e.g., Livingston, Rosette, & Washington, 2012). The stereotype of Black people shifts as it intersects with gender. For example, the Black woman stereotype lists characteristics linked to the stereotype of women such as overly emotional, but the emotion emphasized for Black women is anger, irrationality, and aggressiveness. And the Black man stereotype emphasizes characteristics associated with men, such as agency and assertiveness, but this escalates to violence, criminality, and threat. Thus, as gender and race intersect, stereotyping takes on a distinct nature.

> **Intersectionality:** When a person has more than one social category with which they are identified and evaluated so that multiple (perhaps interlocking) group stereotypes and evaluative responses could be brought to bear on evaluation.

Woodhams, Lupton, and Cowling (2015), as well as Greenman and Xie (2008), found that employees identified as having an intersectional identity had lower salaries than those belonging to a single minority group. Derous, Ryan, and Serlie (2015) found them to be rated as likely to be worse employees. Dupree, Torrez, Obioha, and Fiske (2021) found that people rate Black Americans as also being low-status and likely to hold what are perceived to be low-status jobs, and the greater the belief that such intersectional identities crossing race and status exist, the greater the prejudice, such as in increased rejection rates for job applicants. A series of experiments by Bart-Plange and colleagues focuses on how the cognitive processing of a perceiver is impacted by the intersectionality of the targets of their perception. First, Bart-Plange and Trawalter (2024) replicate the finding of Purdie-Vaughns and Eibach (2008) that categorizing a target according to gender is biased by how gender intersects with race. White women are characterized as women more easily than Black women. Similarly, they show that categorizing a target according to race is biased by how race intersects with gender. Black men are categorized as Black more easily than Black women are. White women are prototypical of "women" and Black men are prototypical of "Black people," making Black women non-prototypical for their race and their gender (thus rendering them somewhat invisible and subject to greater neglect; Purdie-Vaughns & Eibach, 2008; Thomas et al., 2014). Bart-Plange (2022) shows that this bias due to intersectionality also extends to the judgments a perceiver makes. For example, judgments of pain tolerance in medical decision making differ for White people than Black people (who are seen as less likely to experience pain), and differ still as race intersects with gender. Black women were judged especially less likely to be experiencing debilitating pain (and thus less in need of treatment for pain). Bart-Plange, Trawalter, and Pearce (2024) further show stronger stereotype-consistent trait attributions as stereotypes intersect – for example, women are judged to be more "sensitive to the needs of others" than men, but this is especially true for Black women. The more prototypically "Black" a face is perceived to be, the more strongly personality traits are inferred from those faces (e.g., Blair et al., 2002).

Remarkably, Bart-Plange and colleagues not only show how the intersectional nature of one's group memberships impacts social cognition. The goal of this work was to make an additional point – that these stereotypic biases in categorization and judgment are *exaggerated as skin tone becomes darker*. Darker skinned Black women were judged the least likely to be experiencing debilitating pain; biases to rate Black women as more "sensitive to the needs of others" than White women were more pronounced for darker skinned Black women; biases to categorize Black men as Black more easily than Black women were exaggerated for darker skinned Black men. Biases at the intersection of gender and race become more pronounced among darker-skinned people. The impact of having darker skin tone on exaggerating negative stereotypes is known as **colorism** (e.g., Dixon & Telles, 2017; Hunter, 2007). As we saw already, colorism impacts judgment, as Black men with darker skin tone were more likely to be sentenced with the death penalty for a murder conviction (e.g., Eberhardt et al., 2006). Here we see the important ways in which colorism impacts on intersectionality.

> **Colorism:** The impact of having darker skin tone on exaggerating negative stereotypes and prejudice.

These are dramatic disparities in outcomes relating to physical resources. However, the concern of this book is with social cognition, and the focus turns next not to cataloguing the many resource disparities caused by prejudice but to *how* social cognition contributes to disparity.

Implicit Prejudice and Disparate Treatment

One way to illustrate the influence that implicit prejudice has on how we respond is to look at the relationship between disparities in responses and scores on implicit measures of prejudice. For example, evidence was reviewed in Chapter 3 for the idea that prejudice feelings can leak out during cross-race interactions through nonverbal channels of communication (e.g., Dovidio et al., 2002; Richeson & Shelton, 2007). In experiments such as these, the research participants typically take a test that assesses levels of implicit prejudice, such as an IAT, and we can look to see if levels of implicit prejudice predict greater biased behavior. For example, Dovidio et al. found implicit prejudice was related to the amount of racial bias in nonverbal friendliness the White participants exhibited to a Black interaction partner. **Bias leaks out in ways not consciously seen or intended.** Similar findings were shown in the research of Son Hing et al. (2008). If a White job candidate was superior to an Asian candidate on quality *X* but not *Y*, people justified the choice of the White candidate by saying, "it is quality *X* that matters and is why I selected the White candidate." However, when the Asian candidate was superior on quality *X*, the importance of quality *Y* was now seen as obvious and the correct basis for the choice. The bias to shift one's choice so it aligns with an ingroup is predicted by level of implicit prejudice. Support for hiring Asian job candidates was unrelated to explicit prejudice, but it grew weaker as IAT scores (the measure of implicit bias) increased.

> **Bias leaks out in ways not consciously seen or intended:** Evidence for implicit prejudice is shown in the nonverbal behavior through which a person silently communicates their dislike. Prejudice feelings can leak out through nonverbal channels of communication that are difficult to control or monitor.

This same pattern is seen in the medical field when examining disparities to patients. Earlier we reviewed research that showed White doctors are less likely to recommend a preferred treatment (thrombolysis) to Black patients suffering from an apparent coronary syndrome (e.g., Green et al., 2007). What we had not mentioned previously was the fact that the bias in doctors was predicted by their levels of implicit prejudice. As a doctor's pro-White bias on an IAT increased, so did the likelihood of treating White patients and not Black patients with thrombolysis. Further, Blair, Steiner, et al. (2013) report that physicians with high levels of implicit prejudice were rated by Black patients as being lower in communication, trust, positive nonverbal behavior, and medical knowledge. Cooper et al. (2012) similarly showed that physician scores on a measure of implicit prejudice predicted how they behaved during an encounter with a Black patient. Doctors with higher implicit prejudice had a slower pace of dialogue and less patient-centered dialogue (the provider dominated the conversation). Black patients' levels of trust and confidence in their physician was predicted by their physician's level of implicit prejudice.

These are just a sampling of examples illustrating how implicit attitudes—negative associations to a social group—predict biased behavior in ways that explicit prejudice does not. Many of the above examples illustrate the existence of dramatic disparities in outcomes relating to physical resources, such as hiring, promotion, criminal sentencing, drug-related arrests and convictions, salaries, and medical recommendations. The suggestion is that implicit prejudice may contribute to such disparities. The research on intersectionality and colorism reminds us that it is not only disparities in physical resources that may be impacted by implicit prejudice, but social cognition shifts as well. Darker skin tone changes the way people categorize and judge others, with a supposed increase in implicit prejudice mediating the impact of skin tone on these social-cognitive processes. The focus turns next to further exploring *how* social cognition is impacted by implicit prejudice, and in so doing contributes to disparity.

Objectification and Dehumanization

One way in which implicit prejudice affects the targets of that prejudice is it leads them to be seen and treated as less than human (dehumanized)—to be objectified and described in more animalistic and robotic terms (e.g., Harris & Fiske, 2006, 2011; Haslam, Loughnan, Kashima, & Bain, 2008; Leyens et al., 2003; Tipler & Ruscher, 2014). At times this manifests as the target of prejudice being seen as inferior to other humans due to lacking warmth and being unencumbered by emotion (like an automaton). At times this manifests as the target of prejudice being seen as inferior to other humans due to lacking cognitive ability, morality, impulse control, and appropriate levels of cleanliness (evoking feelings of disgust). This creates comparisons to animals and insects, such as calling people from these groups apes, beasts, and cockroaches. They are likened to vermin; associated with disgust and inferiority. At other times it manifests as the target of prejudice being seen as having superhuman ability—as strong as a gorilla, with cat-like speed, immune to pain (or at least with heightened tolerance for it), and posing an unnatural threat as a result. Here, despite positive qualities such as strength and speed being suggested, they are used to describe a negative animalistic or brutish quality.

Haslam, Kashima, Loghnan, Shi, and Suitner (2008) argued that "humanness" is defined not only by attributes that are unique to our species (such as higher-order cognition, civility, culture) but that are typical of our species (warmth, openness, passion, emotionality). **Objectification** occurs when a person, by virtue of their group membership, is denied their humanity by seeing them as possessing fewer of these attributes. However, the type of dehumanization that occurs depends on the type of humanity being denied. When it is typicality as a human being denied, then they argue that dehumanization takes the first form described above: competent, unemotional, lacking warmth, and interchangeable, like machines. When it is human uniqueness being denied, then dehumanization takes the second form described above:

> **Objectification:** When a person is seen and treated as less than human (dehumanized) and is described in more animalistic and robotic terms.

irrational, lacking morality, and animalistic. The "animalistic type" just described would emerge when a group is characterized with low warmth and low competence, resulting in a failure to attribute mental states to such individuals and evoking a disgust response (such as likening a group to vermin and insects and monkeys). "It is often seen in representations of ethnic groups, 'primitive' peoples, immigrants, criminals, and the disabled, and is frequently accompanied by the use of explicit animal labels (e.g., vermin, beasts, apes, cockroaches)" (p. 249). The "robotic" type just described would emerge when a group is characterized with low warmth yet high competence. These groups (for example, Asians and Jews in North America) are often envied for their competence, yet dehumanized for their lack of warmth and apparent omnipresence and interchangeability (Harris & Fiske, 2011; Loughnan & Haslam, 2007). This can lead them to be exploited in the workplace and receive less social support (e.g., Lapka, Kung, Brienza, & Scholer, 2023).

Tipler and Ruscher (2014) argue that the type of metaphor used when dehumanizing a person is associated with the way we might expect bias toward them to manifest. "For example, a perception of outgroup members as parasites—who behave without thought or emotion—prescribes strategies of exterm0ination, whereas a perception of outgroup members as wild animals—who behave with emotion unchecked by reason—prescribes strategies of domestication and domination" (p. 215). Animalistic metaphors, such as referring to a group as similar to monkeys and apes, perhaps allows for more inhuman treatment in addition to being an ugly thing to say. Goff, Eberhardt, Williams, and Jackson (2008) found that subliminally priming White research participants with words related to apes led them to see police violence toward Black men as more justified. This effect did not occur when an animal unrelated to the stereotype (such as a tiger) was primed. There was also no effect of priming with "ape" if the person being subdued by the officers was White. In another experiment looking at real cases tried in the United States, Goff et al. found that newspaper stories concerning Blacks convicted of capital crimes, relative to stories of Whites convicted of capital crimes, contained more language using metaphors to apes. Additionally, the more ape-like the language used in the article, the more likely that person was to receive the death penalty. Glaser et al. (2015) worry that these types of findings can impact verdicts, as well as sentencing (punishment). If Black Americans are seen as less human and unworthy of humane treatment in punishment, then this can mitigate any concern a juror might have over a guilty verdict. While the possibility of extreme punishment may temper desires to convict, this may be less of a concern with White jurors' verdicts toward Black men.

Finally, dehumanizing a person by ascribing them *superhuman qualities* can also have negative consequences. For example, in medical research reviewed above it has been shown that there is a perception that the typical Black person is less sensitive to pain (followed by the typical Hispanic person) when compared to the typical White person (Hoffman, Trawalter, Axt, & Oliver, 2016; Wander et al., 2014). Waytz, Hoffman, and Trawalter (2014) showed that White participants have implicit associations of Black men to superhuman qualities (such as strength), as well as explicit beliefs that link the two. Most importantly, these beliefs predicted the degree to which participants believed a Black man could withstand pain. This can contribute to feeling that they need less treatment, even given greater levels of punishment. While such empirical findings are somewhat new, history is replete with examples of Black men being ascribed greater strength and speed; not as a compliment but as a signal of the need to subdue and control. In a 2014 opinion piece for *Slate* (Bouie, 2014) entitled "Michael Brown Wasn't a Superhuman Demon" (in the wake of the killing of Michael Brown in Ferguson, Missouri), Jamelle Bouie describes a dehumanizing characterization of Brown by the officer who shot him:

[The officer's] physical description of Brown . . . describes the "black brute," a stock figure of white supremacist rhetoric in the lynching era of the late 19th and early 20th centuries. . . . To the white public, the "black brute" was a menacing, powerful creature who could withstand the worst punishment. Likewise, in northern papers, it was easy to find stories of "giant negroes" who "spread terror" and rampaged through urban centers. That image never went away; it lingers in crack-era stories of superpowered addicts and teenaged super-predators as well as rhetoric around other victims of police brutality.

Implicit Prejudice and Arousal

Several lines of research emerging in this century have focused on the arousal that is created by implicit prejudice, and the negative impact of that arousal. One line of work, already reviewed in Chapter 5, looks at an interesting form of arousal that occurs when two people in a cross-race interaction observe a *third person* acting in a prejudiced way. Prejudiced-confirming behavior from a third party is proposed to trigger identity threat in each of the two observers, making their own interaction more fraught. For example, imagine a White woman and a Black woman engaged in an interaction when they together see a third person. What if the third person is a White woman acting in a racist way? What if the third person is a Black woman affirming her group's negative stereotype? There is the possibility that the behavior of this unrelated third person will impact how the interaction among the original two people unfolds. Each member of the interaction can experience arousal over concern with their partner attaching the negative stereotypes embodied by the third person to their own interpersonal exchange. This heightened arousal has been shown to alter behavior so that negative stereotypes are downplayed or negated during the exchange. Importantly, it has also been shown to cause a decrease in the desire to interact again—avoidance of the other-race interaction partner in the future, all because of the behavior of an observed third party (e.g., Taylor et al., 2018; Taylor, Yantis, Bonam, & Hart, 2021; Taylor, Yantis, & Valladares, 2023).

Even without observing a racist act, cross-race interactions are arousing, particularly if at least one member of the interaction is concerned with bias (e.g., Blascovich et al., 2001; Kawakami et al., 2009; Vorauer & Kumhyr, 2001). As Richeson and Shelton (2007) illustrate, the member of the dominant group in the interaction might be aroused over concerns of being perceived in a socially undesirable way and wanting to regulate and monitor their actions so as not to seem biased. Simultaneously, the member of the less powerful group might be concerned about detecting whether their partner is treating them in a biased way and monitoring for disparate or unfair treatment. They might additionally be concerned about whether their own behavior might be affirming any negative stereotypes held toward the group, and thus damaging the group reputation (what was described in Chapter 5 as *stereotype threat*; e.g., Murphy & Taylor, 2012; Spencer et al., 1998; Steele, 1997). The anxiety created in such situations could emerge simply from the act of thinking about the fact that others could be thinking about stereotypes. Vorauer, Main, and O'Connell (1998) use the term *meta-stereotyping* to refer to the fact that people think about the stereotypic ways other people think about them: "a person's beliefs regarding the stereotypes that outgroup members hold about them." Meta-stereotyping is an anxiety unique to cross-group interaction and can create arousal that impacts those interactions specifically. In same-group interactions one feels like an individual, but in cross-group interactions one feels perceived as a group member, and subject to the meta-stereotypes. This heightens the arousal associated with being the target of prejudice (e.g., Frey & Tropp, 2006).

Because meta-stereotypes reflect what one believes others think about one's group, they shape the goals that one adopts in the interaction and how one behaves (e.g., Bergsieker, Shelton, & Richeson, 2010; Dupree & Fiske, 2019; Purdie-Vaughn & Eibach, 2008). For example, Shelton et al. (2005) found that Black participants' meta-stereotypes led them to perform compensatory behaviors—such as an increased disclosure of personal information—designed to counteract the prejudice they presumed to exist in their White interaction partner. One study took advantage of roommate pairings among first-year college students so that same-race versus cross-race roommates could be compared. Each day an electronic diary entry was made and these revealed that members of a minority group engaged in more self-disclosure with a White roommate, hoping that the disclosure would disprove the negative stereotype of the group. Taylor et al. (2018) showed that this motivation to disprove the meta-stereotype is greater when imagining what it would be like to witness stereotypically negative acts from a potential interaction partner. Even if such compensatory attempts to disprove the stereotype are effective as a way to manage a stereotype, it comes at the cost of making the interaction less authentic, making the person feel constantly aroused, and putting one in a chronic state of needing to regulate the arousal, which is difficult (e.g., Richeson, Trawalter, & Shelton, 2005).

WHY ARE STEREOTYPES EASILY ACTIVATED?

We simply do not have the time or capacity to think as deeply as we would like about each person we encounter. There is too much information assaulting the senses from moment to moment. Does this mean we do not think about them? No. We think by using stereotypes that quickly simplify the complexity. Chapters 1 and 2 attempted to establish the normalcy and speed of the cognitive processing through which meaning is produced, with Chapter 3 establishing its automaticity. Chapter 10 established that the activation of stereotypes can occur efficiently, with no nefarious motives. The perceived person is attended to, identified, and categorized as an instance of a concept we have previously encountered, our knowledge of which is stored in memory and retrieved from memory to allow us to understand the person who currently faces us. Thus, our understanding of people and the world around us is dependent on associating each new event with what is stored in memory. *Stereotype activation* occurs well within a second of seeing the person, and usually without realizing we have done so. People low in prejudice and high in prejudice will each pull stereotypes out of memory immediately upon seeing a person, without realizing they have done so. Once this information is activated in our mind, and because it gets there without us realizing *we placed it there*, it appears to us that the information was suggested to us by the person we have encountered. We naturally confuse the qualities that sit ready to be used in our mind with the qualities that the other person possesses. We infer: "If I'm thinking 'athletic,' it must be because he is athletic." We do not realize that spreading activation caused us to think "athletic" merely because we saw a person from a group with the stereotypic quality of athleticism associated with it (e.g., Higginbotham et al., 2021).

Examples of stereotype activation occurring outside awareness and without intent were provided in Chapters 4 and 10.[3] Based on such findings, Devine (1989) proposed that stereotype activation was *automatic*. By this, Devine meant stereotype activation could not be prevented, and occurs given the mere presence of a group member (as illustrated in Chapter 10, Figure 10.3). Devine stated: "[A stereotype] is a well-learned set of associations that is *automatically* activated in the presence of a member (or symbolic equivalent) of the target group. The model holds that this unintentional activation is equally strong and equally inescapable for high- and low-prejudice persons" (p. 6).

However, before settling on the conclusion that the activation of a stereotype is uncontrollable and inevitable, let us remember two important methodological points about Devine's research. First, the experiment only tests to see whether the negative stereotype is activated after exposing people to words that are part of the group stereotype (e.g., "poor," "lazy") in addition to the group label ("Black"). Thus, this is not a case of being in "the presence" of a group member, but of the stereotype itself being directly triggered through the presentation (albeit subliminally) of the very traits comprising the stereotype. It is true that both low-prejudice and high-prejudice people have the stereotype activated, but this does not seem like an adequate test of whether low-prejudice and high-prejudice people *never differ in their implicit processing* whenever they see a group member. It might be that, for low-prejudice people, the presence of a group member would not trigger the negative stereotype but trigger a positive stereotype (and Lepore & Brown, 1997, provide evidence for this). It also might be that while implicit processes require that what is most strongly associated with the group be activated, for a person who is low in prejudice a stereotype may not be what is most strongly associated with the group (as shown by Blair & Banaji, 1996; Moskowitz et al., 1999). There is no reason to assume the cultural stereotype is what is most strongly linked to the category, or that activation of this stereotype is uncontrollable.

A second methodological point is that Devine (1989) concludes that low-prejudice people cannot control stereotype activation based on only one method for identifying such people (the use of what is known as the Modern Racism Scale). This reasoning, however, is flawed. The fact that one group of people (those labeled as low in prejudice by this one scale) do not control this process (or even dozens of illustrations of groups of people who do not exert control) does not mean that stereotype activation can never be controlled, or that this group of people *cannot be taught to*. Hundreds of examples of lack of control do not prove it is uncontrollable, and it would only take one illustration of control to show that the process is not automatic. An illustration of such willful control over stereotype activation was first provided by Moskowitz et al. (1999). We will turn to address this issue of how to control stereotype activation in Chapter 13.

The point being made here is subtle: we are arguing that the activation of a stereotype occurs often, and it occurs efficiently and outside awareness. This can lead it to have many undesired consequences, and we turn to reviewing the pernicious influence of stereotype activation shortly. However, this should not be taken to mean the process is uncontrollable and that we are always doomed to trigger stereotypes each time we see a person. It does not need to be an *automatic* process to be a ubiquitous biasing influence, damaging to many. It simply needs to be an implicit process that we do not intend or see. Rather than continue this subtle debate about whether the process is efficient and unintended versus automatic, let us turn instead to a question that underscores each of these points: Why should stereotype activation occur so easily? We elaborate here on the functional nature of stereotypes as a reason for their implicit activation.

Stereotypes Are Functional: Stereotype Activation as a Tool to Serve an End

Lippmann (1922) introduced the term "stereotype" as a neutral cognitive step required to survive in a complex world, one that throws information toward us at ever-increasing speeds. In his famous 1907 essay on pragmatism, William James called this bombardment of information "a motley which we have to unify by our wits" (p. 76). In a world where the speed of life is overwhelming, and information comes at us in ever-widening forms and needs to be processed and made sense of quickly, how do we deal with the overload? Chapters 2 and 10 revealed that we use schemas and accessible constructs, a view summarized by Bargh and Pietromonaco (1982):

> The social perceiver is continuously confronted with a formidable array of environmental information to interpret. Bruner (1957, 1958) was one of the first to recognize that this information is manageable only by selectively attending to certain features of the stimulus field and by further reducing this limited range of information by assigning it to cognitive *categories*. . . . The relative accessibilities of these categories, therefore, partly determine the selection and interpretation of social information. (p. 437)

We have knowledge awaiting to greet and absorb the bombardment, organizing it, defining it, structuring it, giving it meaning—sense. Stereotypes are one such type of schema, one kind of accessible knowledge, that deliver for a perceiver the experience of sufficient understanding. In this definition, a stereotype is not emotionally charged with any of the negative connotation the word has taken on in the vernacular but described in a way best likened to a tool that people can pull out of a "mental toolbox" to sort out the "sensation overload" that bombards us every second (e.g., Gilbert & Hixon, 1991). One function of stereotypes, therefore, is that they allow us to absorb and organize more information; to produce meaning and expectations from complex stimuli using less effort than when a stereotype does not exist. Of course, they also allow us to fill in the gaps when there is little information, making it a very flexible tool that can serve us at times when information is both overabundant and underwhelming in its informational value.

Macrae, Milne, et al. (1994) provide a nice illustration of how stereotypes allow us to process more information and to remember more information during times of overabundance. They asked research participants to watch a computer monitor and use the traits that were being presented about a person to form an impression of that person. It was arranged so that 10 traits about a person would appear, and then 10 traits about another person would appear, and so on. For each set of traits, half of the traits provided were consistent with a stereotype. For example, all people would be told to form an impression of John and were given the traits *rebellious, aggressive, dangerous, dishonest, untrustworthy,* lucky, observant, modest, optimistic, and curious. The italicized traits were all consistent with the stereotype of a "skinhead." Participants learned many such sets of traits about several different stereotyped groups. The key to this experiment is that the participants were not all given these stereotypic labels. Half of them were told that John was a skinhead (and the stereotyped groups for all the other people they learned about), but half of the participants had to learn this abundance of information without the stereotypic label being provided. Therefore, for half of the participants the category label would serve as an organizing structure to make sense out of the many traits. Macrae, Milne, et al. predicted that, if present, stereotypes would enhance performance on the task and allow people to remember more traits about each person. This is what they found. Accurate memory for the qualities learned about each person (their 10 traits) was better if research participants used stereotypes during impression formation.

Another function of stereotypes is that they allow us to be flexible in resource allocation—that is, even though we can process more information with a stereotype, this processing is also made easier by the use of the stereotype. It requires less cognitive effort. Stereotypes save our limited cognitive resources to be used if needed elsewhere. Tajfel (1969) stated that the effort used to pursue meaning "works within the limits imposed by the capacities of the individual" (p. 79), and "for reasons of cognitive economy [meaning] will tend toward as much simplification as the situation allows for" (p. 92). However, despite it being described as economy seeking, the mind is not like a nation's economy. A national economy can spend more than its resources and exist in a state of debt. The mind must always operate within a balanced budget. We do not have more resources to expend than that which we have, and those resources must be utilized to their fullest extent. Thus, people evolve strategies that tend to work when there is too much information for our limited system to process completely (even if the result is not 100% accurate). They attempt to get solutions and make judgments that are sufficiently good, and to the extent that less effort can accomplish this, less effort is used. But if people are being economical, surely there must be some *savings* that can be observed. The resources that are not being used when one is using a stereotype on a first task must be available and able to aid in the performance of a second task. This is a type of mental economy that is adaptive. Stereotypical thinking on one task would allow one to dedicate greater cognitive effort on another task. For example, when working on two tasks simultaneously, the cognitive load associated with this multi-tasking makes it difficult to succeed on either task. This is a resource allocation problem. If a stereotype is used to work on one of the tasks, making it more economical, this would "free up" energy that could help one perform the other task. One could transfer mental effort saved on one task to the other.

In support of this, Macrae, Milne, et al. (1994) showed that stereotypes not only help people remember more information but the ease of doing so allows perceivers to put greater effort into a second task. As mentioned above, research participants performed a task of forming an impression of a person based on 10 traits presented about that person. What had not been revealed in describing that experiment was that participants also simultaneously performed a *second* task that had them listening to a recorded description of the geography and economy of Indonesia, a topic that they did not know much, if anything, about. Given this set of events two things should occur. First, people with stereotypic labels should be able to remember more traits, and we saw this result above. Second, even though they are doing better on this first task, they should also do better on the second task. The savings in effort from relying on the stereotype can be used to put toward the other task of learning about Indonesia. As predicted, the participants who were provided with a stereotypic label had *both* better memory for the traits and better performance on the test about Indonesia. A savings from using a stereotype was spent on another task that also required mental effort. The stereotype served as a *tool* that facilitated processing of a separate and unrelated task.

Sherman (2001) argued that especially when processing resources are scant and conditions of cognitive load exist, we rely on stereotypes to help process detailed behavioral information about specific individuals. The stereotype functions to make the processing of some information easier: stereotype-consistent information. However, this does not mean it operates as a filter that disregards everything except such consistent information. As with the Macrae, Milne, et al. (1994) research, if stereotypes make the processing of consistent information easier, this should provide a savings that can be applied to other information that is less easily interpreted. Stereotypes allow for the *flexible distribution of resources*, thus creating both stability and plasticity in information processing. By plasticity it is meant that the system is able to update itself. Paradoxically, the time spent easily processing the stereotype-consistent information allows for the processing of inconsistent information. This distribution of processing resources to the inconsistent information allows for that information to be stored in memory for one to return to at a later time, when resources are no longer taxed (e.g., Nosofsky, Palmeri, & McKinley, 1994; Schank, 1982). At that time one can make adjustments to one's concepts and perhaps update a stereotype based on the stored information (e.g., Sherman, Klein, Laskey, & Wyer, 1998). Even though in the moment it may appear as if only the consistent information has been processed, looking deeper can reveal that much attention had also been paid to the stereotype-inconsistent information because the stereotype being used allowed one the flexibility to do so.

To illustrate, consider a series of experiments conducted by Sherman, Lee, et al. (1998). Research participants read stereotypeconsistent and inconsistent information about a target person (Bob Hamilton) who was first identified as belonging to a stereotyped group (e.g., he is identified as a priest). Half of the people read the behavioral descriptions while under cognitive load, while half had full access to their cognitive resources. A first experiment assessed the amount of time participants spent reading the information provided for them. The results revealed no differences when cognitive load did not exist. However, when people were under cognitive load, they spent a greater amount of time reading *inconsistent* (a priest who shoved his way to a center seat in a movie theater) versus consistent information (a priest who gave a stranger a quarter). Participants seemed to be directing attention to the inconsistent information when they were under cognitive load, devoting greater resources to the encoding of inconsistent information. In another experiment, they once again had participants, half of whom were under cognitive load, read stereotypeconsistent and inconsistent information about a priest (e.g., "swore at the salesgirl"). Participants were then asked to identify words flashed very briefly on a computer screen. The extent to which participants had attended to details was measured by their ability to later identify words that had appeared in the sentences they had seen (e.g., identifying the word "salesgirl"). Once again, attention to details of the inconsistent information was evident, even when participants were under cognitive load. In opposition to filtering out the inconsistencies, people were found to have better attention to details for them, even under cognitive load. When resources were taxed in this way, stereotypes eased the processing of consistent information, thus allowing people to *attend carefully* to inconsistent information, and to *more thoroughly encode the details* of the inconsistent information (e.g., Sherman, 2001; Sherman et al., 1998; Sherman & Frost, 2000).

A third function of stereotyping is that they create expectations and predictions that prepare us for action. We see a person, and without knowing it the stereotypes of the group to which that person belongs are triggered in our mind. They are not only seen but immediately seem to have certain qualities that the stereotype dictates. When I say the word "chair" an image or snapshot immediately comes to your mind that contains the features of the chair (it has legs and a back, maybe arms), as well as your beliefs about the uses of a chair (to an adult it can be sat on, to a child jumped on as well). Such knowledge is extremely helpful, since it prevents you from needing to figure out what each and every chair you encounter is, and what it might be used for. Instead, when you see a chair you immediately know what it is and how to act toward it. The same is true of social groups. When we see a French cousin, we can know instinctively to greet her by kissing each cheek, yet know this would be inappropriate as a way to greet her French boss, who is a stranger. If I meet a job candidate who wears a yarmulke, my knowledge of Judaism would lead me to avoid the restaurant that serves largely pork and shellfish when choosing a location for a dinner meeting. To make sense of the world as if we were experiencing it anew each time we encountered it would be a highly inefficient way to build a human. There are features that experience has taught us are associated with a group, and there are customs and rules we believe drive the behavior of group members. Knowing these features and customs, and having them triggered when we encounter a group member is useful; it tells us how to behave appropriately. Just like with a chair. We do not need to (consciously) think what it means to be French, a woman, or Jewish each time we see a person who belongs to one of these groups.

Though serving a function, the stereotype could be wrong. The Jewish job candidate may eat shellfish regularly. But the stereotype can be correct and help to efficiently select appropriate behavior. Stereotypes, like our knowledge of anything, deliver to us beliefs and inferences, a snapshot that is delivered in the blink of an eye, at speeds so fast we do not even know they were delivered. This enables a stereotype to allow us to know what to think and how to act—directing what we do, navigating us through a complex world. As Allport (1954) said, stereotypes "facilitate perception and conduct . . . [they] make our adjustment to life speedy, smooth, and consistent" (p. 21). Though our reactions seem unguided, instinctive, and absent of reason, we were still thinking—we merely were not aware of the ways in which we were thinking. We use stereotypes without consciously intending, without awareness, when hurried, and when overwhelmed by the amount of information present. By efficiently delivering beliefs, we feel confident we have control; that we know what is to be expected and what is appropriate for us to do in a situation.

While the definition of stereotype is not linked to its accuracy, the functionality of any given stereotype hinges on its *accuracy* and the ability to help to prepare us to act appropriately. For example, medical doctors should have categories for types of diseases so they know the associated symptoms to look for, and to know which tests to run. Additionally, as Moskowitz, Stone, and Childs (2012) point out, medical doctors believe it is beneficial to have stereotypes about patient groups since there are medical conditions that have higher prevalence among some social groups than others. Many doctors believe that base rates can be used to factually link specific groups with epidemiological evidence. For example, Moskowitz et al. asked doctors to identify medical conditions that pose a higher threat to African Americans, and more than 75% agreed that hypertension and sickle cell anemia are seen by the medical community as representing an acute threat to African Americans. Moskowitz et al. used a reaction time task to show that stereotypic diseases such as hypertension do come to mind when White medical doctors (their participants) were subliminally exposed to the face of a Black man (but not when exposed to a White man's face). If accurate, it would be functional for a doctor to have this stereotype triggered when they meet with an African American patient so that they are reminded to screen for these known threats that have a genetic link to the group. Unfortunately, Moskowitz et al. also found that along with this epidemiologically accurate information being associated with the group (and triggered upon the subliminal image being presented), the doctors also associated other stereotypically negative qualities with the group that were not medically accurate (such as drug use, obesity, and HIV infection, which while stereotypically associated with Black men, were not statistically more prevalent among them). The stereotype was triggered to serve a function, but this meant increasing the prevalence of not only the accurate beliefs but the inaccurate ones.

Stereotypes Having a Useful Function
Does Not Mean People Function Usefully

When discussing the functions of stereotypes in the classroom, a student will usually object and ask, "but where do we draw the line? How can you say stereotypes are like knowledge about chairs? When have we crossed from having useful knowledge to false beliefs?" The answer is simple: There is no line to cross. A stereotype is like any other category of knowledge you possess—it is just knowledge about a class of people instead of a class of objects, like chairs. The definition of a stereotype says nothing about how good the content of a particular stereotype is, or more specifically, how accurate it is. By definition, a stereotype can be knowledge about that class, which is 100% accurate. Of course, it can also be riddled with half-truths and outright inaccuracies. For example, the stereotype of African Americans is not limited to facts such as members of the group having ancestry linked to Africa, or their large numbers in North America having its origins in brutal and forced immigration through the slave trade, or individuals in this group having a genetic makeup predisposing them to the disease sickle cell anemia. It includes erroneous beliefs such as Blacks are genetically predisposed to having qualities such as inferior intellect, violence, and laziness. Yet we may fail to see these beliefs as wrong, or, further, we may fail to see that we even possess or use these erroneous beliefs, believing instead our stereotypes to be filtered of these inaccuracies (e.g., Moskowitz et al., 2011).

But once again, this is true of any knowledge you have about any category of things, even chairs. You could go to sit on a chair only to learn it (1) could not support your weight, or (2) has a back that is not meant to be leaned against leaving you toppled over backward on the floor, or (3) is not meant to be stood on and jumped on as your schema when a child may have suggested, or (4) was not a chair at all, but a piece of modern art in the museum. Stereotypes have taken on a negative meaning because so many of our stereotypes have developed in inaccurate ways. But this is not the problem of the stereotype as a type of cognitive process but a problem with a perceiver's use of a stereotype; it is a problem with one's goals and motivations. If one could develop more accurate knowledge, the stereotype would be less maligned. Without doubt the stereotype is a shortcut that does not consider the full complexity of an individual member of the category. But the accuracy of the shortcut could still be quite high. The problem is that the accuracy is often quite low—hence, our sense that stereotypes are not good. We have taken a potentially useful tool and turned it into a damaging force.

That is, the reason people are resistant to hearing about how stereotypes are useful is because of the insistent knowledge they have learned about stereotypes being harmful, and the point just made that the stereotypes we learn are often riddled with inaccuracy. The notion that one might be constantly engaging in the harmful activity of inaccurately foisting negative beliefs on another person is difficult to accept or see as useful. Our culture has been telling us we should eradicate stereotypes. This information about stereotypes is also correct. Despite the stereotype *in theory* being a useful tool, *in practice* this tool is often used in a harmful way, one rising to the level of a serious social problem. The harm comes from the *inaccuracy* of certain stereotypes, with incorrect negative, and opportunity-constraining, beliefs about a group being delivered just as efficiently and invisibly as useful and accurate information. Stereotypes serve the same function whether accurate or not, and our reliance on them as a way of making sense of the world presents a somewhat ubiquitous way we can be incorrectly judging and treating people without realizing we are doing so. It remains an unfortunate fact that in most cultures there are power dynamics and economic forces at play that socialize members of the culture to accept inaccurate beliefs about groups within the culture that can then influence how members of the culture think about individuals from these stigmatized groups. This happens both efficiently and invisibly. A stereotype is useful only if the beliefs comprising it are largely true. It represents a ubiquitous threat to the social order when the beliefs are wrong.

This reality that stereotypes are harmful is not inconsistent with their functional nature. These two seemingly contradictory ideas are compatible. Spoiler alert—the movie *2001: A Space Odyssey* begins not in space, but on earth, with primitive creatures discovering tools. The tools help them to dig and hunt and are useful in a variety of ways. Of course, one way is to bludgeon other creatures, and it is not long until the useful tools are being used to kill other members of the species. The movie then cuts to the future where another useful tool that had been created, the computer, is also trying to kill members of the species that created the tool. A stereotype may be a tool that has function, but misuse and inappropriate overuse can lead to danger for members of the species. We turn next to examining *how* the ease of stereotype activation can cause harm.

THE USE OF IMPLICITLY ACTIVATED STEREOTYPES

We have already reviewed many examples showing an accessible stereotype's influence on judgments and attributions. For example, Devine (1989) showed that people judge a person to be more hostile following the activation of the stereotype of African Americans. Darley and Gross (1983) showed a student was judged to be less intelligent when the stereotype of poor people was activated. Duncan (1976) illustrated how the same ambiguous shove is seen differently if the stereotype of Black men is activated (it is seen as an aggressive act) versus the stereotype of White men (it is seen as a playful act). Banaji et al. (1993) showed that men with an implicit stereotype of women triggered through a first task later judged a woman in a more stereotypic way. Inzlicht et al. (2008) showed that emotionally ambiguous facial features in men are interpreted as displaying more contempt when female research participants have accessible stereotypes of men. Using the shooter task, Sadler, Correll, Park, and Judd (2012) showed that when the stereotype of Black men was activated, White research participants (1) felt a greater sense of threat, (2) were more likely to shoot when a man was not holding a gun, and (3) were faster to shoot when a man was holding a gun (vs. an innocuous object). And the more strongly the stereotype is activated, the more powerful the influence can be. Correll et al. (2007) found that the three types of effects on the shooter task just listed were dramatically increased when the activation was strengthened. For example, in one experiment this was done by asking participants to first read a newspaper article describing violent criminals who were all Black men and then perform the task.

All of these illustrations, reviewed with complete detail earlier in the book, reveal how insidious stereotyping can be, even in low-prejudice people. Simply by virtue of knowing a stereotype, a person can have that stereotype triggered by merely seeing a person from the group. They end up judging that person in a stereotype-confirming way, confining them to a box and potentially limiting that person's opportunities, without realizing they have engaged in any biased processing at all. Stereotyping can happen fully outside of awareness with no malicious intent. Before turning to other ways in which stereotypes influence us, we review a few more detailed examples showing an impact on attributional reasoning and judgment.

Taylor and Jaggi (1974) performed what was perhaps the first experimental illustration of how stereotypes are sustained and confirmed by the types of judgments we form. Their Hindu research participants in southern India were asked to evaluate Muslim men performing either positive or negative behavior in four different contexts—such as giving shelter to someone in a rain storm (or failing to do so), or helping someone who was injured (vs. not helping). For each behavior the participants rated what caused the Muslim man in the story to act as they had. Participants could choose from among a list of internal and external causes. The findings reveal a pattern of biased judgments that confirmed the existing negative stereotypes that Hindus in that region held toward Muslims. Judgments that blamed the person were more likely to be used to explain the negative behavior of a Muslim (denying help to an injured person) as opposed to positive behavior (giving shelter in a storm). Thus, negative behavior was seen as caused by the traits and goals of the person, whereas positive behaviors were attributed to external pressures that forced the Muslim to act positively. Pettigrew (1979) called this bias to confirm stereotypes with attributional reasoning the *ultimate attribution error*: a strategic preference for using traits to explain behavior that keeps stereotypic beliefs in place. "Observers often employ external, situational attributions to explain 'away' positive behaviors of members of disliked groups" (p. 464). Just as Heider (1958) described a similar bias to protect self-esteem, here we see a motive to protect positive views held about liked groups and negative views held about disliked groups. If a disliked group engages in positive behavior, or a preferred group engages in negative behavior, we judge it as caused by something external to them, such as luck, or pressure to act that way. We also confirm a stereotype if the behavior is consistent by seeing it as caused by a disposition, such as a disliked group's undesirable traits (see also Sherman et al., 2005).

The courtroom provides a fertile ground for stereotyping to impact attributions. The prosecuting attorney is attempting to convince the jury that they should attribute the cause of the crime to something internal to the person being charged. Judgmental biases in judging the causes for events could play an important role in determining the outcomes of a trial. In Chapter 6 we described how stereotypes about people with baby faces can impact the outcomes of criminal proceedings. Are defendants for whom we have a negative stereotype more likely to be judged harshly or found guilty? Two types of evidence were already presented in this chapter when discussing dehumanization. Goff et al. (2008) showed that priming aspects of a stereotype led to harsher punishments in a criminal case that participants were asked to evaluate. Glaser et al. (2015) showed not only punishment but conviction likelihood was impacted by stereotypes.

When we have strong stereotypes we may no longer be as likely to do our job as jurors and weigh the evidence as carefully as possible, falling prey instead to the bias to rely on judgments based on stereotypes. Bodenhausen and Wyer (1985) examined whether people use stereotypes as a heuristic on which they base their decisions. Decisions in a trial include (1) how to interpret the evidence (which is likely to involve a great deal of ambiguity and be open to interpretation and subjectivity), (2) whether to assign a verdict of guilt or innocence, (3) how to punish the criminal act, (4) the likelihood of recidivism, and (5) the willingness to grant parole. There are at least two broad ways such decisions can be guided by stereotypes. First, the stereotype may be immediately triggered by the group membership of the individual on trial and used from the start as a way of making sense of the individual's action. Second, stereotypes may be turned to only after people thoroughly examined the information in a detailed and effortful way and are still left wanting for an explanation, one the stereotype can then provide (as a last resort).

To examine through what cognitive processes stereotypes are invoked—as confirmatory agents throughout, or as the last resort—Bodenhausen and Wyer (1985) asked participants to judge a defendant who was signaled to be White or Hispanic (via the name and place of birth of the alleged criminal; e.g., Juan from Puerto Rico). The crime committed by this person was also manipulated so that it was either consistent with or inconsistent with cultural stereotypes (embezzlement vs. a violent crime). They found that when a member of a stereotyped group committed an infraction that was consistent with the stereotype of that group (Puerto Rican man and a violent crime), the action was more likely to be seen as a stable quality of that person: The individual was seen as more personally responsible for those acts. The stereotype allowed the perceiver to see the crime as a more natural feature or characteristic of the criminal than when the crime was not relevant to the stereotype (Puerto Rican man and an accounting crime). This pattern suggests that the stereotype was not a last resort but distorting the perception of the evidence, making the consistent evidence seem stronger and worthy of harsher punishment. People did not simply eschew stereotypes because they were asked to be jurors and be fair observers of the evidence. Instead, when a White man and a Hispanic man both get arrested for being in a fight, the Hispanic man is judged as more likely to have been responsible, more likely to be a recidivist, and more likely to get harsher punishment with reduced opportunity for parole.

The influence of an implicitly activated stereotype is not restricted to the explicit judgments we make. Even a spontaneous trait inference (STI) can be biased by an implicit stereotype, as first suggested by Moskowitz and Uleman (1987). People will unintentionally and unknowingly infer that a member of a stereotyped group has a trait that confirms the stereotype. Otten and Moskowitz (2000) provided an illustration of this process even when the inferences being made are about minimal groups. They first assigned participants to arbitrary groups, and then had them read sentences about ingroup and outgroup members that implied negative or positive traits (such as cruel or kind). They assessed the extent to which participants formed STIs from these behaviors. Positive traits inferred about ingroup members and negative traits inferred about outgroup members were labeled as stereotype-consistent STIs. They found evidence for this pattern of implicit stereotype confirmation. Members of one's own group were inferred to have positive qualities when the same behavior from an outgroup member led to no inference.

This influence is exaggerated only when real groups, as opposed to minimal groups, are used. Both Wigboldus, Dijksterhuis, and Van Knippenberg (2003) and Ramos et al. (2012) found that STIs were biased by stereotypes. For example, participants read behaviors that implied traits, and these behaviors also contained information about group stereotypes. The people described in the sentences were identified by their occupation, such as professor, trash collector, and so on. The inference that emerged confirmed the stereotype. Specifically, participants failed to form STIs from behaviors that clearly implied the trait if the trait was inconsistent with the stereotype (such as a professor who was unintelligent). Yet they inferred the trait spontaneously from the behavior if it was consistent with a stereotype (such as a trash collector who was unintelligent). There is resistance to stereotype-inconsistent information, yet traits are easily inferred outside of awareness from the same behavior if those traits are not inconsistent with the stereotype. Yan, Wang, and Zhang (2012) showed similar findings exploring inferences made about gender. They replicated the finding that STIs were less likely to be formed when research participants read about a trait-implying behavior that was inconsistent with gender stereotypes. Together, these results show that stereotypes not only inhibit STIs when the behavior is inconsistent with the activated stereotype, but they enhance STIs when the behavior is consistent with the stereotype.

The Outgroup Homogeneity Effect (Other-Race Bias)

The 1968 movie *Planet of the Apes* attempted to be a not-so-subtle allegory on race relations. In one scene toward the end, there is an escape sequence where the human "fugitive" is told that he might just "get away" since his ape pursuers (being from a different species) will not be able to distinguish one person from the next—"you all look alike."[4] This scene only has the intended effect if most viewers have had some experience with the feeling that people who are not from one's own ethnic group seem to look similar to one another, and are harder to differentiate than people who are from one's own group. People are better at recognizing faces of members of ingroups, especially own-race faces (e.g., Hugenberg, Young, Bernstein, & Sacco, 2010). This bias extends beyond faces—we see more differentiation in our own group when it comes to beliefs. Conservatives may believe that all "liberals think alike, yet we conservatives are a diverse group with wide-ranging beliefs." Lawyers see fine distinctions in the type of law practiced—distinctions they fail to make when thinking about types of psychology practiced by psychologists (who are all seen as clinicians). The French see Americans as being "all alike," yet see themselves as subtle, complex, and highly differentiated. The phenomenon of seeing differentiation and complexity in one's ingroups, contrasted with seeing outgroups in a more undifferentiated and homogeneous manner, is known as **outgroup homogeneity**.

The basic idea is that our categories or schemas about other groups can range from being highly complex to overly simplified. When complex, we can think of many different features or subtypes that can exist within the group. When simple we tend to produce extreme evaluations and see members of the group as the same. People are more familiar with members of their own group and, therefore, have more highly differentiated categories with which to make distinctions between people (e.g., Linville, Salovey, & Fischer, 1986). When we have fewer features incorporated into our thinking about

> **Outgroup homogeneity:** When we have fewer features incorporated into our thinking about a group, and a less complex set of issues that are brought to the processes of evaluation and judgment, we see greater similarity within that group. We tend to see members of the group as homogenous and produce extreme evaluations.

a group, and a less complex set of issues that are brought to the processes of evaluation and judgment, we see greater similarity in that group and we make more extreme judgments about them based on that belief in their uniformity. Allport (1954) summarized this in stating that an outsider sees a Lutheran simply as a Lutheran, "but to an insider it makes a difference whether he is a member of one Synod or another" (p. 134).

One explanation for the outgroup homogeneity effect is that when we simply know more—have more differentiated types of information about groups to which we belong—this leads to a reduced sense of homogeneity. Linville and Jones (1980) illustrate that the amount of information alone can impact perceived extremity of a stimulus. They had research participants focus attention on either two or six features of a stimulus. They found that the participants made less extreme evaluations of the stimulus when attention was focused on six features than when focused on two features associated with the stimulus. Linville and Jones extended this to racial groups by exploring whether such exaggerated similarity among group members occurs. Instead of manipulating whether people are forced to have six versus two features to focus on, they gave participants the same stimuli and looked to see whether people naturally created more complex sets of information out of those stimuli when they believed the stimuli to describe an ingroup member versus an outgroup member. They tested the idea that White research participants have more complex sets of beliefs about White people than about Black people. Research participants each received a set of 40 cards with a trait word printed on it. Participants were asked to sort the cards so that traits that went together would be grouped with one another in the same pile. They were asked to form as many groups as they thought was necessary and to continue until they had formed all the groups they thought were important. Half of the participants were told to think of the groups being formed as representing the characteristics of White people; the other half were asked to think of them as the characteristics of Black people. As predicted, White research participants formed more piles with the cards when thinking about White people. They were able to come up with more dimensions for describing members of their own group than for describing members of the outgroup.

The logical extension of this line of reasoning is that one reason we make more extreme evaluations of members of stereotyped groups, relative to members of our own group, is because we have more simplistic and less differentiated mental representations about other groups. For example, Linville and Jones (1980) reported that people made more extreme ratings of members of an outgroup, for both positive and negative evaluations, relative to members of their own group. Their research participants were asked to play the role of an admission board member and evaluate applications to law school. Applications varied on two dimensions. They were either strong or weak, and were either submitted by a White or a Black applicant. They found that when White participants made judgments of two identical applications, they made more extreme evaluations for Black versus White applicants. A weak application was seen as weaker if submitted by a Black versus a White person, a strong application was seen as stronger. Linville and Jones posited that one reason for this difference when judging identical qualifications from two groups is the degree of complexity with which people think about the groups. Outgroup homogeneity leads White perceivers to see less nuance and more extremity in Black applicants.

Complexity in a person or group is not limited to single evaluations or individual traits. It is not just that perceivers focus on one quality of an outgroup that all members seem to have to some extreme degree, despite differentiation seen in one's own group on that dimension (such as a man's belief that all women are emotional, yet men range on this quality). Linville, Fischer, and Yoon (1996) extend this to the idea that people do not only think about groups in terms of isolated features but as clusters of many features. With this in mind, homogeneity would be represented by seeing much greater covariation among the clusters of features for some groups relative to others. They illustrate that people have greater familiarity with members of their own social groups, and this greater familiarity leads to less covariation being seen among features that describe the group. Yet for outgroups, with which they have less familiarity, there is a greater sense that there is covariation among the traits of group members (students see more covariation among the features of senior citizens, while older people see greater covariation in college students). Research participants overestimate the consistency among the traits of outgroup members. Familiarity exposes perceivers to more and more varied exemplars and counterexamples, which weakens the covariation. Lacking such familiarity with outgroups causes homogeneity being perceived in the form of greater covariation. And, when one has great familiarity with an outgroup, such perceived covariation is reduced. For example, one experiment compared the judgments made by undergraduates against students pursuing a degree as a master of business administration (MBA). The students were asked to make judgments about different types of people who work in organizations—subtypes of the business world. Students who were pursuing an MBA had more experience in the business world than undergraduate students, so they saw less covariation in the subtypes than the undergraduates (who had less experience).

This greater perceived covariation among outgroup traits, and a general lack of familiarity with the outgroup, leads to seeing the group in a more homogeneous and abstract way. The category seems to apply more broadly to all group members. In contrast, greater familiarity with the ingroup, and seeing less covariation among the traits (and more individuality) leads to seeing the ingroup less as a homogeneous category. More subtypes exist, and more emphasis is placed on specific exemplars of the group as opposed to abstractions. Outgroup homogeneity results in information being processed and stored in a category-based manner, making increased stereotyping likely (e.g., Ryan, Judd, & Park, 1996). In contrast, familiarity with the ingroup allows for ingroup information to be processed in an exemplar-based fashion, with ingroup information processed less abstractly (e.g., Ostrom, Carpenter, Sedikides, & Li, 1993; Park & Judd, 1990). This suggests that *ingroup homogeneity* should be expected under circumstances where abstraction is encouraged when processing ingroup information. This is indeed found when one strongly identifies with a group, when there is high group entitativity. This may seem counterintuitive. Given that familiarity with an ingroup usually breeds perceptions of variability, one might expect that a strong identification with an entitative group might cause greater familiarity and hence greater differentiation. Instead, it heightens the goal for affiliation with the group, and seems to cause a greater need to see similarity and homogeneity. The tendency to see ingroup homogeneity—where members of a group are perceived as a unified cluster—is increased when the perceiver is attempting to strengthen ingroup cohesion and has heightened goals of group affiliation (e.g., Castano & Yzerbyt, 1998; De Cremer, 2001; Rubin & Badea, 2012). When contrast between the ingroup and outgroup is made salient, such as when one's team defeats another team during competition, the tendency to see the ingroup as unified and homogeneous is increased (e.g., Badea, Brauer, & Rubin, 2012). Losing, or the group having an unfavorable social position produces less ingroup homogeneity (e.g., Doosje, Spears, Ellemers, & Koomen, 1999). Ingroup homogeneity in these instances reflects not a lack of familiarity but a goal of depersonalization (as described earlier in this chapter)—to see cohesion among self and group.

This perception of complexity versus differentiation is not limited to the beliefs we infer about others. This section started with a discussion of facial similarity—that the faces of outgroup members are more easily confused for one another; they look alike. When perceiving members of other groups we do not process the individuality of each face as well as we do when fixing a gaze on ingroup members. A separate line of research on the homogeneity perceived in outgroup faces, and the better ability to differentiate among ingroup faces, has been called the **other-race effect**. Working in the area of eyewitness testimony, Maclin and Malpass (2001) highlighted the importance of mistaken identification of "criminals" by eyewitnesses, a mistake that occurs more often when attempting to identify a person of another race. Meissner and Brigham (2001) report that people are 1.40 times more likely to *correctly* identify a face of the same race, and are 1.56 times more likely to *falsely* identify a face of a different race.

> **Other-race effect:** A tendency to perceive homogeneity in outgroup faces, and the better ability to differentiate among ingroup faces. We see the faces of members of other groups as similar to one another and we mistake one for the other more readily.

Why do people confuse faces from other groups? One suggested reason for the other-race effect is similar to that just described for outgroup homogeneity in beliefs. It is that people have high-quality experience with an ingroup, and this creates more expertise at differentiating the facial features. This ability is less likely to develop for perceiving outgroups with whom one has less contact (e.g., Brigham & Malpass, 1985; Meissner & Brigham, 2001). By "high-quality experience" it is meant that when people are important to us—such as people who hold power over us or on whom we rely—we not only have more contact with them but we need to differentiate among them. Thus, we rely on them in important ways that requires learning to discriminate among them in ways we do not need to for people who are less relevant to us. How would this lead to the other-race effect? It has been proposed that when we learn to differentiate among faces from our ingroup, the features that help us to distinguish one face from another become identified and relied upon. However, the features that are useful for making discriminations among faces need not be the same (on average) for one race versus another. Thus, if one learns the subtle features to distinguish among faces in one's own racial group, this skill set might leave one ill equipped to differentiate among faces of another group that varies on different features. This is one way familiarity with a group could lead to this bias.

A second potential explanation for the other-race effect is that one uses more complex criteria when engaged in same-race perception. This argues that the bias is caused by people using dimensions for identifying other-race faces that are less well-defined than the dimensions used for same-race faces. This lack of definition causes them to rely on a few stereotypic markers to a greater degree. These markers then distort the perception of the other-race faces to make them seem more uniform. Thus, it is not that they try to use the features for their own group to differentiate the other group, and this is less successful. Instead, this argument is that people develop a different and more limited set of features on which to focus, and this smaller set of features morphs the way the remaining facial features are seen: to produce greater similarity.

To test these two different processing explanations for the perceived similarity of outgroup faces, Maclin and Malpass (2001) showed participants identical faces that were ambiguous as to which group the person belonged (it was unclear if the person was African American or Hispanic). Because the faces are identical, using one set of rules about facial features to attend to the face should not matter. However, a focus on one stereotypical feature could matter tremendously if people are using different rules, and less well-defined rules, for members of outgroups (which would produce greater similarity ratings when the exact same face is labeled as an "other"). Maclin and Malpass manipulated one feature associated with the face: such as hairstyle. If a cue, such as hairstyle, signaled that the person was in an outgroup, would the face seem more similar to other faces from the same outgroup? If a cue, such as hairstyle, signaled the person was in the ingroup, would the same face now be better differentiated from other ingroup faces? They found that despite the same faces being used, a face would be less differentiated when it was thought to be an outgroup face. All that differed was whether a cue (in this case, the hair style accompanying the face) led perceivers to label the face as ingroup (Hispanic) or outgroup (Black). If a cue signaled that a face was in the outgroup, this marker led people to see the face in a stereotypic way and the same as other faces that shared the marker. If the exact same face had a cue that signaled it was an ingroup face it was better differentiated from other faces that also shared this ingroup cue. Similarly, Hugenberg et al. (2010) show that the other-race effect emerges from a perceiver selectively attending to categorical information (skin tone) when processing outgroup faces, but when processing ingroup faces they use greater differentiation.

Brown, Uncapher, Chow, Eberhardt, and Wagner (2017) provide neuroscientific evidence in support of there being greater differentiation in the features attended to when processing same-race faces. They find that memory biases in the perception of other-race (vs. same-race) faces arise from the differential allocation of attention as measured by functional magnetic resonance imaging (fMRI). They examined activity in a large-scale frontoparietal network known to be associated with top-down attention, using fMRI to detect activity in the superior frontal sulcus, superior parietal lobule, and medial intraparietal sulcus. They found that these elements of the frontoparietal network were differentially active when encoding same-race versus other-race faces, and this greater attentional engagement with the face-processing regions to same-race faces predicted better memory for those faces. Their research not only suggests that allocation of attention helps in better memory for same-race faces but suggests that people are less motivated to process other-race faces. They argue that people more superficially process outgroups faces, and that this can be reflected by activity in a different part of the frontoparietal network known to be associated with cognitive control. To explore the role of control they used fMRI to detect activity in the inferior frontal sulcus and lateral intraparietal sulcus. They found that these elements of the frontoparietal network were predictive of memory failure for other-race faces. They conclude that their "results provide novel evidence that failure to encode other-race faces is characterized by reduced engagement of parietal cognitive control resources" (p. 3). People seem to process other-race faces more superficially due to lack of motivation to do otherwise.

In support of the bias being somewhat controllable by attention and goals, Van Bavel et al. (2011) argued that the other-race effect could be produced even when faces were arbitrarily made self-relevant by using a minimal group procedure to label faces as ingroup or outgroup. Goals can be created in the moment that reproduce the effect, presumably by shifting the allocation of attention and control. To test this, they explored the very early stages of face processing by examining an area of the fusiform gyrus that is known as the fusiform face area (FFA), where the cognitive processes involved in facial recognition originate. The FFA is known to be associated with the other-race effect such that greater activity is seen in this brain region when processing faces of the same race as opposed to other-race faces (e.g., Brown et al., 2017; Lieberman, Hariri, Jarcho, Eisenberger, & Bookheimer, 2005). Van Bavel et al. used fMRI to assess activity in the FFA after exposure to faces labeled members of the ingroup or the outgroup (holding race of the face constant). They found greater FFA activity for ingroup faces of minimal groups, mirroring the pattern seen when differentiating among racial groups—that is, Van Bavel et al. argue that just as people tune neurons in the FFA to encode faces of their own motivationally relevant groups, a bias to have less well-defined differentiation of outgroup faces can be seen originating in less FFA activity to such faces, even to minimally defined outgroups. Such data suggest that the bias can be shifted by a person's goals (such as a goal to identify with Group *X*) through altering how attention and cognitive control processes are allocated. Thus, while expertise can produce the bias to favor ingroup faces, the processing mechanism through which expertise likely works can be strategically used to replicate the bias in perceiving faces one is motivated to differentiate.

We end this review of outgroup homogeneity by returning to the impact of differences in facial processing on real-world judgments with great importance, such as eyewitness testimony (where the Innocence Project has reported that eyewitness misidentification contributed to the vast majority of convictions overturned by DNA testing). Vitriol, Appleby, and Borgida (2019) performed a series of studies examining fluctuations in other-race bias as a function of the perceiver's level of implicit bias. The task had White research participants judge faces in a simulated police "lineup" using different types of lineup formats (showing all of the faces in the lineup simultaneously vs. showing them sequentially). During the lineup, the participants with greater levels of racially biased attitudes were more likely to falsely identify the face of a Black man as the earlier observed criminal than they were to falsely identify the face of a White man—that is, although accurate in judging the faces of White people, they showed an extremely damaging form of bias in confusing the faces of Black men. Even among White participants who were not high in racist attitudes, a similar bias was produced when the stereotype of Black men was primed through unconscious exposure to objects relating to crime (guns, handcuffs, etc.). Of course, being at a police station to observe a lineup is likely to trigger such thoughts of crime and enhance the possibility of such other-race confusions, even among people who identify as non-racists. They found this to be especially true in simultaneous lineup presentation formats.

Stereotypic Memory

In Chapters 5 and 6 it was reviewed how not only judgment but memory could be distorted by an existing impression, such as a stereotype. How do stereotypes affect memory? First, there is evidence that while stereotype-consistent information is easily processed (e.g., Hastie & Kumar, 1979), a perceiver may use processing effort and motivated reasoning to explain away stereotype-inconsistent information. This would have the result of, ironically, making the inconsistent information especially memorable (e.g., Bodenhausen & Lichtenstein, 1987; Hastie & Park, 1986; Macrae et al., 1993). Another possibility is that rather than exerting effort to dismiss or "explain away" the inconsistencies, one uses this effort to make sense of it (e.g., Sherman, 2001; Sherman, Lee, et al., 1998). This too would make inconsistent information highly memorable. In Chapter 13 we return to discuss when and why memory for stereotype-inconsistent information is enhanced. However, let us focus here on when and why memory shows a confirmation bias.

Several experiments were reviewed in Chapter 5 that illustrated the ease with which people process information that confirms a first impression or stereotype (e.g., Bargh & Thein, 1985; Rothbart et al., 1979; Zadny & Gerard, 1974). This processing ease makes the information that is consistent with the stereotype more memorable, which helps to reaffirm and strengthen the stereotype. Another stereotype confirmation effect in memory described in Chapter 5 is when people incorrectly recall a correlation between a stereotyped group and the traits that define that stereotype. In such cases, a spurious association known as an *illusory correlation* leads to recall of a greater proportion of stereotype-consistent, compared to stereotype-irrelevant, information (e.g., Hamilton & Rose, 1980). In Chapter 10 we reviewed an experiment by Eberhardt et al. (2003) where memory for faces was distorted in a way that was consistent with a primed stereotype.

Rather than repeat a summary of these experiments that show a stereotype-confirming bias in memory, we examine one new illustration. Earlier in this chapter an experiment by Bodenhausen and Wyer (1985) was described. They explored whether participants were making stereotypic judgments of a defendant as a last resort, or whether they had been using the stereotype all along to bias how each piece of the evidence relating to the trial was perceived. The researchers reasoned that if stereotyping was a last resort, then people should have good recall for the arguments and data about the case, since they would have processed it all in a detailed and unbiased way. However, if using stereotypes all along, then people should not have been making fine-grained analyses of all of this information as it was delivered to them. They would have been processing in a superficial way, as guided by their stereotypes. Memory for these details would then be weak and the ability to detect differences in the quality of the arguments low. To examine this, Bodenhausen and Wyer had research participants read a variety of types of information in the transcripts that summarized the case. First, there was demographic information, irrelevant to why the crime occurred. Second, there was information describing events that happened after the transgression occurred, while the person was in prison. This information had nothing to do with why the transgression happened, but might be relevant to deciding about whether the person was rehabilitated and whether the transgression might occur again. Finally, there was information that described events in the person's life around the time the crime occurred that might be used to provide insight as to why it occurred. This contained some stereotype-consistent and some stereotype-inconsistent facts about the person.

If people were using stereotypes when reading these various types of information, then they should have no preferential recall for one type of information over another because they would not have been scrutinizing the information in enough detail to realize some of it is more relevant for making a good decision. However, if not stereotyping until finally using it as a last resort, then they should have been scrutinizing all the information in fine detail (as the judge instructed). The results suggested that the participants used a stereotype-based approach to evaluate the information. When the crime was consistent with a stereotype (e.g., a Hispanic man committing a violent crime) the participants were not taking the time to scrutinize the information carefully. Memory for the information was lower than when the crime being committed was inconsistent with the stereotype (e.g., a Hispanic man committing an accounting crime). Participants were superficially scanning the materials for some evidence that supports their stereotypes and using that to guide their judgment. This made memory for all the information equally poor.

Stereotyping in Shared Communication

Stereotypes not only influence how we reason about events and what we remember, they influence how we share information with other people. Research on how stereotypes are communicated draws from earlier work on the norms used in communication more generally. Grice (1967) detailed several **norms of communication** that, though not originally meant to describe the socially shared nature of stereotypes, help us to see how stereotypes could be easily shared and accepted by members of a majority group. A first rule specified in Grice's norms of communication deals with issues of *trust and truth*—people tailor communication for optimum understanding and quality, saying things they believe and have evidence to support. This norm leads to a bias to trust what we hear. Therefore, when a person shares stereotype-consistent information with us, there is a bias to believe it is true because of the norm that people generally only communicate things they believe to be true. Another rule specified by Grice enjoins people to not provide too much information or unnecessary amounts of information. Thus, a person might choose to share a stereotype because it is a simple and uncomplicated way to communicate. Schaller and Conway (2001) argue that because stereotypes are abstract and homogeneous, this type of information is easier to transmit and easier to resist being changed during the process of communication. Additionally, this clarity and simplicity makes such stereotype-consistent communication easier to be accepted. In Chapter 5 we reviewed research on *linguistic intergroup bias* (e.g., Maass et al., 1995; Wigboldus et al., 2000) showing that we use abstract language (stable personality traits) to describe behavior that is consistent with a stereotype, and in contrast use more concrete language when describing behavior that is inconsistent with our stereotypes—that is, the stereotype is shared in our communication in a simple way that implies it is descriptive of the group. What other rules, norms, or concerns that arise during communication implicate stereotypes?

> **Norms of communication:** A set of principles providing rules that govern how we speak to one another. For example, we do not expect 50% of the information encountered in newspapers, books, and conversations to be false. We follow an assumption that others are being truthful when speaking to us, and that we should be truthful.

Lyons and Kashima (2003) argue that when information is shared among people in a group there are three concerns about stereotypes that are considered: (1) we make inferences about the degree to which the people in the audience with whom we are communicating share a stereotype among one another, (2) we make inferences about our own stereotypes and how they align with the group with whom we are sharing information, and (3) the recipients of the communication make inferences about the degree to which we share their stereotypes. When there is an assumption of a shared stereotype, the presentation of information to the group is cultivated in a way that more strongly implies that the stereotype is true, and the receiver of the information will be primed to see evidence of a shared stereotype in the communication.

To explore such inferences about stereotypes that are made when communicating about outgroups, Kashima (2000) investigated the situation in which an individual has processed and remembered information inconsistent with a stereotype and how that processing impacts the sharing of that information by the individual. Kashima argues that communication processes can be a mechanism for how stereotypes are maintained, even in the face of contradictory evidence. To examine this, a serial reproduction task was used in which a narrative was communicated in a chain from one person to the next (with five people in the chain). The original information given to the first person is in the form of a narrative and contains information that is consistent with gender stereotypes, as well as information inconsistent with gender stereotypes. The hypothesis was that the first person to receive the narrative might attend to and remember the stereotype-inconsistent information (e.g., Sherman, Klein, et al., 1998). However, in reproducing the narrative to share with others they might be biased to instead emphasize the consistent elements, which are perceived to be easier to communicate based on assumptions of a shared stereotype. Each person in the chain might use a similar form of reasoning, so that as the narrative moves along the chain it becomes less representative of the stereotype-inconsistent elements, and more stereotype consistent. The prediction is that, similar to Bartlett (1932) and Allport and Postman (1947), the narrative will morph to fit the stereotype as it gets transmitted. Results showed that stereotype-inconsistent information was reproduced to a greater degree than the consistent elements at the early stages of the chain. But this pattern reversed in the later stages of the chain. The stereotype-consistent information had the advantage by the time the narrative had reached the final recipient (see Ruscher, 1998, for a review of stereotypic communication).

Lyons and Kashima (2003) point out that a stereotype can only be maintained by communication in this way if the people in the chain all share the same stereotype. Thus, as noted above, each communicator must not only share the same stereotype with the others but believe the others share in their own stereotype when preparing the communication—there must be perceived common ground (e.g., Hardin & Conley, 2001; Schaller & Conway, 1999). If this is the case, stereotype-consistent information takes on the added weight of feeling more trustworthy since it has social consensus to back it up, and inconsistent information would be less confidently held.[5]

Stereotypic Shifts in Attention

Yet another way an activated stereotype effects our cognitive processing is through the focus of attention being placed on features that distinguish a stereotyped group. Kruschke (2003) argues that when a category exists, then the learning of information relevant to a new category requires that attention be focused on the features that distinguish the new category from the original category. For example, if one knows that virus X has symptoms such as sore joints and loss of taste, and later learns about a new virus Z, attention will be focused on features of virus Z that are distinctive to it. If virus Z is marked by loss of taste and blurred vision, people associate loss of taste more with virus X, and focus attention on blurred vision as the marker of virus Z. This focused attention will lead a perceiver to exaggerate that quality and to ignore the similarities among the diseases (taste loss). Sherman et al. (2009) argue that these shifts in attention when learning about new categories explain how learning about a group can contribute to stereotyping. For example, members of the majority group in a given culture learn about the qualities that define their own group first. Typically, since they are the dominant group in the culture, the qualities used to define the group are positive. Sherman et al. argue that as a member of the majority group starts to learn about other groups in the culture—minority groups—there is a natural focus of **attention placed on those features that distinguish the groups**, rather than emphasizing the ways in which the groups overlap, or are similar. Typically, it is the negative behaviors learned about the minority group that distinguish the groups and receive close attention. This process does not require that there be real differences between the groups or

Attention placed on those features that distinguish the groups: When a category exists, learning information about a new category focuses one's attention on features that distinguish the new category from the existing category. Majority group members learn (positive) qualities defining their group first. As they learn about minority groups, there is a natural focus on negative behaviors that distinguish the groups.

that the perceiver is motivated to see the minority group negatively. The groups may share many positive features, yet the perceiver can still form highly differentiated representations of the two groups where the negative qualities of the minority are exaggerated. All that is required is one group being learned about first and being seen positively. This is not to say that people are never motivated to focus their attention differently on a minority group (e.g., Hansen, Rakhshan, Ho, & Pannasch, 2015)—such motivation is just not necessary to produce bias.

Attentional shifts not only help to create stereotypes but once a stereotype exists, attentional shifts can help to maintain and strengthen stereotypes by focusing a perceiver on stereotype-confirming information. Attention is grabbed by elements that are consistent with the stereotype. For example, Allen, Sherman, Conrey, and Stroessner (2009) found that as the strength of a stereotype increased, the focus of attention was shifted more to stereotype-confirming information versus stereotype-disconfirming information. Throughout the book, a wide variety of evidence that the attention of White research participants is unintentionally directed by stereotypes about African Americans was reviewed. One type of evidence used measures of gaze to show that attention was placed on faces of Black men under conditions of perceived threat and arousal (e.g., Bean et al., 2012; Richeson & Trawalter, 2008; Trawalter et al., 2008). Another type of evidence used fMRI data showing that attention is differentially allocated to the processing of same-race versus other-race faces (e.g., Brown et al., 2017; Lieberman et al., 2005; Van Bavel et al., 2011). Yet another type of evidence used reaction time measures to show one had been focused on stereotype-confirming information. For example, Eberhardt et al. (2004) illustrated that triggering the stereotype of African Americans leads to a heightened focus of attention to stimuli that are associated with crime (they found that the attentional threshold for consciously detecting crime-related objects in an impoverished visual environment with degraded visual images of objects was reduced after being primed with faces of Black men). While it is certainly true that when motivated to do so, perceivers can focus attention on inconsistent information (e.g., Fiske, Lin, & Neuberg, 1999), the default seems to be to focus attention on stereotype-consistent information.

THE PSYCHOLOGICAL IMPACT OF PREJUDICE AND STEREOTYPING

When one lives in a culture where stereotyping and prejudice toward one's group is pervasive, discrimination and disparities of the type described above naturally result—mortality rate differences, health differences, disparities in pay and banking loans, harsher treatment under the law, and so on. Our concern with social cognition has focused attention here on other types of disparities—those that pervade how people are judged, what we recall, how we communicate, and where we choose to focus attention. Just as members of stereotyped groups acutely feel the disparities that result from structural inequities, they also experience the impact of social cognitive biases toward their group. As discussed earlier in the book, research by Richeson and Shelton (2007) shows that cross-race interactions create a need to constantly regulate that is quite draining. Other research reviewed in Chapter 5 reveals stereotype threat causes heightened distraction and arousal that interferes with performance in domains where one would otherwise exhibit excellence (e.g., Steele, 1997). Other research shows people engaged in meta-stereotyping that can make them avoidant of being placed in situations where biases might flourish and stereotype threat might be acute (e.g., Taylor et al., 2018). One could even manage such threats—and protect self-esteem—by simply denying they exist and feeling sure that one does not face individual discrimination (e.g., Crosby, 1984).

Crocker and Major (1989) noted that stigmatized groups, as the recipient of biased evaluations, might be expected to have lower self-esteem from the barrage of negativity. Yet they report that, for example, many studies reveal that Black Americans do not have lower levels of global self-esteem than White Americans. One reason they suggest that self-esteem is not diminished in stigmatized groups is because individual members of such groups use the discounting principle as described by Kelley (1972b)—that is, members of stigmatized groups attribute the barrage of negative feedback received not to their personal traits but to the prejudice of the majority group. They discount the feedback, and attribute it to the racism of others. We turn toward examining a sampling of ways people who are the targets of bias attempt to regulate and manage such bias.

Attributional Ambiguity

Much of this book has been about certainty and confidence—perceivers desiring to know others and understand their actions so they can use inferences about others' intent to make predictions about how to respond. The ability to perform this important chain of cognitive events is undermined when the person doing the perceiving suspects that the person whose behavior is trying to be understood may be guided by prejudice and stereotypes. The prejudice and stereotypes of others creates uncertainty in a perceiver, causing the perceiver to question whether the behavior they are observing is genuine. For example, if someone displays kindness to you, one might wonder whether this corresponds with a kind attitude toward you, or whether the person is actually biased and has true feelings of hostility. Perhaps the kindness is simply an expression of social desirability concerns that are masking the person's actual prejudice? In another example, suppose a person acts in a way that is supportive. One might wonder whether this benevolence is indicative of confidence in one's ability, or does it reflect that they perceive you as incompetent and childlike, requiring help due to lack of ability? Many people live under a cloud of such uncertainty, where they can never truly trust the inferences made about others' intentions and traits. If stigmatized, one knows that prejudice and stereotypes in others is pervasive, and sees their bias as an obstacle to basic needs to have meaning, feel in control, and be able to predict.

Crocker, Voelkl, Testa, and Major (1991) argue that the need to protect the self against chronic negativity has the unfortunate consequence of making one generally uncertain as to why others act as they do. A positive response from others might indicate genuine feedback about one's skill, or it could be benevolent bias that reflects a paternalistic form of support. Uncertainty emerges from negative feedback as well. If one is criticized, have they actually performed poorly and need to work harder and fix the flaws, or is the person providing feedback simply a racist? Stigmatization can create this type of uncertainty known as **attributional ambiguity**, where the true cause for a person's behavior is unknown due to the plausibility of bias as an explanation.

> **Attributional ambiguity:** A state where a stigmatized person is unable to form a confident attribution for the actions they observe and the feedback they receive due to multiple plausible causes. The true cause can either be the feedback's accuracy or prejudice. Living in a society where bias is prevalent makes each attribution plausible.

Such ambiguity might lead to an expectation of being treated in a biased way, and perhaps a form of confirmation bias where one sees evidence for bias in the behavior of others. For example, Crocker et al. (1991) had African American students receive feedback from a White evaluator. Half of the participants believed the evaluator knew their race (because they were watching them through a one-way mirror), and half believed the evaluator did not know their race. The participant was then shown either a very favorable or a very unfavorable response from the evaluator. Participants then rated how various factors may have influenced the evaluation, including how much they felt they had been the target of prejudice. The findings revealed that when African American participants thought that they could be seen by the other person they believed the unfavorable feedback was especially likely to have been caused by prejudice. In another experiment members of a stigmatized group (women) were asked to write an essay and then received positive or negative feedback about the essay from an outgroup evaluator (a man), who they either did or did not suspect as being prejudiced (the man had either earlier expressed a sexist view or an anti-sexist view). Attributions were used to protect and bolster self-esteem. If negative feedback was delivered by a man said to be sexist, this feedback was attributed to his sexism, and the woman targeted saw no need to be concerned about her own writing ability. If he was not sexist, there was less ambiguity about the negative feedback being provided; the criticism could be taken to heart and there was less of a need to defend self-esteem by invoking sexism. Major and Crocker (1993) proposed that members of stereotyped groups are placed in a unique conflict when attempting to understand why they are treated as they are by the people in their social world. A member of a stereotyped group is faced with attributional ambiguity because they are unsure whether the feedback received from others reflects a bias against their social group. As a result, important feedback that could lead to self-improvement might be incorrectly disregarded as yet another instance of bias. Of course, equally damaging is if one takes feedback to heart and engages in steps aimed at self-improvement, when the feedback was just racist and never accurate or honest.

Negative Affect from Upward Social Comparison

Aside from attributions to shield self-esteem, how else can one regulate the negative evaluations and emotions of living in a culture rife with stereotyping and prejudice? Tajfel and Turner (1986) propose that people can choose to denigrate the dominant group they are comparing themselves to (feeling better through putting others down)—that is, if one is comparing one's group against a dominant group and that social comparison produces negative feedback about one's own group, one can focus on the flaws of the dominant group as opposed to the ways society says they are superior. Social comparisons that undermine the positivity of the group to which one belongs might be especially likely to be met by derogation of the more dominant group if the stereotyped group identity is central to one's self-concept (e.g., Branscombe et al., 1999; Ellemers, Spears, & Doosje, 1997). As an alternative to denigrating the dominant outgroup, people in the stigmatized group can also take action to change the negative identity suggested about one's group by the social comparison. They can change the outcome of the comparison so they come off positively. What action strategies can change a negative social comparison to a positive one? Tajfel and Turner describe two general approaches: one is called social mobility and the other is social change.

Social mobility is a strategy of individual effort and achievement, where personal success would reflect positively on the group, especially if enough individuals from the group can achieve, and in aggregate shift the negative perception of the group. One believes that "if enough individuals act as I do, the lot of the entire group would be lifted up." For social mobility to help a negative identity it requires conditions be

> **Social mobility:** A strategy to change negative evaluations of one's group through one's individual achievement reflecting positively on the group. This is especially likely if enough group members are able to achieve, and in aggregate shift the negative perception of the group.

in place, such as a possibility for advancement to exist. The borders of society must be construed of as free and open. Tajfel and Turner (1986) state:

> Based on the assumption that the society in which the individuals live is a flexible and permeable one, so that if they are not satisfied, for whatever reason, with the conditions imposed upon their lives by memberships in social groups or social categories to which they belong, it is possible for them (be it through talent, hard work, good luck, or whatever other means) to move individually. (p. 9)

If the borders between groups are perceived to be impermeable, with stratification and lines of group membership clearly drawn, social mobility strategies may give way to **social change** strategies. These are collectivistic strategies people adopt as a reaction to negative social identity, such as organizing one's group to instigate change: a group-based approach aimed at changing status. Whereas social mobility leads to thinking about group members as individuals, social change leads to responding to others in ways that define them in terms of group memberships (e.g., Taylor & Moghaddam, 1987; Wright, Taylor, & Moghaddam, 1990). For example, group members can organize to shift the dimension on which social comparisons between groups are made. If the group comes off negatively when we compare against another group along behavior X, then let us now collectively decide that behavior X is irrelevant and start valuing behavior Y instead, a behavior where the ingroup is better than a comparison group. A second collectivistic strategy is to assign a more positive value to attributes the group already possesses rather than accepting the negative value assigned by others. This is known as *redefining* the attributes associated with the group, such as when the slogan "Black is beautiful" emerged during the civil rights movement in the United States. A third behavioral strategy for altering negative identity is to initiate change in how others think about their group (perhaps altering the negative perceptions that are contributing to negative social identity) by a direct challenge to the views of the dominant group. Moscovici (1985) believed that successful social influence occurs through conflict, not compromise—it is dependent on the minority consistently, persistently, and tenaciously adhering to their "unique" minority view and refusing to yield to the majority: "stringent intransigence often typifies the attitude of individuals who have had a great impact on our ideas and behavior" (p. 29). A fourth behavioral strategy for altering negative identity is to change the group used as the standard of comparison. Rather than comparing against a dominant group that reflects negatively on one's own group, choose a different standard for comparison where one's group is now the superior one (downward social comparison). For example, Boldry and Gaertner (2006) showed how people in low-status groups can flexibly shift the social comparison standard to maintain a positive social identity. Perhaps a cost of such a strategy is it may lead one to raise their esteem by derogating other minority groups. Francophones in Quebec are considered a minority due to the seat of Canadian power being occupied by Anglophones. It is not uncommon to see French Canadians denigrating immigrant groups—a downward social comparison.

Another strategy to manage a negative group identity is to identify individual members of the group who are the cause of the negativity and label them as different: the black sheep of the family. A phenomenon known as the **black-sheep effect** (e.g., Marques et al., 1988) is when ingroup members who deviate from the norms of the group and reflect negatively on

Social change: Collectivistic strategies people adopt as a reaction to negative social identity, such as organizing one's group to instigate change. This is a group-based approach aimed at changing status that leads to responding to others in ways that define them in terms of group memberships, as opposed to as individuals.

the group are derogated by the group. This is most likely to happen when the negative behavior enacted is a violation to a norm that is highly relevant to the group. This helps navigate negative group identity by displacing the blame and shame on a small handful of individual outliers within the group. This bears some similarity to the notion of subtyping (as reviewed in Chapter 5), where a person who behaves in a way that is inconsistent with a stereotype is isolated as somehow different from the rest of the group by a perceiver who wishes to maintain their stereotype of the group. By "fencing them off" from their group, a perceiver can maintain their negative perception of that group. With the black-sheep effect the perceiver is isolating a member of their own group in order to label that person's negative behavior as separate from the group.

> **Black-sheep effect:** When ingroup members who deviate from the norms of the group and reflect negatively on the group are derogated by the group. This is most likely to happen when the negative behavior enacted is a violation of a norm that is highly relevant to the group.

Schmader and Lickel (2006) extend this work to suggest that it is not only negative social comparisons that promote the black-sheep phenomenon but the shame that arises from being the target of negative stereotypes and negative prejudice. When a social identity is important, the shame that arises from confirming negative stereotypes of the group can be triggered by other members of the ingroup, leading one to want to isolate and derogate that individual to protect the group from sharing in that shame. In an experiment where participants reported an instance in which they saw an ingroup member behave stereotypically, Schmader and Lickel showed that participants desired to distance themselves from the person in an attempt to repair the negativity reflected on the group and the shame experienced by those who observed that stereotypical ingroup behavior (see also Schmader, Block, & Lickel, 2015).

CONCLUSIONS

Our concern in this chapter (as it has been throughout this book) is with the processes through which prejudice and stereotypes, as mental representations, can be unintentionally triggered and then bias social cognition. The interest has not been on the content of any one stereotype or on prejudice as it relates to any one group (such as what qualities define the stereotype of women in a particular culture, or what affect does German culture associate with Turkish immigrants). Instead, the study of prejudice and stereotyping in social cognition seeks to identify underlying processes that govern how *any* prejudice or stereotype impacts any individual, regardless of the content that defines the prejudice and stereotypes that exist in that person's culture. Irrespective of whether one is investigating bias arising from Hindu and Muslim religious beliefs, Japanese and Korean national identity, African American and White American ethnic identity, or opposing ideological and political groups, the nature of the bias and the manner it manifests in shaping cognition would be the same. Of course, stereotype content matters; but process does too.

The functional nature of stereotyping and prejudice reveals to us that, as Crosby, Bromley, and Saxe (1980) put it, we are far more likely to be biased than we are apt to admit. This is not solely because we seek to hide our biases from others (out of shame). Additionally, we frequently use stereotypes and prejudice, and hide this fact from ourselves! Because these constructs are often implicitly activated, stereotyping and prejudice may proceed without our awareness, biasing us in ways we vehemently deny, and would never suspect. This is a denial borne of ignorance, not shame. We have a bias blind spot. Many people fail to see bias as much of a problem at all in modern life. Instead, they see bias as largely defeated by the progress in intergroup relations made since the end of the Second World War; it is seen as a relic of the past. It is easy for many of us to now believe that the psychological disease of overt prejudice has been removed almost as thoroughly as such bodily diseases as typhoid and the plague. We convince ourselves that the disease is confined to a minority of hateful people; the culture at large is mostly immune. Yet common cognitive processes can lead us to think and act in ways opposite to how we imagine we would respond, or consciously intend to respond, making us biased in unintended and unseen ways. We may think we lack bias when we do not.

Our mental system has evolved to give us the great benefit of using attitudes and schemas to make sense of the world, and to allow them to operate so quickly and efficiently that we do not even know we are evaluating and reacting to stimuli based on those constructs. Yet, just because the triggering of attitudes and stereotypes is common, outside awareness, and efficient, it does not mean the resulting biases are normative and appropriate. Most people who engage in these silent forms of bias would be ashamed to learn they had caused harm in any way, and in no way endorse such processing as acceptable. The danger in discussing the commonality of implicit forms of bias is that calling it common may communicate that it is unproblematic. But calling it common is meant to have the opposite effect: It is meant to communicate that it is so widespread as to be a serious problem (e.g., Daumeyer, Onyeador, Brown, & Richeson, 2019; Moskowitz & Vitriol, 2022). The common nature of the cognitive processes that can give rise to stereotyping and prejudice produces a serious conundrum that we all face—we have a mind that operates quickly, efficiently, and unknowingly to deliver negative affect and stereotypic beliefs that are often unwarranted (and that arise from associations taught by the culture). Further, we have the separate problem of lacking awareness of precisely when and how we do this. These processes allow incorrect associations to be repeatedly triggered, strengthened, and used.

If stereotypes and prejudice have the function of providing fast and useful information to us, why do we allow them to be riddled with inaccuracies? The short answer is that if an inaccurate stereotype still functions reasonably well as a tool, then there is little reason to modify it. Very few of us have encountered situations where stereotypes, even if they contain wrong information, have made it difficult to interact with someone from another group. A perception that our stereotypes are "accurate enough" is one explanation as to why we have no impetus to alter them, but does not address why they may contain inaccuracies in the first place.

It is here where we see how stereotypes deviate from our knowledge about chairs and other objects. With objects we possess fairly simple motives—we want to accurately know what features an object has and what the object can be used for. There is little impetus to develop anything but the most accurate beliefs, and there is little resistance to updating our beliefs if we learn that something previously thought to be true about the object is false. The simpler the object (such as a pencil, an orange, or a chair), the less room there is for other motives to intervene. However, as objects get more complex, or when accuracy is hard to ascertain, the greater the room for alternative motives to get in the way of how we think and for inaccuracies to filter into the discussion. We can apply this logic to people: They are not simple; they act in ways that are out of our control; they have internal states such as attitudes and goals that we cannot see and can only infer; and they may threaten our need for dominance and may even challenge it. Accuracy is not the only motive that drives how we perceive people. We distort, twist, and filter information about social groups in ways we do not when perceiving chairs.

Even if you are driven by concerns regarding accuracy and objectivity, your knowledge about social groups (stereotypes) is still largely learned from the collective: the culture in which you live. And in that culture, accuracy may be only a minor player in the game of identifying and communicating what the features are that describe a complex group of people. As motives for superiority, hierarchy, hegemony, protection, self-esteem, and bonding with similar others enter the equation, so do inaccuracies and distortions in the knowledge the collective develops, and transmits to you, about social groups. These social motives lead the stereotype to develop in ways that belie accuracy, and provide an additional reason that inaccuracies persist: Forces to justify existing social systems, power distributions, and hierarchies are powerful.

Stereotypes can be bad not only due to the false information they contain but due to the incorrect ways in which people use their stereotypes. Even stereotypes that are 100% accurate can be used in incorrect and harmful ways. For example, in the aftermath of the September 11, 2001, attack against the United States there were retaliatory attacks by Americans against Sikhs living in America. If we pretend that the Americans engaged in this violence had stereotypes of Muslim terrorists that were perfectly true, they still pulled out these stereotypes at the wrong time. They incorrectly labeled someone (a Sikh) as a terrorist and then assigned to that person the stereotype of the group Muslim terrorist, which obviously has no relevance to a person who is a Sikh (and thus not a Muslim, and could not possibly be among the very small percentage of Muslims who are also terrorists).

NOTES

1. As illustrated by their faster responses when ingroup names and pleasant words (and outgroup names and unpleasant words) required the same response on the IAT. People were faster to the compatible than incompatible trials, despite compatibility being defined by a temporarily created minimal group.

2. As just a few examples: (1) the infant mortality rate in the United States, measured in deaths per 1,000 live births, shows a growing discrepancy between White and Black infants. In 1982 the ratio of Black to White infant deaths was almost double, at 1.94. In 2000 the gap had grown to 2.46. (2) The death rate for adult men is more than double for Black men compared to White men. (3) A 2007 survey by the Pew Research Center reported that 67% of Black respondents indicated they often face discrimination and prejudice when applying for a job. (4) A 2004 analysis of U.S. Census data reported by the Economic Policy Institute shows the ratio of Black to White salaries is 62%. (5) Despite being only 13% of the drug-using population, Black people were 35% of the population of people arrested for drug use, 55% of the people convicted for drug use, and 74% of the prison population serving time for drug use.

3. For example, Payne (2006) used a reaction time procedure to illustrate an association held by White people between violence/criminality and Black people. We also saw evidence for stereotype activation when we reviewed the shooter task—as part of playing a video game, White research participants shoot (press a button marked "shoot") a Black person depicted as holding a gun faster than (and with greater accuracy) a White person with a gun (e.g., Correll et al., 2002; Correll, Wittenbrink, Park, Judd, & Goyle, 2011). Both Maddox (2004) and Eberhardt et al. (2003) revealed how physiognomy triggers a stereotype; Macrae, Bodenhausen, et al. (1994) triggered stereotypes of skinheads by presenting the group label during a learning task. And Devine (1989) simply flashed a group label subliminally and triggered the stereotype.

4. Played for comical effect 35 years later, the TV show *Futurama* had a fugitive being pursued. This time it was a human fugitive being pursued by aliens. To appease the aliens, the human was turned in. The joke was that instead of "turning in" the actual human fugitive, an ape was turned in, because, to an alien, humans and apes look alike.

5. One exception would be when a communicator feels as if the audience has such complete understanding of the stereotype that sharing the consistent information would be redundant and uninformative. Under such conditions inconsistent information could be seen as useful new information. Another exception is if a communicator understood that while the audience shared knowledge of the stereotype, they also rejected it. In that instance the communicator would want to emphasize the inconsistencies rather than risk being seen as biased by the people who receive the message. Normative pressures could lead one to communicate what others see as appropriate.

CHAPTER 12

Cognitive Processing Is Flexible, and Processing Types Dissociable

The stream of our thought is like a river. On the whole, easy simple flowing predominates in it, the drift of things is with the pull of gravity, and effortless attention is the rule. But at intervals a log-jam occurs, stops the current, creates an eddy, and makes things temporarily move the other way. If a real river could feel, it would feel these eddies and set-backs as places of effort.
—JAMES (1890/1950, p. 451)

After social cognition emerged in the 1970s it led to the flourishing of a first wave of research that culminated by the 1990s with a set of models that sought to provide an overarching framework on the new discoveries. These were labeled **dual-process models**. This name arises from the fact that human processing seemed to be capable of being somewhat mindless and automatic, where heuristics are followed rather than thinking deeply. Yet it can also be deliberate and systematic, where deep processing and effort are engaged (e.g., Conway & Gawronski, 2013; Payne & Cameron, 2014; Pennycook, 2023; Petty & Briñol, 2014; Strack & Deutsch, 2004). Some take this to mean there are two separate systems (e.g., Kahneman, 2011; Smith & DeCoster, 2000),[1] while others describe a continuum of processing with a single system and processes that engage more versus less effort (e.g., Chaiken et al., 1989). In each case, a metaphor of two types of processes is emphasized, hence the name *dual-process models*. This is an old idea, as seen in the quote that starts the chapter. James (1890/1950) argued effortless, theory-driven processing predominates, but under the appropriate conditions more effortful processing occurs. Dual-process models propose this as well, and detail the conditions that prompt such effort. This chapter reviews the various ways to think about the organization of the vast amount of research reviewed in this book and what type of mental models make sense to structure it all. We start with dual-process models.

> **Dual-process models:** Models arguing that cognitive processing is by default somewhat mindless and automatic, where heuristics are followed. Yet when one is motivated to engage in deep processing, it can also be systematic and deliberate. Some conceive of this as a single system and continuum of processing, others as separate systems.

DUAL-PROCESS MODELS

Dual-process models describe people as having a default strategy in which inferences are formed and impressions are made using heuristics, schemas, stereotypes, and expectancies. The strategy that finds humans residing at the effortless end of the information-processing continuum was described earlier in this book as having evolved out of a need to manage the complexity of the environment using a cognitive system with limited resources. That is, two factors combine to create a preference for less effortful information processing. The first is the limited capacity of the cognitive system to engage in effort. While we can perceive and attend to huge amounts of information effortlessly to place extremely briefly in echoic or iconic memory, only a trivial amount of information is entered into conscious attention (e.g., Treisman & Geffen, 1967; Deutsch & Deutsch, 1963). The ability to effortfully manipulate information receiving such conscious attention is easily overloaded due to having limited capacity for effortful deliberation (e.g., Miller, 1956). The second is the complexity of stimulus information bombarding the perceptual system from conditions in the environment. Such conditions include: working on many tasks at once and thus placing people under cognitive load; working on tasks under a deadline where time pressure limits how long you can deliberate about the qualities of others; and working on tasks that, in and of themselves, are complex and difficult. Bruner (1957) highlighted the importance of this last point when asserting that even when we are not overloaded or pressed for time, interpersonal perception is still complex and difficult. As objects of perception, other people are highly equivocal and would be hard to truly know even after hours (perhaps years) of deliberating. Thus, less effortful strategies also become the norm because we have learned that doing more with such complex stimuli will not yield a better result and is tantamount to a costly waste of effort. Less effort is efficient and economical. However, Bruner paved the way for dual-process models by asserting that people are *sometimes* willing to pay this cost and engage in the effort of what he called a "closer look" at the information. The important psychological questions concern when, why, and how we are willing and able to pay such costs and shift to more complex processing.

The term "dual-process model" was coined by Brewer (1988) in describing a comprehensive theory of the processes involved in impression formation. Brewer's model built an important bridge between research focused on how people use schemas, categories, and heuristics in judging others in an effortless way and earlier research focused on the rational and methodical processes that people employ when forming attributions of others (reviewed in Chapter 7). People use each of these processes in their social cognition. However, the conditions that delineated when social cognition would be marked by an overreliance on categories and effortless processes versus an attention to details and effortful processes had not been established. Many other integrative models emerged between 1986 and 1990 that also attempted to specify the conditions that govern when and why people shift from effortless to more systematic processing (e.g., Chaiken, Liberman, & Eagly, 1989; Devine, 1989; Fazio, 1990a; Fiske & Neuberg, 1990; Gilbert, 1989; Kruglanski, 1990; Kunda, 1987; Martin, 1986; Petty & Cacioppo, 1986; Trope, 1986a; Wyer & Srull, 1989). These models share a set of assumptions in which impression formation is organized according to stages, which occur sequentially, such that the perceiver will not expend resources for further processing unless certain conditions are met.

Brewer's (1988) Dual-Process Model of Impression Formation

The attempt to integrate the two types of cognitive processes that had been the focus of impression formation research helped to reintroduce the notion of motivation to mainstream social psychology, a concept that had been diluted (though not absent altogether) in the cognitive revolution. In research studying the automatic nature of social cognition, goals were often held constant, rendering them almost obsolete. However, when researchers began attempting to integrate different forms of thinking within a given perceiver, they soon rediscovered that motives and goals played a central role that made them essential to any model of social cognition. Sorrentino and Higgins's (1986) *Handbook of Motivation and Cognition* helped to awaken the field to this issue, and dual-process models soon sprung forth. Case in point, Brewer's (1988) dual-process model depicted in Figure 12.1 places the role of motivation central to determining the type of social cognition perceivers will engage in. Brewer states, "the majority of the time, perception of social objects does not differ from nonsocial perception in either structure or process. When it does differ, it is determined by the *perceiver's* purposes and processing goals, not by the characteristics of the target of perception" (p. 4).

Brewer's (1988) model is somewhat arbitrarily singled out here for detailed review, and not because it is the first such model (a wave of them developed in parallel) or my favorite (which is that of my mentor, Shelly Chaiken). It is just a good exemplar of the set (and one that gave us the name). Other books provide a review of all the models (e.g., Chaiken & Trope, 1999). And other models are reviewed elsewhere in this book (Chaiken, 1987, in Chapter 1; Trope, 1986a, in Chapter 8; Kunda, 1987, in Chapter 9; Devine, 1989, in Chapter 10; Fiske & Neuberg, 1990, in Chapter 13). As with other models, Brewer's model specifies automatic and controlled processing that contributes to one's ultimate impression of another person. It describes processing types occurring in stages, and the first type of processing is called identification.

Identification

The model begins with automatic processes of attention and identification. When a person enters our social environment, we must first focus attention on that person and identify the person as being present, as having certain features, and as having performed certain types of behavior. This is accomplished through a feature-matching process that allows us to identify the qualities that the target elicits and to categorize the target in an efficient (if not 100% accurate) way. By comparing its features against existing categories we are able to cue an appropriate category. This process is called *identification*. At times the category we identify using this process of matching observable features of a target to an existing mental representation of "person types" is wrong.[2] As Allport (1954) says: "Sometimes we are mistaken: the event does not fit the category. . . . Yet our behavior was rational. It was based on high probability. Though we used the wrong category, we did the best we could" (p. 20).

The model suggests there are a limited number of social categories that are used often and consistently enough to be triggered automatically—for example, age, ethnicity, race, and sex. Exactly which of these categories becomes a superordinate category label that may organize subsequent impression formation processing depends on features of the context, the perceiver, and the target. Fiske and Neuberg (1990) assert that qualities with "temporal primacy, have physical manifestations, are contextually novel, are chronically or acutely accessible in memory, or are related in particular ways to the perceiver's mood will tend to serve the role of category label" (p. 10).

Determining Relevance

The primary outcome of this initial identification stage is a preconscious decision as to whether further processing is necessary to detect whether the person is relevant or irrelevant to us. If a person we have encountered is irrelevant to our current goals and purpose (e.g.,

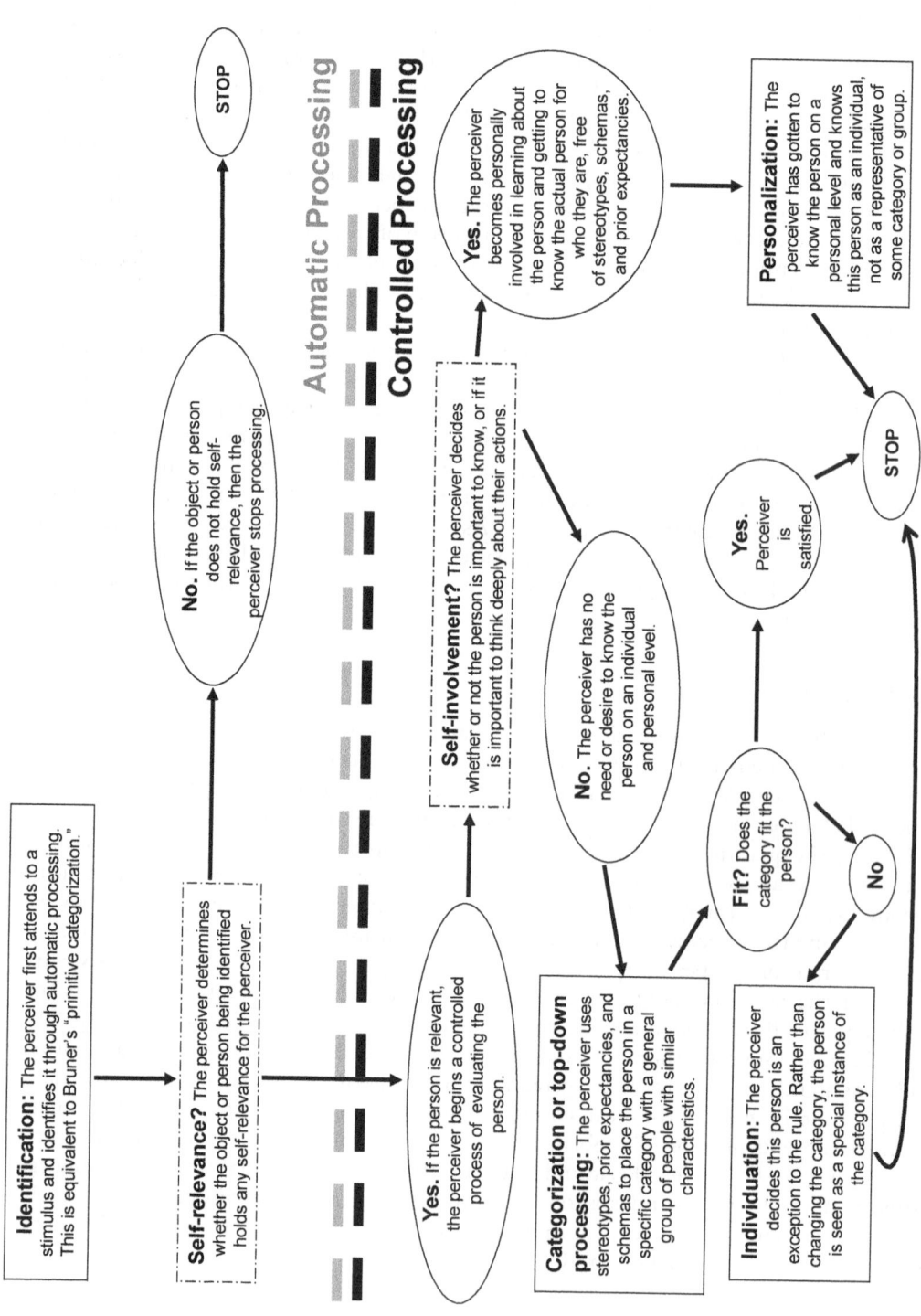

Identification: The perceiver first attends to a stimulus and identifies it through automatic processing. This is equivalent to Bruner's "primitive categorization."

Self-relevance? The perceiver determines whether the object or person being identified holds any self-relevance for the perceiver.

No. If the object or person does not hold self-relevance, then the perceiver stops processing.

STOP

Automatic Processing

Controlled Processing

Yes. If the person is relevant, the perceiver begins a controlled process of evaluating the person.

Self-involvement? The perceiver decides whether or not the person is important to know, or if it is important to think deeply about their actions.

Yes. The perceiver becomes personally involved in learning about the person and getting to know the actual person for who they are, free of stereotypes, schemas, and prior expectancies.

No. The perceiver has no need or desire to know the person on an individual and personal level.

Categorization or top-down processing: The perceiver uses stereotypes, prior expectancies, and schemas to place the person in a specific category with a general group of people with similar characteristics.

Fit? Does the category fit the person?

Yes. Perceiver is satisfied.

No

Individuation: The perceiver decides this person is an exception to the rule. Rather than changing the category, the person is seen as a special instance of the category.

Personalization: The perceiver has gotten to know the person on a personal level and knows this person as an individual, not as a representative of some category or group.

STOP

FIGURE 12.1. Brewer's (1988) dual-process model of impression formation.

416

a stranger passing us on the subway platform, a driver stopped at a red light as we walk down the street, a clerk at the market placing mustard on the shelf), then further processing, and the expenditure of cognitive effort to think about this person, is not necessary. Impression formation processes are halted. However, if the person is deemed relevant (and this can range from a minor degree of relevance, such as a store clerk placing mustard on a shelf when one wants condiments, to a major degree, such as a stranger passing you on the subway platform who attempts to take your wallet), then further processing is triggered.

Thus even the preconscious decision that determines whether we dedicate any energy to thinking about a person and process further information about the person depends on goals (i.e., the relevance of the target). From this point onward, processing can no longer be characterized as automatic since it requires a goal: the goal of needing to know more about the person because of their potential relevance to you. At this point a critical choice is made between two alternative processing modes described in the model: categorization and personalization. This is not to say that such further processing cannot occur with little effort, or without awareness.

Categorization/Typing

Motives do not only determine whether you proceed to think about others but they also determine *how* you proceed to think about them. The decision to gather further information about a person does not mean it will always be an effortful, deliberative, rational, and objective process. We can produce judgments of others in a categorical way, relying on schemas, heuristics, stereotypes, and prior expectations. This relatively effortless type of thinking, that is anchored by and directed exclusively by the categories that have been triggered, is called **categorization**, or **typing**. With categorization processes, judgments about a person are based on available "person types" or schemas that are matched to the information at hand about the person being evaluated. An iterative, pattern-matching process is conducted until an adequate fit is found between one of the person types or categories stored in memory and the stimulus characteristics. The process starts with a rather general category, and if there is no match, subtypes of the general category that provide more specific types are compared against the target person. Brewer (1988) offers a concrete example of the abstract superordinate category and the more concrete

> **Categorization (typing):** A type of impression formation where judgments about a person are based solely on available "person types" or schemas that fit the salient features of the stimulus. If the more general category invoked has inadequate fit, subtypes that provide more specific types are compared against the target person.

subtypes within that category: The superordinate category "old man" is fairly abstract and contains a wide range of features. Within that superordinate category is the more specific category type "the businessman," which is still relatively abstract, but less so than the category label in which it is nested (older men). Moving downward in the category hierarchy we arrive at even more specific subtypes of the category businessman that have fine-grained sets of features, such as the "uptight authoritarian boss who is a tightwad and a stickler for detail" (p. 12).

Given these different levels of category types, Brewer (1988) concluded that the exact manner in which a given person is categorized is dependent not only on the features of that person being matched against a category but on the level of abstraction within the category structure that the feature-matching process begins. Exactly where in the perceiver's category system this process begins can be determined by several factors: what categories were automatically triggered during identification, cues in the current situation, and the processing goals of the perceiver. For example, if a person is identified both according to age as a teenager and according to occupation as a writer for a well-respected news outlet, then a somewhat low-level categorization forms in which a specific subtype of teenager—for example, a whiz kid, genius, or overachiever—is used to structure and organize information about the person. However, if age was not salient in the initial identification, then the category used to structure and organize information about the person is the more abstract category of professional writer, rather than the more concrete whiz kid.

These initial categorizations are important for several reasons. First, category-driven impressions might be the sole contributor to one's final judgment of the person, constituting the entire basis for one's opinion—that is, there are times when perceivers are perfectly happy to rely on their categories to supply them with broad overgeneralizations that can extend from the category level to individual members of the category. Second, even if the impression one forms evolves and gets transformed in later stages of information processing, the category-based judgment will still serve as an input that anchors (serves as a starting point for) any future judgment (e.g., Park, 1989). Finally, categorical processing not only serves as an anchor around which future, effortful judgments shift. It also anchors the effortless processing that occurs during categorization—that is, during the process of trying to match "person types" against a person's characteristics in order to categorize them, the initial categorization, even if inadequate for categorizing the person, impacts how subsequent feature mapping and person typing proceeds. If the initial match between a category and a person's features is not successful, this first attempt is not discarded for a new, irrelevant person type to match against the target. Instead, Brewer (1988) says,

> the search for an appropriate categorization will be directed downward, among subtypes of the original category, rather than horizontally among alternative categories at the same level of abstraction. . . . Thus, initial category activation sets in motion an iterative process that constrains the final category selection. (pp. 18–19)

Individuation

The processes of categorization seem to involve no more motivational impetus than trivial levels of self-involvement. But as the needs and goals of the perceiver dictate, they can engage more detailed, elaborate, and effortful types of cognitive processing while still staying tethered or anchored to their categories.[3] Brewer (1988) calls this fairly effortful, but still category-based processing **individuation**. In this type of processing, information that we receive about a person that is inconsistent with the category label is not disregarded, nor is a more specific instance of the category used to describe the person. Instead, the individual is treated as an isolated case or a specific instance of the category. Thus, qualities of the individual are processed with effort and detail, but not for the purpose of making the person fit the category but to create a specific and detailed novel instance of the category. Brewer used a good example: "the first anchorwoman that appeared on a national television news program was no doubt highly individuated as a member of the category of news broadcasters" (p. 21). In this example, the superordinate category is not woman but anchor. A subtype "anchorwoman" did not exist, and sexism made consideration of others to type in this way unlikely. The category is inadequate, but not abandoned. The person is typed as an exceptional instance of the category.

Individuation: A type of impression formation where the individual is treated as a specific instance of the category. The qualities of the individual are processed in detail, not to make that individual fit well with the category, but to create a specific and detailed novel instance of the category.

Personalization

There are times, however, when no form of category-based processing is deemed appropriate by the perceiver. At such times a wholly different form of processing in both format and organizational structure is suggested by the model. In such processing the category is rejected for the individual as the basis for organizing information. The attributes of the person serve as the organizing framework for understanding them, rather than the features of a category. Brewer (1988) referred to this type of information processing as **personalization**. Brewer asserts that "the new organizational structure is a sort of mental flip-flop of the category-based structure," and provides an example via analysis of the statement "Janet is a nurse" (p. 22). This could be organized and analyzed in a category-based way, with Janet treated as a type of person within the category "nurse." Alternatively, the information could be organized and analyzed in a way that treats nurse as subordinate to, and a feature of, the properties of a person named Janet. In one case the category "nurse" is the organizing structure about which the emerging mental representation is built. In the other case it is the person, Janet. Brewer says, "'nurse' as a feature of Janet would contain only those aspects of nursing that are characteristic of Janet in that role, and would be disassociated from the prototypic representation of nurse as a general category, which may contain many features not applicable to Janet" (p. 22).

> **Personalization:** A type of impression formation where the individual becomes the basis for organizing information. Here, the category label is no longer superordinate, but instead the attributes of the individual serve as the organizing framework for understanding that individual.

Exactly what sort of conditions lead a perceiver to conclude that category-based processing is not appropriate? Brewer (1988) asserts that personalization needs to be motivated, and requires an "*affective* investment on the part of the perceiver" (p. 25, italics in original). For example, a relationship with the person (such as a shared social identity, or a friendship), or a person affording one an opportunity to achieve a desirable goal (e.g., a coworker whose work on a joint project will also determine how you are evaluated, a manager whose evaluation will determine whether you are promoted), will motivate one to personalize rather than categorize. We are more likely to form impressions based on the attributes and features we have taken the time to detect. The complete dual-process model is depicted in Figure 12.1 as a flow chart with decision points. Decisions regarding the motivational relevance of the person being perceived are depicted by boxes with dashed lines.

ALTERNATIVES TO DUAL-PROCESS MODELS

The idea of there being two styles of thinking is appealing. It elegantly explains a history of data showing us that people are at times mindless and seeking only to confirm preexisting theories, stereotypes, and values or goals, yet at other times are tethered to the data and exerting effort to follow the facts. Yet, dual-process models imply a person is engaged in one type of processing at a time, even though able to shift from one to the other as their goals dictate. This conception ignores the possibility that both types of processing can be engaged simultaneously and interact to determine how a person responds. By definition, such models also ignore the possibility that more than two processes are operating. Rather than processing in a serial fashion, a variety of cognitive processes may operate in parallel and in cooperation with one another. Models such as the *associative-propositional evaluation* (APE) model (e.g., Gawronski & Bodenhausen, 2011) reviewed in Chapter 6, process dissociation (PD) models (e.g., Jacoby, 1991), and the quadruple process model (e.g., Sherman,

2006) address a need to assess the unique contribution of multiple processes in any cognitive response, arguing that no response is "process pure," or reflecting only one type of processing at a time.

PD Models

Process dissociation (PD) models argue that any response is influenced by the simultaneous operation of automatic and controlled processes happening in parallel and that math-

> **Process dissociation (PD) models:** Models that focus on the separation and measurement of the distinct automatic and controlled processes contributing to a response, each operating simultaneously, in parallel. Mathematical equations are used to produce estimates of the role of each type of processing in any given response.

ematical equations can be used to produce estimates of the role of each type of processing in any given response (e.g., Jacoby, 1991; Jacoby, Toth, & Yonelinas, 1993; Lindsay & Jacoby, 1994; Payne, 2001; Payne & Jacoby, 2006). For example, if you respond that a piece of information is true, the response can be based on a *gut feeling* emerging because the information feels familiar, as well as based on an *explicit recollection* of having seen the event on which that information is based. The distinct contribution of each to the response can be identified. As another example, if a White police officer decides to shoot a Black man at a crime scene, the response can be based on an *implicit sense* that there is heightened threat, as well as on the conscious detection of a weapon being brandished. The multiple bases for the response can each be assessed separately rather than treating the response as reflecting only one. Recognition memory tasks and stereotyping tasks are two examples of how PD models are used. Burke (2015) provides a summary of a few others.

To study these matters, researchers need to perform experiments that create conditions both of conflict and of compatibility. By **conditions of compatibility** it is meant that the "gut reaction" or implicit response produces the exact same outcome on the task as the

> **Conditions of compatibility:** The trials on a task where the "gut reaction" or implicit response produces the exact same outcome on the task as the explicit reaction.
>
> **Conditions of conflict:** The trials on a task where the "gut reaction" or implicit response produces a different outcome on the task than the explicit reaction.

explicit reaction. In the first example used above, a compatible response would be when you have to identify whether some information shown to you is new or was previously learned, and both the gut reaction and the explicit recollection tell you that it was previously learned. In the second example used above, a compatible response would be when you have to decide whether to shoot someone who is posing a threat in the form of holding a gun, and both the gut reaction and your explicit perception tell you that firing your weapon is appropriate. By **conditions of conflict** it is meant that the "gut reaction" or implicit response produces a different outcome on the task than the explicit reaction. In the first example used above, a conflict would be when you have to identify whether some information shown to you is new or was previously learned, and the gut reaction is that it feels familiar and hence learned, but your explicit recollection tells you that you have not seen this information before. In the second example above, a conflict would be when you have to decide whether to shoot someone who is posing a threat in the form of holding a gun, and your gut reaction is to experience a threat, but your explicit perception tells you that the person has no gun. Designs like this— where there are "trials" of the experiment that have compatibility and "trials" of the experiment that have conflict—allow for a mathematical formula to be applied that can examine how the person has responded on each type of trial as a pattern of responding across the experiment and produce an estimate of the unique contribution of the two influences. The two processes—the automatic and controlled components of one's response—can be dissociated.

There are two general types of PD models. One is called a "late-correction" model because it is used in tasks where it is assumed that automatic processes produce inappropriate or unwanted responses, and part of the conscious response is to edit out or suppress the inappropriate influence on the response made on the task. When control fails, the automatic process influences the person's response. The first example above, estimating the influences of familiarity (the automatic response) and recollection (the controlled response) on recognition memory performance (e.g., Jacoby, 1991), is a late-correction PD procedure. The procedure is borrowed from older research on recognition memory (e.g., Mandler, 1980), which assumes that when performing a task where one has to recognize information as old or new, there are independent effects of recollection and familiarity. As stated above, arranging the task so that there are trials in which the two processes have the same influence on judgment and trials in which they have opposing influences on judgment allows one to derive estimates of the influence of each process separately. The second type of PD model is called an "early-selection" model. This is used on tasks like the IAT, the shooter task, and the Stroop task where the issue is not whether control fails but whether an automatic association guides responding from the outset, serving as a constraining force over what comes to mind (e.g., Lindsay & Jacoby, 1994). The second example above, estimating the influence of both activated stereotypes and conscious detection of a weapon on whether a person decides to shoot, is an early-selection PD procedure. A more detailed examination of the processes being dissociated in the shooter task illustrates how PD models can help us to understand stereotyping, and precisely how/why Americans are faster and more likely to shoot Black men.

In Chapter 4 we reviewed research on the shooter bias, where White participants playing a simulation game were faster to shoot Black men holding a gun than White men holding a gun. The discussion there was focused on how one could use both measures of reaction time and errors to indicate implicit stereotyping. Through PD we can explore the precise nature of the implicit stereotyping seen in that task. *Why* would having a stereotype lead to differences on this shooter task? One possibility is *sensitivity*, a type of processing discussed in Chapter 4. This is the ability to discriminate among the stimuli being presented during a task (to detect a cue from others), which in this case is whether the person is holding a gun or some other object. It is a measure of White research participants' conscious processes of accurately detecting what a person is holding in each trial of this task. Does detection of a weapon differ when a Black person relative to a White person is holding it, thus confirming a stereotypic expectation of what one might see? However, sensitivity to detect a gun is *not* what causes the bias in a shooter task; research shows that *race has little effect on sensitivity*. This is illustrated by the top half of Figure 12.2, where sensitivity in detecting a gun held by a White man (the top left of the figure) is no different than sensitivity in detecting a gun held by a Black man (the top right of the figure). Sensitivity is measured by how far apart the peak of the distribution of responses to a man who is unarmed is from the peak of the distribution of responses to a man who is armed. The less sensitive one is at differentiating among guns and other objects, the more one will mistakenly see a gun when not there (bringing those distributions closer together and overlapping more). If differences existed as a function of race, the results would look like those depicted in the lower half of Figure 12.2, where the distribution peaks are closer together for Black men as compared to White men (indicating less sensitivity, and a greater likelihood of seeing guns regardless of whether one was there or not). Instead, the actual results are similar to the top half of the figure, with no racial bias in sensitivity. Participants easily discriminate between people

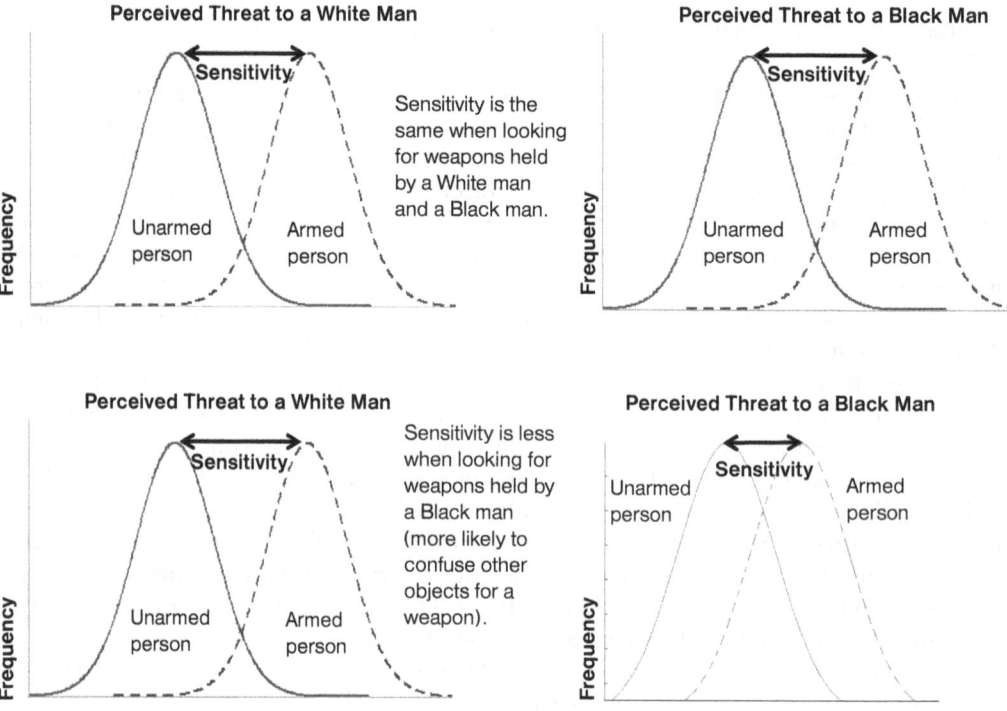

FIGURE 12.2. Two examples of sensitivity in the shooter task.

holding guns and people holding other objects, regardless of the person's race. They associate guns with Black men (e.g., Payne, 2001), but this does not lead to errors in identifying who is holding a gun in the shooter task. Stereotypes cause the shooter bias, but it is not because of errors of sensitivity.

A second possible reason a stereotype would impact the shooter task is a form of shifting standards where the perceiver sets and uses a decision *criterion* differently for men of different racial groups (reviewed in Chapter 4). The criterion is the point during a task where one decides to respond to the stimulus, which in this case is making the decision to shoot *after* one has identified whether the person is holding a gun. While stereotypes do not appear to help one detect whether a gun is present, they do appear to *shape how one responds once a gun is detected*. The stereotype seems to alter the criterion, shifting the standard for the perception of threat that is detected. A lower criterion means that the person is setting a more lenient standard for defining threat and this makes it easier to shoot. A higher criterion means that the person is setting a stricter standard for defining threat and this makes it harder to shoot. The participant will shoot only at targets posing an extreme threat when the criterion is high. In research on bias in a shooter task it has generally been found that race affects the criterion, with a lower criterion set for Black men as targets in comparison to White men. This more lenient criterion creates a greater perception of threat for the identical behavior (holding a gun) and a greater willingness to shoot. This lowered criterion makes the decision to shoot a Black man more accurate and faster (see Chapter 4, Figure 4.7).

PD can help us understand many biases. One further example is the finding that people are more likely to incorrectly attribute uniquely human emotions to an ingroup, and less so to an outgroup. PD shows that no differences emerge in the error rates in attributing more animalistic emotions, telling us that the bias is not to implicitly see more primitive emotional experiences in the outgroup but to show greater control over errors of heightened humanity in the outgroup (Gaunt, Leyens, & Demoulin, 2002). Another example is the bias to have poorer memory for other-race faces. PD analyses show that such effects are not caused by familiarity but by effortful processes when encoding the faces (Meissner, Brigham, & Butz, 2005).

Initial PD models (just reviewed) are able to dissociate automatic from effortful processes based on two variables: trial compatibility (conflict or compatible) and the ultimate response made (e.g., shoot or do not shoot). More recent PD models explore not just the decision made, but how such a binary choice interacts with more dynamical responses made while making the choice. For example, one measure that can also be assessed when making a choice (click on a box marked *A* to shoot, and a box marked *B* to not shoot) is speed of responding. Another measure that can be assessed when making such a choice is indecisiveness. For example, imagine choice *A* (shoot) is on the left of the screen, and choice *B* (do not shoot) is on the right, and the cursor sits at the bottom of the screen, in the middle. To choose to shoot one must move the mouse toward the left. Reaction time measures how quickly the choice is made, but the trajectory of the mouse that is used to click on the choice shows the complexity of the decision process (e.g., Freeman, 2018; Hehman, Stolier, & Freeman, 2015; March & Gaertner, 2021; Stillman, Shen, & Ferguson, 2018). A simple and decisive choice would be indicated by moving the mouse so that the cursor travels in a direct line to box *A*. In contrast, a complex and more indecisive choice would be indicated by moving the mouse so that the cursor travels indirectly to box *A*. It drifts over after initially moving toward box *B*, taking a circuitous rather than direct path. Dynamical models treat the process of selecting a response as one that unfolds over time, making parameters such as time, speed, and trajectory important to use when dissociating the processes contributing to a response (e.g., Pleskac, Cesario, & Johnson, 2018). For example, there may be no bias in the choice to shoot a Black man versus a White man, but this does not mean the response was unbiased. Bias is revealed through the choice being faster and more decisive for one group, which PD reveals through examining these parameters.

The Quad Model

The **quadruple process model** focuses on four types of information processing that can co-occur when a person is engaged in social cognition, and uses mathematical models to determine how much each process contributes to any specific cognitive response. Rather than arguing that a person is either engaged in implicit processing or effortful processing, it asks about the unique contributions of four types of processes in producing a response (e.g., Sherman 2006; Sherman et al., 2008). Why four processes? Because any response can be conceived of as concerning two global issues: choosing how to respond and self-regulation (or control). Within each of these two categories are two types of processes. In choosing how to respond there are first processes of accessibility and spreading activation that shape the response—the triggering of an association from the mere presence of a relevant cue in the environment. Activation upon detection of the cue will shape perception, attention, and inference. In choosing how to respond there are also processes of assessment and validation. These processes are used to weigh the strengths (and the weaknesses) of the available information to assess its value, validity,

> **Quadruple process model:** A model focusing on four types of information processing that can co-occur, and that uses mathematical models to determine how much any specific cognitive response is contributed to by each of the four processes.

and influence. However, in addition to these two processes, are a pair of processes that are concerned with regulating output. In choosing how to regulate a response there are first processes of correction. These processes monitor to see whether a response is inappropriate and are used to overturn or suppress an inappropriate response if detected. Regulation not only concerns correcting for bias in a choice or judgment but processes shaping the initial choice or judgment. For example, when trying to recall whether a piece of information is new or had been previously learned, one might have no explicit memory of having seen it before. An assessment process suggests it is new. However, the information feels familiar. An activation process suggests it is old. A response is not yet made. A self-regulatory process is then invoked to eliminate the uncertainty and apply a theory about how to respond. This could be a guess based on experience, or a heuristic like "if it is familiar, it must be known."

The model assigns a name to each of these four types of responses, and a mathematical formula to calculate the degree to which each process is impacting a response. Rather than detail each formula, and how to calculate the four processes, we instead describe them through a single running example to illustrate each process. We consider the "shooter task"—where the research participant has the goal to shoot (by a button press on the keyboard) if a man is holding a gun, and to not shoot (by another button press) if he is not. The objects held (gun, wallet) can serve as a cue as to how to respond. However, the experiment also introduces another factor aside from what object the man is holding. His race is manipulated so that he is at times a White man and at other times a Black man. The quad model argues that *how* stereotypes impact responses on tasks such as these—faster to make a correct response (a hit), more likely to make an incorrect response (a false alarm)—is determined by four distinct processes.

Association activation (AC) is the name for the process that reflects the degree to which a construct is spontaneously activated by the mere presence of associated attributes in the environment. Using the example of the shooter task, AC is the activation of the association that the person has brought into the task between Black men and the construct of threat. A triggering of this association activates further constructs associated with threat—danger, violence, guns, and so on—that could lead one to respond faster to guns when they appear (due to the readiness to see them). Thus, a portion of the bias emerging in the shooter task could be caused by the activation of a stereotype from an associated cue (AC).

Detection (D) is the process through which a person notices and differentiates between correct versus incorrect responses. The process is aimed at attaining and assessing information that will inform what response is appropriate. With D processes, the person analyzes the stimulus information in order to assess its attributes—Is it a high-quality argument (if part of a persuasive message)?, Is it a verifiable quality (if a quality of a person)? This could be driven by a goal to be accurate and attain the best information possible, or a goal to make a fast decision that is merely good enough. For example, in the shooter task, D indicates one's ability to correctly make a "shoot" decision or a "no-shoot" decision by identifying a gun or a wallet (similar to what we earlier called "sensitivity"). Thus, a portion of the bias that emerges in the shooter task could be caused

> **Association activation (AC):** An effortless process that reflects the degree to which a construct is spontaneously activated (primed) by the mere presence of associated attributes in the environment, and associated constructs are triggered (spreading activation).

> **Detection (D):** Processes through which perceivers differentiate among correct versus incorrect responses. This is often characterized by the person analyzing the stimulus information to accurately assess its attributes and seeking to determine if it is a high-quality argument (if part of a persuasive message) or if it is a verifiable quality (if an attribute of a person).

by an inaccurate assessment of the person—concluding that they have a gun when they do not.

Overturning bias (OB) processes are regulation processes in which a person attempts to suppress or correct for the influence of unwanted information, when one has determined that one's response might be biased (such as having a response assimilated to a triggered stereotype, or confirming an unwanted expectation or affective response). These are often conceptualized as effortful processes that reflect aims to overcome a bias introduced by an effortless process. In the "shooter task," this would be a process where a person recognizes a potential influence from a stereotype. Once bias is detected, one tries to overcome this automatic association between Black men and threat. This would manifest as an attempt to compensate for the tendency to respond "shoot" by making "no-shoot" decisions when encountering an unarmed Black man as a "target."

Overturning bias (OB): A process of self-regulation where a person suppresses or corrects for the influence of unwanted information when one determines a response is biased (such as a response confirming an unwanted stereotype). These are often conceptualized as effortful processes aimed at controlling an effortless process.

Guessing (G) is the existence of a general response bias that the participant brings to the experiment, a bias that is unrelated to the specific demands of the task or the stimuli used. For example, a person might have a bias to say that something that feels familiar is true, which exists for all stimuli, not just the items in the current experiment. Returning to the running example of the "shooter task," a person might

Guessing (G): A process where the perceiver uses a general response bias that existed prior to the experiment (that is untethered to the demands of the task or the stimulus). For example, a bias to respond faster with the right hand, or a bias to say yes when uncertain.

have a bias to respond faster with the right hand, or a bias to say yes. Thus, in the shooter task, G reflects a bias to shoot or to not shoot a Black man for reasons not driven by the associations activated in the mind during decision making for this task. For example, G could be reflected in a person's "general tendency to presume danger in the absence of clear evidence to the contrary" (Sherman et al., 2008, p. 316).

While much of the discussion of the quad model implies that OB and G are effortful processes because they require control or self-regulation, there is the possibility in the model to treat each process as effortless. There is nothing in the model that *requires* consciousness and effort be required elements of control. It is simply that most discussions of these matters are still rooted in the language of consciousness and effort. However, what truly matters to the quad model is not a discussion of whether a particular process is implicit or explicit. What matters for distinguishing among the processes is what they *do*—what Sherman (2006) called "the particular nature of the process" (p. 181), not their relative automaticity. Automaticity is a feature of a process in this model, not a defining element of the process. As such, it is important to also note that nothing in the model requires that automaticity be associated with error. It is not uncommon to hear discussions of automaticity equated with error, such as in the analysis of the shooter task where AC led to a bias.[4] None of the four processes must cause bias, or need be equated with effort (or effortlessness). Calanchini and Sherman (2013) state this well:

> The operation of Detection [D] and Overcoming Bias [OB] demands a more nuanced portrayal of automaticity and control because D and OB possess features of both. For example, though it is clear that their operation can be disrupted, it also is clear that they are sufficiently efficient to influence responses during the performance of implicit tasks. This suggests two important points. First, researchers should resist the temptation to describe processes as either automatic or controlled. . . . Second, we need to broaden the range of processes that may be characterized as automatic. (p. 661)

Propositional Models

In contrast to models that attempt to show multiple processes, other models argue that processing is entirely propositional. The notion of propositional learning was reviewed in the Chapter 6 discussion of Gawronski and Bodenhausen's (2006) APE model. *Propositional learning* refers to the fact that in addition to associations between constructs, processing also includes information about the *relationship* among the content stored in memory. Propositional learning contains information about cause and effect, or proposes a direction to a relationship among associated constructs. This is an important distinction. Using an example detailed in Chapter 6, an association would mean that whenever one had a rash (a negative event) and applied lotion, this would create a link between lotion and the bad outcome (rash)—lotion would then trigger negative thoughts of the rash. Propositional processing would add that the lotion was used to *alleviate* the negative event, to soothe the rash, and was positive.

Some models propose that all processing is propositional in nature, and that there is, therefore, only a single process (not two, or four, or more). Kruglanski, Erb, Pierro, Mannetti, and Chun (2006) argue that the one process responsible for human judgment is based on conditional IF-THEN statements. It is propositional and rule driven. Even processes of association—which are described as merely being conditioned responses (e.g., Bargh, 1990, 1994; Olson & Fazio, 2003)—are also described as propositional because they are guided by IF-THEN rules (if stimulus X is present, activate the associated information A, B, C, etc,). These IF-THEN rules, from this point of view, were necessary for the association to develop and were quite explicit as conditioning was first occurring. However, time and practice has simply habitualized the use of the rule and removed it from conscious awareness with its routinization. Thus, it is not a separate process, just a fast and invisible process of propositional learning. Similarly, this model argues that dual-process models do not truly describe two different processes, but different types of information being subjected to one process. These content differences produce judgments that may look like they were based on different processes (one implicit, the other explicit), but they were merely based on rules of inference. Different content calls on different inferential rules, but not different processes. If stimulus X is a heuristic cue, such as a celebrity endorsing a product, or a majority (consensus of people) expressing an opinion, or a long list of arguments in support of a position, then the rule called upon is the proposition that such information is to be trusted and accepted. If stimulus X is low in relevance to you personally, the proposition might be to form an impression quickly using whatever is presented first or easiest to grab hold of. If stimulus Y is a cue that suggests the situation is complex, ambivalent, or ambiguous, then the rule called upon is the proposition that such information should be examined more closely. If stimulus Y has high relevance to you, then the proposition might be to withhold judgment until diverse types of information have been considered. From this view the difference is not one of process but the nature of the stimulus and the content of the rule that is then applied.

For a "unimodel" to work it needs to specify many parameters, such as how one decides what is relevant and knows which rule to follow, which from among the many cues will become salient and specify its associated rules, when will cognitive demands and limited resources specify whether it will be difficult applying a rule, and will the rule be applied automatically or require conscious effort. In the end, many parameters could be identified to specify how this single process functions. Yet others might argue that specifying parameters is really detailing the many processes involved, and that a single process is untenable. For example, Pryor and Reeder (2006) argue that a basic problem with the unimodel is that it overextends the concept of if-then judgment rules to include all regularity in psychological processes. Any deterministic quality in human behavior, therefore, would follow an "if-then" rule and would imply a rule-based process. . . . At some point, the unimodel's quest for reductionism seems to obscure some important distinctions in psychological processes. (p. 232)

Once again, detailed reviews of such debates are not the goal of this chapter, which merely hopes to illustrate the many ways it is possible to think about the nature of processing. There are those who see it as a single, propositional, rule-based form of learning.

Iterative Processing Models

Some models claim to have a different level of analysis, grounded in neuroscience, that is focused on the actual brain processes that produce human judgment. Though inspired by neuroscience, I would argue that these approaches are not truly pitched at a different level of analysis, since they do not inform us as to *how* these implicated brain regions actually produce the products (judgment, attitude, evaluation, etc.). They simply provide a different metaphor for describing processing than that offered by dual-process systems. The "neuroscientific" evidence described is simply that increased activity in certain brain regions, such as the amygdala, is correlated with performing some types of tasks. Pointing to a brain region does not provide any more of an explanation as to how judgments and evaluations are produced, or a different level of explanation (e.g., Marr, 1982), than models arguing for separate systems. However, it is a different metaphor that provides a unique way of structuring the data about processing.

One such model is the iterative reprocessing (IR) model (e.g., Cunningham & Zelazo, 2007). Rather than discussing separate types of processes or systems to explain judgments and evaluations that appear to be implicit versus explicit, the IR model describes brain areas that are modular in that they are dedicated to certain types of tasks. Processing nodes are divided into functions that have been attributed to human brain regions, and as such these processes are in turn attempted to be mapped onto (largely limbic) brain areas known to be involved in emotional and mnemonic function. Subcortical regions perform largely automatic cognitive tasks, such as pattern recognition, affective associations, and detecting whether a stimulus is salient. The amygdala and ventral striatum are said to compute emotional salience and valence, while the hypothalamus is responsible for behavioral and visceral expression of emotion (e.g., Cunningham & Zelazo, 2007; Cunningham, Zelazo, Packer, & Van Bavel, 2007). These tasks in these brain regions are ongoing, constantly being updated in an iterative fashion, and constantly producing output with each iteration. Cortical regions perform tasks that are associated with control. They describe the orbitofrontal cortex as comparing past and/or expected rewards and punishments. The dorsolateral prefrontal cortex chooses which aspects of stimulus to attend to/evaluate, directing attentional resources to evaluating less immediately salient stimulus information, as well as context. The insula keeps a running tab on how you are feeling (viscerally, emotionally) at any given time. The outcomes of the controlled cortical processes update the automatic subcortical representation. And with each iteration of processing, in each area, comes updating in each area. Thus, there is no true separation of processes, or serial processing, but a constant communication among brain regions with updating with each iteration.

Thus, for example, evaluation in the moment (as distinguished from attitudes, which are more stable) is captured in this model as a spectrum of depth of processing. When time and resources are constrained, processing of stimuli relies on tasks in the subcortical regions. But if there is opportunity and motivation to evaluate more deeply, controlled mechanisms in the cortical regions can be recruited. In these instances, there is an iterative process in which the outputs of earlier, more automatic processing can serve as inputs to later, higher-level, and more reflective processing, but with presumably automatic visceral perception and expression continuously producing the evaluative output. Each cycle begins with lower-order processes including activity in subcortical structures that lead to physiological reactions, but these lower-order structures also get information from relatively higher-order structures in cortical regions modulating attention to further information. Thus, with each cycle the lower-order (faster) processes provide information to higher-order processes through "forward spread of activation," yet are also modulated by the higher-order processes through "backward spread of activation." What we think of as explicit processing corresponds to a greater number of iterations or cycles. Later revisions of the model scale back emphasis on the directionality of the continuum of iterations along an automatic/controlled axis, in order to account for findings that early, time-limited evaluations can be modified by cognitive influences (e.g., context). Emphasis is now on the prediction that evaluations evolve over time, via iterative processing, passing computation between more automatic and more controlled processes throughout.

And of course, this is all metaphorical. No single brain region is actually dedicated to any one task. In this "limbic loop," many of these brain regions are bidirectionally connected, making it very hard to differentiate the role of any of these areas. It is a circuit—brain regions, even those associated with distinct functions, are highly interconnected and argue against real modularity (e.g., Buzsáki, 2006; Forbes & Grafman, 2013). But by the IR model ascribing unique tasks to specific structures, it allows for one type of description of how evaluation and judgment is produced and updated. Yet despite implicating biological processes, it is still purely descriptive and tells us only about the function of cognitive processing (the types of outputs produced), not the manner in which the outputs are produced. To say "computing emotional salience happens in the amygdala" is the same type of explanation as to say "attitudes are propositional," or that there are "systems" implicated. Unfortunately, though interesting in what it proposes, there is, at the moment, no way to differentiate through an experiment what is proposed by the IR model from the processes implicated in other (dual-process) models. The outputs would look the same despite the different stories of why. A strength of the IR model is it imagines a neural implementation, which few other models even attempt. However, it is left to conjecture, as the model does not specify those neural mechanisms but describes a more abstract process. Of course, this is still movement in the right direction since a metaphor that proposes an abstract modular view of neuroscience is more likely to approximate something the brain actually does, instead of purely metaphorical boxes and arrows. Unlike dual-process models, it proposes a single dynamical system in which information is processed repeatedly, in a cycle, in what is described as an iterative fashion, across many interacting brain regions, each with a unique task. But in the end, these are not models that explain the *how of processing*, but provide a different *way of describing functionality* with a new metaphor for processing that relies on neuroscience.

Parallel Distributed Processing: Activation and Inhibition

Anderson and Bower (1973) identified a long set of theories on associationism, all sharing the belief that "ideas, sense data, memory nodes, or similar mental elements are associated together in the mind through experience" (p. 10). The notion of association was introduced in Chapter 2 and described as essential to social cognition in every chapter of this book.

An *associative network* implies that knowledge does not reside in isolation but is linked in memory to other bits of knowledge. In the metaphorical language cognitive psychologists use to describe this network, each isolated piece of knowledge being mentally represented is called a node. Thus, if you say you know (or remember) that the musician John Lennon was murdered in New York on December 8, 1980, it means an association exists in memory between the concepts "New York, "John Lennon," "murder," and "December 8." This would be referred to as a person node. The triggering of this memory activates associated memories, such as the gun-related deaths of other musicians, like Sam Cooke, Marvin Gaye, Tupac Shakur, Kurt Cobain, Selena, Peter Tosh, Jam Master Jay, The Notorious B.I.G., Nipsey Hussle, and Pop Smoke. Perhaps it triggers thoughts of other gun-related deaths, such as those relating to school shootings. Perhaps it triggers thoughts of shots fired at political figures (such as JFK, MLK, RFK, Ronald Reagan, Gerald Ford, Gabby Giffords, Dick Cheney, and Malcolm X). Maybe it triggers beliefs about gun control. Just as a real net consists of knots that are tied together by rope, the mental network is a series of metaphorical knots—nodes—connected through associations.

If you previously did not know who Sam Cooke was, you likely by now have constructed such a node that includes an association to Kurt Cobain, John Lennon, and so on, and includes knowledge that he was a musician who was shot. Thus, new nodes are constructed by creating links to existing nodes in the network, and such is the way in which we build our knowledge (and impressions) of other people. Associated behaviors and traits then get triggered and perhaps linked to the person as well, even if the person did not act in the new ways. Thus, we might infer Sam Cooke was creative even though all we learned about him was that he was murdered. Thus, when one has categorized a stimulus, the activation of that knowledge travels along the associative network, triggering associated concepts and knowledge. This process is called *spreading activation*. In Chapter 2 we illustrated that the stronger the association between concepts, the faster and the more likely that activation will spread. Activation starts at the triggered node, flowing most easily and quickly along the paths that represent stronger associations.

However, we take a moment here to introduce another popular conceptualization of how associative memory processes work that is different from the network models just described. This is known as **parallel distributed processing** (PDP; also *connectionism*). The major difference between network models and PDP is that PDP describes a more systemwide type of association than we have been describing. The network models described thus far posit individual nodes that are organized sets of features and attributes, with some organizing principle being the heart of the node. Thus, we have a person node for "John Lennon" around which all features relating to him are locally linked. With the PDP metaphor of a networked memory system, there is no "John Lennon" node, nor any specific category around which a local organization exists (no "violence" node, no "school shootings" node, etc.). Instead, there are distributed representations (not local ones) in which nodes are dispersed across a vast network of nodes. Rather than our category for "John Lennon" being a set of closely clustered nodes with direct links to one another, it consists of a set of nodes that are simultaneously triggered (triggered in parallel) without them needing to be conceived of as passing through a local system or shared space that has all the nodes along the way triggered.

> **Parallel distributed processing (PDP; connectionism):** A more systemwide type of association than spreading activation describes. With the PDP metaphor of a networked memory system, there is no closely clustered set of nodes with direct links to one another, nor any specific category around which a local organization exists. Instead, there are distributed representations (not local ones) in which nodes are dispersed across a vast network of nodes that are simultaneously triggered (triggered in parallel) without passing through a local system or shared space.

A good metaphor might be to contemplate how we think about an old scoreboard. In the old days a scoreboard functioned by many independent light bulbs turned on simultaneously in order to produce an image, perceptible sentence, or series of numbers. Only the simultaneous (parallel) activation of disparate bulbs among a vast and dispersed set of bulbs allows for the board to work. This is how a connectionist model imagines memory works. A category for "John Lennon" might be best thought of as a pattern of nodes being simultaneously triggered, perhaps node numbers 9 and 1,458 and 56,762 and 457, and so on, all activated in parallel, even though they are not conceived of as being stored in a physically shared space with direct connections, to yield what we then experience as knowledge of "John Lennon." We do not need here to get into a debate about PDP versus other forms of associationism, nor need we review the details of such models (a vast task, one better left for a book dealing with models of categorization or cognitive psychology). Our point is only to illustrate that there are a variety of ways to conceive of how the processing system *associates* mental representations.

A distributed system might better explain how we so easily make sense of cases where there is conflict among associated knowledge (which are somewhat typical). For example, in the Stroop effect (introduced in Chapter 3) there are multiple responses that can be made to a stimulus (the semantic meaning of the word and the color of the font) and those responses are in conflict with one another (the word is "black" but it is written in grey font). An account of the Stroop effect from a PDP perspective, as depicted in Figure 12.3, would suggest that there are associations to both the word meaning and the word color, and one of those responses (word meaning—"black"—is more dominant. However, the context specifies a goal (name the font color) that suggests the simultaneous inhibition of the dominant response and activation of the less-dominant response, so that the response made will match the goal.

As another example, take the word "bank." It has multiple meanings: a place to put money, a metaphorical sense of security or confidence, a river's edge, and so on. If all of these meanings were simultaneously triggered by spreading activation, it might cause

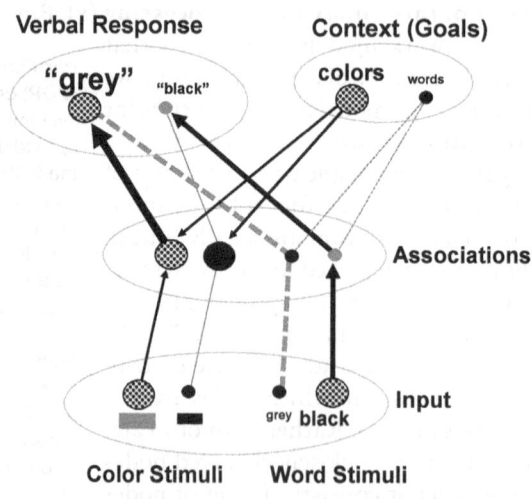

FIGURE 12.3. PDP and the Stroop effect.

competition and conflict among them. In contrast, a system that only triggers the appropriate nodes (as specified by the context and goals) would be more efficient. Thus, if I said "take it to the bank" after I handed you money, it might trigger only those nodes relevant to that context, as would also be the case if we were in a tent in the woods and I handed you a canoe oar and similarly said "take it to the bank." Kunda and Thagard (1996) offer what they call the **parallel-constraint-satisfaction model**, which asserts that not everything in the lexicon associated with a category or stereotype is triggered when we encounter a member of that category, or a behavior that falls in a category. Instead, goals, expectations, and context bolster the activation of some information while simultaneously (in parallel) inhibiting or constraining the activation of other information. Kunda, Sinclair, and Griffin (1997) offer a nice example:

> **Parallel-constraint-satisfaction model:** A model asserting that not everything in the lexicon associated with a category/stereotype is triggered when we encounter cues to that category (such as behavior or a group member's face). Instead, goals, expectations, and context bolster activation of some information while simultaneously (in parallel) inhibiting the activation of other information.

> Aggressive may activate both punch and argue. The context in which aggressive is activated may serve to narrow its meaning. Thus, courtroom may activate argue while deactivating punch . . . a given trait may have a rich and diverse network of associates; only a subset of these is activated on any occasion. (p. 721)

This distributed processing account of association holds that not all information associated with a category is triggered. In fact, the goals of the perceiver and the context one is in inhibit some associations, making them less (rather than more) likely to be accessible and used (thus, when one is in a courtroom, notions of being argumentative are activated, but notions of punching are not). Such processing ideas have been used in my own research on stereotyping. My colleagues and I (Moskowitz, 2002, 2010; Moskowitz et al., 1999; Moskowitz & Li, 2011; Moskowit et al., 2000, 2011; Sassenberg & Moskowitz, 2005; Sassenberg et al., 2022) have investigated whether our goals lead to the strategic activation and inhibition of concepts associated with a stereotype. We review this work later in the chapter, but we find that a stereotype is not always activated when encountering a relevant cue. That same cue can trigger the inhibition of the stereotype and the activation of an alternative construct dependent on the goals the person is pursuing. For example, the semantic content linked to a cultural stereotype ("women") was inhibited following categorization, rather than activated. But only if one had a goal to be egalitarian to women. Other experiments show that when a young, White research participant is given the goal of taking the perspective of a member of a stereotyped group (an older man, a Black man) the stereotype of that group is not triggered (e.g., Galinsky & Moskowitz, 2000b, 2007). A category does not trigger all concepts with which it is associated if one's goals deem a concept incompatible. The stereotype is inhibited instead.

A similar point consistent with a distributed representation is made in research where context rather than goals determines what associations are activated. For example, Macrae et al. (1995) showed that if two opposing stereotypes are relevant to the same stimulus, then context will determine which constructs are activated by the stimulus. Participants observed a Chinese woman in one of two possible contexts: one that triggered stereotypes of women and one that triggered stereotypes of Chinese people. They found that when gender stereotypes were most accessible (by watching a video of a Chinese woman applying makeup), people were likely to have gender stereotypes accessible but not stereotypes of the Chinese (which instead were now inhibited). However, if the Chinese stereotype had been activated (by watching a video of a Chinese woman eating while using chopsticks), it is the stereotype associated with this category that is most accessible, and gender stereotypes were no longer accessible but inhibited. Macrae and MacLeod (1999) examined similar types of interference and inhibition between competing constructs in the domain of memory and forgetting. The inability to remember information may be caused by interference from a competing representation that blocks the desired information from consciousness (the temporary suppression of competing constructs). For example, if one wants to remember the name of a date one is meeting at a restaurant, this is served by the names of past dates taken to the same restaurant being suppressed. Retrieving a specific item from memory leads to the suppression (rather than accessibility) of relevant, but competing items.

Another illustration that is consistent with distributed processing is when information inconsistent with a stereotype is inhibited. Just as one might want to suppress the names of other dates taken to a restaurant to shield the current date from interference, one might want to inhibit thoughts incompatible with a stereotype (that, if activated, would undermine the stereotype) to shield the stereotype. Such inhibition of incompatible constructs was provided in an experiment by Dijksterhuis and van Knippenberg (1996). They illustrated that priming a stereotype (asking participants to imagine a typical "soccer hooligan") facilitated access to stereotype-consistent traits (e.g., aggressive, fanatical, violent, and insolent) yet also inhibited access to stereotype-inconsistent traits (e.g., friendly, intelligent, and understanding) relative to control words. Similarly, Rothbart, Sriram, and Davis-Stitt (1996) illustrated that stereotypes increased the ability to retrieve typical category members while limiting access to atypical members. The more counterstereotypic a category member was, the lower the probability that this member was activated and retrieved when the stereotype was accessible. For example, in a study involving rival fraternities, typical members of a rival fraternity were more likely to be recalled, and atypical ones (members who disconfirmed the stereotype) inhibited and less likely to be recalled. These findings suggest that counterstereotypic traits and exemplars are being inhibited when stereotypes are accessible.

The research just reviewed suggests an alternative to the conception of control offered by dual-process models. Dual-process theories equate control with effort. This is an appealing notion since, intuitively, to pursue a goal, to self-regulate, seems to require consciousness and effort (e.g., Wegner & Bargh, 1998). However, pitting low effort and control as opposites (either in two separate systems, or as opposing ends of a continuum) ignores the fact that control can be effortless and self-regulation can happen outside of conscious awareness (e.g., Aarts, Custers, & Holland, 2007; Bargh, 1990; Gollwitzer & Moskowitz, 1996; Moskowitz, Li, & Kirk, 2004). Controlled processing is not the same as effortful processing. Dual-process models obscure this fact, at great cost. For example, equating control and effort leads to the erroneous belief that stereotyping is a default response, and to control it *requires* conscious awareness and effort. If people lack awareness of bias, or lack the capacity to exert the effort, such models would have us believe stereotype control would not be possible.

We next review evidence for the idea that implicit processes can be controlled from being executed, rather than just corrected after having occurred. As Fiedler and Hütter (2014) stated, "even though organisms certainly profit from a rich repertoire of well-exercised defaults and routine behaviors, an adaptive organism must also have learned to regulate the execution of these routines" (p. 507). For example, stereotype activation can be controlled (Moskowitz et al., 1999), evaluative conditioning effects are malleable (e.g., Spruyt, Hermans, De Houwer, Vandromme, & Eelen, 2007; Fiedler & Unkelbach, 2011; Gawronski, Balas, & Creighton, 2014), and IAT as well as affect misattribution procedure (AMP) responses are subject to self-regulation (e.g., Blair, Ma, & Lenton, 2001; Dasgupta, 2004; Dasgupta & Rivera, 2006; Mann & Ferguson, 2017; Payne, Cheng, Govorun, & Stewart, 2005).

IMPLICIT CONTROL: CONTROL IS NOT ALWAYS EFFORTFUL
AND CAN BE PROACTIVE

"Control" and "goal pursuit" are words that seem synonymous with effort and explicitly "trying" to accomplish something. As Wegner and Bargh (1998) put it, "Intuitively, after all, most people think of control in humans as conscious control, so much so that the term 'unconscious control' doesn't seem right at all" (p. 453). Yet starting in the book's first chapter we have seen research from Bruner (1957) in which low-level, implicit cognitive processes (such as where attention is focused and what is perceived) are shaped by goals that people do not realize they have. This idea is far older than the 1950s. Try to recall the story of Archimedes running naked through the streets of Syracuse yelling "Eureka!" from your early history lessons. While running naked is hardly an implicit response, the epiphany that drew Archimedes to the streets was. Archimedes was grappling with a dense and difficult problem: how to measure the purity of gold. He was stumped and frustrated. So, he consciously decided to place his ruminations on this problem on hold. He abandoned the problem to relax in the bath. Archimedes, as is the case for many of us, had his best idea while relaxing in the tub. Consciousness had vacated the goal of solving the problem for other pastures (a bath), but his nonconscious cognition was still pursuing it. He did not realize he was still working on the problem when a solution hit him. Displacement of the water by his body triggered the answer to the problem he had consciously abandoned. The shock of it appearing out of the blue, springing into consciousness as if delivered from God, led him to his famous shout of exuberance: "Eureka!" And off he streaked.

If you do not know the story of Archimedes, simply think back to the last time you had difficulty retrieving information from memory (e.g., who shot and killed Robert Kennedy?). We often experience a tip-of-the-tongue effect (Brown & McNeill, 1966) where the desired information feels as if it is knowledge you possess and is about to reach consciousness. But despite feeling like it will come to you, the response cannot be produced. Struggling with this for some time ultimately leads you to consciously disengage from the task (assume you did not just google it). Interestingly, that information often comes rushing into consciousness at some later time when you were not consciously trying to retrieve it (e.g., "it was Sirhan Sirhan!"). This is an example of nonconscious goal pursuit. Both the goal and the strategies used to pursue the goal were no longer conscious, and thus the attainment of the goal is delivered to the conscious mind as if by magic (or as if by divine intervention). But divinity and magic are not needed to explain this.

One is not always aware of a goal they are pursuing while pursuing it. Goals can be triggered outside of awareness. Goals can also be consciously selected but then abandoned, leaving them still activated without one being consciously aware of this. Control is not always effortful, and can even be wholly implicit, such as when a goal is implicitly activated and pursued through implicit means (e.g., Bargh, 1990; Moskowitz, 2014). Let us start with two empirical illustrations of the point, picked randomly from hundreds of possible experiments to make the point. First, Koole, Smeets, van Knippenberg, and Dijksterhuis (1999) activated a goal of being intelligent without participants knowing. In a first task, participants received feedback that they lacked intelligence relative to other people performing a task. Even when disengaging from this task, the goal to be intelligent should now be activated, even though participants were no longer thinking consciously about it. They then used a lexical decision task to assess whether the goal to be intelligent was activated when performing an ostensibly unrelated task. Relative to control participants, those with a goal to be intelligent triggered were faster to recognize words related to the goal.

In an early set of experiments, Kurt Lewin and his students set up conditions that blocked goal pursuit. Zeigarnik (1927) undertook a doctoral dissertation where participants worked on tasks (such as solving puzzles) until they were clearly completed. But some of the activities were interrupted before they were completed. The tasks were then removed from sight so participants could no longer work on them. What impact would the blocking of a simple, unimportant goal have? Participants continued to focus on attaining the goal—ruminating on the task outside consciousness—even though its pursuit was blocked. To show this, Zeigarnik later asked the participants to try to recall the tasks that they had worked on. She found that the unfinished tasks were recalled twice as much as the finished ones. Participants used memory as a means to work toward an unmet goal, a phenomenon labeled the **Zeigarnik effect**. Eighty years later a similar result was provided by

Zeigarnik effect: When people continue to work on a goal that is consciously blocked, or from which they are disengaged. Despite conscious operations toward pursuing the goal being eliminated, one uses implicit processing to continue attempts at reaching the desired state, processes such as ruminating on the material to attempt to find a solution.

Deliberation-without-attention effect: A phenomenon where conscious decision-making processes are blocked, yet the factors one should be weighing to produce a decision are weighed outside conscious awareness anyway. The goal to ruminate on the options and produce a decision is continued despite consciousness for this goal having been released.

Dijksterhuis et al. (2006) in what they called a **deliberation-without-attention effect**. As described in Chapter 3, participants were given an explicit goal of ruminating on the qualities of several products. Some participants were allowed to consciously ruminate on the pros and cons of the possible options, other participants were prevented from consciously deliberating over the choices. The goal persisted implicitly, so that participants who were prevented from consciously deliberating about these choices made better decisions than those who were not prevented from deliberating. Many other relevant examples of how control can occur outside awareness were scattered throughout the book: the New Look research of Jerome Bruner and his colleagues discussed in Chapter 1; the *cocktail party effect* in Chapter 3; the discussion of dichotic listening tasks in Chapter 4; the research of Balcetis et al. (2012) reviewed in Chapter 5 showing control over the implicit process of resolving binocular rivalry; the research of Aarts et al. (2004) reviewed in Chapter 6 showing goal contagion; and experiments by Fitzsimons and Bargh (2003) described in Chapter 10 where people had implicit helping goals or implicit achievement goals that could be triggered without one knowing by simply thinking about people associated with those goals.

Proactive Control of Stereotyping

Devine (1989) popularized the notion that because a cultural stereotype is the strongest association to the category, it is *inevitably* activated. Thus, any hope to control stereotyping was said to require overturning these activated thoughts to correct their influence. This is what is known as **reactive control**, where one becomes aware of a biasing influence after it has occurred and then reacts to this knowledge with an attempt to correct or overturn the bias. While reactive models of stereotype control are an important area of study, we also know correction attempts often fail. The notion of implicit control introduced here suggests a complementary way to control stereotypes. Rather than reacting to a stereotype after it has been triggered, one could also control the bias if the triggering was controlled in the first place. This is what is known as **proactive control**, where one's goals direct an initial response so that a bias that might otherwise appear is inhibited or replaced by an

Reactive control: When a stereotype has been activated and has started to impact responding, and one retroactively controls for this by removing its influence and correcting the bias it has exerted.

Proactive control: Controlling a stereotype by willfully inhibiting the stereotype's activation. Rather than being more accessible, goals render this association less accessible prior to it ever being activated. As such, the stereotype cannot ever have influenced the person, due to its removal from the equation altogether.

alternative, nonbiased way of responding. We discuss two distinct ways such proactive control can be initiated.

One is in the manner described by James (1890/1950). James stated, "often-repeated movements follow on their mental cue. An end consented to as soon as conceived innervates directly the centre of the first movement of the chain which leads to its accomplishment, and then the whole chain rattles off *quasi*-reflexly" (p. 519, italics in original).

Practice and repetition associating a goal with a group of people (such as men practicing egalitarianism to women) can lead to, over time, a restructuring of the representation so that the goal becomes the strongest association to the group. At first this requires consciousness, but it ultimately becomes implicit. With time and practice at responding in an unbiased way in the presence of cues associated with a goal to be unbiased, the mere presence of the cues should trigger the control response. Through repetition these steps can become automated so that reactive control is not needed. Rather than responding inappropriately and fixing it, the cues that once led to inappropriate responses can now directly trigger the goal, the means to the goal, the contexts in which means are encountered, and the operations or desired responses.

A second way stereotype control can be proactively initiated is in the manner described by Lewin (1935) and does not require such extensive practice or being the type of person who has developed a chronic goal to control stereotyping. It requires merely a *strong commitment* to the goal in the moment and a *plan of operations* for implementing the goal that can be triggered by cues associated with the goal (e.g., Gollwitzer & Moskowitz, 1996). With some goals, the plan of how to act has been developed over time; at some point in the past a conscious choice was needed to know how to respond, but that response plan becomes associated with the goal and can merely be triggered when the goal is triggered. With other goals, the plan of how to act is set in the moment. The implementation of goaldirected action needs to be prepared through the individual reflecting on *when*, *where*, *how*, and *how long* to act, thus creating a plan for implementing action (e.g., Gollwitzer, 1993). Though consciously formed in the moment, the commitment to the plan and the specific linking of the plan's precise operations to a cue allows the plan to be triggered outside awareness by that cue (e.g., Aarts, Dijksterhuis, & Midden, 1999; Gollwitzer, 1999; Gollwitzer & Brandstaetter, 1997). Such plans for goal pursuit, what Gollwitzer called **implementation intentions**, are merely triggered, like the scripts and frames discussed in Chapter 2. One can plan "when I see a woman, then I will inhibit stereotypes" so that when a woman is encountered, the inhibition rattles off unconsciously, not the stereotype.

> **Implementation intentions:** A specific type of planning where one commits to perform a particular goal-directed response when a specific situation is encountered. The plan links a goal-relevant cue to a response, thus specifying when, where, and how to achieve the goal so action can be rattled off without consciousness when cues are detected.

Proactive Stereotype Control from Chronic Egalitarian Goals

Moskowitz (1993a) proposed that goals that are incompatible with stereotyping can be chronically held by people who have been pursuing the goal across time and contexts. Through this chronic pursuit, a new set of associations that link concepts of fairness and equity to a group form, while cultural stereotypes are repeatedly inhibited. As a result, the mental representation is permanently updated so that the cultural stereotype is not the strongest association. For such people the inhibition rather than activation of the negative elements of the cultural stereotype should be triggered by cues

> **Chronic egalitarian goals:** Personally relevant goals to pursue fairness, equity, and justice toward a specific group to which a person is so strongly committed that the goal is in a state of chronic activation (and pursued across a variety of contexts). Cues signaling group membership will trigger these goals rather than a stereotype.

associated with the group. To illustrate this, Moskowitz et al. (1999) first identified people with **chronic egalitarian goals**. These are personally relevant goals to pursue fairness, equity, justice, and to eliminate bias toward a specific group. The goal to be egalitarian is in a state of chronic accessibility. Once identifying such people, they were recruited as research participants to examine whether, compared to control participants, stereotypes are inhibited.

Moskowitz et al. (1999) recruited male participants who had a chronic goal to be egalitarian to women and nonchronics (these men were not high in sexism, they just were not holding chronic egalitarian goals). Participants performed a task in which words either relevant to the stereotype of women or control words were presented on the screen. Participants had to speak the words aloud into a microphone, with the computer recording their pronunciation speeds. Half of the time these words were preceded by faces of women and half of the time by faces of men. The task measured stereotype activation and inhibition without participants realizing the task was about stereotyping. They found that chronic egalitarians did not have stereotypes activated when cues relating to women were encountered. Instead they *inhibited* the stereotype. Reaction time measures revealed that they were slower to pronounce words relevant to the stereotype of women than to pronounce control words irrelevant to the stereotype. This occurred only when the word was preceded by a picture of a woman and not if preceded by pictures of men. This inhibition of the stereotype did not occur for men who were not chronic egalitarians, who instead showed stereotype activation. Chronic egalitarians inhibited stereotypes. The mental representation was updated—rather than stereotype activation, spreading inhibition is triggered (e.g., Fox, 1995).

If chronic egalitarian goals led to the semantic content linked to a cultural stereotype being inhibited rather than activated, what new associations are triggered in this updated structure? One answer to this question is that people can replace negative stereotypes with positive stereotypes. While this still represents a form of stereotyping, it at least updates the stereotype so that it is less negative (e.g., Lepore & Brown, 1997). Another answer to the question is that one's goals associated with the group are what are activated. Allport (1954) suggested this was possible when he asserted that whatever association to a category that is *most dominant* is what gets triggered. What is most dominant could be the stereotype. But something other than a stereotype might be triggered because it, not the stereotype, is the dominant response. Moskowitz et al. (2000) argued that for chronic egalitarians, rather than automatically trigger the stereotype, a cue associated with a stereotyped group will inhibit the stereotype and instead trigger the goal to be egalitarian. To illustrate this, they performed an experiment similar to Moskowitz et al. (1999), except using African American faces as primes, words relevant to the stereotype of African Americans in the reaction time task, and chronic goals relating to African Americans in recruiting participants. They replicated the finding of stereotype inhibition among chronic egalitarians. A second experiment assessed whether the faces of Black men triggered egalitarian goals. They used a reaction time task that measured speed of responding to words relating to egalitarianism ("fairness," "justice," "equity," etc.). People identified as having chronic egalitarian goals were faster to perceive words relevant to the goal of egalitarianism following faces of Black men (and not White men), but were not faster at perceiving words irrelevant to the goal. Their goals were implicitly triggered by the mere presence of a goal-relevant stimulus.

Proactive Stereotype Control from Momentary Goals

Stereotype activation happens outside awareness and without one's conscious intent, but it is nonetheless a cognitive process used by people *to help attain a goal*—such as the epistemic goal to have fast and efficient knowledge about a person. Because it is a process that serves a specific goal, stereotype activation is controllable if people have goals that are incompatible with stereotyping. These need not be chronic goals. Moskowitz (2001, 2002, 2010, 2014) proposed that one must merely have commitment to a goal that is stronger than the epistemic goals that associate the stereotype with the group. For example, people with the goal of taking the perspective of a stigmatized group member do not show evidence of stereotype activation. The goal triggers a set of cognitive operations associated with achieving that specific goal, and this does not involve recruiting the stereotypes of the group. Rather than overturning an unwanted bias, one proactively minimizes stereotypic thoughts while increasing positive thoughts (e.g., Galinsky & Moskowitz, 2000b; Todd & Galinsky, 2014). The set of cognitive operations triggered in pursuit of this goal render stereotypes irrelevant to the task at hand.

Other research from my lab has similarly shown that a goal that has nothing to do with stereotyping—being creative—also does not lead to one activating a stereotype when a group member is encountered. Sassenberg and Moskowitz (2005) argue that because creativity requires ingenuity, novelty, and innovation, it may lead to seeing group members in more atypical ways that do not involve stereotypes. They hypothesized that creativity goals trigger a specific set of implicit operations: the inhibition of typical associations to whatever concept one is attempting to think creatively about, and the increased accessibility of atypical associates to the same concept. This led to stereotype control because people with a creativity goal implicitly inhibited the typical associations to the category. White research participants who saw the face of a Black man did not have stereotypes activated but instead had these typical associations inhibited—but only if they had a creativity goal implicitly activated. From this perspective, the association of stereotypes with a group is only usefully activated when one's current goals are facilitated by a stereotype being recruited. It is true that our epistemic goals, by default, often make recruiting such thoughts common. This makes stereotyping common. But it is not inevitable. Shifting the goals that are driving one's responding could, even inadvertently, inhibit stereotype activation. Of course, adopting goals whose specific aim is to control stereotypes can also inhibit them.

Moskowitz and Li (2011) show, across four experiments, that when people *temporarily* adopt an egalitarian goal, the stereotype is inhibited by exposure to the group, rather than the stereotype being activated. In this research the egalitarian goal is described as being implicit because although participants have it triggered consciously (by writing about a time they failed at being egalitarian), they are not aware they are pursuing the goal when stereotyping is assessed later in the experiment. The experiment is set up as purportedly being two experiments, one with a task of writing about a goal failure (half writing about egalitarian goals, half about a different goal), and a separate "cognitive" experiment with a reaction time task that participants do not see as related to the first task (or to stereotyping). Thus, conscious thoughts of the egalitarian goal are abandoned as they enter this seemingly unrelated task. However, the goal is only consciously abandoned. The goal's implicit activation is evidenced by the fact the stereotype is inhibited, as measured by a reaction time task that assessed accessibility of words related to the stereotype of Black men versus control words, and, crucially, by manipulating whether those words follow faces of either Black men or White men (as Moskowitz et al., 1999, showed with chronic goals).

Extending this illustration of stereotype inhibition following a temporary goal, Moskowitz and Stone (2012) show that the egalitarian goal is now associated with the group and triggered implicitly. In one experiment they manipulated egalitarian goals in the moment and used a reaction time task to assess the implicit activation of such goals. The words in the reaction time task were words relating to egalitarian goals. Similar to what Moskowitz et al. (2000) showed with chronic goals, White research participants with temporary egalitarian goals were faster to perceive words relevant to the goal of egalitarianism follow-ing faces of Black men (and not White men), but were not faster at perceiving control words.

In a final illustration of the proactive control of stereotype activation, Moskowitz et al. (2011) used an attention task to show the association that develops among egalitarian goals and Black men. The logic was that people with egalitarian goals should be implicitly scanning their environment for opportunities to address their goal. For a White person with an implicitly activated egalitarian goal created during the experiment, a Black man represents just such an opportunity. Thus, the evidence for an implicit association between a group (Black men) and a goal (egalitarianism) would be attention being disrupted from a focal task when (and only when) a face of a Black man is presented as part of a supposed distractor task. Attention would momentarily be drawn to the face of the Black man in the distractor task, and slow (ever so slightly) the response to the focal task. This is precisely what is found, but only in participants with egalitarian goals momentarily triggered.

It should be noted that while we have chosen to focus the discussion on the important topic of stereotype control, these principles hold for any type of self-regulation (e.g., Char-trand & Bargh, 1996). For example, when pursuing the goal of dieting, a piece of cake is a temptation—the goal of eating it is attractive in the short run, but opposed to the long-term goal, which is more important than the momentary pleasure of tasting the cake. Implicit operations associated with a goal pursuit help us to deal with such temptations. If one asso-ciates a dieting goal with cake, then seeing the cake should trigger the goal of dieting and inhibit the eating of the cake. As part of a given goal pursuit selected in a given moment, we often see operations triggered to "shield" or protect the goal from potential distractions to its pursuit (e.g., Fishbach et al., 2003; Kruglanski et al., 2002; Shah, Hall, & Leander, 2009)—just as we saw with the inhibition of stereotypes that were incompatible with egali-tarian goals. The very temptation (in our example, a piece of cake) that should be trigger-ing one behavior often associated with it (in our example, eating cake) is counteracted by a strengthening of and heightened accessibility of the focal goal (in our example, dieting). If strong dieting goals are created, then exposure to cake leads to greater health consciousness in food choices and the dieting goal being more accessible (Fishbach et al., 2003).

The implicit nature of the control described here does not make the response any less willed or driven by one's goals. Goal tending can be an invisible process. A feeling of willing a response or a feeling of determination is not required for the response to be volitional. Given that responses become implicit only after having made a conscious decision to enact and engage them when encountering a specific cue that is related to a goal, this model makes clear that consciousness is not an epiphenomenon. But it also is not required for current goal pursuits.

Context as a Cue

If a change in goals can lead to a change in cognitive processing, it stands to reason that as we have different goals in different situations, and with different people, how we pro-cess will change from one context to the next—that is, specific contexts will trigger the goals associated with those contexts, and the use of stereotypes or the control of stereo-types depend on what the context triggers (e.g., Bargh, 1990; Gollwitzer & Moskowitz, 1996; Kruglanski et al., 2002). We have seen many examples of this principle scattered throughout the book. When in a context where reminded of one's mother, the goals associated with mother are triggered. When in a library, the goals associated with libraries are triggered. When one forms an implementation intention, the goals of the person are associated with a specific contextual cue so that the context can trigger the goal. In this way, contexts trigger stereotype control just as easily as they can trigger stereotype activation. For example, Mendoza, Gollwitzer, and Amodio (2010) had research participants form an implementation intention to not stereotype that was tied to a specific cue in the environment. They found that these cues, when later encountered, triggered a goal to not stereotype, which led to control over stereotype activation (and better conscious control).

Casper, Rothermund, and Wentura (2010) similarly showed that the context determined whether a stereotype was activated or not. Stereotypes that associated Bavarians with beer (a common stereotype in Germany) were triggered in contexts where such associations seemed to fit. However, in contexts where the stereotype was a poor fit (such as if the context was a shop as opposed to a beer garden), then the context did not lead to stereotype activation. Finally, Allen, Sherman, and Klauer (2010) also demonstrated how implicit stereotyping shifts from one context to the next. The bias to rate Black people negatively on implicit measures such as the IAT was shown to be reduced when the context in which the White research participant observed the Black person was a positive one, such as at church. As a form of proactive control, the context could serve as a cue to an implicit goal that associates constructs other than a negative stereotype with the category.

CONCLUSIONS

Dual-process models proposed a motivated social cognition in which by default people rely on the fast triggering of associations, often outside awareness. They are motivated by epistemic needs to get meaning efficiently. Yet, when motivated by stimuli that have personal relevance, people can modify the outputs of fast processing through effortful processing. This has costs: It may be hard to do when time is pressured, it may come up short if one is overloaded, and it may never yield an accurate answer (no matter how closely you scrutinize, some things are just too complex or ambiguous). Perceiving people often incurs such costs. In the 21st century there have been arguments made not only for such a two-process system but for a single-processing system, for there being four essential processes, and for distributed processing. A fundamental problem is that any designation of a specific number of processes is a bit arbitrary (e.g., Sherman, 2006). After all, the processing models offered by social cognition are not pitched at the level of the neuron or brain systems and as such are only metaphors that describe how attitudes, judgments, decisions, and so on are produced. These models are at the level of describing how the mind functions, not attempting to depict how the actual biological mechanisms "churn the gears"—a whole different level of analysis found in neuroscience (e.g., Marr, 1982). Instead, dual-process models are psychological, not biological. They are explanations for behavioral outcomes as opposed to literal descriptions of brain processes (making counting number of processes arbitrary), allowing for theory building and making predictions regarding judgment and action.

Then what metaphor is most apt? How many processes describe social cognition? A 2006 issue of the journal *Psychological Inquiry* was dedicated to debating this issue, and many scholars said that the number of processes is not the relevant question. It depends on level of analysis, the domain being studied, and the context. The more important questions surround issues of what functions are served by processing and how to measure these operations. As Sherman (2006) stated:

> Consider the key distinction between automatic and controlled processes that is central to virtually all dual-process models. In fact, there are a practically limitless number of different controlled processes that can be dissociated from one another both behaviorally and

neurobiologically, including stimulus detection processes, conflict detection processes, resistance to interference processes, cognitive regulation processes, emotional regulation processes, processes for maintaining attention, and processes for switching attention.... Given the seemingly endless possibilities of dividing processes into ever finer distinctions, the goal of obtaining a count of the "real" number of processes is futile. (p. 173)

Dual-process models typically distinguish between goal-directed processes (control) and cue-driven/associative processing (automaticity). This depicts control as the opposite of effortless processing—that it requires effort and conscious intent. Some models are explicit about control being effortful (e.g., Gilbert, 1989), others left it implied (e.g., Payne, 2008). Yet starting around 1990 (e.g., Bargh, 1990; Gollwitzer, 1990) the tide began to turn with the view that control is not synonymous with effort and conscious contemplation of goals and how to implement them. Control can be efficient and implicit (see Moskowitz, 2001, 2010, 2014, for reviews). This opened the door for alternative processing models that were less focused on a duality between implicit and explicit processing, and more focused on understanding how a variety of cognitive processes interact in producing a response. For example, propositional models (e.g., De Houwer, 2007; Gawronski & Bodenhausen, 2011; Kurdi & Banaji, 2023) fully updated the dual-process notion of control as an automatic association followed by a correction. Gone was the idea of control being the product of slow changes to the strength of associations produced over extended periods of learning. This was replaced with the notion of implicit processes being able to shift in the moment as goals, rewards, and new learning within the context dictate (e.g., Kurdi & Banaji, 2017; Kurdi, Morehouse, & Dunham, 2023; Payne, Lambert, & Jacoby, 2002; Spencer, Charbonneau, & Glaser, 2016; Stewart & Payne, 2008; Van Dessel, Ye, & De Houwer, 2019). These models have absorbed what models of proactive control had been saying since 1990, "that implicit social cognition may be amenable to the same basic processes of flexible updating as explicit social cognition" (Kurdi & Banaji, 2023, p. 464). Kurdi and Banaji state that this flexibility arises from embracing the idea that

associations can be sensitive not only to co-occurrences experienced in the environment but also, indirectly, to the relational content of propositions. That is, they are assumed to encode not only the fact that two stimuli are associated with each other and the degree of their relatedness but also the type of relationship that they share with each other. (p. 463)

Daumeyer et al. (2019) show that if we treat implicit bias as if it is uncontrollable, there are consequences. A perceiver who learns that the implicit bias of another person is uncontrollable will not see that person as accountable for their bias, and that person will be less likely to be seen as in need of change or deserving of punishment (compared to a person whose bias is believed to be controllable). Their conclusion is not that we should, therefore, stop talking about implicit bias. It is that "it may be time to revisit the tendency for researchers and others to describe implicit bias as unconscious and/or uncontrollable" (p. 8). Sadly, as we saw in this last section of the chapter, that time actually arrived over 30 years ago when research on the proactive control of implicit bias began. What is sad is that researchers and others have not noticed. That despite a large body of evidence that separates control from consciousness, and that illustrates the many ways that implicit bias can be controlled, our discipline has continued to use this outdated notion of "control as impossible" as a convenient shorthand for the fact that bias can often be implicit. Control of implicit bias does not need to be revisited. The evidence is in. We simply need to shift our metaphor away from the dual-process model's reactive notion of control. This does not mean abandoning its important questions of when and why we are at times trying to be as economical and efficient as possible versus systematic and deliberate. We simply do not need to equate those questions with the question of control.

NOTES

1. One neuroscientific model of two processing systems posits an implicit/procedural processing system based in the striatum, and a frontal-based system responsible for executive control and self-regulation (Ashby, Alfonso-Reese, Turken, & Waldron, 1998; Ashby & Valentin, 2005; Ashby & Waldron, 1999) specifies an "X-system" for automatic processing (that implicates neural regions such as the amygdala, dorsal anterior cingulate cortex, basal ganglia, lateral temporal cortex, and vetromedial prefrontal cortex), and a "C-system" for controlled processing (that implicates the lateral prefrontal cortex, medial prefrontal cortext, right anterior cingulate cortex, medial temporal lobe, and medial parietal cortex). Some models specify separate systems for evaluative versus semantic processing (e.g., Amodio & Ratner, 2011; Amodio et al., 2004).

2. For example, we assume a person who speaks fluent English without an accent is from North America when they are Dutch; we assume a person with what appears to be white skin is White when they identify as African American; we infer that shedding a tear indicates sadness when it is a bug in the eye; we misidentify a person's gender.

3. This is not to say all category-based processing must be relatively effortless. At times we expend quite a good deal of energy and effort to maintain our categories. We have discussed in Chapter 5 how people process information that is inconsistent with (or incongruent with) an expectation or category, often working quite hard to continue to process in a categorical way (because, despite this effort, it is still less effortful than reorganizing one's whole category structure and changing an entire mental representation).

4. It is important to note that the four processes are not limited to describing a shooter task! It is just one example selected for illustrative purposes. For example, Gonsalkorale and Sherman (2007) did a quad analysis of a task where implicit evaluations were assessed after a person received information inconsistent with an expectation they had developed. Vitriol, O'Shea, and Calanchini (2023) performed a quad analysis on the defensive responses people exhibit when they are given negative feedback.

CHAPTER 13

The Updating of Impressions Is Promoted by Diagnostic Stimuli and One's Goals

The updating of first impressions—the regulation of and correction of one's attitudes and judgments—is an important issue because it is at the heart of both intergroup and interpersonal dynamics. When considering interpersonal dynamics, it is equivalent to changing how we see people, especially faulty reactions. As such, it drives reactions such as apology and forgiveness, accountability and blame, and self-awareness and behavior modification. When considering intergroup dynamics, the belief that social ills can be partly addressed by attempting to update faulty impressions of groups is reflected in the explosion since 2015 of workshops and intervention programs aimed at raising awareness (with varying degrees of success) about stereotyping and prejudice (e.g., Axt, Casola, & Nosek, 2018; Carter, Onyeador, & Lewis, 2020; U.S. Department of Justice, 2016; Dobbin & Kalev, 2016; Lipman, 2018; Nordstrom & Goodfriend, 2023; Schmader, Dennehy, & Baron, 2022; Stone, Moskowitz, Zestcott, & Wolsiefer, 2020). Given its importance to both interpersonal and intergroup dynamics, work examining the updating of first impressions is found both in research on stereotyping (and the perception of social groups) and person perception (where individuals are being perceived and judged).

By **updating** we mean that an impression can be altered and changed in light of either new information or a reexamination of old information. This is often triggered either by being confronted in some way by information that calls the initial impression into doubt, or a desire to correct or improve the accuracy of an initial impression by adopting goals that lead to a striving to regulate a first impression. Throughout this book we have highlighted a resistance to updating—that people have a confirmation bias and a motivation to cling to existing attitudes and beliefs. However, we also reviewed times in which updating does occur. Let us consider a few examples.

> **Updating:** When impressions are altered either by learning edifying new information or by reexamining the basis for existing beliefs/attitudes. Such changes are often triggered either by being confronted by new information that calls the initial impression into doubt or by a perceiver's newly adopted goals to alter the impression.

Devine and Elliot (1995) looked at how stereotypes had changed in the United States since the 1930s. Looking at a host of groups, they saw that the traits people use to describe each of those groups were quite different from 1933 to 1995. However, they also found that the *attitudes* had not changed—while new traits were used to describe the group, those traits were still negative. Expanding on this work, Charlesworth, Caliskan, and Banaji (2022) explored the change in attitudes and stereotypes over a 200-year period in the United States. Their research used the novel method of examining the language used in newspapers, books, and magazines to quantify what words were most commonly used when referencing specific groups (e.g., women, the elderly, Black people, Asians, Native Americans, Hispanics, fat people, poor people). This allowed them to catalog how the traits associated with a group changed over the course of 200 years. They found that, looking at 50-year intervals, the traits used to describe a group change. The cultural stereotype is updated. But as with Devine and Elliot, the attitudes did not change. The traits remain *negative* even though the specific traits used to describe a group change. A similar approach of examining change in stereotyping using natural language use was taken by Bhatia and Bhatia (2021). Bhatia (2017) used a method of studying word co-occurrence in natural language (such as examining 100 years of articles from the *Los Angeles Times*) to explore associations among groups and prejudice (as well as stereotypes). Bhatia and Bhatia used this technique to discover that while gender bias still exists, associations among women and stereotypic traits have weakened over the last 100 years.

Eagly and Revelle (2022) discuss how gender prejudice might change as binary notions of gender change and as more people identify as lesbian, gay, bisexual, transgender, queer/questioning (LGBTQ; which they have, as close to 16.0% of millennials identify as LGBTQ and 0.5% of Americans report being nonbinary, according to a 2021 Gallup poll). Eagly, Mladinic, and Otto (1991) noticed that while attitudes toward women are typically described as negative, the traits used to describe women were quite positive (warm, affectionate, sympathetic, kind, nurturing, etc.)—an observation described in Chapter 6 as benevolent sexism. This led Eagly et al. to propose that prejudice should not be defined simply by holding negative attitudes toward a group but by also considering prescriptions toward the group that limit their opportunities in specific contexts. Thus, to think about updating, it is not merely a question of whether traits change, but if prescriptions that limit a group also change. Beliefs that women are expected to be communal but not agentic were shown to have changed from 1970 through 2020 in data reported by Hsu, Badura, Newman, and Speach (2021). While much of the research on attitude change explores explicit attitudes using self-report measures, Charlesworth and Banaji (2022) show updating of implicit attitudes. For many groups implicit attitudes have been changing to become less negative over time (depicted in Figure 13.1).

Despite these important changes in attitudes and beliefs in the culture, the concern in this chapter is not to catalog shifting attitudes at the societal level; it is with the *process* of updating. Rather than showing more examples that change happens with time, and at the level of the culture, we focus instead on a question of social cognition: How does change happen in the individual? What happens to a mental representation when it updates and what triggers this alteration?

Three overarching themes are consistently noted when describing theories of how to update an impression. A first theme relates to awareness. If one is not aware that an impression has been formed (such as an STI or an implicit attitude), or not aware that it has been formed in a biased manner, then updating will fail to occur. A second theme relates to ability. If one is aware of bias, then for updating to occur one must have the ability to update an impression in terms of both efficacy and cognitive capacity. If one lacks efficacy, not

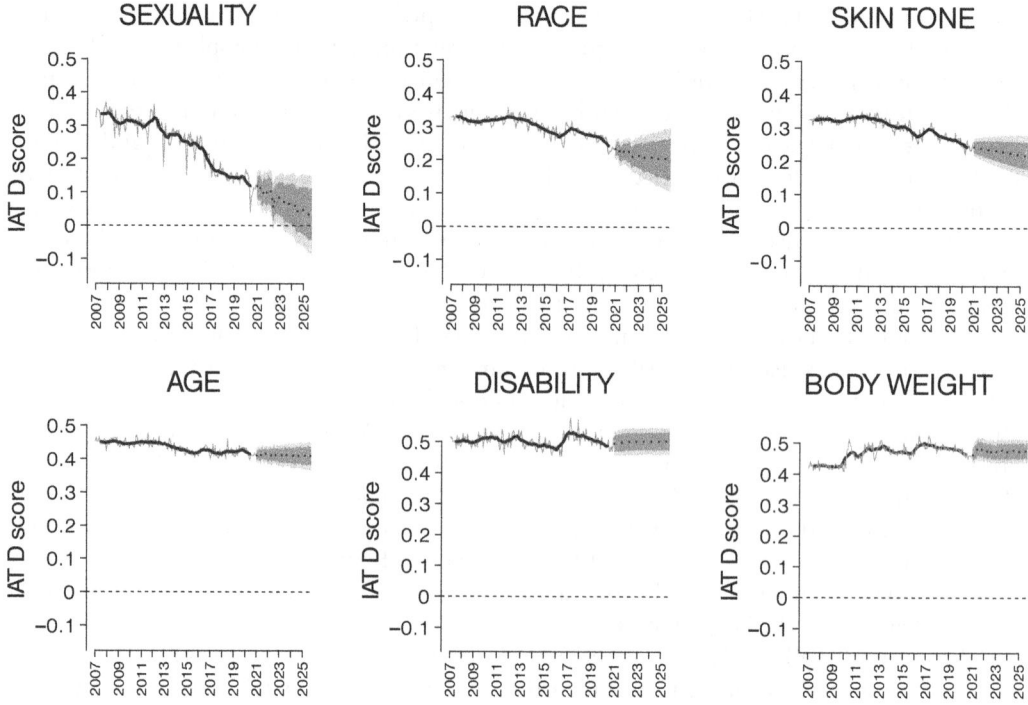

FIGURE 13.1. Implicit attitude change, 2007–2020, from millions of project implicit participants.

knowing what to do or how to appropriately create an unbiased impression, then correction will not occur. Additionally, if the correction requires mental effort, but fatigue or cognitive load have usurped the energy to exert that effort, then updating will fail to occur. A third theme relates to motivation. If one is aware an impression has formed and is biased, and one has the capacity to overturn it but is not motivated to do anything about it (either for fear of disagreeing with others, fear of seeing something distasteful in the self, or because one feels the biased impression is just fine), then updating will fail to occur.

AWARENESS AND CAPACITY

Becoming Aware That an Impression Needs Updating

Despite the many obstacles to awareness that an impression is in need of updating reviewed in Chapters 5 and 6, creating awareness is possible. At times it comes from self-reflection, where one looks inward to assess one's state, generating feedback that change is needed. People often monitor their impressions, they self-reflect on their beliefs and attitudes, to ensure that they reach the standards they hold for themselves. When one self-reflects it may reveal that the first impression is not sufficient (it feels biased, or based on incomplete information). For example, in the research of Monteith et al. (2002) the participants viewed images—faces of people, car crashes, flowers, and so on—while hooked up to an apparatus that revealed their levels of physiological arousal. The apparatus allowed people to reflect on their attitudes toward each of the images—if they find those images arousing and disturbing. The experiment was set up so that White research participants could be led to believe that they had aversive and arousing physiological reactions to faces of Black men (by the apparatus providing false feedback). This feedback created awareness that they had reactions discrepant with the type of person they hoped to be. In another example of self-reflection creating awareness, Moskowitz (2002) asked participants to write about a time in their life where they failed to meet standards they had set for being an egalitarian person. In this way the participants self-reflected, delivering their own feedback about how their behavior was discrepant with their egalitarian goals.

Other times the feedback we receive, and our monitoring of how we are doing in a goal pursuit, comes from feedback from others. In the domain of first impressions this means receiving feedback that one's first impression may be invalid or biased. This feedback can be provided by directly telling someone their impression is wrong, or by providing them with new information that is inconsistent with their existing beliefs or attitudes. If done poorly, providing feedback that a person's impressions need to change can feel like a confrontation (e.g., Chaney, Sanchez, & Remedios, 2023; Czopp et al., 2006; Gulker, Mark, & Monteith, 2013; Stone et al., 2011). Especially given biases to see the self as above average in most domains (Pronin et al., 2002) and to see the self as unbiased (e.g., Crandall et al., 2002; Dovidio & Gaertner, 2000), negative feedback can seem unwarranted and wrong and lead to the "accused" being defensive. But if done well, providing feedback to others can make them aware of a shortcoming and motivate the person to reexamine their beliefs and attitudes to alter them. This makes the issue of how to appropriately deliver feedback, so that it creates a motivation to change and not to be defensive, an extremely important topic—one already reviewed in Chapter 6. Even if one is not defensive when receiving feedback, one may still fail to become aware of one's bias if one forms attributions that dismiss the feedback. This has been illustrated in the domain of moral reasoning—a person believes they are less morally responsible for their behavior if they feel that they lack control over that behavior (e.g., Alicke, 2000; Nadler & McDonnell, 2012; Shaver, 1985). This has also been shown in the domain of implicit bias. Daumeyer et al. (2019) showed that if you read about a person who exhibits bias, attributions made about that person shift dependent on whether you believe their bias is controllable and emerges from explicit prejudice or is uncontrollable and emerges from implicit bias. When learning about a person's implicit bias, a perceiver sees that person as less accountable, less blameworthy, less deserving of punishment, and less requiring of reform. This suggests that if I see myself as fair, that impression is less likely to update if I attribute disconfirming feedback to forces over which I lack control. Thus, interventions that deliver feedback about bias must be careful not to suggest that implicit bias means one lacks control or culpability.

There are other ways in which attributions can interfere with updating. Any behavior, including one for which one has received feedback, needs to be categorized and identified. One can identify it as a certain class of action (such as that was a biased behavior I performed) or one can identify it as an indicator of a disposition (that behavior suggests I am a biased person). The former is something unstable and not expected to repeat (I may act unbiased in the future); the latter is something stable and likely to repeat (I am likely to be biased in the future). If the feedback is that one is biased, one may identify the behavior being challenged as an unstable feature ("my behavior was biased because I lacked control or because of odd circumstances"). One can accept the feedback as true, but designate it as not worthy of concern since it does not indicate something stable about the self that warrants change. In this instance one has not truly become aware of one's bias despite the feedback being heard. The person can dismiss it as a temporary quality, an anomaly that can be assigned to what Asch and Zukier (1984) called a separate sphere of the person. Additionally, the person can dismiss it as being pressured by the situation, and as having an external locus of causality. In doing so, the behavior is not seen as a quality of the "inner person" but is contextualized. By **contextualization** it is meant that the new information is tied to the specific circumstance.[1] However, if the response to the feedback is to identify the behavior in question as a stable feature ("like all people, I have a propensity to respond with bias, and that needs monitoring over time"), then the feedback is internalized and one is aware of having a need to update. This discussion highlights that there are, in fact, different types of "awareness." There is (1) awareness that an action has occurred (such as "I acted rudely to an outgroup member at the airport"), and (2) awareness that the action reflects a disposition for which one is responsible. For updating of a first impression to occur, raising awareness must be done in the second way described above, in a way that creates what Perry et al. (2015) call *bias awareness*. This is more than simply pointing out undesirable action, but awareness that this action reflects a disposition in need of change.

> **Contextualization:** When newly learned information about a person is tied to the specific circumstance in which it occurred, making it unlikely to generalize across contexts and be seen as a basis for changing an already-existing impression. While first impressions typically characterize someone's traits/attitudes, new information is seen as describing the context.

The Ability—Capacity and Efficacy—to Update

Even if aware of a flawed first impression, updating may fail to occur if one lacks the capacity to engage in the operations that will address the bias in, or shortcomings in, one's impressions. For example, one might lack the capacity to perform the response due to cognitive load. Or one might lack the efficacy to update a first impression, without having the skill to do so (e.g., Bandura, 1989; Gollwitzer & Moskowitz, 1996). Several examples of lacking efficacy have been reviewed throughout the book. In Chapters 5 and 6 it was shown that updating fails when one has a flawed theory of correction. In Chapter 11 we saw how attempts to undo stereotyping by pursuing a goal of being colorblind led to a greater use of race (Norton, Vandello, et al., 2008), and that attempts to suppress stereotypes led to increased strength and accessibility of the stereotype rather than its diminishment (e.g., Wegner, 1994). These failures at updating from lack of efficacy inform us that interventions meant to create updated impressions in its attendees must do more than make sure bias awareness has been created. They must also provide people with efficacious strategies to update. If left to their own devices to select a strategy, many strategies that seem intuitive (such as suppressing an unwanted thought) can have the opposite effect. Of course, throughout the book we have also emphasized how cognitive load, even if one feels efficacious, can interfere with updating. In both Figure 8.3 (Chapter 8) and Figure 10.3 (Chapter 10) we see a description of processing occurring in stages, with the second stage being where effortful adjustments to implicit processing are made. When updating requires effort (and proactive control informs us this is not always the case), then cognitive load will interfere with this processing stage.

In contrast, if one has both capacity and a sense of efficacy, bias awareness can promote updating. In one example that explored how people update stereotypes, Taylor et al. (2021) showed that one's processing capacity as well as one's perceived sense of efficacy matters a great deal. In their research, participants observe an ingroup member act in a stereotypic way. As described in Chapter 11, this triggers meta-stereotypes that one wishes to change or update. However, it is easier to just avoid the person who triggers the meta-stereotype (less cognitively demanding) than updating what one thinks of the person through approaching them and regulating the interaction. They argued that efficacy beliefs—having a sense that one is well equipped to cope with this difficult situation—would determine whether one avoided or self-regulated in response. People who have a sense of efficacy should be more willing to embrace the more cognitively demanding response strategy. This is what was found: people who believed they had the ability to deal with such a situation were more motivated to attempt to update the group stereotype, rather than avoid the situation. People with low levels of efficacy chose avoidance.

When people are aware of an impression that is need of updating, and have the capacity to address it, they still must be motivated to engage in the required operations. Such motivation, as described in Chapter 6, often comes from negative feedback loops. When feedback creates awareness of a desired state (to have an impression that is not biased or incomplete) and that desired state is discrepant with one's actual state, this **discrepancy**, this sense of where one stands being insufficient, is unpleasant and creates a feeling of tension or dissonance (e.g., Festinger, 1957). People are motivated to eliminate the negative state. They engage in operations, or **compensatory responses**, which are responses made that are aimed at removing the discrepancy. While it is true that many strategies can eliminate the tension that do not involve updating the first impression, and instead involve rationalizing, trivializing, or dismissing the feedback, there are also many strategies that resolve the tension by updating. Our interest next turns to how to create the motivation that will trigger updating once one is aware that bias exists.

> **Discrepancy:** When feedback (either from others or self-examination) leads one to detect that one's current state is dissonant to or inconsistent with a desired state (goal). It is a sense that where one currently stands is insufficient according to one's standards, which is an aversive feeling one is driven to ameliorate.
>
> **Compensatory responses:** A response initiated with the purpose of reducing or eliminating a discrepancy (in order to eliminate or reduce its aversive tension). It is a type of self-regulation where, to compensate for the thoughts/feelings/actions that give rise to a discrepancy, one responds in ways that counteracts and corrects the discrepant responses.

MOTIVATION TO UPDATE: DOUBT AFTER SEEING INCONSISTENT INFORMATION COMPELS UPDATING

One factor that motivates updating is when one experiences doubt about the validity of a first impression; when one loses confidence that an impression is sufficient to use. This can occur if new evidence is encountered that is inconsistent with the first impression, contradicting the evidence on which the first impression is based. In Chapter 6 this was called a *confidence gap*, where the current level of confidence in one's judgment, based on a first impression, is less than the desired level of confidence because of new information that introduces doubt. This motivates one to update the first impression until a sufficiently good judgment is produced (see Chapter 6, Figure 6.6). It is important to note that this type of motivation to update is externally compelled. The actions of others force a perceiver to reexamine an existing belief, and this would not occur without one being challenged by new information. This asks others to metaphorically shake us from the slumber of our confirmation biases—to articulate and display ideas and behaviors inconsistent with our first impressions. In Allport's (1954) terms, this places a "preponderance of responsibility" (p. 384) on others to act in ways that initiate doubt in what we know and change how we think. However, research reviewed on confirmation bias throughout Chapters 5 and 6 told us that the judgments people form after receiving such inconsistent information still align with a first impression—it appears as if updating is not motivated. Some of the research found that information that disconfirms a stereotype or expectation is simply ignored. Other research found that even when people do not ignore the inconsistent information, they try to explain it away. The mental energy required to dismiss it was said to make it especially likely to be attended to and remembered (e.g., Bargh & Thein, 1985; Hastie & Kumar, 1979; Sherman, Klein, et al., 1998). Yet other research shows how people use attributions to protect a first impression, such as identifying inconsistent information as not relevant to the perceived person's disposition (e.g., Crocker, Hannah, & Weber, 1983; Sherman et al., 2005). After completing that review of confirmation biases, it was promised that we would revisit this issue since, as we all know, updating does at times occur. *When* does new information that is inconsistent with a first impression motivate updating as opposed to being ignored or explained away? We turn to this issue now.

The Relative Strength of the First Impression

Stangor and Ruble (1989) argue that one factor determining whether a first impression will be updated after learning **stereotype-inconsistent information** is how well developed the first impression is. Stronger, better-developed impressions, may have the ability to reject inconsistent information altogether, or at least rationalize it away with relatively little effort needed. For example, one may be better able to discount such information, or make attributions to the situation (e.g., Crocker et al., 1983). As Stangor and Ruble put it, "strong expectations will lead perceivers to 'filter' or ignore inconsistent information, in an attempt to maintain the established expectancy intact . . . they rely on 'top down'

Stereotype-inconsistent information: Information that calls a stereotype into doubt. If such information were to be accepted as true it would create a confidence gap regarding the validity of and use of that stereotype because it is new evidence that contradicts the evidence on which the stereotype is based.

rather than 'bottom up' processes to guide impression formation" (p. 20). However, if an impression is weak, not well formed, or still developing, it is more vulnerable to updating. It is not easy to simply disregard the inconsistent information. Thus, for weakly held first impressions we might see inconsistent information dominant in memory because of the effort one has to exert to either incorporate it into the impression or to explain it away. Evidence that weak impressions are easily updated was provided in Chapter 6 when reviewing the research of Gregg et al. (2006). They had research participants learn information about two fictional groups and form first impressions about them (the Niffites were described as barbaric, savage, authoritarian, brutal; the Luupites were described as benevolent, accommodating, civilized). After forming these first impressions the experimenter reports that a programming error caused the computer to have reversed the originally learned information about the Niffites and Luupites. It was shown that participants easily updated the explicit impressions of the person to reflect the correct, newer information that was inconsistent with the first impression. Wyer (2010) showed a similar type of reversal by first telling participants a person was a skinhead, and they inferred he had anarchic and violent qualities. Then participants learned this information was wrong and that the person's bald head was not an ideological choice made by a skinhead but a reaction to cancer medication. Once again, the impression changed. In both of these examples it was the explicitly reported impression that was updated. The implicitly formed first impression was more resistant to change, but we will return to that shortly.

Stangor and Ruble (1989) explored updating as a function of a first impression's strength by manipulating this in the experiment. Some participants formed impressions of two fictitious groups based on reading a set of 60 behaviors that suggested one group was predominantly extroverted and the other predominantly introverted. These were relatively weak impressions. Other participants had stronger impressions by first reading a separate set of behaviors strongly suggesting that one group were extroverts, the other introverts (after having formed the strong impression they then read and evaluated the set of 60 behaviors). Thus, some participants were developing their impression as they were reading the 60 behaviors, the other participants already formed a strong impression before exposure to these behaviors. According to the logic outlined above, participants with a more developed impression should be more likely to show a confirmation bias in memory. This is what was found: Participants who formed an impression prior to reading the target information recalled proportionately more extroverted than introverted behaviors of a group that was extroverted (and more introverted behaviors about an introverted group). However, when there was not an impression developed beforehand, they showed no confirmation bias. Weaker stereotypes that were still developing were easier to update.

A variety of factors can make a first impression strong. These include it being (1) embedded in a rich network of associations, (2) about a group with high entitativity, (3) linked to important goals and one's vested interests, (4) related to a chronic pursuit of the individual so that it becomes frequently triggered, and (5) learned from others in the culture and thus consensually shared. Rather than review all the things that make impressions strong, let us focus on one illustrative example of how the strength of a first impression (attitude or stereotype) is shaped by one of these factors, and in turn impacts updating. Entitativity is the extent to which a group is perceived as a coherent social entity (e.g., Allison & Messick, 1988; Hamilton, 1991). In Chapter 7 entitativity was defined as the "groupiness" of the group; how closely tied together it seems to be, and how much the members seem to share a common fate (e.g., Yzerbyt, Rogier, & Fiske, 1998). This suggests that people expect similarity among a "groupier" group, and impressions formed about entitative groups will be more strongly formed and harder to overturn. If updating is to occur, one way to promote this is to undermine the degree to which the group is defined in such a coherent and clannish fashion. This would allow stereotype-inconsistent information that was previously disregarded by such stereotype strength to have the power to instigate updating. Another way to promote updating with an entitative group would be to increase the strength of the stereotype-inconsistent information that challenges it. As discussed in the next section, diagnosticity can have this effect.

This summary of the impact of a first impression's strength does not mean that strongly held impressions and stereotypes are unalterable. In the experiments just reviewed the impression formed was about a group for which there is a strong first impression. Perhaps when learning about groups there is an impulse to see this impression as particularly stable since it is shared among many people. It may be that a strongly held first impression of an individual person (as opposed to a social group) is more likely to be updated. Consistent with this, Srull (1981) showed that perceivers who observe individual targets (as opposed to groups) have greater memory for items inconsistent with their initial impressions of those targets as compared to information that is consistent.[2]

We now return to the interesting point reported above that even a weak first impression is not updated by inconsistent information if those impressions are measured using *implicit* tests. A growing body of research suggests that implicit impressions may be more resistant to change than explicit ones (see Moskowitz, Olcaysoy Okten, & Schneid, 2023; Shen & Ferguson, 2023, for reviews). Even if this were true, and both (1) strong explicit impressions and (2) all types of implicit impressions are more resistant to updating, it would *not mean that they cannot* be updated. For such impressions to be updated the new information being learned may need to be especially strong. Research has shown that several features of newly learned information can create doubt about an original impression and impact whether updating occurs. These include a single piece of highly diagnostic information that contradicts a first impression (e.g., he is a child molester), hitting people over the head with a barrage of inconsistent (but not extreme) information, introducing a contingency or ulterior motive that reinterprets the first impression (he is a liar, but he lied to deceive Nazis to save a Jewish family he hid in his home), and through the additional information changing the meaning of the act entirely (he was screaming at the child, but to prevent her from touching a hot stove; the meaning of screaming shifts from cruel to protective). We shift now from considering the strength of the impression held by the perceiver in promoting updating to the strength of the inconsistent information the perceiver learns.

Updating Following the Learning of Highly Diagnostic New Behaviors

Even implicit evaluations can be updated by certain information that is inconsistent with the first impression (e.g., Brannon & Gawronski, 2017; Cone & Ferguson, 2015; Cone, Flaharty, & Ferguson, 2019; Cone, Mann, & Ferguson, 2017; Mann & Ferguson, 2015, 2017; Olcaysoy Okten et al., 2019). One circumstance where this happens is when learning **diagnostic information**, or information about a person that by virtue of its strength and extremity is taken to be indicative of the person's "true nature"—it is unlikely to be dismissed or tied to a situational constraint, but compels the perceiver to incorporate it into the impression. For example, if one learns "Bob mutilated a small defenseless animal," it is both extreme and negative. It is hard to say that the situation forced him to do this. In one set of experiments (of six in total), Cone and Ferguson had research participants learn 100 behaviors performed by the same person (Bob), all of the same valence (some learned positive behaviors, others negative). At this point they used an implicit measure to assess the participant's attitude toward Bob. Next, participants were provided with a single inconsistent behavior by Bob that was highly diagnostic. They then again used an implicit measure to assess the attitude toward Bob. These experiments show that updating occurs if the single piece of information is highly diagnostic—the evaluation reverses, even though measured implicitly. Updating is especially likely when the initial impression was positive and the new behavior was thought to be immoral (e.g., Cone & Ferguson, 2015; Peters & Gawronski, 2011; Rydell, McConnell, Mackie, & Strain, 2006).

> **Diagnostic information:** Behavior learned about a person that by virtue of its strength and extremity, is taken to be indicative of the person's "true nature." Such information is unlikely to be contextualized or dismissed, but compels the perceiver to incorporate this information into their impression of the person.

A similar illustration of implicit updating following diagnostic behavior is provided by Ferguson et al. (2024). Participants learned about a set of behaviors from a person named Jack whose face was placed in a specific context (such as an office setting) as each behavior was learned. The statements describe Jack's positive behavior. After the learning task is over, participants' explicit and implicit evaluations of Jack were measured. Next, they learn one more piece of diagnostic information: Jack was convicted of child molestation. The context for this information was manipulated to be either the same as (the office) or different from (at home) the context used when learning the initial behaviors. After learning this diagnostic behavior, explicit and implicit evaluations were measured again. Both of these initial positive impressions of Jack were reversed. And the context did not matter for this updating; contextualization of the new information (linking their impression to the situation where it was learned) was overcome.

While these findings were somewhat new in regard to the updating of *implicit* impressions, a long history of research had already shown that *explicit* impressions will update following exposure to diagnostic information. For example, Locksley and colleagues (1980; Locksley, Hepburn, & Ortiz, 1982) found evidence that people update their impressions by discarding a stereotype, and instead embrace the specific and counterstereotypic qualities of a person learned about during the experiment. This updating of the impression occurred if the new behavior being learned was highly diagnostic—unambiguous and strongly positive behavior that was inconsistent with the existing negative stereotype. Locksley et al. (1980) showed participants a transcript of a conversation between two people. One person describes themselves as having acted clearly and strongly assertively (or passively) in three separate situations. No other information about the individual was provided. The people having the conversation also had their names stated to signal gender to participants. The results show that the participants overturned the use of a gender stereotype when making judgments of how aggressive the person was, and relied instead on the diagnostic information provided. A woman who has acted assertively on three separate occasions just cannot be described as passive, no matter what the stereotype says. Locksley et al. (1980, 1982) claim that practically any time you provide people with diagnostic information that signals a person is behaving in a nonstereotypic way, they abandon the stereotype in favor of the stereotype-inconsistent information.[3]

In another example we see that one piece of diagnostic and stereotype-inconsistent information can lead to updating even if it is accompanied by additional stereotype-consistent information. Locksley et al. (1982) gave participants information about 12 men and 12 women that provided four past behaviors relevant to assertiveness. Participants were then asked to guess how assertive each of the men and women would act in a fifth situation. Instead of providing participants with four instances of assertive behavior, this factor was manipulated. Some of the men and women read about had three assertive prior responses and one passive one. Some were passive in half of the situations and assertive in the other half. Some were passive in three of the behaviors and assertive in the fourth. Finally, some were entirely assertive or entirely passive. The results showed people did not rely on gender stereotypes when at least one piece of diagnostic, stereotype-inconsistent behavior was included among the four.

A similar finding is seen in studies that look at memory for stereotype-consistent versus stereotype-inconsistent information. In a review of the illusory correlation research, Stroessner and Plaks (2001) report that the bias to ignore and discard stereotype-inconsistent information is overcome when that information is diagnostic, distinct, and salient. When they are diagnostic, stereotype-inconsistent behaviors can capture attention and this will trigger elaborate processing, making the stereotype-inconsistent behaviors more memorable than the stereotype-consistent behaviors (e.g., McConnell, Sherman, & Hamilton, 1994). The representation is updated to include strong associations to the new and inconsistent behaviors. While such results seem contradictory to the pervasive influence of stereotypes described up until now, it must be kept in mind that the stereotypic biases reviewed in Chapter 11 were from the start explained to be most likely in ambiguous situations. Here we see that when a person from a stereotyped group unambiguously acts in a nonstereotypic way, then we do not try to force a stereotyped interpretation on them. If the data are so dominant (diagnostic of being counterstereotypic), it forces people to abandon a first impression, even a stereotype (e.g., Deaux & Lewis, 1984). Updating following diagnostic information could be a very limiting condition, where the only reason it occurs is because the newly learned behavior is so extreme, and makes it obvious that a decision to ignore it would be a clear case of stereotyping. We examine updating after exposure to less extreme inconsistent information next.

Hitting Over the Head: A Barrage of Inconsistent Information

In the United States, part of the rationale for desegregating schools in the 1950s and for the 1954 *Brown v. Board of Education of Topeka, Kansas* case (Warren & Supreme Court of The United States, 1953) was that contact among members of disparate groups would expose them to counterstereotypic behavior. Separate schools based on race were not in fact equal, and even if resources could be held equal among them, bias would still exist and be exaggerated by such separation. By eliminating separation based on race, it was believed that people would not only have equal access to schools of the same quality, but due to contact among people of different groups now being possible, stereotypes would change (along with dis-criminatory behavior). That in addition to updating being initiated by a single diagnostic behavior, updating is also able to occur through exposure, over time, to a repeated barrage of stereotype-inconsistent behavior. Though not the focus here, the **contact hypothesis** proposes that prejudice and ste-reotyping can be undermined and undone by repeated expo-sure to (contact with) members of previously isolated groups. This is because our biased expectations and impressions will be shattered by the observed behavior, behavior that is incon-sistent with the group stereotypes (e.g., Allport, 1954; Petti-grew, 1997; Uluǧ & Tropp, 2021; Zhou, Page-Gould, Aron, Moyer, & Hewstone, 2019). We explore next the impact of exposure to repeated, stereotype-inconsistent actions by a group.[4]

Contact hypothesis: Belief that stereotyping/prejudice is undone by repeated exposure to members of stigmatized/stereotyped groups. Such contact—by virtue of observed behavior that is inconsistent with group stereotypes—will shatter biased expectations and impressions. How-ever, several specified ingredients need to be present for such contact to have these positive effects.

One research domain already reviewed in Chapter 3 has provided evidence for the impact of a consistent barrage of unexpected and expectation-violating behavior. In exam-ining *minority influence*, Moscovici (1976, 1985) highlighted the importance of a minority consistently and steadfastly acting in ways that are inconsistent with the stereotypes that hold them in disfavor. Such a violation of what is expected (where the minority view is repeat-edly clung to despite enormous pressure to conform) can create doubt regarding whether the negative impression that one has about the minority is sufficient. This doubt triggers a reappraisal of the negative impression that one has about the minority, and this reappraisal could lead to the impression being updated (e.g., Moskowitz, 1996). In Chapter 3 the type of minority influence examined was updating of one's perceptual experience (e.g., Moscovici, Lage, & Naffrechoux, 1969; Moscovivi & Personnaz, 1980; Nemeth, 1986). Yet a barrage of information inconsistent with an expectation held about a minority can impact more than color perception, but impressions held about the group as well. Indeed, it was the updating of stereotypes about groups in the "real world"—women, Quakers, African Americans—that fueled Moscovici's theorizing about how minority behavior triggers updating. For example, Moskowitz and Chaiken (2001) showed that when research participants learned statements that repeatedly *disconfirmed* an expected minority position, the motivation to pay closer attention to the minority view and abandon the initial expectations emerged. This height-ened assessment led to doubt regarding one's own views (e.g., Eagly & Chaiken, 1993), which in turn led to updating of the initial impression of the minority, instead of categorical rejec-tion of the minority as wrong (e.g., Baker & Petty, 1994; Bohner, Erb, Reinhard, & Frank, 1996; Crano & Chen, 1998; De Dreu & De Vries, 1996; Jung, Bramson, Crano, Page, & Miller, 2021; Kruglanski & Mackie, 1990; Nemeth, Mayseles, Sherman, & Brown, 1990; Pérez, Falomir, & Mugny, 1995; Trost, Maass, & Kenrick, 1992; Wood, Pool, Leck, & Purvis, 1996).

Repeated contact with information inconsistent with a first impression is not only responsible for the updating of explicit impressions but has been shown to update implicit impressions as well (e.g., Brannon & Gawronski, 2017; Gawronski, Rydell, Vervliet, & De Houwer, 2010; Olcaysoy Okten & Moskowitz, 2020a; Petty et al., 2006; Rydell & Gawron-ski, 2009; Rydell & McConnell, 2006; Rydell, McConnell, Strain, Claypool, & Hugenberg, 2007). Experiments illustrating this follow a similar format: The research participant first forms an impression of a person by learning a large number of behaviors that have the same valence (all positive or all negative). Their implicit evaluation is then assessed using procedures such as the IAT or the affect misattribution procedure (AMP). They then learn a set of new behaviors with an opposite valence to the first impression. Results show that learning many new inconsistent behaviors does lead to the implicit evaluation overturning and updating. For example, Rydell and McConnell showed that increasing the number of behaviors learned that are inconsistent with the initial impression formed leads to increased updating of that implicit impression (see also Rydell et al., 2007). As new information is learned that is inconsistent with the first impression there is an increase in the strength of the new association. The impression comes to increasingly rely on the ever-strengthening new association instead of the original association (the association between person X and "good" becomes stronger than the first impression that associated person X with "bad").

In another example, repeated learning of information inconsistent with a first impression not only led to updating, but was able to overcome contextualization. Brannon and Gawronski (2017) showed people new information that was inconsistent with their first impression, but also manipulated whether that information was learned in the same context in which the initial impression was formed or in a different context. A contextualization account (as described above) would lead us to expect that information learned in a different context would potentially be tied to that context, and hence the impression would not be updated. However, they found that the implicit impression *was updated irrespective of context*. Such research on implicit impressions supplements that reviewed above so that we see it is not only quality of inconsistent information (is it diagnostic) but its quantity (is it repeated sufficiently) that can lead to updating.

Updating from Reinterpretation

The total evaluative reversal of an impression is not the only way to update. Sometimes inconsistent information can serve to reinterpret the original information, altering what we believe we have seen by changing the meaning of the initial act. Consider two examples. First, imagine you have been brought by a friend to a dinner at the home of someone you have never met. Upon arrival you hear the host screaming at his toddler in another room. His supposed anger leads you to form a very negative impression of him. However, you later learn the child was about to knock over a pot of boiling water and get severely burned, and the man's yelling saved the child from a horrific accident. In a second example, imagine you learn a man broke into a stranger's house and damaged many precious things and removed some others in the process. However, you later learn the house was on fire and the man saved both a toddler trapped on the second floor and the toddler's injured parents on the first floor. In this second example updating occurs because the new information changes the inferred intentions of the person. He is still seen as damaging and removing items, but the reason why has shifted from stealing to helping, with the impression updated from thief to hero. In the first example updating occurs because the newly learned information changes the meaning of the original behavior (scream means to protect not harm). There are no new behaviors, just additional information that alters the way a behavior is categorized and understood. Research has explored these two types of updating.

Mann and Ferguson (2015, 2017), for example, used the exact scenario described above of learning about a person who damages a home, and then later learning it was because they were rescuing the inhabitants from a fire. To show that the original behavior gets reinterpreted and the impression updated they presented two types of positive behavior. One was relevant to the original behavior in that it offered a reinterpretation (heroism) and the other was irrelevant and was simply a random inconsistent behavior (such as the person volunteers at a soup kitchen). A single inconsistent behavior does not lead to updating *unless* that single inconsistent behavior is relevant to the original behavior and offers a reinterpretation. An implicit measure reveals that the impression updates from negative to positive when the inconsistent behavior changes the implied intention of the person.

Although the impression is measured using implicit tests, their experiments also suggest that the participant needs to actively think about the implications of the new information through deliberation and effort (see also Wyer, 2010).

Returning to the first example, Olcaysoy Okten et al. (2019) showed that when a person's initial behavior (screaming at the toddler) was supplemented by later learning that it was contingent on a specific event (the child being in extreme danger), the implicit evaluation was updated. They found that the implicit impression shifted from negative to positive when a reinterpretation was provided, despite there being no new behaviors, just additional information that alters the way the behavior (screaming) is categorized and understood. In another experiment, Olcaysoy Okten and Moskowitz (2020a) show that reinterpretation can happen when an implicit inference shifts from one about the traits of the person to one about the person's goals. For example, if one learns about a negative behavior of a stranger one might make an inference about their negative traits. However, if one later learns the person is a member of a group with which one closely identifies, the quality inferred might be reinterpreted as a temporary goal rather than a long-standing trait of the person. For example, if they were said to be lying during a job interview, one might infer a somewhat permanent trait—they are dishonest. But if one later learns they are a member of one's fraternity, one might now infer that they had a temporary goal of getting a summer internship.

Three Types of Updating:
Addition, Negation, Reactivation and Reconsolidation

We have now reviewed several types of evidence that updating is often triggered by being confronted by new information that calls the initial impression into doubt. However, through what mechanisms specifically is the impression altered and changed? What has actually happened to the memory structure as the new impression is encoded? There are three ways—not at all in conflict—that updating has been said to alter the memory structure (see Figure 13.2).

Addition

Perhaps the most commonly described way that updating changes the encoded impression is by the **addition** of new associations—associations to behaviors performed by, and to inferences about, the person—that leave the original associations intact. For example, imagine a set of behaviors lead one to infer that a person is cruel (e.g., mocked an older teacher in front of the entire class). However, imagine one later learns the same person also acted kindly (e.g.,

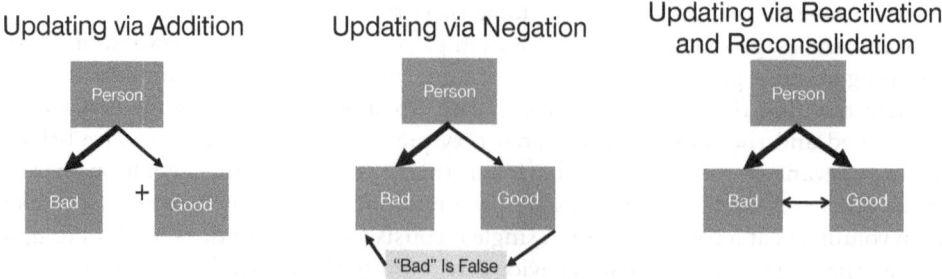

FIGURE 13.2. Updating via addition, negation, and reactivation and reconsolidation.

went out of the way to help a person with whom they worked). An association might form that links the new behaviors and the inference of "kindness" to them. Yet, the inference "cruel" might also remain associated to the person, unchanged. Both inferences, through a process of addition, would be associated with the person and each is capable of guiding how one reacts toward them. From the many associations that could potentially be tied to a representation due to processes of addition, the one used when making an explicit judgment of the person could be dependent upon which association is accessible at that point in time, the context, or the relative strength of each association (e.g., Cone & Ferguson, 2015; Gawronski et al., 2010, 2018; Gawronski, Hu, Rydell, Vervliet, & De Houwer, 2015; Olcaysoy Okten et al., 2019; Petty & Briñol, 2010; Rydell & McConnell, 2006; Rydell et al., 2007).

> **Addition:** A proposed mechanism for updating in which changes to the encoded impression occur with the addition of new associations to recently learned behaviors performed by the person and new inferences about the person (while leaving the original associations intact).

Negation

Negation processes occur when updating to the memory structure involves falsification or invalidation of the original associations (e.g., Boucher & Rydell, 2012; Rydell, McConnell, & Mackie, 2008; Winter, Scholl, & Sassenberg, 2021; Wyer, 2016). Some models argue that this happens through the association of a "tag" to the original inference about the person that labels it as false (e.g., Gilbert et al., 1990; Petty & Briñol, 2010; Petty et al., 2007). Thus, the association stays intact but is marked as incorrect. While the associations to this tag are initially weak and might not be strong enough to alter the impression that is expressed, repeated negation via learning information inconsistent with the first impression strengthens the tag and ultimately allows for updating of the impression. Other models do not argue for such a *validity tag*, but through the meaning of the initial inference being altered so that its original meaning is negated by a new quality essentially replacing the original one in the association (e.g., Calanchini, Gonsalkorale, Sherman, & Klauer, 2013; Kawakami, Young, & Dovidio, 2002; Mann & Ferguson, 2015, 2017; Wyer, 2010).

> **Negation:** A proposed mechanism for updating in which changes to the encoded impression occur due to the falsification or invalidation of the original associations.

Reactivation and Reconsolidation

Memory updating models in cognitive psychology (e.g., Hupbach et al., 2007, 2009; Nader, Schafe, & LeDoux, 2000) argue that when memory enters a state of plasticity it is temporarily open to behavioral and physiological interference. To enter such a state, the memory must be reactivated, where the original memory and its associations are triggered. If new learning occurs while the old memory is reactivated, the new information can be absorbed into the old memory structure, altering it. A restructuring of memory occurs so that, once complete, the original associations that had existed in memory are permanently changed. However, this restructuring will not become a permanent part of memory unless it has time to reconsolidate, which often occurs during sleep. Hupbach (2013) argues that this is one manner by which false memories emerge. An originally correct memory is merged, over time, with false information learned when the memory had been reactivated, leading a new and incorrect memory to emerge after **reconsolidation**; a memory one feels

> **Reconsolidation:** When a stable ("consolidated") long-term memory is reactivated, it enters a state of plasticity where it is modifiable and its content changed, strengthened, weakened, or erased, thus changing the memory to include new components that were not part of the original learning episode. Reconsolidation refers to processes that restabilize these altered memories.

confident is real. There is very little research that explores whether impressions of people can be updated through reconsolidation (e.g., Bray, Armenta, & Zarate, 2023; Olcaysoy Okten & Moskowitz, 2020a). The possibility exists that a first impression is overwritten during reconsolidation by the new associations learned when the memory was in a plastic state. The original memory would no longer be able to be reinstated; it has been replaced. A first attempt to explore this type of updating was made by Olcaysoy Okten and Moskowitz by manipulating whether a first impression was reactivated or not prior to learning inconsistent, new information. They additionally manipulated whether there was time for reconsolidation to occur (bringing participants back to the lab the next day, after a night's sleep, to have their implicit impression assessed). They found support for reconsolidation leading to updating. This offers a promising new direction for changing first impressions, especially unwanted stereotypes. It suggests that reactivating the first impression and then presenting new information that is inconsistent with the stereotype could lead the structure to be updated.

Detecting If Updating Has Occurred: Judgment versus Memory Measures

The judgments that people report are not the only way psychologists assess the impressions a person has formed. As Chapter 4 reviewed, it is also typical to use memory measures as a more subtle or implicit measure of impression formation. However, we have seen that memory measures do not always suggest the same conclusions as judgment measures. Chapters 5 and 11 provided illustrations of how people react to new learning that is inconsistent with a first impression by having very strong memory for the inconsistencies, yet a judgment that confirms the first impression. For example, Sherman, Klein, et al. (1998) measured both the judgments and memory of research participants. They found that while participants still *judged* the person in a stereotypic way, *memory* favored the stereotype-inconsistent acts. There was encoding of the details about a person's stereotype-inconsistent behaviors (such as a priest who did bad things) even though attaching them to one's memory structure did not cause one to rearrange the abstract way in which that person as a whole was judged. As another example, one way to preserve a first impression is to attribute to the situation any new behaviors learned that are inconsistent. The perceiver can deem such information not dispositionally relevant (e.g., Crocker et al., 1983) since the behavior was constrained by the situation. Despite not being attributed to the person's personality, or likely to be used when expressing an impression of the person, such information is not ignored. It is stored along with other information about the person, and stored in a way that makes it highly memorable. Finally, we reviewed other research that suggested that because the use of stereotypes and other types of schemas are functional, they allow us to specifically focus on inconsistent information. New behaviors that confirm a first impression are easy to process, and this creates a resource savings that can be used to make sense out of the inconsistent information. Rather than ignore it, or try to dismiss it, the new information is simply attended to more deeply to attempt to comprehend it (e.g., Macrae, Milne, et al., 1994; Sherman, Klein, et al., 1998).

Is this updating, even if the judgment made does not reflect a change of opinion? One could argue it is, because there is a change to the memory structure so that it now includes details about the inconsistent information about a person or group. This strong memory for the details inconsistent with the first impression might impact the judgment that is expressed at some *later point in time* even if it does not impact one's judgment at that moment. If one way that updating occurs is that new information initiates doubt regarding the validity of the first impression, then any time the new information is not ignored or dismissed it creates an opportunity for such doubt to occur. When we see that memory for inconsistent information is stronger than memory for the consistent information, the possibility for updating of judgment exists. But this creates an interesting question about when and if updating has occurred. Has updating occurred if a perceiver *reports that they judge* a person in a way that ignores the inconsistent information (and that their impression is consistent with the first impression), but that same perceiver has clearly *altered their memory representation* so that it now includes the inconsistent information? Is updating about what people expect, report, and do in the present moment, or is it about the changing of one's mental representations so that what one expects, reports, and does in the future might be different and incompatible with the original learning? The answer to this is one for which there is no agreement among scholars and reflects a choice in how to define updating.

The review of how to promote updating thus far has been on how inconsistent behavior can challenge a first impression, casting it into doubt. If it is strong enough, diagnostic enough, or encountered frequently enough, behavior that is inconsistent with a first impression will reduce the confidence the perceiver has in relying on that first impression, and in so doing trigger updating. While these strategies of challenging the first impression with inconsistent behavior can be successful to produce updating, they do place the burden for updating a stereotype (or any flawed first impression) on the person who is the target of that impression. If their behavior strategically disconfirms the stereotype, it will prompt updating in the perceiver. Of course, this is only one way to trigger the overturning of a flawed first impression. One other method shifts the burden off the person who is targeted by the first impression and places it on the perceiver who is incorrectly holding such an impression. A perceiver can adopt the goal of achieving greater confidence in their judgment. Goals that motivate perceivers to update (rather than being compelled to do so by the behaviors of others that violate an expectation) are reviewed next.

UPDATING BY ADOPTING GOALS TO OVERTURN BIAS (GOALS THAT TRIGGER CORRECTION)

People can be motivated to update a first impression not only when their confidence in the impression drops when challenged but because they desire greater certainty in their judgments than "least-effort" processing will allow. They are flexible enough to raise the threshold for how strong their impressions must be and to want to make certain that the judgments they form are not insufficient or marred by inaccuracies (such as stereotypes). When one has adopted goals that increase the level of confidence they require from their judgments, they have made a reliance on a first impression less likely to be acceptable. Let us review such goals that promote updating.

Accountability Goals

One goal that leads to a desire for judgmental confidence and increased effort is the goal of taking public responsibility for one's thoughts and actions, where those thoughts and actions are subjected to the scrutiny and evaluation of others. This is known as an **accountability goal**. For example, when reading about a topic for a public presentation one might attend closely to the material and be more careful in the conclusions one reaches than if one were reading the same material for private consumption. In another example, if a supervisor evaluates your work, the amount of time and effort put into what you produce will likely be greater than if not being scrutinized, and the work might be directed toward what you

Accountability goal: The goal of taking public responsibility for one's thoughts/actions and accept that one will be subjected to the evaluation of others. This leads to the kind of thoughts/actions that either satisfy a goal to be more accurate, or to conform to what one believes is desired by those holding you accountable.

subjectively think the supervisor hopes to see and hear (e.g., Tetlock, 1983, 1985, 1992; Tetlock & Kim, 1987). Accountability does not always lead to more accurate thinking but it leads to the kind of thinking desired by the audience to whom one is accountable. One is either updating one's impressions to reflect what is objectively correct, or to reflect what is subjectively desired by those holding you accountable.

Tetlock (1983) examined the degree to which accountability goals lead people to abandon their reliance on a first impression and update that impression. The focus was on **primacy effects**—when early information has a greater impact on judgment than information learned later. Thus, one's beliefs about a person are formed quickly from the initial information one receives, and later information is not given the appropriate weight and effort required to incorporate it fully into one's final judgment. The key assumption of the study is that participants with accountability goals would be less susceptible to primacy effects and more cautious about drawing inferences from incomplete evidence. This should lead them to attend to more information and analyze that information more carefully (compared to people without such goals). Tetlock found that unaccountable people exhibited primacy effects in forming impressions, placing greater emphasis on information presented early. However, people told that they would be accountable for their impressions were not influenced by the order in which that information was presented. Additionally, accountability led to better memory for all of the information, indicating that the first impression exerted no more weight on one's processing than information that was learned later in the sequence. Tetlock (1985) turned the focus from updating a primacy effect to correspondent inference. In the classic correspondence bias effect, a speechwriter's position is attributed to their true beliefs, even if forced to write the speech. Tetlock found accountability goals update this impression, leading the perceiver to not rely on traits and attitudes as the explanation. The accountability goal created a more discriminating perceiver whose extra processing effort made them consider information that overturned the first impression. Similarly, Thompson et al. (1994) found such goals updated a *priming effect*—rather than using accessible constructs, people think more deeply if accountable.

> **Primacy effects:** When information learned early has a greater impact on judgment than information learned later. Thus, one's beliefs about a person are formed quickly from the initial information one receives, and later information is not given the appropriate weight and effort required to incorporate it fully into one's final judgment.

Accuracy Goals

Another goal that leads people to raise their sufficiency thresholds is the goal of being accurate. Sometimes the situation explicitly calls for one to be accurate, such as when one serves as a juror (where a judge might instruct you to pay close attention and to be objective and accurate) or works as a teacher (where evaluating students requires an accurate assessment of exams). Other situations merely suggest (imply) accuracy is important, such as when one works with other people to attain some mutual goal (e.g., you have a partner for a joint project and being rewarded depends on the performance of your partner). When one is dependent on another individual to obtain the outcomes one desires, and those outcomes cannot be attained through individual effort alone, one is said to be in a state of **outcome dependency**. When outcome dependent, it is useful to form accurate judgments about what your partner is able to contribute so you can best utilize those skills; you need to accurately assess the partner.

> **Outcome dependency:** When the outcomes one desires cannot be attained through individual effort alone, making one dependent on another individual. Such goals typically require one to attempt to be more accurate in forming impressions about the people on whom one is dependent since attaining the desired outcomes requires relying upon them.

Neuberg and Fiske (1987) examined how outcome dependency updates an impression so that a stereotype is no longer applied. They reasoned that when a negative expectation is associated with a particular group, people evaluate members of that group using the negative stereotype. For example, most people hold negative expectations about what it would be like to interact with a person who is schizophrenic. They are likely to form judgments that are fairly negative, despite not thinking too carefully about or attending much to that person's behavior. However, updating such a judgment could occur if the perceiver had a goal to do so. Neuberg and Fiske created such a goal by placing participants in a state of outcome dependency. They asked participants to interact with another person as part of a purported program on "the reintegration of hospital patients" to start preparing patients for life in the community after a period of hospitalization. For some participants these were said to be schizophrenic patients, and thus negative stereotypes were triggered. Other participants were given no label regarding their partner, and hence had no expectations. Some participants were next made outcome dependent on their partner by telling them that their joint performance with their partner could win them a cash prize if their team performed better than other teams. Other participants were left independent of the partner. As the primary measures of interest, they assessed whether participants exerted more effort in learning about their partner and overturned (vs. relied upon) stereotypes. They did so by providing them with "personal information" about the partner before working together with them. Do they evaluate the information they receive about others more closely, and in so doing update their stereotypic impression, when outcome dependent? They do—when people were dependent on a partner with schizophrenia they took twice as much time to read the "personal information" and form their evaluation of that person than participants who were not outcome dependent. This led to updating—the judgments made about the partner with schizophrenia were less negative as compared to participants who were not outcome dependent.

Neuberg (1989) found similar findings when directly telling people to adopt the goal of being accurate. A job interview is a forum for gathering information and testing hypotheses about a person, so stereotyping and relying on first impressions may be acute in those situations. They can not only lead to the interviewer forming a stereotypic judgment but asking questions that elicit answers and behaviors affirming negative expectations: a self-fulfilling prophecy that strengthens the stereotype. However, Neuberg illustrated that the bias exerted by a first impression in a job interview is updated if the interviewer has accuracy goals—people updated by gathering more comprehensive and less biased information. They spent more time listening to the person for whom they had a negative expectation, were more encouraging in the questions asked, and asked more open-ended, novel, and positively framed questions. These responses led applicants to act in ways that were more positive, and for the negative first impression to then be updated. Accuracy concerns can be created in many ways (from being dependent, from being directly asked, from being paid, even from being held accountable), and applied to many situations. Recent interest has been on the question of whether the spread of and belief in misinformation might be mitigated if people adopt accuracy goals. Research on judgments of politically charged issues shows that financial incentives to be accurate can reduce the biases shown by partisans (e.g., Bullock & Lenz, 2019; Prior, Sood, & Khanna, 2015). Such incentives even reduce the differences among partisans of opposing groups over what news is true versus false. Partisans who were given accuracy goals showed an increased belief in news that they might otherwise dismiss as misinformation because it is inconsistent with their political views. They can better identify stories they disagree with as, nonetheless, true (Rathje, Van Bavel, & van der Linden, 2021).

Perspective-Taking Goals

In Chapter 9 we briefly reviewed another goal that was shown to update a correspondent inference. Storms (1973) showed that if the perceiver's perspective was changed so that the perceiver saw what the person being perceived saw—so the perceiver's focus was on the situation impacting the person being perceived rather than focused on that person and their behavior—this bias was eliminated. It was while teaching this research in my first year at Princeton University (as a new assistant professor) that I had an epiphany. My research at the time was focused on how to disrupt the activation of stereotypes. The epiphany was to connect the two ideas. If changing one's physical perspective could alter how impressions were formed, so that a bias to focus on the personality of the person being perceived could be mitigated, could it also update impressions so that a stereotype on which one was focused as an explanation for behavior was overturned? What if instead of literally taking their perspective so that visual attention was now focused on the salient situational pressures

> **Perspective taking:** Contemplating or seeing the world as if in another's shoes, to consider their views and barricades/obstacles/constraints. The ability to understand that people not only have goals separate from one's own, but beliefs different from one's own, and to consider that person's goals/beliefs/obstacles when trying to understand that person's behavior and feelings.
>
> **Self–other merging:** When one's own self-concept is combined with the attitudes and beliefs of others, spreading one's positive self-evaluation to them. The overlap of self and other leads one to desire greater accuracy when judging them (as one would want when evaluating the self), and promotes a more favorable view of them.

they faced, one instead simulated taking that person's perspective and imagined the obstacles they faced? I soon pitched this idea to my graduate student colleague, and he decided to change his dissertation topic: Instead of exploring whether accountability goals update stereotypes, we embarked on an exploration of **perspective taking** and stereotype control. Two decades of research on this topic has since emerged (e.g., Epley, Keysar, Van Boven, & Gilovich, 2004; Eyal, Steffel, & Epley, 2018; Galinsky & Moskowitz, 2000b; Todd & Galinsky, 2014; Todd, Bodenhausen, Richeson, & Galinsky, 2011).

How does the goal of taking another person's perspective promote updating of a stereotype? There are several answers. One is that it promotes what is known as **self–other merging**, where the self-concept is combined with the attitudes and beliefs about the group, spreading one's positive self-evaluation to the group. The overlap of self and other leads one to desire greater accuracy when judging the person (as one would want when evaluating the self), and it promotes a more favorable view of them (as one would want for the self). These ideas were explored by Galinsky and Moskowitz (2000b), who had participants take the perspective of an older man (or not). Perspective-taking participants were shown to be associating their own positive qualities with the older man in a way not seen in participants not taking his perspective. The characteristics associated with the self were used to describe the target, reflecting a *merging of the self and the other*. Taking perspective allows one to see how others are like you (e.g., Todd & Burgmer, 2013; Todd, Bodenhausen, & Galinsky, 2012). Similarly, Davis, Conklin, Smith, & Luce (1996) found that perspective taking leads one to perceive greater overlap between the self and the target: one sees more self-descriptive traits in the target.

A second way that perspective taking can lead to updating uses the attributional logic of the research of Storms (1973) discussed above. Taking the perspective of another person would require considering the situation the person is in, causing one to see and consider influences on that person that are separate from the stereotype, perhaps challenging the stereotype. In so doing this might inhibit stereotypic associations, while also creating new associations. Galinsky and Moskowitz (2000b) illustrated that although perceivers use stereotypes when responding to members of stereotyped groups, people taking the perspective of those individuals failed to show a reliance on stereotypes. To illustrate this, they contrasted the responses of people asked to take the perspective of others with those explicitly asked to suppress any stereotypic thoughts. Macrae, Bodenhausen, et al. (1994) had shown that thought suppression leads to the stereotype to initially be removed from how people respond, but ultimately it comes back and is even more strongly activated and likely to be used (as reviewed in Chapter 8). Galinsky and Moskowitz added a perspective-taking group to the Macrae, Bodenhausen, et al. research design. When asked to write an essay about a day in the life of a person belonging to a stereotyped group (an older man), participants who took the perspective of that person did not use stereotypes in their essays. Neither did people asked to suppress stereotypes. Additionally, when an implicit measure was used to see whether the stereotype of older adults was accessible in the participants, the results showed that for those asked to suppress the stereotype, the stereotype was now hyperaccessible. But for participants asked to take the person's perspective, stereotyping was controlled. Todd et al. (2011) showed that these same findings occur with a measure of implicit prejudice, as opposed to stereotypes. Using the IAT they found that perspective taking led to fewer automatic racial biases than a control condition.

A third way that perspective taking can lead to updating is by promoting greater empathy with the targets of bias. Research has shown that there are two distinct types of empathy that could promote updating. One is the experience of parallel empathy, where the perspective taker will feel the same emotions as the outgroup whose perspective is being adopted. A second type is known as reactive empathy and involves experiencing concern for another's well-being, which in turn leads to updating negative impressions (e.g., Todd & Galinsky, 2014). For example, Clore and Jeffery (1972) had research participants take the perspective of a person in a wheelchair by having them engage in role-playing exercises that required them to use a wheelchair on their college campus. These participants reported more reactive empathy and more positive attitudes toward individuals with physical disabilities. Todd and Galinsky suggest that as more detail about the person or group is provided, then perspective taking is more likely to lead to updating through attributional and empathy mechanisms (see also Vescio, Sechrist, & Paolucci, 2003).

The Goal to Counterstereotype

One strategy of suppressing a stereotype has already been discussed as one that backfires. Rather than asking people to avoid stereotypes, we can give people goals that teach them new ways of thinking—such as to develop new expectations or to generate counterstereotypic associations to the group (e.g., Burns, Monteith, & Parker, 2017). For example, Blair and Banaji (1996) manipulated the expectations that people had regarding gender stereotypes. Participants were told they were going to see a series of names that would be preceded by a personal trait, and the task was to simply identify whether the name was "male" or "female." Stereotyping is illustrated by people responding faster when the name is preceded by a stereotypic trait. However, some of the research participants were also led to expect that the traits they would be seeing were counterstereotypic. They expected that traditionally "male" traits would precede female names (e.g., ambitious Betty) and traditionally "female" traits would precede male names (e.g., sensitive Brian). People without expectations show a classic stereotyping effect—such as being faster to classify female names when preceded by stereotypically female traits. But when people had the expectation they would see counterstereotypic pairings, they no longer showed this facilitation: Stereotype activation was disrupted.

Dasgupta and Asgari (2004) showed that counterstereotypic expectations could be created in a perceiver by exposure to other people who are exemplars representing the counterstereotype. Some of their female research participants rated their identification with well-known female leaders (and in another experiment they contemplated examples of actual exposure to counterstereotypic women). Other participants were in a control group where such examples were not considered. Such counterstereotypic expectations led to control over stereotype activation. The same is found with implicit prejudice. Dasgupta and Greenwald (2001) found that exposure to admirable exemplars of African Americans led to control over implicit prejudice.

Kawakami et al. (2000) took a slightly different tack in examining whether stereotype activation could be controlled. They reasoned that if stereotype activation is a case of association, with concepts linked to a category triggered, perhaps people could be trained to have associations to a counterstereotypic category. They provided people with *counterstereotype association training*. Participants completed a lengthy training session in which nonstereotypic associations to an outgroup were learned through repeated pairings. The training forced people to practice responding "no" each time they saw a stereotypic trait being paired with a member of a stereotyped group. For example, the participants had to press a button marked "no" on the keyboard each time they saw a picture of a skinhead paired with a trait that is stereotypic of skinheads (e.g., malicious). Additionally, they pressed a key marked "yes" if they saw a picture of a skinhead paired with a counterstereotypic trait (e.g., timid). They practiced developing these new associations for 45 minutes, training themselves to embrace the counterstereotype. They found that despite a lifetime of having learned to associate the stereotype with the group, the training created new associations that led to stereotype activation being disrupted.

The notion that training can be used to disrupt implicit bias has also been shown in research using the first-person shooter task (FPST). Research participants allowed to practice performing the task over several days did not show the classic bias—White participants were not more likely to incorrectly "shoot" Black men in the task (Correll et al., 2007; Sim et al., 2013). Similarly, Correll et al. found that police officers who receive extensive training are able to control the bias when asked to perform the FPST. This effect has been replicated many times, though shown to vary dependent on factors such as fatigue, cognitive load, and whether one's training is as a "beat" officer or special forces (gang-unit) officer (e.g., Ma et al., 2013; Sim et al., 2013). Correll et al. (2014) argue that training can teach a person how to exert control over the bias. While not exactly the same as adopting a goal to counterstereotype, such training does focus the person on learning not to use race in such situations. Whereas tasks such as the FPST illustrate a prepotent tendency to rely on race and racial stereotypes, this bias can be controlled by learning to ignore race as a relevant cue, though bias returns in cases of fatigue and cognitive load.

Multicultural and Colorblind Goals

An early social psychological finding was that there are multiple ways to attain the same goal, and one route to goal completion can substitute for another (Lissner, 1933; Mahler, 1933). In modern times, this is called **equifinality** (e.g., Kruglanski et al., 2002). When it comes to stereotyping, there are, as with other goal pursuits, multiple means that satisfy the same goal of not stereotyping (e.g., Plaut, Thomas, Hurd, & Romano, 2018)—there are two broad goals people often adopt when trying to not stereotype. One is a strategy of **colorblindness** that emphasizes ignoring or denying that there are differences that exist among

Equifinality: When there are multiple ways to attain the same goal, and one route to goal completion can substitute for another. For example, there are multiple means that satisfy the same goal of not stereotyping (one can ignore categories, one can suppress stereotypes, one can value differences, etc.).

groups, and instead embrace the ideology of equality that states we should simply see all people as equal and interacting with one another on a level playing field irrespective of race or gender or other group differences. The claim is that if we are to be unbiased and evaluate people purely on the "content of their character," then we must ignore group membership. The other is a strategy of **multiculturalism** that emphasizes the differences that are known to exist between groups (e.g., diversity), with an appreciation for the positive differences. The claim is that if we are to be unbiased and evaluate people purely on the "content of their character"—and hope for eradicating the disparities that social biases and systemic injustice inflict—then we must not ignore group membership, since our group identity shapes the nature of the "playing field," which is not level. Multicultural goals suggest embracing group membership and keeping group identity in consideration as a possible source of valuable input: that people draw identity from multiple groups, recognizing the distinctive qualities of each group (e.g., Brewer, 1991). This inclusiveness yields an abstractness to how one thinks about a person, where a perceiver considers a wider range of characteristics relating to the person. Many now believe that the assimilation of a minority group into a dominant group allows for the perpetuation of inequality rather than a fairer society (e.g., Hahn, Banchefsky, Park, & Judd, 2015; Knowles, Lowery, Hogan, & Chow, 2009; Whitley & Webster, 2019). Within this philosophy there is more recently a debate about whether positive distinctiveness is best achieved by multiculturalism, **polyculturalism** (focusing on how cultures intermix and change one another through contact), or **interculturalism** (emphasizing intergroup dialogue, contact, and shared unity; e.g., Yogeeswaran, Verkuyten, & Ealam, 2021).

> **Colorblindness:** A goal/strategy for stereotype control that emphasizes ignoring differences among groups. The claim is that if we are to be unbiased and evaluate people purely on the "content of their character" then we must ignore group membership. It embraces the ideology that we should see all people as equal.
>
> **Multiculturalism:** A goal/strategy for stereotype control that emphasizes positive differences existing between groups. The claim is that if we are to be unbiased and evaluate people purely on the "content of their character" then group identity must be considered as a source of valuable input, and accept that diversity has value.
>
> **Polyculturalism:** A goal/strategy for stereotype control that takes a historical view, focusing on how cultures have always intermixed and changed each other through contact. This presumably leads people to realize that culture has always been shifting and amorphous.
>
> **Interculturalism:** A goal/strategy for stereotype control that emphasizes intergroup contact and communication to promote an appreciation of diversity as well as an identification of commonalities and areas of unity. It also prescribes contact between cultures so that cultural mixing can be normalized.

There are costs and benefits to each goal. For example, Norton, Vandello, et al. (2008) show that each of us likely has adopted each of these strategies, but often under different circumstances. Seventy percent of their research participants felt that a multicultural strategy was essential when discussing differences among groups in the abstract—such as when determining the composition of an incoming college class and being sure that it reflected a diverse group of people. However, at the same time, 90% of their research participants felt that a colorblind strategy was essential when thinking about specific individuals at a concrete level—such as when determining whether a given person should be admitted to a college. What is the impact of selecting one of these equifinal means to the goal over the other? Wolsko, Park, Judd, and Wittenbrink (2000) had White research participants adopt one of these goals (a third group was in a control condition) and then they performed a task where they estimated the percentage of White people and Black people who possessed a set of traits and rated their feelings toward the groups. They found that adopting a multicultural goal led to less favoritism for the ingroup in ratings of feelings toward each group: The control group and colorblind group felt more positively about a group of White people. However, there were also differences in how people stereotyped, this time with the multicultural strategy revealing greater perceived group differences in traits. Participants in the multicultural group showed both greater positive stereotyping of Black people than of White people, and greater negative stereotyping. In a second experiment the researchers created the same three groups and had participants assess values associated with each group. They also performed a task that tapped the accuracy of their stereotypes (comparing responses to actual census data). Once again, colorblind and multicultural strategies led to different effects on information processing. A colorblind approach led to greater perceived similarity in the values of White people and Black people. However, the perception of greater group differences by people with a multicultural strategy was accompanied by greater accuracy. Based on comparisons to census data, a multicultural strategy allowed people to better detect real differences that exist in the data that describe the groups.

Richeson and Nussbaum (2003) explored how adopting a colorblind versus a multicultural strategy affected implicit prejudice using a race IAT. As might be expected, White research participants showed a strong pro-White bias regardless of whether they had a multicultural or colorblind goal. However, the participants in the colorblind group showed a greater bias. Adopting a colorblind approach to being nonprejudiced generated greater automatic race bias than adopting a multicultural approach. Without a control group it is impossible to know whether the colorblind strategy led to more bias than is typical, or whether the multicultural strategy led to less bias than is typical. Research on *thought suppression* suggests that it is likely the case that colorblind strategies enhance implicit bias. In Chapter 8 it was reviewed that specifically asking people to not stereotype leads them to attempt to search for stereotypic thoughts in order to then control expressing them. Ironically, this search for stereotypic words with the purpose of being less biased leads to an increased accessibility of the very stereotypic thoughts one is trying to avoid. A colorblind approach can be thought of as akin to thought suppression. In this way, the research on stereotype suppression complements the findings of Richeson and Nussbaum on implicit bias and colorblindness versus multiculturalism. However, while colorblind goals may lead to more implicit bias than multicultural goals, this does not mean multicultural goals reduce prejudice. In some cases, they even increase prejudice (e.g., Yogeeswaran & Dasgupta, 2014).

There is a widening consensus that while multiculturalism has many positive effects, it can also promote stereotyping. It does so not merely by incorporating positive stereotypes along with negative stereotypes, but by implying groups have traits. By promoting thinking about groups in terms of traits, multiculturalism implies a sense of essentialism: that other groups are different from us (e.g., Wilton, Apfelbaum, & Good, 2019), and since the difference is in their traits, these differences will not change, thus promoting segregation of groups (e.g., Hahn et al., 2015) and feelings of exclusion among majority group members (e.g., Plaut, Garnett, Buffardi, & Sanchez-Burks, 2011). Thus, these findings taken together reveal that the manner with which one attempts to not be biased will alter the type of bias that is manifested. Moskowitz and Vitriol (2022) argued that this is a real danger for those who attempt to run interventions aimed at reducing bias. A well-intentioned organization can unintentionally heighten bias if the strategies they introduce to try to reduce it lead people to use race more, rather than less.

Goals with Vested Interests and Heightened Personal Importance

Having a vested interest or increased personal involvement in the outcome of a judgment will also lead to increased goals to process more deeply and to updating. For example, Borgida and Howard-Pitney (1983) focused on how having a vested interest impacts the effects of perceptual salience. Salient things attract our attention. We assume things on which we focus are likely to be the cause of what goes on around us (Taylor, Crocker, Fiske, Sprinzen, & Winkler, 1979) and we place more causal weight on (and are more influenced by) people on whom we focus attention. But these effects of attention and salience are updated when personal relevance is involved. Borgida and Howard-Pitney had perceivers listen to a debate on a topic they believed was either not relevant or relevant to them personally (a proposed change in undergraduate course requirements), with attention focused on one person in the debate who they heard argue for one side of the issue. If personal involvement was low, students rated the salient person more favorably regardless of whether that person argued in favor of or against the proposed changes. When involvement was high, the ratings of the person depended on what position the person took regarding the curriculum changes rather than simply where attention was focused. Thus, when a perceiver had heightened motivational concerns, an initial impression based on salience effects was updated by broadening attention to include information inconsistent with the first impression (that might otherwise be ignored).

Another example of personal relevance impacting updating is seen in research that explores when a person is vested in the goal to reduce personal prejudice. Fazio (1990a; see also Fazio & Olson, 2014) argues that people need both *motivation* and *opportunity* to update, striking the same themes reviewed at the start of this chapter. In their research, motivation is provided by manipulating the personal relevance of the goal to reduce prejudice. Opportunity is provided by manipulating whether conditions of cognitive load and fatigue serve as an obstacle to effortful control (e.g., Towles-Schwen & Fazio, 2006). If either element is absent, control fails; if both are present, updating should occur. An example is provided by Olson and Fazio (2004) in an experiment where some of the participants had a personally relevant goal to control prejudice (and some did not). All their participants saw pictures of people in a variety of occupations who also varied regarding their race. Participants provided their impressions of them, which allowed for the computation of a positivity score by aggregating across all the Black individuals and all the White individuals rated, to compare against one another. In addition to these explicit ratings, they also assessed implicit prejudice. They found that when a person was low in the motivation to control prejudice the impressions explicitly reported aligned with the implicit prejudice—they had negative attitudes. However, when participants had a personally relevant goal to control prejudice, the impression that was reported was updated; it no longer aligned with implicit prejudice. They reported positive explicit attitudes despite having negative implicit attitudes.

In a third example, Devine (1989) manipulated the relevance of the goal to control prejudice in the experiment. As part of an experiment ostensibly about how people informally talk about groups, White participants were asked to list as many labels for the group "Blacks" as they could, even slang words and negative words. This task forces people to say things they do not endorse, and creates a motivation in the moment to prove that being unprejudiced is personally important to them (to compensate for the bias they were forced to show). Devine found that participants subsequently expressed far more positive beliefs about Black Americans than a control group. However, tricking one into doing or saying reprehensible things is not a particularly pragmatic way to create heightened relevance of one's egalitarian goals. One popular way to heighten the personal relevance of a goal is through directly providing feedback that one is not meeting desired standards (as described earlier in this chapter). Devine, Monteith, Zuwerink, and Elliot (1991) did so by relying on self-discrepancy theory. Participants were asked to state how they should act when encountering a member of a minority group, and then to state how they actually would act. When these two differ, an "ought discrepancy" (as defined in Chapter 9) is experienced. This then provides feedback to the participant that they have failed to meet a desired goal to be nonprejudiced. This negative feedback creates a heightened personal relevance of the goal, which motivates the person to reduce the discrepancy, to align how one would act with the unprejudiced way that one should act. The motivation, in turn, leads to deeper processing that will update and overturn one's biased initial reactions. Monteith (1993) and colleagues (e.g., Monteith et al., 1993, 1998, 2002) have used negative feedback to motivate the control of prejudice. Let us review several examples.

Monteith (1993) had heterosexual research participants play the role of a law school admissions officer and review applicants. They were provided with negative feedback that they had shown bias against gay applicants. Rather than continue to use stereotypes, the participants responded by a heightened focus on controlling bias. When next asked to read an essay about how gay people are targeted by bias, the experimenters recorded the amount of time participants dedicated to working on this task and had participants track their thoughts while working on the task. Negative feedback triggered motivation to be unbiased, which produced more controlled and careful responding. In a second experiment they also found that the participants were not only more careful when working on the task, but also were more effective at inhibiting prejudiced responding on a subsequent task (rating jokes that had homosexuals as the target of the humor). Negative feedback about prejudice heightens the personal relevance of the goal to be unbiased, which triggers control—compensating by expressing a problem with jokes invoking stereotypes.

In the experiment just described, the motivation is created in the moment by negative feedback. Can the personal relevance of this goal be "automated" over time, so that it is triggered even when negative feedback is no longer present? Earlier, when discussing proactive control, it was suggested that goals can be triggered by relevant cues in the environment. Goals are not just conscious tools we effortfully deploy, but they are cognitively explicated, represented in memory, and capable of being implicitly activated, like any other representation (e.g., Bargh, 1990; Bargh & Gollwitzer, 1994; Gollwitzer & Moskowitz, 1996): No consciousness needed. For example, if a White person is provided feedback that they have bias against Black men, this not only increases the personal relevance of the goal to be unbiased and motivates control, it also leads to developing an association between increased personal relevance of the goal and a cue associated with the feedback, such as the presence of a Black man. If such associations develop, then merely seeing a Black man would subsequently trigger one's motivation to be unbiased and increase control efforts. The cues (people who may potentially be evaluated in a biased way) serve as a warning that the bias one has shown in the past needs to be controlled from surfacing in this moment. Over time this process becomes automated. A cue can prospectively trigger the control response—without feedback, and without awareness of either the cue or the response.

To illustrate this, Monteith et al. (2002) had participants take the IAT. Being informed of their (actual) implicit bias served as the negative feedback and increased the relevance of their egalitarian goals. Shortly after receiving this feedback, participants completed a task that involved viewing words on a monitor and then indicating whether they liked or disliked the words. The items they saw were both filler words, as well as words from the IAT that they had earlier categorized as associated with Black people. The rationale was that if one received negative feedback about their IAT performance, then encountering words from the IAT task presented in the new task would serve as cues that would trigger the goal (since these words would have been associated with the goal from taking the IAT). There were two ways in which responses on the like–dislike task could indicate updating of one's biased response. First, the choice of whether they liked or disliked the word would become more positive. Second, people would respond more slowly when making that choice, indicating their greater processing effort and deliberation about their response. Each of these responses were found to occur.

In fact, across the experiments reviewed in this section a consistent pattern is shown where participants respond more slowly (ratings of liking vs. disliking, labeling jokes as not funny, expressing positive beliefs about the group). This is a signal of a specific type of control that Gray (1982) called **behavioral inhibition**. Behavioral inhibition is described as a self-regulatory response where there is a momentary pausing or interruption of one's current behavior. This brief stoppage of action allows one to increase attention to stimuli that are relevant to one's current goal and to determine what might have caused one to fall short of reaching that goal to help one prepare a response. Monteith and Voils (2001) summarize a model of updating as a case of behavioral inhibition of unwanted responses (see Figure 13.3):

> **Behavioral inhibition:** Self-regulatory response where one momentarily pauses or interrupts current behavior. This brief stoppage of action allows one to increase attention to stimuli relevant to one's current goal and to determine what might have caused one to fall short of reaching that goal. This helps one prepare an appropriate compensatory response.

1. Negative feedback about goal pursuit occurs (in this case the goal to be unbiased).
2. Associations form between pursuing this goal and cues relating to the negative feedback.
3. When those cues for control are subsequently encountered, behavioral inhibition occurs.
4. This causes a slowing of ongoing behavior and more careful processing.
5. Responses are made to help achieve the goal and to update the biased response that had originally been triggered—control is exerted.

We have noted throughout this book that rather than being motivating, such feedback can be threatening, and perceivers may dismiss it instead. Perceivers may attribute any bias suggested by the feedback to uncontrollable forces that make them less concerned about

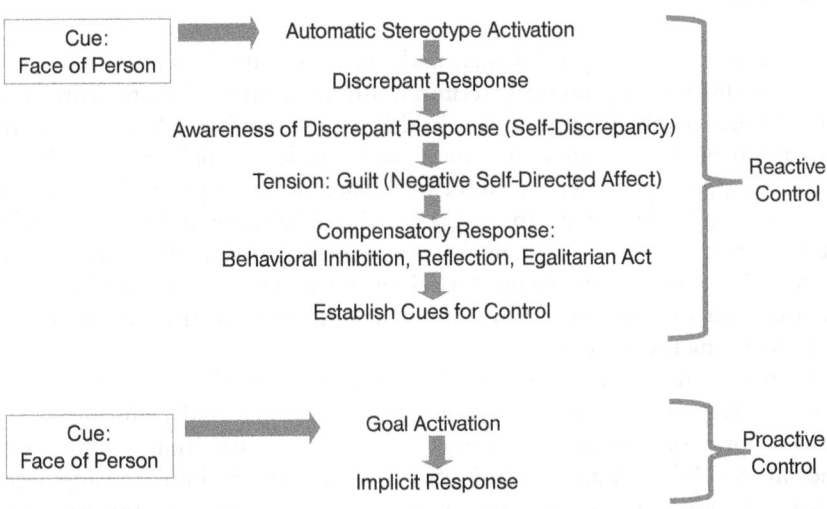

FIGURE 13.3. From explicit and reactive control to implicit and proactive control.

bias (e.g., Cameron, Payne, & Knobe, 2010; Daumeyer et al., 2019; Redford & Ratliff, 2016; Vitriol & Moskowitz, 2021). Yet, raising awareness of a discrepancy in a goal pursuit (in this case, being more biased than one intends) *can* be done in a way that mitigates such threat and motivates control.

Control is not limited to behavioral inhibition and greater attention. People compensate for bias by seeking out interventions to learn how to reduce bias (e.g., Plant & Devine, 2009). They compensate for their biases with a reduction in their potentially discriminatory behavior (e.g., Cooley, Lei, & Ellerkamp, 2018). As reviewed in Chapter 12, they also engage in proactive control (e.g., Moskowitz, 2010, 2014) as depicted in the bottom of Figure 13.3. Unfortunately, the concept of proactive control introduced in 1990 did not gain much mention at all in discussions of impression updating for almost 2 decades. It was not until Vohs and Baumeister (2004) published the *Handbook of Self-Regulation* that we began to see broader acknowledgment within the discipline that rather than control requiring consciousness, control could also be described as happening outside conscious awareness. Gregg, Seibt, and Banaji (2006) noted that in the study of attitudes, a body of work had been accumulating that showed despite prejudiced attitudes being implicit, they are malleable and controllable (e.g., Amodio et al., 2003; Blair, 2001; Dasgupta & Greenwald, 2001; Lowery et al., 2001; Olson & Fazio, 2003; Richeson & Ambady, 2003; Rydell & Jones, 2009). For example, Turner and Crisp (2010) showed that implicit attitudes as measured by an IAT were malleable such that imagining a goal of intergroup contact led to more positive responses on the IAT. A non-Muslim research participant who imagined a conversation with a Muslim stranger had less-negative implicit attitudes than a control group. As another example, earlier findings of proactive updating in stereotyping (e.g., Blair & Banaji, 1996; Gilbert & Hixon, 1991; Lepore & Brown, 1997; Moskowitz et al., 1999) soon began to be more broadly acknowledged and incorporated into modern research (e.g., Amodio, 2009; Amodio, Devine, & Harmon-Jones, 2008; Amodio & Swencionis, 2018). The malleability of stereotype activation and the central role that *implicit control* processes play in updating is finally being more widely discussed.

CONCLUSIONS

What prescription should a psychologist make to a person who needs to change behavior to meet the threat of a potentially terminal illness? Reading the literature on behavior change might proactively motivate a new health regimen and save lives. It may also be so threatening that people trivialize the disease and attack the credentials of the scientists. How should we approach gender bias in the workplace? Workshops that heighten awareness might motivate egalitarian people to change individual behavior and institutional practice. It might also create a backlash where the environment worsens. How should politicians convince constituents that a policy needs to change? Change can motivate hope for a better future, but it can also create uncertainty and fear that leads to striking out against scapegoats and preserving the status quo.

Failure to update has important implications for how we live our lives and how organizations (medical communities, governments, legal professionals, educators, etc.) try to regulate behavior. People and organizations see social disparities that exist in their world—disparities in the United States toward African Americans include housing access, judicial verdicts, medical decision making, policing, incarceration, and unemployment (e.g., Eberhardt et al., 2006; Green et al., 2007; Pager & Shepherd, 2008; Sabin & Greenwald, 2012; Smith & Holmes, 2003; Stone et al., 2020; Terrill & Reisig, 2003; West & Sabol, 2009). People and organizations understand that justice may require regulation of such biases (at least as a component of how disparities can be reduced). Failure is a powerful motivator, and negative feedback is a popular tool used in workshops and interventions to attempt to address bias and disparity. We fail, and we react to feedback about our failure with stepped-up efforts and increased goal commitment. However, raising awareness via such feedback also induces threat that drives the worst of the human condition. Negative feedback can demotivate us, scare us, and threaten us, and it shines a negative light on self-esteem (that we are also motivated to protect and defend). Psychological research reveals an updating conundrum. To achieve our goals—be it egalitarian pursuits, weight loss, work achievement, relationship success, or a health goal (such as quitting smoking, running a marathon, or taking our pills regularly)—and to alter unwanted behavior and bad habits, we need to fail, and respond to negative feedback with stepped-up goal pursuit. But it may instead threaten and demotivate us. One solution to the conundrum is for our science to develop a better understanding of when and how feedback leads to updating. To better understand the mechanisms of reactive control and how conscious effort can help people overturn bias. we must understand when new learning will motivate updating versus defensiveness and when inconsistent information will be dismissed versus incorporated into our mental representations. Interventions based on such science will have a better chance to succeed (e.g., Moskowitz et al., 2023; Moskowitz & Vitriol, 2022).

We have also seen that negative feedback is not the only way to motivate updating. People can also adopt goals that render confirming a first impression undesirable. Especially in domains where people have a vested interest, they may value the updating of, and correcting for, an inaccuracy over the ease of confirming what was initially believed. However, attempts to motivate people can also fail to lead to updating if people lack efficacy or capacity to update. At times, motivating them to hold a goal as personally relevant might, ironically, make them defensive or avoidant. This could happen if they begin to worry that the goal is of such importance, that failing to meet it will be embarrassing and socially damning (as others condemn one for failing at such an important goal). Another solution is to embrace the scientific findings that tell us that control can be nonconscious. This is true of how we select and activate goals to pursue, and of how we pursue and implement those goals. Huang and Bargh (2014) argued for the brain regions that engage implicit processes to be more ancient, with consciousness being a more recent addition to the evolution of the human brain. With this argument came a belief that implicit processes were, therefore, efficient and able to operate despite limitations that derail conscious processing. Some biases made when consciously pursuing a goal are avoided when not "trying" but using implicit processes (e.g., Sassenberg, Moskowitz, Fetterman, & Kessler, 2017). This is not to say effortless control is better than reactive control—just that we need to understand when updating is achieved by proactive and implicit forms of control versus reactive and effortful forms of control. Each type of control can allow us to update unwanted impressions, and for our mental representations to be altered and made more accurate. Despite being creatures of bias, we are also creatures who are goal driven and able to update our thoughts and feelings according to our goals.

NOTES

1. We all know that behavior can change in different contexts—for example, a person may be serious at work but fun at a bar. Feedback about an impression being biased or wrong can be dismissed if the person sees their original impression as a quality that is broad and generalizes across contexts, but is motivated to see the inconsistent new behavior as tied to the situation.

2. Of course, it is possible that the better memory for the inconsistent information does not reflect updating but the fact that the perceiver was trying to keep their first impression intact and in doing so was explaining away the inconsistencies in a manner that made them memorable.

3. They also raise the possibility that such updating is an error—that base rates (such as those suggested by stereotypes) *should be* used in favor of recently learned and highly salient information. Why throw probabilities out the window for recently encountered examples? For example, if you know that 80% of the people at a party are librarians, and you are asked to guess if a woman at the party is a librarian, you should guess yes, regardless of whether she exhibited a behavior that was not typical of the librarian stereotype (such as telling loud, crude jokes).

4. However, contact, and exposure to stereotype-inconsistent behavior, does not guarantee stereotyping will diminish. As Allport (1954) noted, the case is not so simple as merely bringing people together. Contact between people at a superficial level may do little to reduce prejudice and stereotypes, and can even, at times, lead to increased prejudice (even if behavior inconsistent with the stereotype is routinely performed and seen). Several other ingredients need to be in place to promote positive effects due to contact (Allport, 1954; Pettigrew, 1997): (1) the people in contact must have meaningful (not superficial) interactions with each other, (2) they must have equal status in these contact situations, (3) they should pursue common goals, and (4) the situation they are in should promote a norm of equality between groups (there should be social support that sanctions all groups as equals).

References

Aaker, J. L., & Lee, A. Y. (2001). "I" seek pleasures and "we" avoid pains: The role of self-regulatory goals in information processing and persuasion. *Journal of Consumer Research, 28*(1), 33–49.

Aarts, H., Custers, R., & Holland, R. W. (2007). The nonconscious cessation of goal pursuit: When goals and negative affect are coactivated. *Journal of Personality and Social Psychology, 92,* 165–178.

Aarts, H., & Dijksterhuis, A. (2003). The silence of the library: Environment, situational norm, and social behavior. *Journal of Personality and Social Psychology, 84*(1), 18–28.

Aarts, H., Dijksterhuis, A. P., & Midden, C. (1999). To plan or not to plan? Goal achievement of interrupting the performance of mundane behaviors. *European Journal of Social Psychology, 29,* 971–979.

Aarts, H., Gollwitzer, P. M., & Hassin, R. R. (2004). Goal contagion: Perceiving is for pursuing. *Journal of Personality and Social Psychology, 87*(1), 23–37.

Abelson, R. (1981). Psychological status of the script concept. *American Psychologist, 36,* 715–729.

Acorn, D. A., Hamilton, D. L., & Sherman, S. J. (1988). Generalization of biased perceptions of groups based on illusory correlations. *Social Cognition, 6,* 345–372.

Adams, E. A., Kurtz-Costes, B. E., & Hoffman, A. J. (2016). Skin tone bias among African Americans: Antecedents and consequences across the life span. *Developmental Review, 40,* 93–116.

Adorno, T. W., Frenkel-Brunswik, E., Levinson, D. J., & Sanford, R. N. (1950). *The authoritarian personality.* New York: Harper & Row.

Ahler, D. J., Citrin, J., Dougal, M. C., & Lenz, G. S. (2017). Face value? Experimental evidence that candidate appearance influences electoral choice. *Political Behavior, 39,* 77–102.

Alba, J. W., & Hasher, L. (1983). Is memory schematic? *Psychological Bulletin, 93,* 203–231.

Albarracin, D., Johnson, B. T., & Zanna, M. P. (Eds.). (2005). *The handbook of attitudes and attitude change.* Hillsdale, NJ: Erlbaum.

Albright, L., Kenny, D. A., & Malloy, T. E. (1988). Consensus in personality judgments at zero acquaintance, *Journal of Personality and Social Psychology, 55*(3), 387–395.

Alicke, M. D. (1985). Global self-evaluation as determined by the desirability and controllability of trait adjectives. *Journal of Personality and Social Psychology, 49*(6), 1621–1630.

Alicke, M. D. (2000). Culpable control and the psychology of blame. *Psychological Bulletin, 126,* 556–574.

Alicke, M. D., Klotz, M. L., Breitenbecher, D. L., Yurak, T. J., & Vredenburg, D. S. (1995). Personal contact, individuation, and the better-than-average effect. *Journal of Personality and Social Psychology, 68*(5), 804–825.

Allen, T. J., Sherman, J. W., Conrey, F. R., & Stroessner, S. J. (2009). Stereotype strength and attentional bias: Preference for confirming versus disconfirming information depends on processing capacity. *Journal of Experimental Social Psychology, 45*(5), 1081–1087.

Allen, T. J., Sherman, J. W., & Klauer, K. C. (2010). Social context and the self-regulation of implicit bias. *Group Processes and Intergroup Relations, 13*(2), 137–149.

Allison, S. T., & Messick, D. M. (1988). The feature-positive effect, attitude strength, and degree of perceived consensus. *Personality and Social Psychology Bulletin, 14*(2), 231–241.

Allport, F. H., & Lepkin, M. (1945). Wartime rumors of waste and special privilege: Why some people believe them. *Journal of Abnormal and Social Psychology, 40*(1), 3–36.

Allport, G. W. (1937). *Personality: A psychological interpretation.* New York: Holt.

Allport, G. W. (1954). *The nature of prejudice.* Reading, MA: Addison-Wesley.

Allport, G. W., & Postman, L. (1947). *The psychology of rumor.* New York: Henry Holt.

Alves, H., Koch, A., & Unkelbach, C. (2017). The "common good" phenomenon: Why similarities are positive and differences are negative. *Journal of Experimental Psychology: General, 146*(4), 512–528.

Ambady, N., Hallahan, M., & Conner, B. (1999). Accuracy of judgments of sexual orientation from thin slices of behavior. *Journal of Personality and Social Psychology, 77*(3), 538–547.

Ambady, N., & Rosenthal, R. (1992). Thin slices of expressive behavior as predictors of interpersonal consequences: A meta-analysis. *Psychological Bulletin, 111*(2), 256–274.

Ambady, N., & Rosenthal, R. (1993). Half a minute: Predicting teacher evaluations from thin slices of nonverbal behavior and physical attractiveness. *Journal of Personality and Social Psychology, 64*(3), 431–441.

Amodio, D. M. (2009). Intergroup anxiety effects on the control of racial stereotypes: A psychoneuroendocrine analysis. *Journal of Experimental Social Psychology, 45*(1), 60–67.

Amodio, D. M. (2019). Social Cognition 2.0: An interactive memory systems account. *Trends in Cognitive Science, 23*(1), 21–33.

Amodio, D. M., & Devine, P. G. (2006). Stereotyping and evaluation in implicit race bias: Evidence for independent constructs and unique effects on behavior. *Journal of Personality and Social Psychology, 91*(4), 652–661.

Amodio, D. M., Devine, P. G., & Harmon-Jones, E. (2008). Individual differences in the regulation of intergroup bias: The role of conflict monitoring and neural signals for control. *Journal of Personality and Social Psychology, 94*(1), 60–74.

Amodio, D. M., Harmon-Jones, E., & Devine, P. G. (2003). Individual differences in the activation and control of affective race bias as assessed by startle eyeblink response and self-report. *Journal of Personality and Social Psychology, 84*(4), 738–753.

Amodio, D. M., Harmon-Jones, E., Devine, P. G., Curtin, J. J., Hartley, S. L., & Covert, A. E. (2004). Neural signals for the detection of unintentional race bias. *Psychological Science, 15*(2), 88–93.

Amodio, D. M., & Ratner, K. G. (2011). A memory systems model of implicit social cognition. *Current Directions in Psychological Science, 20*, 143–148.

Amodio, D. M., & Swencionis, J. K. (2018). Proactive control of implicit bias: A theoretical model and implications for behavior change. *Journal of Personality and Social Psychology, 115*(2), 255–275.

Andersen, S. M., & Cole, S. W. (1990). Do I know you? The role of significant others in general social perception. *Journal of Personality and Social Psychology, 59*, 384–399.

Andersen, S. M., Glassman, N. S., & Gold, D. A. (1998). Mental representations of the self, significant others, and nonsignificant others: Structure and processing of private and public aspects. *Journal of Personality and Social Psychology, 75*(4), 845–861.

Andersen, S. M., & Klatzky, R. L. (1987). Traits and social stereotypes: Levels of categorization in person perception. *Journal of Personality and Social Psychology, 53*, 235–246.

Anderson, C. A., & Deuser, W. E. (1993). The primacy of control in causal thinking and attributional style: An attributional functionalism perspective. In G. Weary, F. Gleicher, & K. L. Marsh (Eds.), *Control motivation and social cognition* (pp. 94–121). New York: Springer-Verlag.

Anderson, C. A., Horowitz, L. M., & French,

R. (1983). Attributional style of lonely and depressed people. *Journal of Personality and Social Psychology, 45,* 127–136.

Anderson, C. A., & Sedikides, C. (1991). Thinking about people: Contributions of a typological alternative to associationistic and dimensional models of person perception. *Journal of Personality and Social Psychology, 60,* 203–217.

Anderson, J. R., & Bower, G. H. (1973). *Human associative memory.* Oxford, UK: Routledge.

Anderson, N. H. (1965a). Adding versus averaging as a stimulus combination rule in impression formation. *Journal of Experimental Psychology, 70,* 394–400.

Anderson, N. H. (1965b). Primacy effects in personality impression formation using a generalized order effect paradigm. *Journal of Personality and Social Psychology, 2,* 1–9.

Ansfield, M. E., & Wegner, D. M. (1996). The feeling of doing. In P. M. Gollwitzer & J. A. Bargh (Eds.), *The psychology of action: Linking cognition and motivation to behavior* (pp. 482–506). New York: Guilford Press.

Arndt, A., & Henderson, M. (2022). O brother, O sister, who art thou? Inferring the gender of others in ambiguous situations. In E. Balcetis & G. B. Moskowitz (Eds.), *Handbook of impression formation: A social psychological approach* (pp. 54–72). New York: Routledge.

Arndt, J., Greenberg, J., Pyszczynski, T., Solomon, S., & Simon, L. (1997). Suppression, accessibility of death related thoughts, and cultural worldview defense: Exploring the psychodynamics of terror management. *Journal of Personality and Social Psychology, 73,* 5–18.

Aron, A., Aron, E. N., Tudor, M., & Nelson, G. (1991). Close relationships as including other in the self. *Journal of Personality and Social Psychology, 60*(2), 241–253.

Aronson, E. (1968). The theory of cognitive dissonance: A current perspective. In L. Berkowitz (Ed.), *Advances in experimental social psychology* (Vol. 4, pp. 1–34). New York: Academic Press.

Aronson, E. (1988). *The social animal.* Oxford, UK: Freeman.

Asch, S. E. (1946). Forming impressions of personality. *Journal of Abnormal and Social Psychology, 41,* 258–290.

Asch, S. E. (1948). The doctrine of suggestion, prestige and imitation in social psychology. *Psychological Review, 55*(5), 250–276.

Asch, S. E. (1952). *Social psychology.* New York: Prentice-Hall.

Asch, S. E., & Zukier, H. (1984). Thinking about persons. *Journal of Personality and Social Psychology, 46,* 1230–1240.

Ashburn-Nardo, L., Voils, C. I., & Monteith, M. J. (2001). Implicit associations as the seeds of intergroup bias: How easily do they take root? *Journal of Personality and Social Psychology, 81*(5), 789–799.

Ashby, F. G., Alfonso-Reese, L. A., Turken, A. U., & Waldron, E. M. (1998). A neuropsychological theory of multiple systems in category learning. *Psychological Review, 105*(3), 442–481.

Ashby, F. G., & Valentin, V. V. (2005). Multiple systems of perceptual category learning: Theory and cognitive tests. In H. Cohen & C. Lefebvre (Eds.), *Handbook of categorization in cognitive science* (pp. 547–572). Berkeley, CA: Elsevier Science.

Ashby, F. G., & Waldron, E. M. (1999). On the nature of implicit categorization. *Psychonomic Bulletin & Review, 6*(3), 363–378.

Ashmore, R. D., & Del Boca, F. K. (1981). Conceptual approaches to stereotypes and stereotyping. In D. L. Hamilton (Ed.), *Cognitive processes in stereotyping and intergroup behavior* (pp. 1–35). Hillsdale, NJ: Erlbaum.

Atkinson, J. W. (1964). *An introduction to motivation.* Princeton, NJ: Van Nostrand.

Avnet, T., & Higgins, E. T. (2003). Locomotion, assessment, and regulatory fit: Value transfer from "how" to "what." *Journal of Experimental Social Psychology, 39*(5), 525–530.

Axt, J. R., Casola, G. M., & Nosek, B. A. (2018). Reducing social judgment biases may require identifying the potential source of bias. *Personality and Social Psychology Bulletin, 45*(8), 1232–1251.

Badea, C., Brauer, M., & Rubin, M. (2012). The effects of winning and losing on perceived group variability. *Journal of Experimental Social Psychology, 48*(5), 1094–1099.

Bago, B., Rand, D. G., & Pennycook, G. (2020). Fake news, fast and slow: Deliberation reduces belief in false (but not true) news headlines. *Journal of Experimental Psychology: General, 149*(8), 1608–1613.

Baker, S. M., & Petty, R. E. (1994). Majority and minority influence: Source–position imbalance as a determinant of message scrutiny. *Journal of Personality and Social Psychology, 67,* 5–19.

Balcetis, E., & Dunning, D. (2006). See what you want to see: Motivational influences on visual perception. *Journal of Personality and Social Psychology, 91*(4), 612–625.

Balcetis, E., & Dunning, D. (2007). Cognitive dissonance and the perception of natural environments. *Psychological Science, 18*(10), 917–921.

Balcetis, E., & Dunning, D. (2010). Wishful seeing: Motivational influences on visual perception of the physical environment. In E. Balcetis & G. D. Lassiter (Eds.), *Social psychology of visual perception* (pp. 77–101). London: Psychology Press.

Balcetis, E., Dunning, D., & Granot, Y. (2012). Subjective value determines initial dominance in binocular rivalry. *Journal of Experimental Social Psychology, 48*(1), 122–129.

Baldwin, M. W. (1992). Relational schemas and the processing of information. *Psychological Bulletin, 112*, 461–484.

Baldwin, M. W., Carrell, S. E., & Lopez, D. F. (1990). Priming relationship schemas: My advisor and the Pope are watching me from the back of my mind. *Journal of Experimental Social Psychology, 26*, 435–454.

Ballew, C. C., & Todorov, A. (2007). Predicting political elections from rapid and unreflective face judgments. *Proceedings of the National Academy of Sciences, 104*, 17948–17953.

Banaji, M. R., & Greenwald, A. G. (1995). Implicit gender stereotyping in judgments of fame. *Journal of Personality and Social Psychology, 68*, 181–198.

Banaji, M. R., & Greenwald, A. G. (2013). *Blindspot: Hidden biases of good people.* New York: Delacorte Press.

Banaji, M. R., Hardin, C. D., & Rothman, A. J. (1993). Implicit stereotyping in person judgment. *Journal of Personality and Social Psychology, 65*, 272–281.

Bandura, A. (1989). Self-regulation of motivation and action through internal standards and goal systems. In L. A. Pervin (Ed.), *Goal concepts in personality and social psychology* (pp. 19–85). Hillsdale, NJ: Erlbaum.

Barberá, P., Jost, J. T., Nagler, J., Tucker, J. A., & Bonneau, R. (2015). Tweeting from left to right: Is online political communication more than an echo chamber? *Psychological Science, 26*(10), 1531–1542.

Bargh, J. A. (1982). Attention and automaticity in the processing of self-relevant information. *Journal of Personality and Social Psychology, 43*, 425–436.

Bargh, J. A. (1984). Automatic and conscious processing of social information. In R. S. Wyer & T. K. Srull (Eds.), *Handbook of social cognition* (Vol. 3, pp. 1–44). Hillsdale, NJ: Erlbaum.

Bargh, J. A. (1989). Conditional automaticity: Varieties of automatic influence in social perception and cognition. In J. S. Uleman & J. A. Bargh (Eds.), *Unintended thought* (pp. 3–51). New York: Guilford Press.

Bargh, J. A. (1990). Auto-motives: Preconscious determinants of social interaction. In E. T. Higgins & R. M. Sorrentino (Eds.), *Handbook of motivation and cognition: Foundations of social behavior* (Vol. 2, pp. 93–130). New York: Guilford Press.

Bargh, J. A. (1992). Does subliminality matter to social psychology? Awareness of the stimulus versus awareness of its influence. In R. F. Bornstein & T. S. Pittman (Eds.), *Perception without awareness* (pp. 236–255). New York: Guilford Press.

Bargh, J. A. (1994). The four horseman of automaticity: Awareness, intention, efficiency, and control in social cognition. In R. S. Wyer, Jr., & T. K. Srull (Eds.), *Handbook of social cognition* (2nd ed., pp. 1–40). Hillsdale, NJ: Erlbaum.

Bargh, J. A. (1997). The automaticity of everyday life. In R. S. Wyer, Jr. (Ed.), *Advances in social cognition* (Vol. 10, pp. 1–62). Hillsdale, NJ: Erlbaum.

Bargh, J. A. (2017). *Before you know it: The unconscious reasons we do what we do.* New York: Touchstone.

Bargh, J. A., & Barndollar, K. (1996). Automaticity in action: The unconscious as repository of chronic goals and motives. In P. M. Gollwitzer & J. A. Bargh (Eds.), *The psychology of action: Linking cognition and motivation to action* (pp. 457–481). New York: Guilford Press.

Bargh, J. A., Bond, R. N., Lombardi, W. J., & Tota, M. E. (1986). The additive nature of chronic and temporary sources of construct accessibility. *Journal of Personality and Social Psychology, 50*, 869–878.

Bargh, J. A., Chaiken, S., Govender, R., & Pratto, F. (1992). The generality of the automatic attitude activation effect. *Journal of Personality and Social Psychology, 62*, 893–912.

Bargh, J. A., Chen, M., & Burrows, L. (1996). Automaticity of social behavior: Direct effects of trait construct and stereotype activation on action. *Journal of Personality and Social Psychology, 71*, 230–244.

Bargh, J. A., & Gollwitzer, P. M. (1994). Environmental control of goal-directed action: Automatic and strategic contingencies between situations and behavior. In W. D. Spaulding (Ed.), *Integrative views of motivation, cognition, and emotion* (pp. 71–124). Lincoln: University of Nebraska Press.

Bargh, J. A., Gollwitzer, P. M., Lee-Chai, A., Barndollar, K., & Troetschel, R. (2001). The automated will: Nonconscious activation and pursuit of behavioral goals. *Journal of Personality and Social Psychology, 81*, 1014–1027.

Bargh, J. A., Lombardi, W. J., & Higgins, E. T. (1988). Automaticity of chronically accessible constructs in person × situation effects on person perception: It's just a matter of time. *Journal of Personality and Social Psychology, 55*, 599–605.

Bargh, J. A., & Pietromonaco, P. (1982). Automatic information processing and social perceptions: The influence of trait information presented outside of conscious awareness on impression formation. *Journal of Personality and Social Psychology, 43*, 437–444.

Bargh, J. A., & Pratto, F. (1986). Individual construct accessibility and perceptual selection. *Journal of Experimental Social Psychology, 22*, 293–311.

Bargh, J. A., & Shalev, I. (2012). The substitutability of physical and social warmth in daily life. *Emotion, 12*(1), 154–162.

Bargh, J. A., & Thein, R. D. (1985). Individual construct accessibility, person memory, and the recall-judgment link: The case of information overload. *Journal of Personality and Social Psychology, 49*, 1129–1146.

Bargh, J. A., & Tota, M. E. (1988). Context-dependent processing in depression: Accessibility of negative constructs with regard to self but not others. *Journal of Personality and Social Psychology, 54*, 924–939.

Barreto, M., & Ellemers, N. (2003). The effects of being categorised: The interplay between internal and external social identities. In W. Stroebe & M. Hewstone (Eds.), *European review of social psychology* (Vol. 14, pp. 139–170). Hove, UK: Psychology Press/Taylor & Francis.

Barsalou, L. (2010). Grounded cognition: Past, present, and future. *Topics in Cognitive Science, 2*, 716–724.

Barsalou, L. W., & Medin, D. L. (1986). Concepts: Static definitions or context-dependent representations? *Cahiers de Psychologie: Context and Cognition, 6*(2), 187–202.

Bartlett, F. (1932). *Remembering.* Cambridge, UK: Cambridge University Press.

Bart-Plange, D.-J. (2022). *On the psychology of gendered colorism.* Unpublished thesis, University of Virginia, Graduate School of Arts and Sciences, Charlottesville, VA.

Bart-Plange, D.-J., & Trawalter, S. (2024). *Gendered colorism: Evidence from social categorization studies.* Princeton, NJ: Princeton University Press.

Bart-Plange, D.-J., Trawalter, S., & Pearce, L. (2024). *Gendered colorism: Evidence from trait attributions.* Princeton, NJ: Princeton University Press.

Bassili, J. N. (1989). Trait encoding in behavior identification and dispositional inference. *Personality and Social Psychology Bulletin, 15*(3), 285–296.

Baumeister, R. F., Bratslavsky, E., Finkenauer, C., & Vohs, K. D. (2001). Bad is stronger than good. *Review of General Psychology, 5*(4), 323–370.

Baumeister, R. F., Bratslavsky, E., Muraven, M., & Tice, D. M. (1998). Ego depletion: Is the active self a limited resource? *Journal of Personality and Social Psychology, 74*(5), 1252–1265.

Baumeister, R. F., & Leary, M. R. (1995). The need to belong: Desire for interpersonal attachments as a fundamental human motivation. *Psychological Bulletin, 117*, 497–529.

Baumeister, R. F., & Steinhilber, A. (1984). Paradoxical effects of supportive audiences on performance under pressure: The home field disadvantage in sports championships. *Journal of Personality and Social Psychology, 47*(1), 85–93.

Bean, M. G., Slaten, D. G., Horton, W. S., Murphy, M. C., Todd, A. R., & Richeson, J. A. (2012). Prejudice concerns and race-based attentional bias: New evidence from eyetracking. *Social Psychological and Personality Science, 3*(6), 722–729.

Bean, M. G., Stone, J., Badger, T. A., Focella, E. S., & Moskowitz, G. B. (2013). Evidence of nonconscious stereotyping of Hispanic patients by nursing and medical students. *Nursing Research, 62*(5), 362–367.

Beck, A. T. (1976). *Cognitive therapy and the emotional disorders.* New York: International Universities Press.

Begg, I. M., Anas, A., & Farinacci, S. (1992). Dissociation of processes in belief: Source recollection, statement familiarity, and the illusion of truth. *Journal of Experimental Psychology: General, 121*(4), 446–458.

Begg, I., Armour, V., & Kerr, T. (1985). On believing what we remember. *Canadian Journal of Behavioral Science, 23,* 195–213.

Bempechat, J., London, P., & Dweck, C. S. (1991). Children's conceptions of ability in major domains: An interview and experimental study. *Child Study Journal, 21*(1), 11–36.

Berglas, S., & Jones, E. E. (1978). Drug choice as a self-handicapping strategy in response to noncontingent success. *Journal of Personality and Social Psychology, 36,* 405–417.

Bergsieker, H. B., Shelton, J. N., & Richeson, J. A. (2010). To be liked versus respected: Divergent goals in interracial interactions. *Journal of Personality and Social Psychology, 99*(2), 248–264.

Bernstein, M. J., Young, S. G., & Hugenberg, K. (2007). The cross-category effect—Mere social categorization is sufficient to elicit an own-group bias in face recognition. *Psychological Science, 18*(8), 706–712.

Bezjak, S., Clyburne-Sherin, A., Conzett, P., Fernandes, P., Görögh, E., Helbig, K., et al. (2018). *Open science training handbook.* Retrieved from *https://book.fosteropenscience.eu.*

Bhatia, N., & Bhatia, S. (2021). Changes in gender stereotypes over time: A computational analysis. *Psychology of Women Quarterly, 45*(1), 106–125.

Bhatia, S. (2017). The semantic representation of prejudice and stereotypes. *Cognition, 164,* 46–60.

Biernat, M., & Kobrynowicz, D. (1997). Gender- and race-based standards of competence: Lower minimum standards but higher ability standards for devalued groups. *Journal of Personality and Social Psychology, 72*(3), 544–557.

Biernat, M., & Manis, M. (1994). Shifting standards and stereotype-based judgments. *Journal of Personality and Social Psychology, 66,* 5–20.

Biernat, M., Manis, M., & Nelson, T. E. (1991). Stereotypes and standards of judgment. *Journal of Personality and Social Psychology, 60,* 485–499.

Biernat, M., & Thompson, E. R. (2002). Shifting standards and contextual variation in stereotyping. *European Review of Social Psychology, 12,* 103–137.

Bivens, R., & Haimson, O. L. (2016). Baking gender into social media design: How platforms shape categories for users and advertisers. *Social Media + Society, 2*(4).

Blair, I. (2001). Implicit stereotypes and prejudice. In G. B. Moskowitz (Ed.), *Cognitive social psychology: The Princeton symposium on the legacy and future of social cognition* (pp. 359–374). Mahwah, NJ: Erlbaum.

Blair, I. V., & Banaji, M. R. (1996). Automatic and controlled processes in stereotype priming. *Journal of Personality and Social Psychology, 70,* 1142–1163.

Blair, I. V., Chapleau, K. M., & Judd, C. M. (2005). The use of Afrocentric features as cues for judgment in the presence of diagnostic information. *European Journal of Social Psychology, 35,* 59–68.

Blair, I. V., Havranek, E. P., Price, D. W., Hanratty, R., Fairclough, D. L., Farley, T., et al. (2013). Assessment of biases against Latinos and African Americans among primary care providers and community members. *American Journal of Public Health, 103*(1), 92–98.

Blair, I. V., Judd, C. M., & Chapleau, K. M. (2004). The influence of Afrocentric facial features in criminal sentencing. *Psychological Science, 15,* 674–679.

Blair, I. V., Judd, C. M., Sadler, M. S., & Jenkins, C. (2002). The role of Afrocentric facial features in person perception: Judging by features and categories. *Journal of Personality and Social Psychology, 83,* 5–25.

Blair, I. V., Ma, J. E., & Lenton, A. P. (2001). Imagining stereotypes away: The moderation of implicit stereotypes through mental imagery. *Journal of Personality and Social Psychology, 81*(5), 828–841.

Blair, I. V., Steiner, J. F., Fairclough, D. L., Hanratty, R., Price, D. W., Hirsh, H. K., et al. (2013). Clinicians' implicit ethnic/racial bias and perceptions of care among Black and Latino patients. *Annals of Family Medicine, 11*(1), 43–52.

Blascovich, J., Mendes, W. B., Hunter, S. B., Lickel, B., & Kowai-Bell, N. (2001). Perceiver threat in social interactions with stigmatized others. *Journal of Personality and Social Psychology, 80*(2), 253–267.

Block, J., & Block, J. (1951). An investigation of the relationship between intolerance of ambiguity and ethnocentrism. *Journal of Personality, 19*(3), 303–311.

Bobo, L., Kluegel, J. R., & Smith, R. A. (1997). Laissez-faire racism: The crystallization of a kinder, gentler antiblack ideology. In S. A. Tuch & J. K. Martin (Eds.), *Racial attitudes in the 1990s: Continuity and change* (pp. 15–44). Westport, CT: Praeger.

Bodenhausen, G. V., & Lichtenstein, M. (1987). Social stereotypes and information-processing strategies: The impact of task complexity. *Journal of Personality and Social Psychology, 52*(5), 871–880.

Bodenhausen, G. V., & Wyer, R. S. (1985). Effects of stereotypes on decision making and information-processing strategies. *Journal of Personality and Social Psychology, 48,* 267–282.

Bohner, G., Erb, H. P., Reinhard, M. A., & Frank, E. (1996). Distinctiveness across topics in minority and majority influence: An attributional analysis and preliminary data. *British Journal of Social Psychology, 35*(1), 27–46.

Bohnet, I. (2016). *What works: Gender equality by design.* Cambridge, MA: Belknap Press/Harvard University Press.

Boldry, J. G., & Gaertner, L. (2006). Separating status from power as an antecedent of intergroup perception. *Group Processes and Intergroup Relations, 9*(3), 377–400.

Bonam, C., Taylor V. J., & Yantis, C. (2017). Racialized physical space as cultural product. *Social and Personality Psychology Compass, 11*(9), 1–12.

Bonam, C., Yantis, C., & Taylor, V. J. (2020). Invisible middle-class Black space: Asymmetrical person and space stereotyping at the race-class nexus. *Group Processes and Intergroup Relations, 23*(1), 24–47.

Borgida, E., & Howard-Pitney, B. (1983). Personal involvement and the robustness of perceptual salience effects. *Journal of Personality and Social Psychology, 45,* 560–570.

Boring, E. G. (1953). A history of introspection. *Psychological Bulletin, 50,* 169–189.

Boucher, K. L., & Rydell, R. J. (2012). Impact of negation salience and cognitive resources on negation during attitude formation. *Personality and Social Psychology Bulletin, 38*(10), 1329–1342.

Bouie, J. (2014, November 26). "Michael Brown wasn't a superhuman demon: But Darren Wilson's racial prejudice told him otherwise." *Slate, News and Politics Section.*

Bousfield, W. A. (1953). The occurrence of clustering in the recall of randomly arranged associates. *Journal of General Psychology, 49,* 229–240.

Bradley, G. W. (1978). Self-serving biases in the attribution process: A reexamination of the fact or fiction question. *Journal of Personality and Social Psychology, 36*(1), 56–71.

Brambilla, M., Carraro, L., Castelli, L., & Sacchi, S. (2019). Changing impressions: Moral character dominates impression updating. *Journal of Experimental Social Psychology, 82,* 64–73.

Brambilla, M., & Leach, C. W. (2014). On the importance of being moral: The distinctive role of morality in social judgment. *Social Cognition, 32*(4), 397–408.

Brandone, A. C., Horwitz, S. R., Aslin, R. N., & Wellman, H. M. (2014). Infants' goal anticipation during failed and successful reaching actions. *Developmental Science, 17*(1), 23–34.

Brandone, A. C., & Wellman, H. M. (2009). You can't always get what you want: Infants understand failed goal-directed actions. *Psychological Science, 20*(1), 85–91.

Brannon, S. M., & Gawronski, B. (2017). A second chance for first impressions? Exploring the context-(in)dependent updating of implicit evaluations. *Social Psychological and Personality Science, 8*(3), 275–283.

Branscombe, N. R., Ellemers, N., Spears, R., & Doosje, B. (1999). The context and content of social identity threats. In N. Ellemers, R. Spears, & B. Doosje (Eds.), *Social identity: Context, commitment, content* (pp. 35–58). Oxford, UK: Blackwell.

Bray, J. R., Armenta, A. D., & Zarate, M. A. (2023). Memory consolidation: The cornerstone for gauging spontaneous impression longevity. In E. Balcetis & G. B. Moskowitz (Eds.), *Handbook of impression formation: A social psychological approach* (pp. 416–434). New York: Routledge.

Brescoll, V. L. (2011). Who takes the floor and why: Gender, power, and volubility in organizations. *Administrative Science Quarterly, 56*(4), 622–641.

Brewer, M. B. (1988). A dual process model of impression formation. In T. K. Srull & R. S. Wyer (Eds.), *Advances in social cognition* (Vol. 1, pp. 1–36). Hillsdale, NJ: Erlbaum.

Brewer, M. B. (1991). The social self: On being

the same and different at the same time. *Personality and Social Psychology Bulletin, 17,* 475–482.

Brewer, M. B. (1999). The psychology of prejudice: Ingroup love and outgroup hate? *Journal of Social Issues, 55,* 429–444.

Brewer, M. B., & Gardner, W. (1996). Who is this "we"? Levels of collective identity and self-representations. *Journal of Personality and Social Psychology, 71*(1), 83–93.

Brewer, M. B., & Kramer, R. M. (1986). Choice behavior in social dilemmas: Effects of social identity, group size, and decision framing. *Journal of Personality and Social Psychology, 50*(3), 543–549.

Brigham, J. C., & Malpass, R. S. (1985). The role of experience and contact in the recognition of faces of own- and other-race persons. *Journal of Social Issues, 41*(3), 139–155.

Brinkman, L., Todorov, A., & Dotsch, R. (2017). Visualising mental representations: A primer on noise-based reverse correlation in social psychology. *European Review of Social Psychology, 28*(1), 333–361.

Brock, T. C., & Balloun, J. L. (1967). Behavioral receptivity to dissonant information. *Journal of Personality and Social Psychology, 6*(4, Pt.1), 413–428.

Brown, R., & McNeill, D. (1966). The "tip of the tongue" phenomenon. *Journal of Verbal Learning and Verbal Behavior 5,* 325–337.

Brown, T. I., Uncapher, M. R., Chow, T. E., Eberhardt, J. L., & Wagner, A. D. (2017). Cognitive control, attention, and the other race effect in memory. *PLOS One, 12*(3), e0173579.

Bruner, J. S. (1957). On perceptual readiness. *Psychological Review, 64,* 123–152.

Bruner, J. S., & Goodman, C. D. (1947). Value and need as organizing factors in perception. *Journal of Abnormal Social Psychology, 42,* 33–44.

Bruner, J. S., Goodnow, J. G., & Austin, G. A. (1956). *A study of thinking.* New York: Wiley.

Bruner, J. S., & Postman, L. (1948). Symbolic value as an organizing factor in perception. *Journal of Social Psychology, 27,* 203–208.

Bruner, J. S., & Tagiuri, R. (1954). The perception of people. In G. Lindzey (Ed.), *Handbook of social psychology* (Vol. 2, pp. 634–654). Reading, MA: Addison-Wesley.

Bullock, J. G., & Lenz, G. (2019). Partisan bias in surveys. *Annual Review of Political Science, 22,* 325–342.

Burke, C. T. (2015). Process dissociation models in racial bias research: Updating the analytic method and integrating with signal detection approaches. *Group Processes and Intergroup Relations, 18*(3), 402–434.

Burns, M. D., Monteith, M. J., & Parker, L. R. (2017). Training away bias: The differential effects of counterstereotype training and self-regulation on stereotype activation and application. *Journal of Experimental Social Psychology, 73,* 97–110.

Buzsáki, G. (2006). *Rhythms of the brain.* New York: Oxford University Press.

Byrne, S., & Hart, P. (2009). The boomerang effect: A synthesis of findings and a preliminary theoretical framework. *Annals of the International Communication Association, 33,* 3–37.

Cacioppo, J. T., Hawkley, L. C., Crawford, L. E., Ernst, J. M., Burleson, M. H., Kowalewski, R. B., et al. (2002). Loneliness and health: Potential mechanisms. *Psychosomatic Medicine, 64*(3), 407–417.

Cacioppo, J. T., & Petty, R. E. (1982). The need for cognition. *Journal of Personality and Social Psychology, 42,* 116–131.

Calanchini, J., Gonsalkorale, K., Sherman, J., & Klauer, K. (2013). Counter-prejudicial training reduces activation of biased associations and enhances response monitoring. *European Journal of Social Psychology, 43,* 321–325.

Calanchini, J., & Sherman, J. W. (2013). Implicit attitudes reflect associative, non-associative, and non-attitudinal processes. *Social and Personality Psychology Compass, 7*(9), 654–667.

Call, J., & Tomasello, M. (2008). Does the chimpanzee have a theory of mind? 30 years later. *Trends in Cognitive Science, 12*(5), 187–192.

Cameron, C. D., Payne, B. K., & Knobe, J. (2010). Do theories of implicit race bias change moral judgments? *Social Justice Research, 23,* 272–289.

Campbell, D. T. (1963). Social attitudes and other acquired behavioral dispositions. In S. Koch (Ed.), *Psychology: A study of a science. Study II. Empirical substructure and relations with other sciences. Vol. 6. Investigations of man as socius: Their place in psychology and the social sciences* (pp. 94–172). New York: McGraw-Hill.

Campbell, M. R., & Brauer, M. (2021). Is discrimination widespread? Testing assumptions about bias on a university campus. *Journal of Experimental Psychology: General, 150*(4), 756–777.

Campbell, W. K., & Sedikides, C. (1999). Self-threat magnifies the self-serving bias: A meta-analytic integration. *Review of General Psychology, 3,* 23–43.

Cantor, N., & Fleeson, W. (1991). Life tasks and self-regulatory processes. In M. Maehr & P. Pintrich (Eds.), *Advances in motivation and achievement* (Vol. 7, pp. 327–369). Greenwich, CT: JAI Press.

Cantor, N., & Fleeson, W. (1994). Social intelligence and intelligent goal pursuit: A cognitive slice of motivation. In W. D. Spaulding (Ed.), *Integrative views of motivation, cognition, and emotion* (pp. 125–179). Lincoln, NE: University of Nebraska Press.

Cantor, N., & Kihlstrom, J. F. (1987). *Personality and social intelligence.* Englewood Cliffs, NJ: Prentice-Hall.

Cantor, N., & Mischel, W. (1977). Traits as prototypes: Effects on recognition memory. *Journal of Personality and Social Psychology, 35,* 38–48.

Cantor, N., & Mischel, W. (1979). Prototypes in person perception. In L. Berkowitz (Ed.), *Advances in experimental social psychology* (Vol. 12, pp. 3–52). New York: Academic Press.

Carli, L. L. (2001). Gender and social influence. *Journal of Social Issues, 57*(4), 725–741.

Carli, L. L., & Eagly, A. H. (2007). Overcoming resistance to women leaders: The importance of leadership style. In B. Kellerman & D. L. Rhode (Eds.), *Women and leadership: The state of play and strategies for change* (pp. 127–148). San Francisco: Jossey-Bass.

Carli, L. L., & Leonard, J. B. (1989). The effect of hindsight on victim derogation. *Journal of Social and Clinical Psychology, 8*(3), 331–343.

Carlston, D. E. (1980). The recall and use of traits and events in social inference processes. *Journal of Experimental Social Psychology, 16,* 303–328.

Carlston, D. E., & Skowronski, J. J. (1994). Savings in the relearning of trait information as evidence for spontaneous inference generation. *Journal of Personality and Social Psychology, 66,* 840–856.

Carlston, D. E., & Skowronski, J. J. (1995). Savings in relearning: II. On the formation of behavior-based trait associations and inferences. *Journal of Personality and Social Psychology, 69*(3), 429–436.

Carlston, D. E., & Skowronski, J. J. (2005). Linking versus thinking: Evidence for the different associative and attributional bases of spontaneous trait transference and spontaneous trait inference. *Journal of Personality and Social Psychology, 89*(6), 884–898.

Carney, D., Cuddy, A., & Yap, A. (2010). Power posing: Brief nonverbal displays affect neuroendocrine levels and risk tolerance. *Psychological Science, 21,* 1363–1368.

Carpenter, M., Akhtar, N., & Tomasello, M. (1998). Fourteen- through 18-month-old infants differentially imitate intentional and accidental actions. *Infant Behavior & Development, 21*(2), 315–330.

Carpenter, W. G. (1884). *Principles of mental physiology, with their applications to the training and discipline of the mind and study of its morbid conditions.* New York: Appleton.

Carter, E. R., Onyeador, I. N., & Lewis, N. A. (2020). Developing & delivering effective anti-bias training: Challenges and recommendations. *Behavioral Science and Policy, 6*(1), 57–70.

Carver, C. S., & Scheier, M. F. (1978). Self-focusing effects of dispositional self-consciousness, mirror presence, and audience presence. *Journal of Personality and Social Psychology, 36,* 324–332.

Carver, C. S., & Scheier, M. F. (1981). *Attention and self-regulation: A control theory approach to human behavior.* New York: Springer.

Carver, C. S., & Scheier, M. F. (1982). Outcome expectancy, locus of attribution for expectancy, and self-directed attention as determinants of evaluations and performance. *Journal of Experimental Social Psychology, 18,* 184–200.

Casper, C., Rothermund, K., & Wentura, D. (2010). Automatic stereotype activation is context dependent. *Social Psychology, 41*(3), 131–136.

Castano, E., & Yzerbyt, V. Y. (1998). The highs and lows of group homogeneity. *Behavioural Processes, 42*(2–3), 219–238.

Cesario, J., Grant, H., & Higgins, E. T. (2004). Regulatory fit and persuasion: Transfer from "feeling right." *Journal of Personality and Social Psychology, 86*(3), 388–404.

Cesario, J., Higgins, E., & Scholer, A. (2007). Regulatory fit and persuasion: Basic principles and remaining questions. *Social and Personality Psychology Compass, 2,* 444–463.

Cesario, J., Jonas, K. J., & Carney, D. R. (2017). Power poses: What was the point and what did we learn? *Comprehensive Results in Social Psychology, 2*(1), 1–5.

Chaiken, S. (1980). Heuristic versus systematic information processing and the use of source versus message cues in persuasion. *Journal of Personality and Social Psychology, 39,* 752–766.

Chaiken, S. (1987). The heuristic model of persuasion. In M. P. Zanna, J. M. Olson, & C. P. Herman (Eds.), *Social influence: The Ontario symposium* (Vol. 5, pp. 3–39). Hillsdale, NJ: Erlbaum.

Chaiken, S., Liberman, A., & Eagly, A. H. (1989). Heuristic and systematic information processing within and beyond the persuasion context. In J. S. Uleman & J. A. Bargh (Eds.), *Unintended thought* (pp. 212–252). New York: Guilford Press.

Chaiken, S., & Trope, Y. (Eds.). (1999). *Dual-process theories in social psychology.* New York: Guilford Press.

Chan, J. C. K., & LaPaglia, J. A. (2013). Impairing existing declarative memory in humans by disrupting reconsolidation. *Proceedings of the National Academy of Sciences of the USA, 110*(23), 9309–9313.

Chaney, K. E., Sanchez, D. T., & Remedios, J. D. (2023). Confronting first impressions: Motivating self-regulation of stereotypes and prejudice through prejudice confrontation. In E. Balcetis & G. B. Moskowitz (Eds.), *Handbook of impression formation: A social psychological approach* (pp. 435–458). New York: Routledge.

Chapman, L. J. (1967). Illusory correlation in observational report. *Journal of Verbal Learning and Verbal Behavior, 6,* 151–155.

Charlesworth, T. E. S., & Banaji, M. R. (2021). Patterns of implicit and explicit attitudes: II. Long-term change and stability, regardless of group membership. *American Psychologist, 76*(6), 851–869.

Charlesworth, T. E. S., & Banaji, M. R. (2022). Patterns of implicit and explicit attitudes: IV. Change and stability from 2007 to 2020. *Psychological Science, 33*(9), 1347–1371.

Charlesworth, T. E. S., Caliskan, A., & Banaji, M. R. (2022). Historical representations of social groups across 200 years of word embeddings from Google Books. *Proceedings of the National Academy of Sciences of the USA, 119*(28), e2121798119.

Chartrand, T. L., & Bargh, J. A. (1996). Automatic activation of impression formation goals: Nonconscious goal priming reproduces effects of explicit task instructions.

Journal of Personality and Social Psychology, 71, 464–478.

Chartrand, T. L., & Bargh, J. A. (1999). The chameleon effect: The perception–behavior link and social interaction. *Journal of Personality and Social Psychology, 76*(6), 893–910.

Chartrand, T. L., & van Baaren, R. (2009). Human mimicry. In M. P. Zanna (Ed.), *Advances in experimental social psychology* (Vol. 41, pp. 219–274). Cambridge, MA: Elsevier Academic Press.

Chase, W. G., & Simon, H. A. (1973). Perception in chess. *Cognitive Psychology, 4,* 55–81.

Chawla, P., & Krauss, R. M. (1994). Gesture and speech in spontaneous and rehearsed narratives. *Journal of Experimental Social Psychology, 30*(6), 580–601.

Chen, J. M. (2019). An integrative review of impression formation processes for multiracial individuals. *Social and Personality Psychology Compass, 13*(1), e12430.

Chen, J. M., Banerji, I., Moons, W. G., & Sherman, J. W. (2014). Spontaneous social role inferences. *Journal of Experimental Social Psychology, 55,* 146–153.

Chen, J. M., Pauker, K., Gaither, S. E., Hamilton, D. L., & Sherman, J. W. (2018). Black + White = Not White: A minority bias in categorizations of Black–White multiracials. *Journal of Experimental Social Psychology, 78,* 43–54.

Chen, J. M., Quinn, K. A., & Maddox, K. B. (2022). Bridging the gap between spontaneous behavior- and stereotype-based impressions. In E. Balcetis & G. B. Moskowitz (Eds.), *Handbook of impression formation: A social psychological approach* (pp. 93–115). New York: Routledge.

Chen, M., & Bargh, J. A. (1999). Consequences of automatic evaluation: Immediate behavioral predispositions to approach or avoid the stimulus. *Personality and Social Psychology Bulletin, 25*(2), 215–224.

Chen, S. (2001). The role of theories in mental representation and their use in social perception: A theory-based approach to significant-other representations and transference. In G. B. Moskowitz (Ed.), *Cognitive social psychology: The Princeton symposium on the legacy and future of social cognition* (pp. 125–142). Mahwah, NJ: Erlbaum.

Chen, S. (2003). Psychological-state theories about significant others: Implications for the content and structure of significant-other representations. *Personality and Social Psychology Bulletin, 29*(10), 1285–1302.

Cheng, P. W., & Novick, L. R. (1990). A probabilistic contrast model of causal induction. *Journal of Personality and Social Psychology, 58,* 545–567.

Cheng, P. W., & Novick, L. R. (1992). Covariation in natural causal induction. *Psychological Review, 99*(2), 365–382.

Chernev, A. (2004). Goal orientation and consumer preference for the status quo. *Journal of Consumer Research, 31*(3), 557–565.

Chiao, J. Y., Heck, H. E., Nakayama, K., & Ambady, N. (2006). Priming race in biracial observers affects visual search for Black and White faces. *Psychological Science, 17*(5), 387–392.

Chiu, C. Y., Hong, Y. Y., & Dweck, C. S. (1997). Lay dispositionism and implicit theories of personality. *Journal of Personality and Social Psychology, 73*(1), 19–30.

Chomsky, N., Roberts, I., & Watumull, J. (2023, March 8). "Noam Chomsky: The false promise of ChatGPT." *New York Times*, p. A19.

Chun, W. Y., Kruglanski, A. W., Sleeth-Keppler, D., & Friedman, R. S. (2011). Multifinality in implicit choice. *Journal of Personality and Social Psychology, 101*(5), 1124–1137.

Cialdini, R. B. (2007). *Influence: The psychology of persuasion*. New York: Harper Collins.

Cialdini, R. B., Borden, R. J., Thorne, A., Walker, M. R., Freeman, S., & Sloan, L. R. (1976). Basking in reflected glory: Three (football) field studies. *Journal of Personality and Social Psychology, 34,* 366–375.

Cikara, M., Botvinick, M. M., & Fiske, S. T. (2011). Us versus them: Social identity shapes neural responses to intergroup competition and harm. *Psychological Science, 22*(3), 306–313.

Cinelli, M., Morales, G. D. F., Galeazzi, A., Quattrociocchi, W., & Starnini, M. (2021). The echo chamber effect on social media. *Proceedings of the National Academy of Sciences of the USA, 118*(9), e2023301118.

Clore, G. L. (1992). Cognitive phenomenology: Feelings and the construction of judgment. In L. L. Martin & A. Tesser (Eds.), *The construction of social judgments* (pp. 133–163). Hillsdale, NJ: Erlbaum.

Clore, G. L., & Jeffrey, K. M. (1972, July). Emotional role playing, attitude change, and attraction toward a disabled person. *Journal of Personality and Social Psychology, 23*(1), 105–111.

Clore, G. L., Schwarz, N., & Conway, M. (1994). Affective causes and consequences of social information processing. In R. S. Wyer, Jr., & T. K. Srull (Eds.), *Handbook of social cognition: Basic processes* (2nd ed., Vol. 1, pp. 323–417). Hillsdale, NJ: Erlbaum.

Cohen, A. R. (1961). Cognitive tuning as a factor affecting impression formation. *Journal of Personality, 29,* 235–245.

Cole, E. R. (2009). Intersectionality and research in psychology. *American Psychologist, 64,* 170–180.

Cole, S., Balcetis, E., & Dunning, D. (2013). Affective signals of threat increase perceived proximity. *Sage Journals, 24*(1), 34–40.

Collins, A., & Loftus, E. (1975). A spreading-activation theory of semantic processing. *Psychological Review, 82,* 407–428.

Collins, A. M., & Quillian, M. R. (1969). Retrieval time from semantic memory. *Journal of Verbal Learning and Verbal Behavior, 8*(2), 240–247.

Collins, M. A., & Zebrowitz, L. A. (1995). The contributions of appearance to occupational outcomes in civilian and military settings. *Journal of Applied Social Psychology, 25*(2), 129–163.

Cone, J., & Ferguson, M. J. (2015). He did what? The role of diagnosticity in revising implicit evaluations. *Journal of Personality and Social Psychology, 108*(1), 37–57.

Cone, J., Flaharty, K., & Ferguson, M. J. (2019). Believability of evidence matters for correcting social impressions. *Proceedings of the National Academy of Sciences, 116*(20), 9802–9807.

Cone, J., Mann, T. C., & Ferguson, M. J. (2017). Changing our implicit minds: How, when, and why implicit evaluations can be rapidly revised. *Advances in Social Psychology, 56,* 131–199.

Conway, P., & Gawronski, B. (2013). Deontological and utilitarian inclinations in moral decision making: A process dissociation approach. *Journal of Personality and Social Psychology, 104,* 216–235.

Cooley, E., Lei, R. F., & Ellerkamp, T. (2018). The mixed outcomes of taking ownership for implicit racial biases. *Personality and Social Psychology Bulletin, 44,* 1424–1434.

Cooper, J., & Fazio, R. H. (1984). A new look at dissonance theory. *Advances in Experimental Social Psychology, 17*, 229–266.

Cooper, L. A., Roter, D. L., Carson, K. A., Beach, M. C., Sabin, J. A., Greenwald, A. G., et al. (2012). The associations of clinicians' implicit attitudes about race with medical visit communication and patient ratings of interpersonal care. *American Journal of Public Health, 102*(5), 979–987.

Corneille, O., & Hütter, M. (2020). Implicit? What do you mean? A comprehensive review of the delusive implicitness construct in attitude research. *Personality and Social Psychology Review, 24*(3), 212–232.

Correll, J., Hudson, S. M., Guillermo, S., & Ma, D. S. (2014). The police officer's dilemma: A decade of research on racial bias in the decision to shoot. *Social and Personality Psychology Compass, 8*, 201–213.

Correll, J., Park, B., Judd, C. M., & Wittenbrink, B. (2002). The police officer's dilemma: Using ethnicity to disambiguate potentially threatening individuals. *Journal of Personality and Social Psychology, 83*(6), 1314–1329.

Correll, J., Park, B., Judd, C. M., Wittenbrink, B., Sadler, M. S., & Keesee, T. (2007). Across the thin blue line: Police officers and racial bias in the decision to shoot. *Journal of Personality and Social Psychology, 92*(6), 1006–1023.

Correll J., Wittenbrink B., Park B., Judd C. M., & Goyle, A. (2011). Dangerous enough: Moderating racial bias with contextual threat cues. *Journal of Experimental Social Psychology, 47*, 184–189.

Cotton, J. L., & Hieser, R. A. (1980). Selective exposure to information and cognitive dissonance. *Journal of Research in Personality, 14*(4), 518–527.

Craik, F. I. M., & Lockhart, R. S. (1972). Levels of processing: A framework for memory research. *Journal of Verbal Learning and Verbal Behavior, 11*, 671–676.

Crandall, C. S., Eshleman, A., & O'Brien, L. (2002). Social norms and the expression and suppression of prejudice: The struggle for internalization. *Journal of Personality and Social Psychology, 82*(3), 359–378.

Crano, W. D., & Chen, X. (1998). The leniency contract and persistence of majority and minority influence. *Journal of Personality and Social Psychology, 74*, 1437–1450.

Crano, W. D., & Prislin, R. (2006). Attitudes and persuasion. *Annual Review of Psychology, 57*, 345–374.

Crocker, J., Hannah, D. B., & Weber, R. (1983). Person memory and causal attributions. *Journal of Personality and Social Psychology, 44*, 55–66.

Crocker, J., & Luhtanen, R. (1990). Collective self-esteem and ingroup bias. *Journal of Personality and Social Psychology, 58*(1), 60–67.

Crocker, J., & Major, B. (1989). Social stigma and self-esteem: The self-protective properties of stigma. *Psychological Review, 96*(4), 608–630.

Crocker, J., Thompson, L. L., McGraw, K. M., & Ingerman, C. (1987). Downward comparison, prejudice, and evaluations of others: Effects of self esteem and threat. *Journal of Personality and Social Psychology, 52*, 907–916.

Crocker, J., Voelkl, K., Testa, M., & Major, B. (1991). Social stigma: The affective consequences of attributional ambiguity. *Journal of Personality and Social Psychology, 60*(2), 218–228.

Crosby, F. (1984). The denial of personal discrimination. *American Behavioral Scientist, 27*(3), 371–386.

Crosby, F., Bromley, S., & Saxe, L. (1980). Recent unobtrusive studies of Black and White discrimination and prejudice: A literature review. *Psychological Bulletin, 87*, 546–563.

Crowe, E., & Higgins, E. T. (1997). Regulatory focus and strategic inclinations: Promotion and prevention in decision-making. *Organizational Behavior and Human Decision Processes, 69*(2), 117–132.

Cuddy, A. J. C., Fiske, S. T., & Glick, P. (2008). The BIAS map: Behaviors from intergroup affect and stereotypes. *Journal of Personality and Social Psychology, 92*(4), 631–648.

Cuddy, A. J. C., Schultz, S. J., & Fosse, N. E. (2018). P-curving a more comprehensive body of research on postural feedback reveals clear evidential value for power-posing effects: Reply to Simmons and Simonsohn (2017). *Psychological Science, 29*(4), 656–666.

Cunningham, W. A., & Zelazo, P. D. (2007). Attitudes and evaluations: A social cognitive neuroscience perspective. *Trends in Cognitive Sciences, 11*, 97–104.

Cunningham, W. A., Zelazo, P. D., Packer, D. J., & Van Bavel, J. J. (2007). The iterative reprocessing model: A multilevel framework for attitudes and evaluation. *Social Cognition, 25*(5), 736–760.

Czopp, A. M., Monteith, M., & Mark, A. Y. (2006). Standing up for change. Reducing bias through interpersonal confrontation. *Journal of Personality and Social Psychology, 90*(5), 784–803.

Dalton, A. N., Chartrand, T. L., & Finkel, E. J. (2010). The schema-driven chameleon: How mimicry affects executive and self-regulatory resources. *Journal of Personality and Social Psychology, 98*(4), 605–617.

Darley, J. M., & Fazio, R. H. (1980). Expectancy confirmation processes arising in the social interaction sequence. *American Psychologist, 35*, 867–881.

Darley, J. M., & Gross, P. H. (1983). A hypothesis-confirming bias in labelling effects. *Journal of Personality and Social Psychology, 44*, 20–33.

Darley, J. M., & Latane, B. (1970). *The unresponsive bystander: Why doesn't he help?* Englewood Cliffs, NJ: Prentice-Hall.

Darwin, C. (1872/1998). *The expression of emotions in man and animal.* Oxford, UK: Murray.

Dasgupta, N. (2004). Implicit ingroup favoritism, outgroup favoritism, and their behavioral manifestations. *Social Justice Research, 17*, 143–169.

Dasgupta, N. (2013). Implicit attitudes and beliefs adapt to situations: A decade of research on the malleability of implicit prejudice, stereotypes, and the self-concept. In P. Devine & A. Plant (Eds.), *Advances in experimental social psychology* (Vol. 47, pp. 233–279).

Dasgupta, N., & Asgari, S. (2004). Seeing is believing: Exposure to counterstereotypic women leaders and its effect on the malleability of automatic gender stereotyping. *Journal of Experimental Social Psychology, 40*(5), 642–658.

Dasgupta, N., & Greenwald, A. G. (2001). On the malleability of automatic attitudes: Combating automatic prejudice with images of liked and disliked individuals. *Journal of Personality and Social Psychology, 81*, 800–814.

Dasgupta, N., Greenwald, A. G., & Banaji, M. R. (2003). The first ontological challenge to the IAT: Attitude or mere familiarity? *Psychological Inquiry, 14*(3–4), 238–243.

Dasgupta, N., & Rivera, L. M. (2006). From automatic antigay prejudice to behavior: The moderating role of conscious beliefs about gender and behavioral control. *Journal of Personality and Social Psychology, 91*(2), 268–280.

Daumeyer, N., Onyeador, I., Brown, X., & Richeson, J. (2019). Consequences of attributing discrimination to implicit vs. explicit bias. *Journal of Experimental Social Psychology, 84*, e103812.

Davis, M. H., Conklin, L., Smith, A., & Luce, C. (1996). Effect of perspective taking on the cognitive representation of persons: A merging of self and other. *Journal of Personality and Social Psychology, 70*, 713–726.

De Cremer, D. (2001). Perceptions of group homogeneity as a function of the social comparison context: The mediating role of group identity. *Current Psychology, 20*, 138–146.

De Dreu, C. K. W., & De Vries, N. K. (1996). Differential processing and attitude change following majority versus minority arguments. *British Journal of Social Psychology, 35*(1), 77–90.

De Dreu, C. K. W., Nijstad, B. A., Bechtoldt, M. N., & Baas, M. (2011). Group creativity and innovation: A motivated information processing perspective. *Psychology of Aesthetics, Creativity, and the Arts, 5*(1), 81–89.

De Houwer, J. (2007). A conceptual and theoretical analysis of evaluative conditioning. *The Spanish Journal of Psychology, 10*(2), 230–241.

De Houwer, J. (2009). The propositional approach to associative learning as an alternative for association formation models. *Learning and Behavior, 37*(1), 1–20.

De Houwer, J. (2014a). Why a propositional single-process model of associative learning deserves to be defended. In J. W. Sherman, B. Gawronski, & Y. Trope (Eds.), *Dual processes in social psychology* (pp. 530–541). New York: Guilford Press.

De Houwer, J. D. (2014b). A propositional model of implicit evaluation. *Social and Personality Psychology Compass, 8*, 342–353.

De Houwer, J. (2018). Propositional models of evaluative conditioning. *Social Psychological Bulletin, 13*(3), 1–21.

De Houwer, J., & Hughes, S. (2016). Evaluative conditioning as a symbolic phenomenon: On the relation between evaluative conditioning, evaluative conditioning via instructions, and persuasion. *Social Cognition, 34*(5), 480–494.

De Soto, C. B., Hamilton, M. M., & Taylor, R. B. (1985). Words, people, and implicit personality theory. *Social Cognition, 3*(4), 369–382.

Deaux, K., & Lewis, L. (1984). Structure of gender stereotypes: Interrelations among components and gender label. *Journal of Personality and Social Psychology, 5*, 991–1004.

Deci, E. L., & Ryan, R. M. (2000). The "what"

and "why" of goal pursuits: Human needs and the self-determination of behavior. *Psychological Inquiry, 11*(4), 227–268.

DeCoster, J., Banner, M. J., Smith, E. R., & Semin, G. R. (2006). On the inexplicability of the implicit: Differences in the information provided by implicit and explicit tests. *Social Cognition, 24*(1), 5–21.

DePaulo, B. M., Kashy, D. A., Kirkendol, S. E., Wyer, M. M., & Epstein, J. A. (1996). Lying in everyday life. *Journal of Personality and Social Psychology, 70*(5), 979–995.

DePaulo, B. M., Lanier, K., & Davis, T. (1983). Detecting the deceit of the motivated liar. *Journal of Personality and Social Psychology, 45*, 1096–1103.

Derous, E., Ryan, A. M., & Serlie, A. W. (2015). Double jeopardy upon resumé screening. *Personnel Psychology, 68*(3), 659–696.

Deutsch, J. A., & Deutsch, D. (1963). Attention: Some theoretical considerations. *Psychological Review, 70*, 80–90.

Devine, P. G. (1989). Stereotypes and prejudice: Their automatic and controlled components. *Journal of Personality and Social Psychology, 56*, 5–18.

Devine, P. G., & Elliot, A. J. (1995). Are racial stereotypes really fading? The Princeton trilogy revisited. *Personality and Social Psychology Bulletin, 21*, 1139–1150.

Devine, P. G., Forscher, P. S., Austin, A. J., & Cox, W. T. L. (2012). Long-term reduction in implicit race bias: A prejudice habit-breaking intervention. *Journal of Experimental Social Psychology, 48*(6), 1267–1278.

Devine, P. G., Monteith, M. J., Zuwerink, J. R., & Elliot, A. J. (1991). Prejudice with and without compunction. *Journal of Personality and Social Psychology, 60*, 817–830.

Diehl, M. (1990). The minimal group paradigm: Theoretical explanations and empirical findings. *European Review of Social Psychology, 1*(1), 263–292.

Dijksterhuis, A., & Bargh, J. A. (2001). The perception–behavior expressway: Automatic effects of social perception on social behavior. In M. P. Zanna (Ed.), *Advances in experimental social psychology* (Vol. 33, pp. 1–40). San Diego, CA: Academic Press.

Dijksterhuis, A., Bos, M. W., Nordgren, L. F., & van Baaren, R. B. (2006). On making the right choice: The deliberation-without-attention effect. *Science, 311*(5763), 1005–1007.

Dijksterhuis, A., & Nordgren, L. F. (2006). A theory of unconscious thought. *Perspectives on Psychological Science, 1*(2), 95–109.

Dijksterhuis, A., Spears, R., Postmes, T., Stapel, D. A., Koomen, W., van Knippenberg, A., et al. (1998). Seeing one thing and doing another: Contrast effects in automatic behavior. *Journal of Personality and Social Psychology, 75*(4), 862–871.

Dijksterhuis, A., & van Knippenberg, A. (1996). The knife that cuts both ways: Facilitated and inhibited access to traits as a result of stereotype activation. *Journal of Experimental Social Psychology, 32*, 271–288.

Dijksterhuis, A., & van Knippenberg, A. (1998). The relation between perception and behavior, or how to win a game of Trivial Pursuit. *Journal of Personality and Social Psychology, 74*, 865–877.

Dik, G., & Aarts, H. (2008). I want to know what you want: How effort perception facilitates the motivation to infer another's goal. *Social Cognition, 26*(6), 737–754.

Dion, K., Berscheid, E., & Walster, E. (1972). What is beautiful is good. *Journal of Personality and Social Psychology, 24*(3), 285–290.

DiTomaso, N. (2015). Racism and discrimination versus advantage and favoritism: Bias for versus bias against. *Research in Organizational Behavior, 35*, 57–77.

Ditto, P. H., & Lopez, D. F. (1992). Motivated skepticism: Use of differential decision criteria for preferred and nonpreferred conclusions. *Journal of Personality and Social Psychology, 63*, 568–584.

Ditto, P. H., Scepansky, J. A., Munro, G. D., Apanovitch, A. M., & Lockhart, L. K. (1998). Motivated sensitivity to preference-inconsistent information. *Journal of Personality and Social Psychology, 75*, 53–69.

Dixon, A. R., & Telles, E. E. (2017). Skin color and colorism: Global research, concepts, and measurement. *Annual Review of Sociology, 43*, 405–424.

Dobbin, F., & Kalev, A. (2016). Why diversity programs fail. *Harvard Business Review, 94*(7).

Donovan, P. (2024, January 21). The economic indicator we need? A candy bar. *The New York Times*, p. 9: Section SR.

Doosje, B., Spears, R., Ellemers, N., & Koomen, W. (1999). Perceived group variability in intergroup relations: The distinctive role of social identity. *European Review of Social Psychology, 10*(1), 41–74.

Doriscar, J. E., Perry, S. P., & Gardner, W. L. (2024, February). *The psychology of white fragility experiences.* Poster presented at the Society for Personality and Social Psychology annual convention, San Diego.

Dotsch, R., Wigboldus, D. H. J., Langner, O., & van Knippenberg, A. (2008). Ethnic outgroup faces are biased in the prejudiced mind. *Psychological Science, 19*(10), 978–980.

Dovidio, J. F., Evans, N., & Tyler, R. B. (1986). Racial stereotypes: The contents of their cognitive representations. *Journal of Experimental Social Psychology, 22*, 22–37.

Dovidio, J. F., & Fiske, S. T. (2012). Under the radar: How unexamined biases in decision-making processes in clinical interactions can contribute to health care disparities. *American Journal of Public Health, 102*(5), 945–952.

Dovidio, J. F., & Gaertner, S. L. (1986). Prejudice, discrimination, and racism: Historical trends and contemporary approaches. In J. F. Dovidio & S. L. Gaertner (Eds.), *Prejudice, discrimination, and racism* (pp. 1–34). New York: Academic Press.

Dovidio, J. F., & Gaertner, S. L. (2000). Aversive racism and selection decisions: 1989 and 1999. *Psychological Science, 11*(4), 315–319.

Dovidio, J. F., Kawakami, K., & Gaertner, S. L. (2002). Implicit and explicit prejudice and interracial interaction. *Journal of Personality and Social Psychology, 82*(1), 62–68.

Dovidio, J., Kawakami, K., Johnson, C., Johnson, B., & Howard, A. (1997). The nature of prejudice: Automatic and controlled processes. *Journal of Experimental Social Psychology, 33*, 510–540.

Duda, J. L., & Nicholls, J. G. (1992). Dimensions of achievement motivation in schoolwork and sport. *Journal of Educational Psychology, 84*(3), 290–299.

Dudai, Y. (2012). The restless engram: Consolidations never end. *Annual Review of Neuroscience, 35*, 227–247.

Duguid, M. M., & Thomas-Hunt, M. C. (2015). Condoning stereotyping? How awareness of stereotyping prevalence impacts expression of stereotypes. *Journal of Applied Psychology, 100*(2), 343–359.

Duncan, B. L. (1976). Differential social perception and attribution of intergroup violence: Testing the lower limits of stereotyping of Blacks. *Journal of Personality and Social Psychology, 34*, 590–598.

Duncker, K. (1945). On problem-solving (L. S. Lees, Trans.). *Psychological Monographs, 58*(5), i–113.

Dunning, D. (1995). Trait importance and modifiability as factors influencing self-assessment and self-enhancement motives. *Personality and Social Psychology Bulletin, 21*, 1297–1306.

Dunning, D. (2011). The Dunning–Kruger effect: On being ignorant of one's own ignorance. In M. P. Zanna & J. M. Olson (Eds.), *Advances in experimental social psychology* (vol. 44, pp. 247–296). New York: Academic Press.

Dunning, D., & Balcetis, E. (2013). Wishful seeing: How preferences shape visual perception. *Current Directions in Psychological Science, 22*(1), 33–37.

Dunning, D., & Helzer, E. G. (2014). Beyond the correlation coefficient in studies of self-assessment accuracy: Commentary on Zell and Krizan (2014). *Perspectives on Psychological Science, 9*(2), 126–130.

Dunning, D., Leuenberger, A., & Sherman, D. A. (1995). A new look at motivated inference: Are self-serving theories of success a product of motivational forces? *Journal of Personality and Social Psychology, 69*(1), 58–68.

Dupree, C. H. (2022). Forming and managing impressions across racial divides. In E. Balcetis & G. B. Moskowitz (Eds.), *Handbook of impression formation: A social psychological approach* (pp. 256–275). New York: Routledge.

Dupree, C. H., & Fiske, S. T. (2019). Self-presentation in interracial settings: The competence downshift by White liberals. *Journal of Personality and Social Psychology, 117*(3), 579–604.

Dupree, C. H., Torrez, B., Obioha, O., & Fiske, S. T. (2021). Race–status associations: Distinct effects of three novel measures among White and Black perceivers. *Journal of Personality and Social Psychology, 120*(3), 601–625.

Dutton, D. G., & Aron, A. P. (1974). Some evidence for heightened sexual attraction under conditions of high anxiety. *Journal of Personality and Social Psychology, 30*(4), 510–517.

Duval, S., & Wicklund, R. A. (1972). *A theory of objective self-awareness.* New York: Academic Press.

Dweck, C. S. (1995). Implicit theories as organizers of goals and behavior. In P. M. Gollwitzer & J. A. Bargh (Eds.), *The psychology of action: Linking cognition and motivation to action* (pp. 69–90). New York: Guilford Press.

Dweck, C. S. (2006). *Mindset: The new psychology of success.* Random House.

Dweck, C. S. (2017). From needs to goals and representations: Foundations for a unified theory of motivation, personality, and development. *Psychological Review, 124*(6), 689–719.

Dweck, C. S., & Elliott, E. S. (1983). Achievement motivation. In P. H. Mussen (Gen. Ed.) & E. M. Hetherington (Ed.), *Handbook of child psychology* (Vol. 4, pp. 643–691). New York: Wiley.

Dweck, C. S., & Leggett, E. L. (1988). A social-cognitive approach to motivation and personality. *Psychological Review, 95,* 256–273.

Dweck, C. S., & Sorich, L. A. (1999). Mastery-oriented thinking. In C. R. Snyder (Ed.), *Coping: The psychology of what works* (pp. 232–251). New York: Oxford University Press.

Eagly, A. H., Ashmore, R. D., Makhijani, M. G., & Longo, L. C. (1991). What is beautiful is good, but . . . a meta-analytic review of research on the physical attractiveness stereotype. *Psychological Bulletin, 110*(1), 109–128.

Eagly, A. H., & Chaiken, S. (1993). *The psychology of attitudes.* Fort Worth, TX: Harcourt Brace Jovanovich.

Eagly, A. H., & Karau, S. J. (2002). Role congruity theory of prejudice toward female leaders. *Psychological Review, 109*(3), 573–598.

Eagly, A. H., Mladinic, A., & Otto, S. (1991). Are women evaluated more favorably than men? An analysis of attitudes, beliefs, and emotions. *Psychology of Women Quarterly, 15*(2), 203–216.

Eagly, A. H., & Revelle, W. (2022). Understanding the magnitude of psychological differences between women and men requires seeing the forest and the trees. *Perspectives on Psychological Science, 17*(5), 1339–1358.

Eaton, A. A., Majka, E. A., & Visser, P. S. (2008). Emerging perspectives on the structure and function of attitude strength. *European Review of Social Psychology, 19,* 165–201.

Eberhardt, J. L. (2020). *Biased: Uncovering the hidden prejudice that shapes what we see, think, and do.* New York: Penguin.

Eberhardt, J. L., Dasgupta, N., & Banaszynski, T. L. (2003). Believing is seeing: The effects of racial labels and implicit beliefs on face perception. *Personality and Social Psychology Bulletin, 29*(3), 360–370.

Eberhardt, J. L., Davies, P. G., Purdie-Vaughns, V. J., & Johnson, S. L. (2006). Looking deathworthy: Perceived stereotypicality of Black defendants predicts capital-sentencing outcomes. *Psychological Science, 17*(5), 383–386.

Eberhardt, J. L., Goff, P. A., Purdie, V. J., & Davies, P. G. (2004). Seeing Black: Race, crime, and visual processing. *Journal of Personality and Social Psychology, 87*(6), 876–893.

Eden, A., Maloney, E., & Bowman, N. (2010). Gender attribution in online video games. *Journal of Media Psychology: Theories, Methods, and Applications, 22*(3), 114–124.

Ehrlinger, J., Johnson, K., Banner, M., Dunning, D., & Kruger, J. (2008). Why the unskilled are unaware: Further explorations of (absent) self-insight among the incompetent. *Organizational Behavior and Human Decision Processes, 105*(1), 98–121.

Einhorn, H. J., & Hogarth, R. M. (1986). Judging probable cause. *Psychological Bulletin, 99*(1), 3–19.

Eitam, B., & Higgins, E. T. (2010). Motivation in mental accessibility: Relevance of a representation (ROAR) as a new framework. *Social and Personality Psychology Compass, 4*(10), 951–967.

Ekman, P., & Friesen, W. V. (1969). Nonverbal leakage and clues to deception. *Psychiatry, 32,* 88–106.

Ekman, P., & Friesen, W. V. (1974). Detecting deception from the body or face. *Journal of Personality and Social Psychology, 29*(3), 288–298.

Ekman, P., & Rosenberg, E. L. (Eds.). (2005). *What the face reveals: Basic and applied studies of spontaneous expression using the facial action coding system (FACS)* (2nd ed.). Oxford University Press.

Ellemers, N., & Haslam, S. A. (2012). Social identity theory. In P. A. M. Van Lange, A. W. Kruglanski, & E. T. Higgins (Eds.), *Handbook of theories of social psychology* (pp. 379–398). Thousand Oaks, CA: Sage.

Ellemers, N., Spears, R., & Doosje, B. (1997). Sticking together or falling apart: In-group identification as a psychological determinant of group commitment versus individual mobility. *Journal of Personality and Social Psychology, 72*(3), 617–626.

Ellemers, N., & van den Bos, K. (2012). Morality in groups: On the social–regulatory functions of right and wrong. *Social and Personality Psychology Compass, 6,* 878–889.

Elliot, A. J., & Devine, P. G. (1994). On the motivational nature of cognitive dissonance: Dissonance as psychological discomfort. *Journal of Personality and Social Psychology, 67*(3), 382–394.

Elliot, A. J., McGregor, H. A., & Gable, S. (1999). Achievement goals, study strategies, and exam performance: A mediational analysis. *Journal of Educational Psychology, 91*(3), 549–563.

Elliott, E. S., & Dweck, C. S. (1988). Goals: An approach to motivation and achievement. *Journal of Personality and Social Psychology, 54*, 5–12.

Epley, N., & Dunning, D. (2000). Feeling "holier than thou": Are self-serving assessments produced by errors in self- or social prediction? *Journal of Personality and Social Psychology, 79*(6), 861–875.

Epley, N., Keysar, B., Van Boven, L., & Gilovich, T. (2004). Perspective taking as egocentric anchoring and adjustment. *Journal of Personality and Social Psychology, 87*(3), 327–339.

Erdelyi, M. H. (1974). A new look at the new look: Perceptual defense and vigilance. *Psychological Review, 81*(1), 1–25.

Eyal, T., Steffel, M., & Epley, N. (2018). Perspective mistaking: Accurately understanding the mind of another requires getting perspective, not taking perspective. *Journal of Personality and Social Psychology, 114*(4), 547–571.

Fazio, R. H. (1986). How do attitudes guide behavior? In R. M. Sorrentino & E. T. Higgins (Eds.), *Handbook of motivation and cognition* (Vol. 1, pp. 204–243). New York: Guilford Press.

Fazio, R. H. (1990a). The MODE model as an integrative framework. *Advances in Experimental Social Psychology, 23*, 75–109.

Fazio, R. H. (1990b). A practical guide of the use of response latency in social psychological review. In C. Hendrick & M. S. Clark (Eds.), *Research methods in personality and social psychology* (pp. 74–97). Newbury Park, CA.: Sage.

Fazio, R. H. (2007). Attitudes as object-evaluation associations of varying strength. *Social Cognition, 25*, 603–637.

Fazio, R. H., & Dunton, B. C. (1997). Categorization by race: The impact of automatic and controlled components of racial prejudice. *Journal of Experimental Social Psychology, 33*, 451–470.

Fazio, R. H., Jackson, J. R., Dunton, B. C., & Williams, C. J. (1995). Variability in automatic activation as an unobtrusive measure of racial attitudes: A bona fide pipeline? *Journal of Personality and Social Psychology, 69*(6), 1013–1027.

Fazio, R. H., & Olson, M. A. (2003). Implicit measures in social cognition research: Their meaning and use. *Annual Review of Psychology, 54*(1), 297–327.

Fazio, R. H., & Olson, M. A. (2014). The MODE model: Attitude–behavior processes as a function of motivation and opportunity. In J. W. Sherman, B. Gawronski, & Y. Trope (Eds.), *Dual-process theories of the social mind* (pp. 155–171). New York: Guilford Press.

Fazio, R. H., Sanbonmatsu, D. M., Powell, M. C., & Kardes, F. R. (1986). On the automatic activation of attitudes. *Journal of Personality and Social Psychology, 50*, 229–238.

Fein, S., Hilton, J. L., & Miller, D. T. (1990). Suspicion of ulterior motivation and the correspondence bias. *Journal of Personality and Social Psychology, 58*, 753–764.

Fein, S., & Spencer, S. J. (1997). Prejudice as self-image maintenance: Affirming the self through negative evaluations of others. *Journal of Personality and Social Psychology, 73*, 31–44.

Feldman, S., & Huddy, L. (2018). Racially motivated reasoning. In H. Lavine & C. S. Taber (Eds.), *The feeling, thinking citizen: Essays in honor of Milton Lodge* (pp. 171–193). New York: Routledge.

Feldman Barrett, L. (2009). Understanding the mind by measuring the brain: Lessons from measuring behavior (Commentary on Vul et al., 2009). *Perspectives on Psychological Science, 4*(3), 314–318.

Fenigstein, A., Scheier, M. F., & Buss, A. H. (1975). Public and private self-consciousness: Assessment and theory. *Journal of Consulting and Clinical Psychology, 43*, 522–527.

Ferguson, M. J., & Bargh, J. A. (2004). Liking is for doing: The effects of goal pursuit on automatic evaluation. *Journal of Personality and Social Psychology, 87*(5), 557–572.

Ferguson, M., Carter, T., & Hassin, R. (2009). On the automaticity of nationalist ideology: The case of the USA. In J. T. Jost, A. C. Kay, & H. Thorisdottir (Eds.), *Social and psychological bases of ideology and system justification* (pp. 53–82). New York: Oxford University Press.

Ferguson, M., Korkmaz, A. Moskowitz, G. B., Hupbach, A., Olcaysoy Okten, I., & Krosch, A. (2024). *Using behavioral, computational, and neural approaches to understand correction of first impressions.* Manuscript under review.

Festinger, L. (1954). A theory of social comparison processes. *Human Relations, 7,* 117–140.

Festinger, L. (1957). *A theory of cognitive dissonance* (pp. 1–31). Stanford, CA: Stanford University Press.

Festinger, L., & Carlsmith, J. M. (1959). Cognitive sequences of forced compliance. *Journal of Abnormal and Social Psychology, 58,* 203–210.

Festinger, L., Riecken, H. W., & Schachter, S. (1956). *When prophecy fails.* Minneapolis: University of Minnesota Press.

Fiedler, K., & Hütter, M. (2014). The limits of automaticity. In J. W. Sherman, B. Gawronski, & Y. Trope (Eds.), *Dual-process theories of the social mind* (pp. 497–513). New York: Guilford Press.

Fiedler, K., & Schenck, W. (2001). Spontaneous inferences from pictorially presented behaviors. *Personality and Social Psychology Bulletin, 27*(11), 1533–1546.

Fiedler, K., Schenck, W., Watling, M., & Menges, J. I. (2005). Priming trait inferences through pictures and moving pictures: The impact of open and closed mindsets. *Journal of Personality and Social Psychology, 88*(2), 229–244.

Fiedler, K., & Unkelbach, C. (2011). Evaluative conditioning depends on higher order encoding processes. *Cognition and Emotion, 25*(4), 639–656.

Finke, R. A. (1996). Imagery, creativity, and emergent structure. *Consciousness and Cognition, 5*(3), 381–393.

Finkel, E., Campbell, W. K., Brunell, A., Dalton, A., Scarbeck, S., & Chartrand, T. (2006). High-maintenance interaction: Inefficient social coordination impairs self-regulation. *Journal of Personality and Social Psychology, 91,* 456–475.

Fischhoff, B., & Beyth, R. (1975). "I knew it would happen": Remembered probabilities of once-future things. *Organizational Behavior and Human Performance, 13*(1), 1–16.

Fishbach, A., Dhar, R., & Zhang, Y. (2006). Subgoals as substitutes or complements: The role of goal accessibility. *Journal of Personality and Social Psychology, 91*(2), 232–242.

Fishbach, A., Friedman, R. S., & Kruglanski, A. W. (2003). Leading us not unto temptation: Momentary allurements elicit overriding goal activation. *Journal of Personality and Social Psychology, 84,* 296–309.

Fisher, E. L., & Borgida, E. (2012). Intergroup disparities and implicit bias: A commentary. *Journal of Social Issues, 68*(2), 385–398.

Fiske, S. T. (1980). Attention and weight in person perception: The impact of negative and extreme behavior. *Journal of Personality and Social Psychology, 38,* 889–906.

Fiske, S. T. (1993a). Controlling other people. *American Psychologist, 48,* 621–628.

Fiske, S. T. (1993b). Social cognition and social perception. *Annual Review of Psychology, 44,* 155–194.

Fiske, S. T., Bersoff, D. N., Borgida, E., Deaux, K., & Heilman, M. E. (1991). Social science research on trial: Use of sex stereotyping research in Price Waterhouse v. Hopkins. *American Psychologist, 46,* 1049–1060.

Fiske, S. T., Cuddy, A. J., & Glick, P. (2007). Universal dimensions of social cognition: Warmth and competence. *Trends in Cognitive Sciences, 11,* 77–83.

Fiske, S. T., Cuddy, A. J. C., Glick, P., & Xu, J. (2002). A model of (often mixed) stereotype content: Competence and warmth respectively follow from perceived status and competition. *Journal of Personality and Social Psychology, 82*(6), 878–902.

Fiske, S. T., Lin, M., & Neuberg, S. L. (1999). The continuum model: Ten years later. In S. Chaiken & Y. Trope (Eds.), *Dual-process theories in social psychology* (pp. 231–254). New York: Guilford Press.

Fiske, S. T., & Linville, P. W. (1980). What does the schema concept buy us? *Personality and Social Psychology Bulletin, 6,* 543–557.

Fiske, S. T., & Neuberg, S. L. (1990). A continuum model of impression formation, from category based to individuating processes: Influences of information and motivation on attention and interpretation. In M. P. Zanna (Ed.), *Advances in experimental social psychology* (Vol. 23, pp. 1–74). New York: Academic Press.

Fiske, S. T., & Taylor, S. E. (1984). *Social cognition.* Reading, MA: Addison-Wesley.

Fiske, S. T., & Taylor, S. E. (1991). *Social cognition* (2nd ed.). New York: McGraw Hill.

Fitzsimons, G. M., & Bargh, J. A. (2003). Thinking of you: Nonconscious pursuit of interpersonal goals associated with relationship partners. *Journal of Personality and Social Psychology, 84,* 148–164.

Flowe, H. D., & Humphries, J. E. (2011). An examination of criminal face bias in a random sample of police lineups. *Applied Cognitive Psychology, 25*(2), 265–273.

Foersterling, F. (1992). The Kelley model as an analysis of variance analogy: How far can it be taken? *Journal of Experimental Social Psychology, 28*(5), 475–490.

Forbes, C. E., & Grafman, J. (2013). Social neuroscience: The second phase. *Frontiers in Human Neuroscience, 7.*

Ford, B. Q., Green, D. J., & Gross, J. J. (2022). White fragility: An emotion regulation perspective. *American Psychologist, 77*(4), 510–524.

Ford, T. E., Boxer, C. F., Armstrong, J., & Edel, J. R. (2008). More than "just a joke": The prejudice-releasing function of sexist humor. *Personality and Social Psychology Bulletin, 34*(2), 159–170.

Ford, T. E., & Ferguson, M. A. (2004). Social consequences of disparagement humor: A prejudiced norm theory. *Personality and Social Psychology Review, 8*(1), 79–94.

Forscher, P. S., & Devine, P. G. (2014). Breaking the prejudice habit: Automaticity and control in the context of a long-term goal. In J. W. Sherman, B. Gawronski, & Y. Trope (Eds.), *Dual-process theories of the social mind* (pp. 468–482). New York: Guilford Press.

Förster, J., Higgins, E. T., & Idson, L. C. (1998). Approach and avoidance strength during goal attainment: Regulatory focus and the "goal looms larger" effect. *Journal of Personality and Social Psychology, 75*, 1115–1131.

Fortin, C., Rousseau, R., Bourque, P., & Kirouac, E. (1993). Time estimation and concurrent nontemporal processing: Specific interference from short-term-memory demands. *Perception and Psychophysics, 53*, 536–548.

Fotuhi, O., Fong, G. T., Zanna, M. P., Borland, R., Yong, H., & Cummings, K. M. (2013). Patterns of cognitive dissonance-reducing beliefs among smokers: A longitudinal analysis from the International Tobacco Control (ITC) Four Country Survey. *Tobacco Control, 22*, 52–58.

Fox, E. (1995). Negative priming from ignored distractors in visual selection: A review. *Psychonomic Bulletin and Review, 2*(2), 145–173.

Frantz, C. M., Cuddy, A. J. C., Burnett, M., Ray, H., & Hart, A. (2004). A threat in the computer: The race Implicit Association Test as a stereotype threat experience. *Personality and Social Psychology Bulletin, 30*(12), 1611–1624.

Freeman, J. B. (2018). Doing psychological science by hand. *Current Directions in Psychological Science, 27*(5), 315–323.

Freeman, J. B., & Johnson, K. L. (2016). More than meets the eye: Split-second social perception. *Trends in Cognitive Sciences, 20*(5), 362–374.

Freitas, A. L., Liberman, N., & Higgins, E. T. (2002). Regulatory fit and resisting temptation during goal pursuit. *Journal of Experimental Social Psychology, 38*(3), 291–298.

Frenkel-Brunswik, E. (1949). Intolerance of ambiguity as an emotional and perceptual personality variable. *Journal of Personality, 18*, 108–143.

Frenkel-Brunswik, E., & Sanford, R. N. (1945). Some personality factors in anti-Semitism. *Journal of Psychology, 20*, 271–291.

Frey, F. E., & Tropp, L. R. (2006). Being seen as individuals versus as group members: Extending research on metaperception to intergroup contexts. *Personality and Social Psychology Review, 10*(3), 265–280.

Friedrich, F., Henik, A., & Tzelgov, J. (1991). Automatic processes in lexical access and spreading activation. *Journal of Experimental Psychology—Human Perception and Performance, 17*(3), 792–806.

Fujita, K., Henderson, M. D., Eng, J., Trope, Y., & Liberman, N. (2006). Spatial distance and mental construal of social events. *Psychological Science, 17*(4), 278–282.

Fujita, K., Trope, Y., Liberman, N., & Levin-Sagi, M. (2006). Construal levels and self-control. *Journal of Personality and Social Psychology, 90*(3), 351–367.

Funder, D. C. (1995). On the accuracy of personality judgment: A realistic approach. *Psychological Review, 102*(4), 652–670.

Funk, F., & Todorov, A. (2013). Criminal stereotypes in the courtroom: Facial tattoos affect guilt and punishment differently. *Psychology, Public Policy, and Law, 19*(4), 466–478.

Gaertner, S. L. (1973). Helping behavior and racial discrimination among liberals and conservatives. *Journal of Personality and Social Psychology, 25*(3), 335–341.

Gaertner, S. L., & Dovidio, J. F. (1977). The subtlety of White racism, arousal, and helping behavior. *Journal of Personality and Social Psychology, 35*(10), 691–707.

Gaertner, S. L., & Dovidio, J. (1986). The aversive form of racism. In J. Dovidio & S. Gaertner (Eds.), *Prejudice, discrimination, and racism* (pp. 61–89). New York: Academic Press.

Gaertner, S. L., & McLaughlin, J. P. (1983). Racial stereotypes: Associations and ascriptions of positive and negative characteristics. *Social Psychology Quarterly, 46*(1), 23–30.

Gagné, F. M., & Lydon, J. E. (2004). Bias and accuracy in close relationships: An integrative review. *Personality and Social Psychology Review, 8*(4), 322–338.

Gailliot, M. T., Plant, E. A., Butz, D. A., & Baumeister, R. F. (2007). Increasing self-regulatory strength can reduce the depleting effect of suppressing stereotypes. *Personality and Social Psychology Bulletin, 33*(2), 281–294.

Galinsky, A. D., & Moskowitz, G. B. (2000a). Counterfactuals as behavioral primes: Priming the simulation heuristic and consideration of alternatives. *Journal of Experimental Social Psychology, 36,* 384–409.

Galinsky, A. D., & Moskowitz, G. B. (2000b). Perspective taking: Decreasing stereotype expression, stereotype accessibility and ingroup favoritism. *Journal of Personality and Social Psychology, 78,* 708–724.

Galinsky, A. D., & Moskowitz, G. B. (2007). Further ironies of suppression: Stereotype and counterstereotype accessibility. *Journal of Experimental Social Psychology, 43*(5), 833–841.

Galinsky, A. D., Moskowitz, G. B., & Skurnik, I. (2000). Counterfactuals as self-generated primes: The effects of prior counterfactual activation on person perception judgments. *Social Cognition, 18*(3), 252–280.

Ganzach, Y., & Schul, Y. (1995). The influence of quantity of information and goal framing on decision. *Acta Psychologica, 89*(1), 23–36.

Gast, A., & Rothermund, K. (2011). I like it because I said that I like it: Evaluative conditioning effects can be based on stimulus-response learning. *Journal of Experimental Psychology: Animal Behavior Processes, 37*(4), 466–476.

Gaunt, R., Leyens, J.-P., & Demoulin, S. (2002). Intergroup relations and the attribution of emotions: Control over memory for secondary emotions associated with the ingroup and outgroup. *Journal of Experimental Social Psychology, 38,* 508–514.

Gawronski, B., Balas, R., & Creighton, L. A. (2014). Can the formation of conditioned attitudes be intentionally controlled? *Personality and Social Psychology Bulletin, 40*(4), 419–432.

Gawronski, B., & Bodenhausen, G. V. (2006). Associative and propositional processes in evaluation: An integrative review of implicit and explicit attitude change. *Psychological Bulletin, 132*(5), 692–731.

Gawronski, B., & Bodenhausen, G. V. (2011). The associative–propositional evaluation model: Theory, evidence, and open questions. In J. M. Olson & M. P. Zanna (Eds.), *Advances in experimental social psychology* (Vol. 44, pp. 59–127). New York: Academic Press.

Gawronski, B., & Bodenhausen, G. V. (2014). Implicit and explicit evaluation: A brief review of the associative–propositional evaluation model. *Social and Personality Psychology Compass, 8*(8), 448–462.

Gawronski, B., & Bodenhausen, G. V. (2018). Evaluative conditioning from the perspective of the associative–propositional evaluation model. *Social Psychological Bulletin, 13*(3), 1–33.

Gawronski, B., De Houwer, J., & Sherman, J. W. (2020). Twenty-five years of research using implicit measures. *Social Cognition, 38,* S1–S25.

Gawronski, B., Geschke, D., & Banse, R. (2003). Implicit bias in impression formation: Associations influence the construal of individuating information. *European Journal of Social Psychology, 33*(5), 573–589.

Gawronski, B., Hu, X., Rydell, R. J., Vervliet, B., & De Houwer, J. (2015). Generalization versus contextualization in automatic evaluation revisited: A meta-analysis of successful and failed replications. *Journal of Experimental Psychology: General, 144*(4), e50–e64.

Gawronski, B., Rydell, R. J., De Houwer, J., Brannon, S. M., Ye, Y., Vervliet, B., et al. (2018). Contextualized attitude change. *Advances in Experimental Social Psychology, 55,* 1–52.

Gawronski, B., Rydell, R. J., Vervliet, B., & De Houwer, J. (2010). Generalization versus contextualization in automatic evaluation. *Journal of Experimental Psychology: General, 139*(4), 683–701.

Geller, V., & Shaver, P. (1976). Cognitive consequences of self-awareness. *Journal of Experimental Social Psychology, 12,* 99–108.

Gerber, J., Wheeler, L., & Suls, J. (2018). A social comparison theory meta-analysis 60+ years on. *Psychological Bulletin, 144*(2), 177–197.

Gergely, G., Nádasdy, Z., Csibra, G., & Bíró, S. (1995). Taking the intentional stance at 12 months of age. *Cognition, 56*(2), 165–193.

Gibson, J. J. (1979). *The ecological approach to visual perception.* Boston: Houghton Mifflin.

Gil, S., & Droit-Volet, S. (2011). "Time flies in the presence of angry faces" . . . depending on the temporal task used! *Acta Psychologica, 136*(3), 354–362.

Gilbert, D. T. (1989). Thinking lightly about others: Automatic components of the social inference process. In J. S. Uleman & J. A. Bargh (Eds.), *Unintended thought* (pp. 189–211). New York: Guilford Press.

Gilbert, D. T. (1998). Ordinary personology. In D. T. Gilbert, S. T. Fiske, & G. Lindzey (Eds.), *The handbook of social psychology* (4th ed., Vol. 2, pp. 89–150). New York: McGraw Hill.

Gilbert, D. T., & Hixon, J. G. (1991). The trouble of thinking: Activation and application of stereotypic beliefs. *Journal of Personality and Social Psychology, 60,* 509–517.

Gilbert, D. T., Krull, D. S., & Malone, P. S. (1990). Unbelieving the unbelievable: Some problems in the rejection of false information. *Journal of Personality and Social Psychology, 59,* 601–613.

Gilbert, D. T., & Osborne, R. E. (1989). Thinking backward: Some curable and incurable consequences of cognitive busyness. *Journal of Personality and Social Pscychology, 57,* 940–949.

Gilbert, D. T., Pelham, B. W., & Krull, D. S. (1988). On cognitive business: When person perceivers meet person perceived. *Journal of Personality and Social Psychology, 54,* 733–740.

Gilbert, D. T., Pinel, E. C., Wilson, T. D., Blumberg, S. J., & Wheatley, T. P. (1998). Immune neglect: A source of durability bias in affective forecasting. *Journal of Personality and Social Psychology, 75,* 617–638.

Gilbert, D. T., Tafarodi, R. W., & Malone, P. S. (1993). You can't not believe everything you read. *Journal of Personality and Social Psychology, 65*(2), 221–233.

Gilovich, T. (1991). *How we know what isn't so: The fallibility of human reason in everyday life.* New York: Free Press

Gilovich, T., Jennings, D. L., & Jennings, S. (1983). Causal focus and estimates of consensus: An examination of the false-consensus effect. *Journal of Personality and Social Psychology, 45*(3), 550–559.

Gilovich, T., Medvec, V. H., & Savitsky, K. (2000).

The spotlight effect in social judgment: An egocentric bias in estimates of the salience of one's own actions and appearance. *Journal of Personality and Social Psychology, 78*(2), 211–222.

Gilovich, T., Savitsky, K., & Medvec, V. H. (1998). The illusion of transparency: Biased assessments of others' ability to read our emotional states. *Journal of Personality and Social Psychology, 75,* 332–346.

Glaser, J., Martin, K. D., & Kahn, K. B. (2015). Possibility of death sentence has divergent effect on verdicts for Black and White defendants. *Law and Human Behavior, 39*(6), 539–546.

Glaser, J., Spencer, K. B., & Charbonneau, A. (2014). Racial bias and public policy. *Policy Insights from Behavioral and Brain Sciences, 1,* 88–94.

Glick, P., & Fiske, S. (1996). The ambivalent sexism inventory. *Journal of Personality and Social Psychology, 70,* 491–512.

Glick, P., & Fiske, S. T. (2001a). Ambivalent sexism. *Advances in Experimental Social Psychology, 33,* 115–188.

Glick, P., & Fiske, S. T. (2001b). An ambivalent alliance: Hostile and benevolent sexism as complementary justifications for gender inequality. *American Psychologist, 56*(2), 109–118.

Glucksberg, S., & Weisberg, R. W. (1966). Verbal behavior and problem solving: Some effects of labeling in a functional fixedness problem. *Journal of Experimental Psychology, 71*(5), 659–664.

Goff, P. A. (2016). Identity traps: How to think about race and policing. *Behavioral Science and Policy, 2*(2), 11–22.

Goff, P. A., Eberhardt, J. L., Williams, M. J., & Jackson, M. (2008). Not yet human: Implicit knowledge, historical dehumanization, and contemporary consequences. *Journal of Personality and Social Psychology, 94,* 292–306.

Goff, P. A., Jackson, M. C., Di Leone, B. A. L., Culotta, C. M., & DiTomasso, N. A. (2014). The essence of innocence: Consequences of dehumanizing Black children. *Journal of Personality and Social Psychology, 106*(4), 526–545.

Goff, P. A., & Kahn, K. B. (2013). How psychological science impedes intersectional thinking. *Du Bois Review, 10,* 365–384.

Goff, P. A., Steele, C. M., & Davies, P. G. (2008).

The space between us: Stereotype threat and distance in interracial contexts. *Journal of Personality and Social Psychology, 94*(1), 91–107.

Gollwitzer, A., Olcaysoy Okten, I., Pizarro, A. O., & Oettingen, G. (2022). Discordant knowing: A social cognitive structure underlying fanaticism. *Journal of Experimental Psychology: General, 151*(11), 2846–2878.

Gollwitzer, P. M. (1990). Action phases and mind-sets. In E. T. Higgins & R. M. Sorrentino (Eds.), *Handbook of motivation and cognition* (Vol. 2, pp. 53–92). New York: Guilford Press.

Gollwitzer, P. M. (1993). Goal achievement: The role of intentions. In W. Stroebe & M. Hewstone (Eds.), *European review of social psychology* (Vol. 4, pp. 141–185). Chichester, UK: Wiley.

Gollwitzer, P. M. (1999). Implementation intentions: Strong effects of simple plans. *American Psychologist, 54*, 493–503.

Gollwitzer, P. M., & Brandstaetter, V. (1997). Implementation intentions and effective goal pursuit. *Journal of Personality and Social Psychology, 73*, 186–199.

Gollwitzer, P. M., Heckhausen, H., & Steller, B. (1990). Deliberative vs. implemental mind-sets: Cognitive tuning toward congruous thoughts and information. *Journal of Personality and Social Psychology, 59*, 1119–1127.

Gollwitzer, P. M., & Moskowitz, G. B. (1996). Goal effects on action and cognition. In E. T. Higgins & A. W. Kruglanski (Eds.), *Social psychology: Handbook of basic principles* (pp. 361–399). New York: Guilford Press.

Gollwitzer, P. M., Wicklund, R. A., & Hilton, J. L. (1982). Admission of failure and symbolic self-completion: Extending Lewinian theory. *Journal of Personality and Social Psychology, 43*, 358–371.

Gonsalkorale, K., & Sherman, J. W. (2007). *Altering newly formed implicit attitudes: An examination of the underlying mechanisms.* Unpublished raw data.

Goodwin, G. P., & Darley, J. M. (2012). Why are some moral beliefs perceived to be more objective than others? *Journal of Experimental Social Psychology, 48*(1), 250–256.

Gopnik, A., & Wellman, H. M. (1994). The theory theory. In L. A. Hirschfeld & S. A. Gelman (Eds.), *Mapping the mind: Domain specificity in cognition and culture* (pp. 257–293). New York: Cambridge University Press.

Gosling, P., Denizeau, M., & Oberlé, D. (2006). Denial of responsibility: A new mode of dissonance reduction. *Journal of Personality and Social Psychology, 90*(5), 722–733.

Graham, J., Haidt, J., & Nosek, B. A. (2009). Liberals and conservatives rely on different sets of moral foundations. *Journal of Personality and Social Psychology, 96*(5), 1029–1046.

Grant, H., & Dweck, C. S. (1999). Content versus structure in motivation and self-regulation. In R. S. Wyer, Jr. (Ed.), *Perspectives on behavioral self-regulation: Advances in social cognition* (Vol. 7, pp. 161–174). Mahwah, NJ: Erlbaum.

Grant, H., & Dweck, C. S. (2003). Clarifying achievement goals and their impact. *Journal of Personality and Social Psychology, 85*, 541–553.

Grant, P. R., & Holmes, J. G. (1981). The integration of implicit personality theory schemas and stereotype images. *Social Psychology Quarterly, 44*(2), 107–115.

Gray, J. A. (1982). *The neuropsychology of anxiety: An enquiry into the functions of the septo-hippocampal system.* New York: Oxford University Press.

Green, A. R., Carney, D. R., Pallin, D. J., Ngo, L. H., Raymond, K. L., Lezzoni, L. I., et al. (2007). Implicit bias among physicians and its prediction of thrombolysis decisions for black and white patients. *Journal of General Internal Medicine, 22*, 1231–1238.

Greenberg, J., Pyszczynski, T., Solomon, S., Rosenblatt, A., Veeder, M., Kirkland, S., & Lyon, D. (1990). Evidence for terror management theory II: The effects of mortality salience on reactions to those who threaten or bolster the cultural worldview. *Journal of Personality and Social Psychology, 58*(2), 308–318.

Greenberg, J., Pyszczynski, T., Solomon, S., Simon, L., & Breus, M. (1994). Role of consciousness and accessibility of death-related thoughts in mortality salience effects. *Journal of Personality and Social Psychology, 67*(4), 627–637.

Greenberg, J. R., Solomon, S., & Pyszczynski, T. (1997). Terror management theory of self-esteem and cultural worldviews: Empirical assessments and conceptual refinements. In M. P. Zanna (Ed.), *Advances in experimental social psychology* (Vol. 29, pp. 61–139). San Diego, CA: Academic Press.

Greenman, E., & Xie, Y. (2008). Double jeopardy? The interaction of gender and race on earnings in the United States. *Social Forces, 86,* 1217-1244.

Greenwald, A. G. (1968). Cognitive learning, cognitive responses to persuasion, and attitude change. In A. G. Greenwald, T. C. Brock, & T. M. Ostrom (Eds.), *Psychological foundations of attitudes* (pp. 147-170). New York: Academic Press.

Greenwald, A. G. (1980). The totalitarian ego: Fabrication and revision of personal history. *American Psychologist, 35,* 603-618.

Greenwald, A. G. (1981). Self and memory. In G. H. Bower (Ed.), *The psychology of learning and motivation* (Vol. 12, pp. 201-236). Orlando, FL: Academic Press.

Greenwald, A. G., McGhee, D. E., & Schwartz, J. L. K. (1998). Measuring individual differences in implicit cognition: The Implicit Association Test. *Journal of Personality and Social Psychology, 74,* 1464-1480.

Greenwald, A. G., Poehlman, T. A., Uhlmann, E. L., & Banaji, M. R. (2009). Understanding and using the Implicit Association Test: III. Meta-analysis of predictive validity. *Journal of Personality and Social Psychology, 97*(1), 17-41.

Gregg, A. P., Seibt, B., & Banaji, M. R. (2006). Easier done than undone: Symmetry in the malleability of implicit preferences. *Journal of Personality and Social Psychology, 90*(1), 1-20.

Greifeneder, R., Jaffé, M., Newman, E., & Schwarz, N. (Eds.). (2020). *The psychology of fake news: Accepting, sharing, and correcting misinformation.* London: Routledge.

Grice, H. M. (1967). *The logic of conversation.* William James Lectures. Cambridge, MA: Harvard University Press.

Grice, H. P. (1975). Logic and conversation. The William James lectures, Harvard University, 1967-68. In P. Cole & J. Morgan (Eds.), *Syntax and semantics 3: Speech arts* (pp. 41-58). New York: Academic Press.

Gulker, J. E., Mark, A. Y., & Monteith, M. J. (2013). Confronting prejudice: The *who, what,* and *why* of confrontation effectiveness. *Social Influence, 8*(4), 280-293.

Hafer, C. L. (2000). Do innocent victims threaten the belief in a just world? Evidence from a modified Stroop task. *Journal of Personality and Social Psychology, 79,* 165-173.

Hahn, A., Banchefsky, S., Park, B., & Judd, C. M. (2015). Measuring intergroup ideologies: Positive and negative aspects of emphasizing versus looking beyond group differences. *Personality and Social Psychology Bulletin, 41*(12), 1646-1664.

Hahn, A., Judd, C. M., Hirsh, H. K., & Blair, I. V. (2014). Awareness of implicit attitudes. *Journal of Experimental Psychology: General, 143*(3), 1369-1392.

Haidt, J., & Graham, J. (2007). When morality opposes justice: Conservatives have moral intuitions that liberals may not recognize. *Social Justice Research, 20*(1), 98-116.

Haidt, J., & Joseph, C. (2008). The moral mind: How five sets of innate intuitions guide the development of many culture-specific virtues, and perhaps even modules. In P. Carruthers, S. Laurence, & S. Stich (Eds.), *The innate mind Vol. 3. Foundations and the future* (pp. 367-391). New York: Oxford University Press.

Ham, J., & Vonk, R. (2003). Smart and easy: Co-occurring activation of spontaneous trait inferences and spontaneous situational inferences. *Journal of Experimental Social Psychology, 39*(5), 434-447.

Hamilton, D. L. (1981). Cognitive representations of persons. In E. T. Higgins, C. P. Herman, & M. P. Zanna (Eds.), *Social cognition: The Ontario symposium* (Vol. 1, pp. 135-159). Hillsdale, NJ: Erlbaum.

Hamilton, D. L. (1991, August). *Perceiving persons and groups: A social cognitive perspective.* Paper presented at the 99th annual convention of the American Psychological Association, San Francisco, CA.

Hamilton, D. L., Chen, J. M., Ko, D. M., Winczewski, L., Banerji, I., & Thurston, J. A. (2015). Sowing the seeds of stereotypes: Spontaneous inferences about groups. *Journal of Personality and Social Psychology, 109*(4), 569-588.

Hamilton, D. L., Dugan, P. M., & Trolier, T. K. (1985). The formulation of stereotypic beliefs: Further evidence for distinctiveness-based illusory correlations. *Journal of Personality and Social Psychology, 48,* 5-17.

Hamilton, D. L., & Gifford, R. K. (1976). Illusory correlation in interpersonal perception: A cognitive basis of stereotypic judgments. *Journal of Experimental Social Psychology, 12,* 392-407.

Hamilton, D. L., Katz, L. B., & Leirer, V. O. (1980a). Cognitive representation of personality impressions: Organizational processes in first impression formation. *Journal of Personality and Social Psychology, 39,* 1050–1063.

Hamilton, D. L., Katz, L. B., & Leirer, V. O. (1980b). Organizational processes in impression formation. In R. Hastie, T. M. Ostrom, E. B. Ebbesen, R. S. Wyer, Jr., D. L. Hamilton, & D. E. Carlston (Eds.), *Person memory: The cognitive basis of social perception* (pp. 121–153). Hillsdale, NJ: Erlbaum.

Hamilton, D. L., & Rose, T. L. (1980). Illusory correlation and the maintenance of stereotypic beliefs. *Journal of Personality and Social Psychology, 39,* 832–845.

Hamilton, D. L., & Sherman, J. W. (1994). Stereotypes. In R. S. Wyer, Jr., & T. K. Srull (Eds.), *Handbook of social cognition: Basic processes; Applications* (pp. 1–68). Hillsdale, NJ: Erlbaum.

Hamilton, D. L., & Trolier, T. K. (1986). Stereotypes and stereotyping: An overview of the cognitive approach. In J. F. Dovidio & S. L. Gaertner (Eds.), *Prejudice, discrimination, and racism* (pp. 127–163). Orlando, FL: Academic Press.

Hamlin, J. K., Newman, G. E., & Wynn, K. (2009). Eight-month-old infants infer unfulfilled goals, despite ambiguous physical evidence. *Infancy, 14*(5), 579–590.

Hamlin, J. K., Wynn, K., & Bloom, P. (2007). Social evaluation in preverbal infants. *Nature, 450*(7169), 557–559.

Hansen, B. C., Rakhshan, P. J., Ho, A. K., & Pannasch, S. (2015). Looking at others through implicitly or explicitly prejudiced eyes. *Visual Cognition, 23*(5), 612–642.

Hansen, F. (2003). Diversity's business case doesn't add up. *Workforce, April,* 28–32.

Hardin, C. D., & Conley, T. D. (2001). A relational approach to cognition: Shared experience and relationship affirmation in social cognition. In G. B. Moskowitz (Ed.), *Cognitive social psychology: The Princeton symposium on the legacy and future of social cognition* (pp. 3–17). Mahwah, NJ: Erlbaum.

Hare, B. (2011). From hominoid to hominid mind: What changed and why? *Annual Review of Anthropology, 40,* 293–309.

Harmon-Jones, E., & Mills, J. (2019). An introduction to cognitive dissonance theory and an overview of current perspectives on the theory. In E. Harmon-Jones (Ed.), *Cognitive dissonance: Reexamining a pivotal theory in psy-* *chology* (pp. 3–24). Washington, DC: American Psychological Association.

Harris, J. R. (2010). Explaining individual differences in personality: Why we need a modular theory. In D. M. Buss & P. H. Hawley (Eds.), *The evolution of personality and individual differences* (pp. 121–153). New York: Oxford University Press.

Harris, L. T., & Fiske, S. T. (2006). Dehumanizing the lowest of the low: Neuroimaging responses to extreme out-groups. *Psychological Science, 17*(10), 847–853.

Harris, L. T., & Fiske, S. T. (2011). Dehumanized perception: A psychological means to facilitate atrocities, torture, and genocide? *Journal of Psychology, 219*(3), 175–181.

Hart, H. L. A., & Honoré, T. (1959). *Causation in the law.* Oxford, UK: Clarendon Press.

Harvey, O. J. (1963). *Motivation and Social interaction: Cognitive determinants.* New York: Ronald Press.

Hasher, L., Goldstein, D., & Toppino, T. (1977). Frequency and the conference of referential validity. *Journal of Verbal Learning and Verbal Behavior, 16,* 107–112.

Hasher, L., & Zacks, R. T. (1979). Automatic and effortful processes in memory. *Journal of Experimental Psychology: General, 108*(3), 356–388.

Haslam, N., Kashima, Y., Loughnan, S., Shi, J., & Suitner, C. (2008). Subhuman, inhuman, and superhuman: Contrasting humans with nonhumans in three cultures. *Social Cognition, 26,* 248–258.

Haslam, N., Loughnan, S., Kashima, Y., & Bain, P. (2008). Attributing and denying humanness to others. *European Review of Social Psychology, 19,* 55–85.

Haslam, S. A., Oakes, P. J., McGarty, C., Turner, J. C., Reynolds, K. J., & Eggins, R. A. (1996). Stereotyping and social influence: The mediation of stereotype applicability and sharedness by the views of in-group and out-group members. *British Journal of Social Psychology, 35,* 369–397.

Hassin, R. R., Aarts, H., & Ferguson, M. J. (2005). Automatic goal inferences. *Journal of Experimental Social Psychology, 41*(2), 129–140.

Hastie, R., & Kumar, P. A. (1979). Person memory: Personality traits as organizing principles in memory for behavior. *Journal of Personality and Social Psychology, 37,* 25–38.

Hastie, R., Ostrom, T. M., Ebbesen, E. B., Wyer,

R. S., Hamilton, D. L., & Carlston, D. E. (1980). *Person memory: The cognitive basis of social perception.* Hillsdale, NJ: Erlbaum.

Hastie, R., & Park, B. (1986). The relationship between memory and judgment depends on whether the judgment task is memory-based or on-line. *Psychological Review, 93*(3), 258–268.

Hastorf, A. H., & Cantril, H. (1954). They saw a game: A case study. *Journal of Abnormal and Social Psychology, 49,* 129–134.

Hastorf, A. H., Schneider, D. J., & Polefka, J. (1970). *Person perception.* Reading, MA: Addison-Wesley.

Hausmann, L. R. M., & Ryan, C. S. (2004). Effects of external and internal motivation to control prejudice on implicit prejudice: The mediating role of efforts to control prejudiced responses. *Basic and Applied Social Psychology, 26*(2–3), 215–225.

Hebl, M., Foster, J., Mannix, L., & Dovidio, J. (2002). Formal and interpersonal discrimination: A field study of bias toward homosexual applicants. *Personality and Social Psychology Bulletin, 28,* 815–825.

Hehman, E., Stolier, R. M., & Freeman, J. B. (2015). Advanced mouse-tracking analytic techniques for enhancing psychological science. *Group Processes and Intergroup Relations, 18*(3), 384–401.

Heider, F. (1944). Social perception and phenomenal causality. *Psychological Review, 51,* 358–374.

Heider, F. (1958). *The psychology of interpersonal relations.* New York: Wiley.

Heilman, M. E. (2001). Description and prescription: How gender stereotypes prevent women's ascent up the organizational ladder. *Journal of Social Issues, 57*(4), 657–674.

Heilman, M. E., & Okimoto, T. G. (2007). Why are women penalized for success at male tasks? The implied communality deficit. *Journal of Applied Psychology, 92*(1), 81–92.

Heilman, M. E., Wallen, A. S., Fuchs, D., & Tamkins, M. M. (2004). Penalties for success: Reactions to women who succeed at male gender-typed tasks. *Journal of Applied Psychology, 89*(3), 416–427.

Hennes, E. P., Ruisch, B. C., Feygina, I., Monteiro, C. A., & Jost, J. T. (2016). Motivated recall in the service of the economic system: The case of anthropogenic climate change. *Journal of Experimental Psychology: General, 145*(6), 755–771.

Henry, P. J., & Sears, D. (2002). The Symbolic Racism Scale. *Political Psychology, 23,* 253–283.

Herr, P. M. (1986). Consequences of priming: Judgment and behavior. *Journal of Personality and Social Psychology, 51,* 1106–1115.

Herr, P. M., Sherman, S. J., & Fazio, R. H. (1983). On the consequences of priming: Assimilation and contrast effects. *Journal of Experimental Social Psychology, 19,* 323–340.

Hess, T. M., & Pullen, S. M. (1994). Adult age differences in impression change processes. *Psychology and Aging, 9*(2), 237–250.

Higginbotham, G. D., Shropshire, J., & Johnson, K. L. (2021). You play a sport, right? A persistent and pernicious intersectional bias in categorization of students vs. student-athletes. *Personality and Social Psychology Bulletin, 48*(11), 1531–1547.

Higgins, E. T. (1989). Self-discrepancy theory: What patterns of self-beliefs cause people to suffer? In L. Berkowitz (Ed.), *Advances in experimental social psychology* (Vol. 22, pp. 93–136). New York: Academic Press.

Higgins, E. T. (1996a). Knowledge activation: Accessibility, applicability, and salience. In E. T. Higgins & A. W. Kruglanski (Eds.), *Social psychology: Handbook of basic principles* (pp. 133–168). New York: Guilford Press.

Higgins, E. T. (1996b). The "self digest": Self-knowledge serving self-regulatory functions. *Journal of Personality and Social Psychology, 71,* 1062–1083.

Higgins, E. T. (2002). How self-regulation creates distinct values: The case of promotion and prevention decision making. *Journal of Consumer Psychology, 12*(3), 177–191.

Higgins, E. T., Bargh, J. A., & Lombardi, W. (1985). Nature of priming effects on categorization. *Journal of Experimental Psychology: Learning, Memory, and Cognition, 11,* 59–69.

Higgins, E. T., & Brendl, C. M. (1995). Accessibility and applicability: Some "activation rules" influencing judgment. *Journal of Experimental Social Psychology, 31,* 218–243.

Higgins, E. T., & Chaires, W. M. (1980). Accessibility of interrelational constructs: Implications for stimulus encoding and creativity. *Journal of Experimental Social Psychology, 16*(4), 348–361.

Higgins, E. T., Idson, L. C., Freitas, A. L., Spiegel, S., & Molden, D. C. (2003). Transfer of value from fit. *Journal of Personality and Social Psychology, 84*(6), 1140–1153.

Higgins, E. T., King, G. A., & Mavin, G. H. (1982). Individual construct accessibility and subjective impressions and recall. *Journal of Personality and Social Psychology, 43*(1), 35–47.

Higgins, E. T., Rholes, W. S., & Jones, C. R. (1977). Category accessibility and impression formation. *Journal of Experimental Social Psychology, 13,* 141–154.

Higgins, E. T., Roney, C., Crowe, E., & Hymes, C. (1994). Ideal versus ought predilections for approach and avoidance: Distinct self-regulatory systems. *Journal of Personality and Social Psychology, 66,* 276–286.

Hillard, A. L., Ryan, C. S., & Gervais, S. J. (2013). Reactions to the Implicit Association Test as an educational tool: A mixed methods study. *Social Psychology of Education, 16*(3), 495–516.

Hilton, D. J., & Slugoski, B. R. (1986). Knowledge-based causal attribution: The abnormal conditions focus model. *Psychological Review, 93,* 75–88.

Hilton, D. J., Smith, R. H., & Kim, S. H. (1995). Processes of causal explanation and dispositional attribution. *Journal of Personality and Social Psychology, 68*(3), 377–387.

Hinzman, L., & Maddox, K. B. (2017). Conceptual and visual representations of racial categories: Distinguishing subtypes from subgroups. *Journal of Experimental Social Psychology, 70,* 95–109.

Hodson, G., Dovidio, J. F., & Gaertner, S. L. (2002). Processes in racial discrimination: Differential weighting of conflicting information. *Personality and Social Psychology Bulletin, 28*(4), 460–471.

Hoffman, C., Mischel, W., & Mazze, K. (1981). The role of purpose in the organization of information about behavior: Trait-based versus goal-based categories in person cognition. *Journal of Personality and Social Psychology, 40*(2), 211–225.

Hoffman, K. M., Trawalter, S., Axt, J. R., & Oliver, M. N. (2016). Racial bias in pain assessment and treatment recommendations, and false beliefs about biological differences between Blacks and Whites. *PNAS Proceedings of the National Academy of Sciences of the USA, 113*(16), 4296–4301.

Hofmann, W., De Houwer, J., Perugini, M., Baeyens, F., & Crombez, G. (2010). Evaluative conditioning in humans: A meta-analysis. *Psychological Bulletin, 136*(3), 390–421.

Hogg, M. A. (2000). Subjective uncertainty reduction through self-categorization: A motivational theory of social identity processes. *European Review of Social Psychology, 11,* 223–255.

Hogg, M. A. (2007). Uncertainty-identity theory. In M. P. Zanna (Ed.), *Advances in experimental social psychology* (vol. 39, pp. 69–126). Cambridge, MA: Elsevier Academic Press.

Hogg, M. A. (2014). From uncertainty to extremism: Social categorization and identity processes. *Current Directions in Psychological Science, 23,* 338–342.

Hogg, M. A., & Blaylock, D. L. (Eds.). (2012). *Extremism and the psychology of uncertainty.* Boston: Wiley-Blackwell.

Hogg, M. A., & Reid, S. A. (2006). Social identity, self-categorization, and group norms. *Communication Theory, 16,* 7–30.

Holland, R. W., Hendriks, M., & Aarts, H. (2005). Smells like clean spirit: Nonconscious effects of scent on cognition and behavior. *Psychological Science, 16,* 689–693.

Holmes, D. S. (1970). Differential change in affective intensity and the forgetting of unpleasant personal experiences. *Journal of Personality and Social Psychology, 15,* 234–239.

Holmes, J., & Cameron, J., (2005). An integrative review of theories of interpersonal cognition: An interdependence theory perspective. In M. Baldwin (Ed.), *Interpersonal cognition* (pp. 415–447). New York: Guilford Press.

Hong, Y.-Y., Chiu, C.-Y., Dweck, C. S., Lin, D. M.-S., & Wan, W. (1999). Implicit theories, attributions, and coping: A meaning system approach. *Journal of Personality and Social Psychology, 77*(3), 588–599.

Hornsey, M. J. (2008). Social identity theory and self-categorization theory: A historical review. *Social and Personality Psychology Compass, 2*(1), 204–222.

Hornsey, M. J., & Jetten, J. (2004). The individual within the group: Balancing the need to belong with the need to be different. *Personality and Social Psychology Review, 8*(3), 248–264.

Howell, J. L., Collisson, B. D., Crysel, L., Garrido, C. O., Newell, S. M., Cottrell, C. A., et al. (2013). Managing the threat of impending implicit attitude feedback. *Social Psychological and Personality Science, 4,* 714–720.

Howell, J. L., Gaither, S. E., & Ratliff, K. A. (2015). Caught in the middle: Defensive responses to IAT feedback among Whites, Blacks, and biracial Black/Whites. *Social Psychological and Personality Science, 6*(4), 373–381.

Howell, J. L., & Ratliff, K. A. (2017). Not your average bigot: The better-than-average effect and defensive responding to Implicit Association Test feedback. *British Journal of Social Psychology, 56*(1), 2–21.

Howell, J. L., Redford, L., Pogge, G., & Ratliff, K. A. (2017). Defensive responding to IAT feedback. *Social Cognition, 35*(5), 520–562.

Howerton, D. M., Meltzer, A. L., & Olson, M. A. (2012). Honeymoon vacation: Sexual-orientation prejudice and inconsistent behavioral responses. *Basic and Applied Social Psychology, 34*(2), 146–151.

Hsu, N., Badura, K., Newman, D., & Speach, M. E. (2021). Gender, "masculinity," and "femininity": A meta-analytic review of gender differences in agency and communion. *Psychological Bulletin, 147*(10), 987–1011.

Hu, X., Gawronski, B., & Balas, R. (2017). Propositional versus dual-process accounts of evaluative conditioning: I. The effects of co-occurrence and relational information on implicit and explicit evaluations. *Personality and Social Psychology Bulletin, 43*(1), 17–32.

Huang, J. Y., & Bargh, J. A. (2014). The selfish goal: Autonomously operating motivational structures as the proximate cause of human judgment and behavior. *Behavioral and Brain Sciences, 37*(2), 121–135.

Hudson, S. T. J., & Ghani, A. (2021). *Sexual orientation and race mute the prescriptive nature of gender stereotypes.* Unpublished manuscript, Yale University, New Haven, CT.

Hugenberg, K., & Bodenhausen, G. V. (2003). Facing prejudice: Implicit prejudice and the perception of facial threat. *Psychological Science, 14*(6), 640–643.

Hugenberg, K., Young, S. G., Bernstein, M. J., & Sacco, D. F. (2010). The categorization-individuation model: An integrative account of the other-race recognition deficit. *Psychological Review, 117*(4), 1168–1187.

Hume, D. (1748/1961). An enquiry concerning human understanding. In S. Buckle (Ed.), *The empiricists.* New York: Dolphin Books.

Hunter, M. (2007). The persistent problem of colorism: Skin tone, status, and inequality. *Sociology Compass, 1*(1), 237–254.

Hupbach, A. (2013). When forgetting preserves memory. *Frontiers in Psychology, 4*(32), 1–9.

Hupbach, A. (2018). Long-term effects of directed forgetting. *Memory, 26*(3), 321–329.

Hupbach, A., Gomez, R., Hardt, O., & Nadel, L. (2007). Reconsolidation of episodic memories: A subtle reminder triggers integration of new information. *Learning and Memory, 14,* 47–53.

Hupbach, A., Gomez, R., & Nadel, L. (2009). Episodic memory reconsolidation: Updating or source confusion? *Memory, 17,* 502–510.

Hupbach, A., Gomez, R., & Nadel, L. (2015). Memory reconsolidation (invited chapter). In M. Barense, D. R. Addis, & A. Duarte (Eds.), *The cognitive neuroscience of human memory* (pp. 244–264). Hoboken, NJ: Wiley-Blackwell.

Hupbach, A., Olcaysoy Okten, I., & Horn, P. (2022). Directed forgetting in the social domain: Forgetting behaviors but not inferred traits. *Journal of Applied Research in Memory and Cognition, 11*(4), 522–533.

Ichheiser, G. (1943). Misinterpretations of personality in everyday life and the psychologist's frame of reference. *Character and Personality; A Quarterly for Psychodiagnostic and Allied Studies, 12,* 145–160.

Ijzerman, H., Gallucci, M., Pouw, W., Weißgerber, S., Van Doesum, N., & Williams, K. (2012). Cold-blooded loneliness: Social exclusion leads to lower skin temperatures. *Acta Psychologica, 140*(3), 283–288.

IJzerman, H., & Semin, G. R. (2009). The thermometer of social relations: Mapping social proximity on temperature. *Psychological Science, 20*(10), 1214–1220.

IJzerman, H., & Semin, G. R. (2010). Temperature perceptions as a ground for social proximity. *Journal of Experimental Social Psychology, 46,* 867–873.

Inzlicht, M., Kaiser, C. R., & Major, B. (2008). The face of chauvinism: How prejudice expectations shape perceptions of facial affect. *Journal of Experimental Social Psychology, 44*(3), 758–766.

Jacoby, L. L. (1991). A process dissociation framework: Separating automatic from intentional uses of memory. *Journal of Memory and Language, 30,* 513–541.

Jacoby, L. L., & Dallas, M. (1981). On the relationship between autobiographical memory and perceptual learning. *Journal of Experimental Psychology: General, 110,* 306–340.

Jacoby, L. L., Kelley, C., Brown, J., & Jasechko, J. (1989). Becoming famous overnight: Limits on the ability to avoid unconscious influences of the past. *Journal of Personality and Social Psychology, 56*(3), 326–338.

Jacoby, L. L., Toth, J. P., & Yonelinas, A. P. (1993). Separating conscious and unconscious influences of memory: Measuring recollection. *Journal of Experimental Psychology: General, 122,* 139–154.

Jacoby, L. L., & Whitehouse, K. (1989). An illusion of memory: False recognition influenced by unconscious perception. *Journal of Experimental Psychology: Learning, Memory, and Cognition, 20,* 304–317.

Jacoby, L. L., Woloshyn, V., & Kelley, C. M. (1989). Becoming famous without being recognized: Unconscious influences of memory provided by dividing attention. *Journal of Experimental Psychology: General, 118,* 115–125.

Jaeger, B., Todorov, A. T., Evans, A. M., & van Beest, I. (2020). Can we reduce facial biases? Persistent effects of facial trustworthiness on sentencing decisions. *Journal of Experimental Social Psychology, 90,* 104004.

James, W. (1890/1950). *The principles of psychology* (Vol. I & II). New York: Dover.

James, W. (1907/1991). *Pragmatism.* New York: Prometheus.

Janis, I. L. (1972). *Victims of groupthink: A psychological study of foreign-policy decisions and fiascoes.* Boston: Houghton Mifflin.

Janoff-Bulman, R., Sheikh, S., & Hepp, S. (2009). Proscriptive versus prescriptive morality: Two faces of moral regulation. *Journal of Personality and Social Psychology, 96*(3), 521–537.

Jarvis, W. B. G., & Petty, R. E. (1996). The need to evaluate. *Journal of Personality and Social Psychology, 70,* 172–194.

Jaspars, J., Hewstone, M., & Fincham, F. D. (1983). Attribution theory and research: The state of the art. In J. M. F. Jaspars, F. D. Fincham, & M. R. C. Hewstone (Eds.), *Attribution theory: Conceptual, developmental and social dimensions* (pp. 3–26). San Diego, CA: Academic Press.

Jerónimo, R., Garcia-Marques, L., Ferreira, M. B., & Macrae, C. N. (2015). When expectancies harm comprehension: Encoding flexibility in impression formation. *Journal of Experimental Social Psychology, 61,* 110–119.

Jetten, J., Hogg, M. A., & Mullin, B. A. (2000). Ingroup variability and motivation to reduce subjective uncertainty. *Group Dynamics: Theory, Research, and Practice, 4,* 184–198.

Jetten, J., Spears, R., & Manstead, A. S. R. (1996). Intergroup norms and intergroup discrimination: Distinctive self-categorization and social identity effects. *Journal of Personality and Social Psychology, 71,* 1222–1233.

Johnson, H. M., & Seifert, C. M. (1994). Sources of the continued influence effect: When misinformation in memory affects later inferences. *Journal of Experimental Psychology: Learning, Memory, and Cognition, 20*(6), 1420–1436.

Johnson, K. L., Lick, D. J., & Carpinella, C. M. (2015). Emergent research in social vision: An integrated approach to the determinants and consequences of social categorization. *Social and Personality Psychology Compass, 9*(1), 15–30.

Johnson, K. L., & Tassinary, L. G. (2005). Perceiving sex directly and indirectly: Meaning in motion and morphology. *Psychological Science, 3,* 890–897.

Johnson, K. L., & Tassinary, L. G. (2007). The functional significance of the WHR in judgments of attractiveness. In V. Swami & A. Furnham (Eds.), *Body beautiful: Evolutionary and socio-cultural perspectives* (pp. 159–184). New York: Palgrave MacMillan.

Johnson, M. K. (1988). Reality monitoring: An experimental phenomenological approach. *Journal of Experimental Psychology, 117*(4), 390–394.

Johnson, M. K., Hashtroudi, S., & Lindsay, D. S. (1993). Source monitoring. *Psychological Bulletin, 114,* 3–28.

Johnson, M. K., & Raye, C. L. (1981). Reality monitoring. *Psychological Review, 88,* 67–85.

Jonas, E., Fritsche, I., & Greenberg, J. (2005). Currencies as cultural symbols—An existential psychological perspective on reactions of Germans toward the euro. *Journal of Economic Psychology, 26*(1), 129–146.

Jones, E. E. (1979). The rocky road from acts to dispositions. *American Psychologist, 34,* 107–117.

Jones, E. E. (1990). *Interpersonal perception.* New York: Macmillan.

Jones, E. E., & Berglas, S. (1978). Control of attributions about the self through self-handicapping strategies: The appeal of alcohol and the role of underachievement. *Journal of Personality and Social Psychology, 4,* 200–206.

Jones, E. E., & Davis, K. E. (1965). From acts to dispositions: The attribution process in person perception. In L. Berkowitz (Ed.), *Advances in experimental social psychology* (Vol. 2, pp. 219–266). New York: Academic Press.

Jones, E. E., Davis, K. E., & Gergen, K. J. (1961). Role playing variations and their informational value for person perception. *Journal of Abnormal and Social Psychology, 63,* 302–310.

Jones, E. E., & Harris, V. A. (1967). The attribution of attitudes. *Journal of Experimental Social Psychology, 3,* 1–24.

Jones, E. E., & Nisbett, R. E. (1972). The actor and the observer: Divergent perceptions of the causes of behavior. In E. E. Jones, D. E. Kanouse, H. H. Kelley, R. E. Nisbett, S. Valins, & B. Weiner (Eds.), *Attribution: Perceiving the causes of behavior* (pp. 79–84). Hillsdale, NJ: Erlbaum.

Jost, J. T. (2019a). A quarter century of system justification theory: Questions, answers, criticisms, and societal applications. *British Journal of Social Psychology, 58*(2), 263–314.

Jost, J. T. (2019b). The IAT is dead, long live the IAT: Context-sensitive measures of implicit attitudes are indispensable to social and political psychology. *Current Directions in Psychological Science, 28*(1), 10–19.

Jost, J. T. (2020). *A theory of system justification.* Cambridge, MA: Harvard University Press.

Jost, J. T., & Banaji, M. R. (1994). The role of stereotyping in system-justification and the production of false consciousness. *British Journal of Social Psychology, 33*(1), 1–27.

Jost, J. T., Glaser, J., Kruglanski, A. W., & Sulloway, F. J. (2003). Political conservatism as motivated social cognition. *Psychological Bulletin, 129*(3), 339–375.

Jost, J. T., & Hunyady, O. (2005). Antecedents and consequences of system-justifying ideologies. *Current Directions in Psychological Science, 14,* 260–265.

Jost, J. T., Ledgerwood, A., & Hardin, C. D. (2008). Shared reality, system justification, and the relational basis of ideological beliefs. *Social and Personality Psychology Compass, 2,* 171–186.

Jost, J. T., Rudman, L. A., Blair, I. V., Carney, D. R., Dasgupta, N., Glaser, J., et al. (2009). The existence of implicit bias is beyond reasonable doubt: A refutation of ideological and methodological objections and executive summary of ten studies that no manager should ignore. *Research in Organizational Behavior, 29,* 39–69.

Judd, C. M., James-Hawkins, L., Yzerbyt, V., & Kashima, Y. (2005). Fundamental dimensions of social judgment: Understanding the relations between judgments of competence and warmth. *Journal of Personality and Social Psychology, 89*(6), 899–913.

Jung, J., Bramson, A., Crano, W., Page, S., & Miller, J. H. (2021). Cultural drift, indirect minority influence, network structure, and their impacts on cultural change and diversity. *American Psychologist, 76,* 1039–1053.

Kahneman, D. (1973). *Attention and effort.* Englewood Cliffs, NJ: Prentice-Hall.

Kahneman, D. (2011). *Thinking, fast and slow.* New York: Farrar, Straus & Giroux.

Kahneman, D., & Miller, D. (1986). Norm theory: Comparing reality to its alternatives. *Psychological Review, 93,* 136–153.

Kahneman, D., & Snell, J. (1992). Predicting a changing taste: Do people know what they will like? *Journal of Behavioral Decision Making, 5,* 187–200.

Kahneman, D., & Tversky, A. (1979). Prospect theory: An analysis of decision under risk. *Econometrica, 47*(2), 263–291.

Kahneman, D., & Tversky, A. (1982). The simulation heuristic. In D. Kahneman, P. Slovic, & A. Tversky (Eds.), *Judgment under uncertainty: Heuristics and biases* (pp. 201–208). New York: Cambridge University Press.

Kahneman, D., & Tversky, A. (1984). Choices, values, and frames. *American Psychologist, 39*(4), 341–350.

Kaiser, C. R., & Miller, C. T. (2001). Reacting to impending discrimination: Compensation for prejudice and attributions to discrimination. *Personality and Social Psychology Bulletin, 27*(10), 1357–1367.

Kanouse, D. E., & Hanson, L. R., Jr. (1972). Negativity in evaluations. In E. E. Jones, D. E. Kanouse, H. H. Kelley, R. E. Nisbett, S. Valins, & B. Weiner (Eds.), *Attribution: Perceiving the causes of behavior* (pp. 47–62). Hillsdale, NJ: Erlbaum.

Kant, I. (1781/1990). *Critque of pure reason* (J. M. D. Meidlejohn, Trans.). Buffalo, NY: Prometheus Books.

Kashima, Y. (2000). Maintaining cultural stereotypes in the serial reproduction of narratives. *Personality and Social Psychology Bulletin, 26,* 594–604.

Kassin, S. M., & Kiechel, K. L. (1996). The social psychology of false confessions: Compliance, internalization, and confabulation. *Psychological Science, 7*(3), 125–128.

Kassin, S. M., & Sukel, H. (1997). Coerced confessions and the jury: An experimental test of the "harmless error" rule. *Law and Human Behavior, 21*(1), 27–46.

Katz, D., & Braly, K. W. (1933). Racial stereotypes of 100 college students. *Journal of Abnormal and Social Psychology, 28*, 280–290.

Kawakami, K., Dovidio, J., Moll, J., Hermsen, S., & Russin, A. (2000). Just say no (to stereotyping): Effects of training in the negation of stereotype associations on stereotype activation. *Journal of Personality and Social Psychology, 78*, 871–888.

Kawakami, K., Dunn, E., Karmali, F., & Dovidio, J. F. (2009). Mispredicting affective and behavioral responses to racism. *Science, 323*(5911), 276–278.

Kawakami, K., Young, H., & Dovidio, J. F. (2002). Automatic stereotyping: Category, trait, and behavioral activations. *Personality and Social Psychology Bulletin, 28*(1), 3–15.

Kelley, H. H. (1967). Attribution theory in social psychology. In D. Levine (Ed.), *Nebraska Symposium on Motivation* (Vol. 15, pp. 192–238). Lincoln: University of Nebraska Press.

Kelley, H. H. (1972a). Attribution in social interaction. In E. E. Jones, D. E. Kanouse, H. H. Kelley, R. E. Nisbett, S. Valens, & B. Weiner (Eds.), *Attribution: Perceiving the causes of behavior* (pp. 1–26). Morristown, NJ: General Learning Press.

Kelley, H. H. (1972b). Causal schemata and the attribution process. In E. E. Jones, D. E. Kanouse, H. H. Kelley, R. E. Nisbett, S. Valins, & B. Weiner (Eds.), *Attribution: Perceiving the causes of behavior* (pp. 151–174). Morristown, NJ: General Learning Press.

Kelley, H. H. (1973). Processes of causal attribution. *American Psychologist, 28*, 107–128.

Kelley, H. H., & Michela, J. L. (1980). Attribution theory and research. *Annual Review of Psychology, 31*, 457–501.

Kelly, G. (1955). *A theory of personality: The psychology of personal constructs*. New York: Norton.

Kenny, D. A. (1994). *Interpersonal perception: A social relations analysis*. New York: Guilford Press.

Kenny, D. A., Horner, C., Kashy, D. A., & Chu, L. (1992). Consensus at zero acquaintance: Replication, behavioral cues, and stability. *Journal of Personality and Social Psychology, 62*(1), 88–97.

Kihlstrom, J. F., & Klein, S. B. (1994). The self as a knowledge structure. In R. S. Wyer, Jr., & T. K. Srull (Eds.), *Handbook of social cognition: Applications* (2nd ed., Vol. 2, pp. 153–208). Hillsdale, NJ: Erlbaum.

Kille, D. R., Forest, A. L., & Wood, J. V. (2013). Tall, dark, and stable: Embodiment motivates mate selection preferences. *Psychological Science, 24*(1), 112–114.

Kleiman, T., & Hassin, R. R. (2013). When conflicts are good: Nonconscious goal conflicts reduce confirmatory thinking. *Journal of Personality and Social Psychology, 105*, 374–387.

Kleiman, T., Stern, C., & Trope, Y. (2016). When the spatial and ideological collide: Metaphorical conflict shapes social perception. *Psychological Science, 27*(3), 375–383.

Klein, S. B., Loftus, J., Trafton, J. G., & Fuhrman, R. W. (1992). Use of exemplars and abstractions in trait judgments: A model of trait knowledge about the self and others. *Journal of Personality and Social Psychology, 63*, 739–753.

Knowles, E. D., Lowery, B. S., Hogan, C. M., & Chow, R. M. (2009). On the malleability of ideology: Motivated construals of color blindness. *Journal of Personality and Social Psychology, 96*, 857–869.

Knowles, E. D., Lowery, B. S., & Schaumberg, R. L. (2010). Racial prejudice predicts opposition to Obama and his health care reform plan. *Journal of Experimental Social Psychology, 46*(2), 420–423.

Koole, S. L., Smeets, K., van Knippenberg, A., & Dijksterhuis, A. (1999). The cessation of rumination through self-affirmation. *Journal of Personality and Social Psychology, 77*(1), 111–125.

Korman, J., & Malle, B. F. (2016). Grasping for traits or reasons? How people grapple with puzzling social behaviors. *Personality and Social Psychology Bulletin, 42*(11), 1451–1465.

Krieglmeyer, R., & Sherman, J. W. (2012). Disentangling stereotype activation and stereotype application in the stereotype misperception task. *Journal of Personality and Social Psychology, 103*(2), 205–224.

Kruglanski, A. W. (1990). Motivations for judging and knowing: Implications for causal attribution. In E. T. Higgins & R. M. Sorrentino (Eds.), *Handbook of motivation and cogni-*

tion (Vol. 2, pp. 333–368). New York: Guilford Press.

Kruglanski, A. W., Erb, H. P., Pierro, A., Mannetti, L., & Chun, W. Y. (2006). On parametric continuities in the world of binary either ors. *Psychological Inquiry, 17,* 153–165.

Kruglanski, A. W., & Freund, T. (1983). The freezing and unfreezing of lay inferences: Effects on impressional primacy, ethnic stereotyping, and numerical anchoring. *Journal of Experimental Social Psychology, 19,* 448–468.

Kruglanski, A. W., & Mackie, D. M. (1990). Majority and minority influence: A judgmental process analysis. In W. Stroebe & M. Hewstone (Eds.), *European review of social psychology* (Vol. 1, pp. 229–261). Chichester, UK: Wiley.

Kruglanski, A. W., Shah, J. Y., Fishbach, A., Friedman, R., Chun, W. Y., & Sleeth-Keppler, D. (2002). A theory of goal systems. In M. P. Zanna (Ed.), *Advances in experimental social psychology* (Vol. 34, pp. 331–378). San Diego, CA: Academic Press.

Kruschke, J. K. (2003). Attention in learning. *Current Directions in Psychological Science, 12*(5), 171–175.

Kubota, J., Banaji, M., & Phelps, E. (2012). The neuroscience of race. *Nature Neuroscience, 15,* 940–948.

Kugler, M., Jost, J. T., & Noorbaloochi, S. (2014). Another look at moral foundations theory: Do authoritarianism and social dominance orientation explain liberal–conservative differences in "moral" intuitions? *Social Justice Research, 27*(4), 413–431.

Külpe, O. (1904). Versuche über abstraktion. *Berlin International Congress of Experimental Psychology,* 56–68.

Kunda, Z. (1987). Motivated inference: Self-serving generation and evaluation of causal theories. *Journal of Personality and Social Psychology, 53*(4), 636–647.

Kunda, Z., & Oleson, K. C. (1995). Maintaining stereotypes in the face of disconfirmation: Constructing grounds for subtyping deviants. *Journal of Personality and Social Psychology, 68,* 565–579.

Kunda, Z., Sinclair, L., & Griffin, D. (1997, April). Equal ratings but separate meanings: Stereotypes and the construal of traits. *Journal of Personality and Social Psychology, 72*(4), 720–734.

Kunda, Z., & Thagard, P. (1996). Forming impressions from stereotypes, trait, and behaviors: A parallel constraint satisfaction theory. *Psychological Review, 103,* 284–308.

Kurdi, B., & Banaji, M. R. (2017). Repeated evaluative pairings and evaluative statements: How effectively do they shift implicit attitudes? *Journal of Experimental Psychology: General, 146*(2), 194–213.

Kurdi, B., & Banaji, M. R. (2019). Attitude change via repeated evaluative pairings versus evaluative statements: Shared and unique features. *Journal of Personality and Social Psychology, 116*(5), 681–703.

Kurdi, B., & Banaji, M. R. (2023). Implicit person memory: Domain-general and domain-specific processes of learning and change. In E. Balcetis & G. B. Moskowitz (Eds.), *Handbook of impression formation: A social psychological approach* (pp. 459–488). New York: Routledge.

Kurdi, B., Morehouse, K. N., & Dunham, Y. (2023). How do explicit and implicit evaluations shift? A preregistered meta-analysis of the effects of co-occurrence and relational information. *Journal of Personality and Social Psychology, 124*(6), 1174–1202.

Kurdi, B., Seitchik, A. E., Axt, J. R., Carroll, T. J., Karapetyan, A., Kaushik, N., et al. (2019). Relationship between the Implicit Association Test and intergroup behavior: A meta-analysis. *American Psychologist, 74*(5), 569–586.

Lakoff, G., & Johnson, M. (1999). *Philosophy in the flesh: The embodied mind and its challenge to Western thought.* New York: Basic Books.

Lambert, A. J., Cronen, S., Chasteen, A. L., & Lickel, B. (1996). Private vs public expressions of racial prejudice. *Journal of Experimental Social Psychology, 32*(5), 437–459.

Lambert, W. E., & Klineberg, O. (1967). *Children's views of foreign people's.* New York: Appleton.

Lamer, S. A., Dvorak, P., Biddle, A., Pauker, K., & Weisbuch, M. (2022). The transmission of gender stereotypes through televised patterns of nonverbal emotion. *Journal of Personality and Social Psychology, 123*(6), 1315–1335.

Lamer, S. A., & Weisbuch, M. (2019). Men over women: The social transmission of gender stereotypes through spatial elevation. *Journal of Experimental Social Psychology, 84,* 103828.

Landau, M. J., Meier, B. P., & Keefer, L. A. (2010). A metaphor-enriched social cognition. *Psychological Bulletin, 136*(6), 1045–1067.

Langer, E., Blank, A., & Chanowitz, B. (1978). The mindlessness of ostensibly thoughtful action: The role of "placebic" information in interpersonal interaction. *Journal of Personality and Social Psychology, 3*(6), 635–642.

Lapka, S. P., Kung, F. Y. H., Brienza, J. P., & Scholer, A. A. (2023). Determined yet dehumanized: People higher in self-control are seen as more robotic. *Social Psychological and Personality Science, 14*(2), 117–129.

Latane, B., & Darley, J. M. (1970). *The unresponsive bystander: Why doesn't he help?* Englewood Cliffs, NJ: Prentice-Hall.

Leander, P., Chartrand, T., & Bargh, J. (2012). You give me the chills: Embodied reactions to inappropriate amounts of behavioral mimicry. *Psychological Science, 23*(7), 772–779.

Lee, A. Y., & Aaker, J. L. (2004). Bringing the frame into focus: The influence of regulatory fit on processing fluency and persuasion. *Journal of Personality and Social Psychology, 86*(2), 205–218.

Lee, H., Shimizu, Y., Masuda, T., & Uleman, J. S. (2017). Cultural differences in spontaneous trait and situational inferences. *Journal of Cross Cultural Psychology, 48*(5), 627–643.

Lefcourt, H. M. (1976). Locus of control and the response to aversive events. *Ontario Psychologist, 8*(5), 41–49.

Legault, L., Gutsell, J. N., & Inzlicht, M. (2011). Ironic effects of antiprejudice messages: How motivational interventions can reduce (but also increase) prejudice. *Psychological Science, 22*(12), 1472–1477.

Lenz, G. S., & Lawson, C. (2011). Looking the part: Television leads less informed citizens to vote based on candidates' appearance. *American Journal of Political Science, 55*(3), 574–589.

Lepore, L., & Brown, R. (1997). Category and stereotype activation: Is prejudice inevitable? *Journal of Personality and Social Psychology, 72,* 275–287.

Lerner, M. J. (1965). The effect of responsibility and choice on a partner's attractiveness following failure. *Journal of Personality, 33,* 178–187.

Lerner, M. J., & Miller, D. T. (1978). Just world research and the attribution process: Looking back and ahead. *Psychological Bulletin, 85*(5), 1030–1051.

Levin, D. T., & Banaji, M. R. (2006). Distortions in the perceived lightness of faces: The role of race categories. *Journal of Experimental Psychology: General, 135*(4), 501–512.

Lewandowsky, S., Ecker, U. K., Seifert, C. M., Schwarz, N., & Cook, J. (2012). Misinformation and its correction: Continued influence and successful debiasing. *Psychological Science in the Public Interest, 13*(3), 106–131.

Lewin, K. (1935). *A dynamic theory of personality: Selected papers* (D. K. Adams & K. E. Zener, Trans.). New York: McGraw Hill.

Leyens, J. P., Cortes, B. P., Demoulin, S., Dovidio, J. F., Fiske, S. T., & Gaunt, R. (2003). Emotional prejudice, essentialism, and nationalism. *European Journal of Social Psychology, 33,* 704–717.

Leyens, J., & Fiske, S. T. (1994). Impression formation: From recitals to symphonie fantastique. In P. G. Devine, D. L. Hamilton, & T. M. Ostrom (Eds.), *Social cognition: Impact on social psychology* (pp. 39–75). San Diego, CA: Academic Press.

Liberman, N., Molden, D. C., Idson, L. C., & Higgins, E. T. (2001). Promotion and prevention focus on alternative hypotheses: Implications for attributional functions. *Journal of Personality and Social Psychology, 80*(1), 5–18.

Liberman, N., Sagristano, M. D., & Trope, Y. (2002). The effect of temporal distance on level of mental construal. *Journal of Experimental Social Psychology, 38*(6), 523–534.

Lick, D. J., & Johnson, K. L. (2016). Straight until proven gay: A systematic bias toward straight categorizations in sexual orientation judgments. *Journal of Personality and Social Psychology, 110,* 801–817.

Lieberman, M. (2007). Social cognitive neuroscience: A review of core processes. *Annual Review of Psychology, 58,* 259–289.

Lieberman, M. D., Hariri, A., Jarcho, J. M., Eisenberger, N. I., & Bookheimer, S. Y. (2005). An fMRI investigation of race-related amygdala activity in African-American and Caucasian-American individuals. *Nature Neuroscience, 8*(6), 720–722.

Lin, C., Keles, U., & Adolphs, R. (2021). Four dimensions characterize attributions from faces using a representative set of English trait words. *Nature Communications, 12,* 51–68.

Lin, S.-Y. (2017). *White Americans' legitimizing reasoning of police violence: In defense of America's moral image and maintenance of racial hierarchy.* Unpublished doctoral thesis, Lehigh University, Bethlehem, PA.

Lindsay, D. S., & Jacoby, L. L. (1994). Stroop process dissociations: The relationship between facilitation and interference. *Journal of Experimental Psychology: Human Perception and Performance, 20*(2), 219–234.

Lingle, J. H., Altom, M. W., & Medin, D. L. (1984). Of cabbages and kings: Assessing the extendibility of natural object concepts models to social things. In R. S. Wyer & T. K. Srull (Eds.), *Handbook of social cognition* (Vol. 1, pp. 71–118). Hillsdale, NJ: Erlbaum.

Linville, P. W., Fischer, G. W., & Yoon, C. (1996). Perceived covariation among the features of ingroup and outgroup members: The outgroup covariation effect. *Journal of Personality and Social Psychology, 70*(3), 421–436.

Linville, P. W., & Jones, E. E. (1980). Polarized appraisals of outgroup members. *Journal of Personality and Social Psychology, 38*, 689–703.

Linville, P. W., Salovey, P., & Fischer, G. W. (1986). Stereotyping and perceived distributions of social characteristics: An application to ingroup–outgroup perception. In J. F. Dovidio & S. L. Gaertner (Eds.), *Prejudice, discrimination, and racism* (pp. 165–208). New York: Academic Press.

Lipman, J. (2018). How diversity training infuriates men and fails women. *Time.* Retrieved from *https://time.com/5118035/diversity-training-infuriates-men-fails-women.*

Lippmann, W. (1922). *Public opinion.* New York: Harcourt, Brace, Jovanovitch.

Lissner, K. (1933). Die entspannung von bedürfnissen durch ersatzhandlungen [The relaxation of needs through substitutive acts]. *Psychologische Forschung, 18*, 218–250.

Livingston, R. W., & Brewer, M. B. (2002). What are we really priming? Cue-based versus category-based processing of facial stimuli. *Journal of Personality and Social Psychology, 82*(1), 5–18.

Livingston, R. W., Rosette, A. S., & Washington, E. F. (2012). Can an agentic Black woman get ahead? The impact of race and interpersonal dominance on perceptions of female leaders. *Psychological Science, 23*(4), 354–358.

Locke, J. (1690/1961). An essay concerning human understanding. In D. Hume (Ed.), *The empiricists.* New York: Dolphin Books.

Locksley, A., Borgida, E., Brekke, N., & Hepburn, C. (1980). Sex stereotypes and social judgment. *Journal of Personality and Social Psychology, 39*, 821–831.

Locksley, A., Hepburn, C., & Ortiz, V. (1982). Social stereotypes and judgments of individuals: An instance of the base-rate fallacy. *Journal of Experimental Social Psychology, 18*, 23–42.

Logan, G. D. (1989). Automaticity and cognitive control. In J. S. Uleman & J. A. Bargh (Eds.), *Unintended thought* (pp. 52–74). New York: Guilford Press.

Lombardi, W. J., Higgins, E. T., & Bargh, J. A. (1987). The role of consciousness in priming effects on categorization. *Personality and Social Psychology Bulletin, 13*, 411–429.

Lord, C. G., Ross, L., & Lepper, M. R. (1979). Biased assimilation and attitude polarization: The effects of prior theories on subsequently considered evidence. *Journal of Personality and Social Psychology, 37*, 2098–2109.

Lorge, I., & Curtiss, C. C. (1936). Prestige, suggestion, and attitudes. *Journal of Social Psychology, 7*, 386–402.

Loughnan, S., & Haslam, N. (2007). Animals and androids: Implicit associations between social categories and nonhumans. *Psychological Science, 18*(2), 116–121.

Lowery, B. S., Hardin, C. D., & Sinclair, S. (2001). Social influence effects on automatic racial prejudice. *Journal of Personality and Social Psychology, 81*, 842–855.

Lyons, A., & Kashima, Y. (2003). How are stereotypes maintained through communication? The influence of stereotype sharedness. *Journal of Personality and Social Psychology, 85*(6), 989–1005.

Lyubomirsky, S. (2022). *The how of happiness: A scientific approach to getting the life you want.* New York: Penguin Press.

Ma, D. S., Correll, J., & Wittenbrink, B. (2015). The Chicago Face Database: A free stimulus set of faces and norming data. *Behavior Research Methods, 47*(4), 1122–1135.

Ma, D. S., Correll, J., Wittenbrink, B., Bar-Anan, Y., Sriram, N., & Nosek, B. A. (2013). When fatigue turns deadly: The association between fatigue and racial bias in the decision to shoot. *Basic and Applied Social Psychology, 35*(6), 515–524.

Ma, N., Vandekerckhove, M., Baetens, K., Van Overwalle, F., Seurinck, R., & Fias, W. (2012). Inconsistencies in spontaneous and intentional trait inferences. *Social Cognitive and Affective Neuroscience, 7*(8), 937–950.

Maass, A., Milesi, A., Zabbini, S., & Stahlberg,

D. (1995). Linguistic intergroup bias: Differential expectancies or in-group protection? *Journal of Personality and Social Psychology, 68,* 116–126.

MacDonald, T. K., & Zanna, M. P. (1998). Cross-dimension ambivalence towards social groups: Can ambivalence affect intentions to hire feminists? *Personality and Social Psychology Bulletin, 24,* 427–441.

MacLin, O. H., & Malpass, R. S. (2001). Racial categorization of faces: The ambiguous race face effect. *Psychology, Public Policy, and Law, 7*(1), 98–118.

Macrae, C. N., Bodenhausen, G. V., & Milne, A. B. (1995). The dissection of selection in person perception: Inhibitory processes in social stereotyping. *Journal of Personality and Social Psychology, 69,* 397–407.

Macrae, C. N., Bodenhausen, G. V., Milne, A. B., & Jetten, J. (1994). Out of mind but back in sight: Stereotypes on the rebound. *Journal of Personality and Social Psychology, 67,* 808–817.

Macrae, C. N., Hewstone, M., & Griffiths, R. J. (1993). Processing load and memory for stereotype-based information. *European Journal of Social Psychology, 23,* 77–87.

Macrae, C. N., & MacLeod, M. D. (1999). On recollections lost: When practice makes imperfect. *Journal of Personality and Social Psychology, 77,* 463–473.

Macrae, C. N., & Martin, D. (2007). A boy primed Sue: Feature-based processing and person construal. *European Journal of Social Psychology, 37*(5), 793–805.

Macrae, C. N., Milne, A. B., & Bodenhausen, G. V. (1994). Stereotypes as energy-saving devices: A peek inside the cognitive toolbox. *Journal of Personality and Social Psychology, 66,* 37–47.

Maddox, K. B. (2004). Perspectives on racial phenotypicality bias. *Personality and Social Psychology Review, 8*(4), 383–401.

Maddox, K. B., & Chase, S. G. (2004). Manipulating subcategory salience: Exploring the link between skin tone and social perception of Blacks. *European Journal of Social Psychology, 34*(5), 533–546.

Maddox, K. B., & Dukes, K. N. (2008). Social categorization and beyond: How facial features impact social judgment. In N. Ambady & J. J. Skowronski (Eds.), *First impressions* (pp. 205–233). New York: Guilford Press.

Maddox, K. B., & Gray, S. A. (2002). Cognitive representations of Black Americans: Reexploring the role of skin tone. *Personality and Social Psychology Bulletin, 28*(2), 250–259.

Maddox, K. B., Rapp, D. N., Brion, S., & Taylor, H. A. (2008). Social influences on spatial memory. *Memory and Cognition, 36*(3), 479–494.

Maheswaran, D., & Chaiken, S. (1991). Promoting systematic processing in low motivation settings: The effect of incongruent information on processing and judgment. *Journal of Personality and Social Psychology, 61,* 13–25.

Mahler, W. (1933). Ersatzhandlungen verschiedenen Realitaetsgrades. Untersuchungen zur Handlungs- und Affektpsychologie XV. Herausgegeben von K. Lewin. *Psychologische Forschung, 18,* 27–89.

Maio, G. R., Greenland, K., Bernard, M., & Esses, V. M. (2001). Effects of intergroup ambivalence on information processing: The role of physiological arousal. *Group Processes and Intergroup Relations, 4,* 355–372.

Maio, G. R., & Haddock, G. (2004). *The psychology of attitudes and attitude change.* London: Sage.

Major, B. (1994). From social inequality to personal entitlement: The role of social comparisons, legitimacy appraisals, and group membership. In M. P. Zanna (Ed.), *Advances in experimental social psychology* (Vol. 26, pp. 293–348). San Diego, CA: Academic Press.

Major, B., & Crocker, J. (1993). Social stigma: The consequences of attributional ambiguity. In D. M. Mackie & D. L. Hamilton (Eds.), *Affect, cognition, and stereotyping: Interactive processes in group perception* (pp. 345–370). San Diego, CA: Academic Press.

Malle, B. F. (1999). How people explain behavior: A new theoretical framework. *Personality and Social Psychology Review, 3*(1), 23–48.

Malle, B. F., & Holbrook, J. (2012). Is there a hierarchy of social inferences? The likelihood and speed of inferring intentionality, mind, and personality. *Journal of Personality and Social Psychology, 102*(4), 661–684.

Mandel, D. R., & Lehman, D. R. (1996). Counterfactual thinking and ascriptions of cause and preventability. *Journal of Personality and Social Psychology, 71*(3), 450–463.

Mandler, G. (1980). Recognizing: The judgment of previous occurrence. *Psychological Review, 87*(3), 252–271.

Manis, M., Nelson, T. E., & Shedler, J. (1988).

Stereotypes and social judgment: Extremity, assimilation, and contrast. *Journal of Personality and Social Psychology, 55,* 28–36.

Mann, T. C., & Ferguson, M. J. (2015). Can we undo our first impressions? The role of reinterpretation in reversing implicit evaluations. *Journal of Personality and Social Psychology, 108*(6), 823–849.

Mann, T. C., & Ferguson, M. J. (2017). Reversing implicit first impressions through reinterpretation after a two-day delay. *Journal of Experimental Social Psychology, 68,* 122–127.

Mann, T. C., Kurdi, B., & Banaji, M. R. (2020). How effectively can implicit evaluations be updated? Using evaluative statements after aversive repeated evaluative pairings. *Journal of Experimental Psychology: General, 149*(6), 1169–1192.

Maoz, I., Ward, A., Katz, M., & Ross, L. (2002). Reactive devaluation of an "Israeli" vs. "Palestinian" peace proposal. *Journal of Conflict Resolution, 46*(4), 515–546.

March, D. S., & Gaertner, L. (2021). A method for estimating the time of initiating correct categorization in mouse-tracking. *Behavior Research Methods, 53*(6), 2439–2449.

March, D. S., Gaertner, L., & Olson, M. A. (2021). Danger or dislike: Distinguishing threat from negative valence as sources of automatic anti-Black bias. *Journal of Personality and Social Psychology, 121*(5), 984–1004.

Marciq, A. V., Roberts, S., & Church, R. M. (1981). Methamphetamine and time estimation. *Journal of Experimental Psychology: Animal Behavior Processes, 7,* 18–30.

Markman, K. D., Lindberg, M. J., Kray, L. J., & Galinsky, A. D. (2007). Implications of counterfactual structure for creative generation and analytical problem solving. *Personality and Social Psychology Bulletin, 33*(3), 312–324.

Markus, H. (1977). Self-schemata and processing information about the self. *Journal of Personality and Social Psychology, 35,* 63–78.

Markus, H. R., & Kitayama, S. (1991). Culture and the self: Implications for cognition, emotion, and motivation. *Psychological Review, 98,* 224–253.

Markus, H., & Zajonc, R. B. (1985). The cognitive perspective in social psychology. In G. Lindzey & E. Aronson (Eds.), *The handbook of social psychology* (3rd ed., pp. 137–230). New York: Random House.

Marques, J., Yzerbyt, V., & Leyens, J-P. (1988).

The "black sheep effect": Extremity of judgments towards ingroup members as a function of group identification. *European Journal of Social Psychology, 18,* 1–16.

Marr, D. (1982). *Vision: A computational investigation into the human representation and processing of visual information.* London: Freeman.

Marsh, R. L., Bink, M. L., & Hicks, J. L. (1999). Conceptual priming in a generative problem-solving task. *Memory and Cognition, 27*(2), 355–363.

Marsh, R. L., Landau, J. D., & Hicks, J. L. (1996). How examples may (and may not) constrain creativity. *Memory and Cognition, 24*(5), 669–680.

Marsh, R. L., Landau, J. D., & Hicks, J. L. (1997). Contributions of inadequate source monitoring to unconscious plagiarism during idea generation. *Journal of Experimental Psychology: Learning, Memory, and Cognition, 23*(4), 886–897.

Marsh, R. L., Ward, T. B., & Landau, J. D. (1999). The inadvertent use of prior knowledge in a generative cognitive task. *Memory and Cognition, 27,* 94–105.

Martin, J. (1986). The tolerance of injustice. In J. M. Olson, C. P. Herman, & M. P. Zanna (Eds.), *Relative deprivation and social comparison: The Ontario symposium* (Vol. 4, pp. 157–175). Hillsdale, NJ: Erlbaum.

Martin, L. L. (1986). Set/reset: Use and disuse of concepts in impression formation. *Journal of Personality and Social Psychology, 51,* 493–504.

Martin, L. L., Seta, J. J., & Crelia, R. A. (1990). Assimilation and contrast as a function of people's willingness and ability to expend effort in forming an impression. *Journal of Personality and Social Psychology, 59,* 27–37.

Martin, L., & Tesser, A. (1996). Some ruminative thoughts. In R. S. Wyer (Ed.), *Advances in social cognition* (Vol. 9, pp. 1–48). Hillsdale, NJ: Erlbaum.

Martin, L. L., & Tesser, A. (2009). Five markers of motivated behavior. In G. B. Moskowitz & H. Grant (Eds.), *The psychology of goals* (pp. 257–276). New York: Guilford Press.

Maslow, A. H. (1943). The authoritarian character structure. *Journal of Social Psychology, 18,* 401–411.

Mather, M., & Johnson, M. K. (2000). Choice-supportive source monitoring: Do our decisions seem better to us as we age? *Psychology and Aging, 15*(4), 596–606.

McArthur, L. Z. (1972). The how and what of why: Some determinants and consequences of causal attribution. *Journal of Personality and Social Psychology, 22,* 171–193.

McArthur, L. Z. (1981). What grabs you? The role of attention in impression formation and causal attribution. In E. T. Higgins, C. P. Herman, & M. P. Zanna (Eds.), *Social cognition: The Ontario symposium* (Vol. 1, pp. 201–246). Hillsdale, NJ: Erlbaum.

McArthur, L. Z., & Apatow, K. (1983). Impressions of baby-faced adults. *Social Cognition, 2*(4), 315–342.

McArthur, L. Z., & Baron, R. (1983). Toward an ecological theory of social perception. *Psychological Review, 90,* 215–238.

McArthur, L. Z., & Berry, D. S. (1987). Cross-cultural agreement in perceptions of baby-faced adults. *Journal of Cross-Cultural Psychology, 18*(2), 165–192.

McArthur, L. Z., & Ginsberg, E. (1981). Causal attribution to salient stimuli: An investigation of visual fixation mediators. *Personality and Social Psychology Bulletin, 7*(4), 547–553.

McArthur, L. Z., & Post, D. L. (1977). Figural emphasis and person perception. *Journal of Experimental Social Psychology, 13,* 520–535.

McClure, J., & Hilton, D. (1997). For you can't always get what you want: When preconditions are better explanations than goals. *British Journal of Social Psychology, 36*(2), 223–240.

McConahay, J. B. (1982). Self-interest versus racial attitudes as correlates of anti-busing attitudes in Louisville: Is it the buses or the Blacks? *The Journal of Politics, 44*(3), 692–720.

McConahay, J. B. (1986). Modern racism, ambivalence, and the Modern Racism Scale. In J. F. Dovido & S. L. Gaertner (Eds.), *Prejudice, discrimination, and racism* (pp. 91–125). Orlando, FL: Academic Press.

McConahay, J. B., & Hough, J. C. (1976). Symbolic racism. *Journal of Social Issues, 32,* 23–45.

McConnell, A. R., & Leibold, J. M. (2001). Relations among the Implicit Association Test, discriminatory behavior, and explicit measures of racial attitudes. *Journal of Experimental Social Psychology, 37*(5), 435–442.

McConnell, A. R., Sherman, S. J., & Hamilton, D. L. (1994). Illusory correlation in the perception of groups: An extension of the distinctiveness-based account. *Journal of Personality and Social Psychology, 67,* 414–429.

McGill, A. L. (1989). Context effects in judgments of causation. *Journal of Personality and Social Psychology, 57*(2), 189–200.

McGinnies, E. (1949). Emotionality and perceptual defense. *Psychological Review, 56,* 244–251.

McGrath, A. (2017). Dealing with dissonance: A review of cognitive dissonance reduction. *Social and Personality Psychology Compass, 11*(12), 1–17.

McMaster, C., & Lee, C. (1991). Cognitive dissonance in tobacco smokers. *Addictive Behaviors, 16*(5), 349–353.

Meck, W. H. (1983). Selective adjustment of the speed of internal clock and memory processes. *Journal of Experimental Psychology: Animal Behavioral Processes, 9,* 171–201.

Medin, D. L. (1989). Concepts and conceptual structure. *American Psychologist, 44,* 1469–1481.

Medin, D. L., Altom, M. W., & Murphy, T. D. (1984). Given versus induced category representations: Use of prototype and exemplar information in classification. *Journal of Experimental Psychology: Learning, Memory, and Cognition, 10*(3), 333–352.

Meissner, C. A., & Brigham, J. C. (2001). Thirty years of investigating the own-race bias in memory for faces: A meta-analytic review. *Psychology, Public Policy, and Law, 7*(1), 3–35.

Meissner, C. A., Brigham, J. C., & Butz, D. A. (2005). Memory for own- and other-race faces: A dual-process approach. *Applied Cognitive Psychology, 19,* 545–567.

Melnikoff, D. E., & Bargh, J. A. (2023). Impression formation, right side up. In E. Balcetis & G. B. Moskowitz (Eds.), *Handbook of impression formation: A social psychological approach* (pp. 185–198). New York: Routledge.

Mendes, W. B., Blascovich, J., Hunter, S. B., Lickel, B., & Jost, J. T. (2007). Threatened by the unexpected: Physiological responses during social interactions with expectancy-violating partners. *Journal of Personality and Social Psychology, 92*(4), 698–716.

Mendoza, S. A., Gollwitzer, P. M., & Amodio, D. M. (2010). Reducing the expression of implicit stereotypes: Reflexive control through implementation intentions. *Personality and Social Psychology Bulletin, 36*(4), 512–523.

Meyer, D. E., & Schvandeveldt, R. W. (1971). Facilitation in recognizing pairs of words:

Evidence of a dependence between retrieval operations. *Journal of Experimental Psychology, 90,* 227–234.

Michotte, A. (1963). *The perception of causality* (T. R. Miles & E. Miles, Trans.). London: Methuen.

Miller, D. T. (1976). Ego involvement and attributions for success and failure. *Journal of Personality and Social Psychology, 34*(5), 901–906.

Miller, D. T., & Prentice, D. A. (1999). Some consequences of a belief in group essence: The category divide hypothesis. In D. A. Prentice & D. T. Miller (Eds.), *Cultural divides: Understanding and overcoming group conflict* (pp. 213–238). New York: Russell Sage Foundation.

Miller, G. A. (1956). The magical number seven, plus or minus two: Some limits on our capacity for processing information. *Psychological Review, 63*(2), 81–97.

Miller, G. A., Galanter, E., & Pribram, K. H. (1960). *Plans and the structure of behavior.* New York: Holt, Rinehart & Winston.

Miller, J. G. (1984). Culture and the development of everyday social explanation. *Journal of Personality and Social Psychology, 46,* 961–978.

Minsky, M. (1975). A framework for representing knowledge. In P. H. Winston (Ed.), *The psychology of computer vision* (pp. 211–277). New York: McGraw Hill.

Mogg, K., & Bradley, B. P. (1999). Orienting of attention to threatening facial expressions presented under conditions of restricted awareness. *Cognition and Emotion, 13*(6), 713–740.

Mogg, K., & Bradley, B. P. (2002). Selective orienting of attention to masked threat faces in social anxiety. *Behaviour Research and Therapy, 40*(12), 1403–1414.

Mogg, K., Bradley, B. P., & Williams, R. (1995). Attentional bias in anxiety and depression: The role of awareness. *British Journal of Clinical Psychology, 34*(1), 17–36.

Mogg, K., Mathews, A., & Weinman, J. (1987). Memory bias in clinical anxiety. *Journal of Abnormal Psychology, 96*(2), 94–98.

Monin, B., & Miller, D. T. (2001). Moral credentials and the expression of prejudice. *Journal of Personality and Social Psychology, 81*(1), 33–43.

Monteith, M. J. (1993). Self-regulation of prejudiced responses: Implications for progress in prejudice reduction efforts. *Journal of Personality and Social Psychology, 65,* 469–485.

Monteith, M. J., Ashburn-Nardo, L., Voils, C. I., & Czopp, A. M. (2002). Putting the brakes on prejudice: On the development and operation of cues for control. *Journal of Personality and Social Psychology, 83,* 1029–1050.

Monteith, M. J., Devine, P. G., & Zuwerink, J. R. (1993). Self-directed versus other-directed affect as a consequence of prejudice-related discrepancies. *Journal of Personality and Social Psychology, 64*(2), 198–210.

Monteith, M. J., Mark, A. Y., & Ashburn-Nardo, L. (2010). The self-regulation of prejudice: Toward understanding its lived character. *Group Processes and Intergroup Relations, 13*(2), 183–200.

Monteith, M. J., Sherman, J. W., & Devine, P. G. (1998). Suppression as a stereotype control strategy. *Personality and Social Psychology Review, 2,* 63–82.

Monteith, M. J., & Voils, C. I. (2001). Exerting control over prejudiced responses. In G. B. Moskowitz (Ed.), *Cognitive social psychology: The Princeton symposium on the legacy and future of social cognition* (pp. 375–388). Mahwah, NJ: Erlbaum.

Morris, M. W., & Peng, K. (1994). Culture and cause: American and Chinese attributions for social and physical events. *Journal of Personality and Social Psychology, 67,* 949–971.

Moscovici, S. (1976). *Social influence and social change.* New York: Academic Press.

Moscovici, S. (1980). Toward a theory of conversion behavior. In L. Berkowitz (Ed.), *Advances in experimental social psychology* (Vol. 13, pp. 209–239). New York: Academic Press.

Moscovici, S. (1985). Innovation and minority influence. In S. Moscovici, G. Mugny, & E. Van Avermaet (Eds.), *Perspectives on minority influence* (pp. 9–51). Cambridge, UK: Cambridge University Press.

Moscovici, S., Lage, S., & Naffrechoux, M. (1969). Influence of a consistent minority on the responses of a majority in a color perception task. *Sociometry, 32,* 365–380.

Moscovici, S., & Personnaz, B. (1980). Studies in social influence: V. Minority influence and conversion behavior in a perceptual task. *Journal of Experimental Social Psychology, 16*(3), 270–282.

Moskowitz, G. B. (1993a). Individual differences in social categorization: The effects of personal need for structure on spontaneous trait inferences. *Journal of Personality and Social Psychology, 65,* 132–142.

Moskowitz, G. B. (1993b). Person organization with a memory set: Are spontaneous trait inferences personality characterizations or behavior labels? *European Journal of Personality, 7,* 195–208.

Moskowitz, G. B. (1996). The mediational effects of attributions and information processing in minority social influence. *British Journal of Social Psychology, 35,* 47–66.

Moskowitz, G. B. (Ed.). (2001). Preconscious control and compensatory cognition. In G. B. Moskowitz (Ed.), *Cognitive social psychology: The Princeton symposium on the legacy and future of social cognition* (pp. 333–358). Mahwah, NJ: Erlbaum.

Moskowitz, G. B. (2002). Preconscious effects of temporary goals on attention. *Journal of Experimental Social Psychology, 38,* 397–404.

Moskowitz, G. B. (2009). The compensatory nature of goal pursuit: From explicit action to implicit cognition. In G. B. Moskowitz, & H. Grant (Eds.), *The psychology of goals* (pp. 304–336). New York: Guilford Press.

Moskowitz, G. B. (2010). On the control over stereotype activation and stereotype inhibition. *Social and Personality Psychology Compass, 4*(2), 140–158.

Moskowitz, G. B. (2014). The implicit volition model: The unconscious nature of goal pursuit. In J. Sherman, B. Gawronski, & Y. Trope (Eds.), *Dual-process theories of the social mind* (pp. 400–422). New York: Guilford Press.

Moskowitz, G. B., & Chaiken, S. (2001). Mediators of minority social influence: Cognitive processing mechanisms revealed through a persuasion paradigm. In C. K. W. de Dreu & N. K. de Vries (Eds.), *Group consensus and minority influence* (pp. 60–90). Oxford, UK: Blackwell.

Moskowitz, G. B., Gollwitzer, P. M., Wasel, W., & Schaal, B. (1999). Preconscious control of stereotype activation through chronic egalitarian goals. *Journal of Personality and Social Psychology, 77,* 167–184.

Moskowitz, G. B., & Li, P. (2011). Egalitarian goals trigger stereotype inhibition: A proactive form of stereotype control. *Journal of Experimental Social Psychology, 47*(1), 103–116.

Moskowitz, G. B., Li, P., Ignarri, C., & Stone, J. (2011). Compensatory cognition associated

with egalitarian goals. *Journal of Experimental Social Psychology, 47*(2), 365–370.

Moskowitz, G. B., Li, P., & Kirk, E. (2004). The implicit volition model: On the preconscious regulation of temporarily adopted goals. In M. Zanna (Ed.), *Advances in experimental social psychology* (Vol. 36, pp. 317–413). San Diego, CA: Academic Press.

Moskowitz, G. B., & Olcaysoy Okten, I. (2016). Spontaneous goal inference (SGI). *Social and Personality Psychology Compass, 10*(1), 64–80.

Moskowitz, G. B., Olcaysoy Okten, I., & Gooch, C. M. (2015). On race and time. *Psychological Science, 26*(11), 1783–1794.

Moskowitz, G. B., Olcaysoy Okten, I., & Gooch, C. M. (2017). Distortion in time perception as a result of concern about appearing biased. *PLOS One, 12*(8), e0182241.

Moskowitz, G. B., Olcaysoy Okten, I., & Schneid, E. (2023). The updating of first impressions. In E. Balcetis & G. B. Moskowitz (Eds.). *Handbook of impression formation: A social psychological approach* (pp. 348–392). New York: Routledge.

Moskowitz, G. B., & Roman, R. J. (1992). Spontaneous trait inferences as self-generated primes: Implications for conscious social judgment. *Journal of Personality and Social Psychology, 62,* 728–738.

Moskowitz, G. B., Salomon, A. R., & Taylor, C. M. (2000). Implicit control of stereotype activation through the preconscious operation of egalitarian goals. *Social Cognition, 18,* 151–177.

Moskowitz, G. B., & Skurnik, I. W. (1999). Contrast effects as determined by the type of prime: Trait versus exemplar primes initiate processing strategies that differ in how accessible constructs are used. *Journal of Personality and Social Psychology, 76,* 911–927.

Moskowitz, G. B., & Stone, J. (2012). The proactive control of stereotype activation: Implicit goals to *not* stereotype. *Journal of Psychology, 220*(3), 172–179.

Moskowitz, G. B., Stone, J., & Childs, A. (2012). Implicit stereotyping and medical decisions: Unconscious stereotype activation in practitioners' thoughts about African Americans. *American Journal of Public Health, 102*(5), 996–1001.

Moskowitz, G. B., & Uleman, J. S. (1987). *The facilitation and inhibition of spontaneous trait inferences at encoding.* Poster presented at the 95th annual convention of the American Psychological Association, New York.

Moskowitz, G. B., & Vitriol, J. A. (2022). A social cognition model of bias reduction. In A. Nordstrom & W. Goodfriend (Eds.), *Innovative stigma and discrimination reduction programs* (pp. 1–39). Oxon, UK: Taylor & Francis.

Mosleh, M., Martel, C., Eckles, D., & Rand, D. G. (2021). Shared partisanship dramatically increases social tie formation in a Twitter field experiment. *Proceedings of the National Academy of Sciences, 118*(7), e2022761118.

Mullen, B., & Johnson, C. (1990). Distinctiveness-based illusory correlations and stereotyping: A meta-analytic integration. *British Journal of Social Psychology, 29,* 11–28.

Murphy, G. L., & Medin, D. L. (1985). The role of theories in conceptual coherence. *Psychological Review, 92,* 289–316.

Murphy, M. C., & Taylor, V. J. (2012). The role of situational cues in signaling and maintaining stereotype threat. In M. Inzlicht & T. Schmader (Eds.), *Stereotype threat: Theory, process, and application* (pp. 17–33). New York: Oxford University Press.

Murphy, S. T., & Zajonc, R. B. (1993). Affect, cognition, and awareness: Affective priming with optimal and suboptimal stimulus exposures. *Journal of Personality and Social Psychology, 64,* 723–739.

Murray, S. L., & Holmes, J. G. (1993). Seeing virtues in faults: Negativity and the transformation of interpersonal narratives in close relationships. *Journal of Personality and Social Psychology, 65*(4), 707–722.

Murray, S. L., Holmes, J. G., & Collins, N. L. (2006). Optimizing assurance: The risk regulation system in relationships. *Psychological Bulletin, 132*(5), 641–666.

Nader, K., Schafe, G. E., & LeDoux, J. E. (2000). Fear memories require protein synthesis in the amygdala for reconsolidation after retrieval. *Nature, 406,* 722–726.

Nadler, J., & McDonnell, M. H. (2012). Moral character, motive, and the psychology of blame. *Cornell Law Review, 97,* 255–304.

Nemeth, C. J. (1986). Differential contributions of majority and minority influence. *Psychological Review, 93,* 23–32.

Nemeth, C. J., Mayseles, O., Sherman, J., & Brown, Y. (1990). Exposure to dissent and recall of information. *Journal of Personality and Social Psychology, 58,* 429–437.

Nemeth, C. J., Swedlund, M., & Kanki, G. (1974). Patterning of the minority's responses and their influence on the majority. *European Journal of Social Psychology, 4,* 53–64.

Neuberg, S. L. (1989). The goal of forming accurate impressions during social interactions: Attenuating impact of negative expectancies. *Journal of Personality and Social Psychology, 56,* 374–386.

Neuberg, S. L., & Fiske, S. T. (1987). Motivation influences on impression formation: Outcome dependency, accuracy-driven attention, and individuating processes. *Journal of Personality and Social Psychology, 53,* 431–444.

Neuberg, S. L., & Newsom, J. T. (1993). Individual differences in chronic motivation to simplify: Personal need for structure and social-cognitive processing. *Journal of Personality and Social Psychology, 65,* 113–131.

Newell, A., & Simon, H. A. (1972). *Human problem solving.* Englewood Cliffs, NJ: Prentice-Hall.

Newman, L. S. (1993). How individualists interpret behavior: Idiocentrism and spontaneous trait inference. *Social Cognition, 11,* 243–269.

Newman, L. S., & Marsden, A. (2023). Around the world in 80 milliseconds (or less): Spontaneous trait inference across cultures. In E. Balcetis & G. B. Moskowitz (Eds.), *Handbook of impression formation: A social psychological approach* (pp. 324–347). New York: Routledge.

Newman, L. S., & Uleman, J. S. (1990). Assimilation and contrast effects in spontaneous trait inferences. *Personality and Social Psychology Bulletin, 16,* 224–240.

N'gbala, A., & Branscombe, N. R. (1995). Mental simulation and causal attribution: When simulating an event does not affect fault assignment. *Journal of Experimental Social Psychology, 31*(2), 139–162.

Niedenthal, P. M., Barsalou, L. W., Winkielman, P., Krauth-Gruber, S., & Ric, F. (2005). Embodiment in attitudes, social perception, and emotion. *Personality and Social Psychology Review, 9,* 184–211.

Niedenthal, P. M., Halberstadt, J. B., & Setterlund, M. B. (1997). Being happy and seeing "happy": Emotional state facilitates visual encoding. *Cognition and Emotion, 11,* 403–432.

Nisbett, R. E., & Ross, L. (1980). *Human inference.* Englewood Cliffs, NJ: Prentice Hall.

Nisbett, R. E., & Wilson, T. D. (1977). Telling more than we can know: Verbal reports on mental processes. *Psychological Review, 84,* 231–259.

Nolen-Hoeksema, S., Girgus, J. S., & Seligman, M. E. P. (1992). Predictors and consequences of childhood depressive symptoms. *Journal of Abnormal Psychology, 101,* 405–422.

Nordstrom, A., & Goodfriend, W. (2023). *Innovative stigma and discrimination reduction programs.* Oxon, UK: Taylor & Francis.

Norem, J. K., & Cantor, N. (1986). Defensive pessimism: "Harnessing" anxiety as motivation. *Journal of Personality and Social Psychology, 55,* 1208–1217.

Norton, M. I., Aknin, L. B., & Dunn, E. W. (2008). Spending money on others promotes happiness. *Science, 319*(5870), 1687–1688.

Norton, M. I., Vandello, J. A., Biga, A., & Darley, J. M. (2008). Colorblindness and diversity: Conflicting goals in decisions influenced by race. *Social Cognition, 26*(1), 102–111.

Nosek, B. A., Banaji, M. R., & Jost, J. T. (2009). The politics of intergroup attitudes. In J. T. Jost, A. C. Kay, & H. Thorisdottir (Eds.), *Social and psychological bases of ideology and system justification* (pp. 480–506). New York: Oxford University Press.

Nosofsky, R. M., Palmeri, T. J., & McKinley, S. C. (1994). Rule-plus-exception model of classification learning. *Psychological Review, 101,* 53–79.

O'Brien, L. T., Crandall, C. S., Horstman-Reser, A., Warner, R., Alsbrooks, A., & Blodorn, A. (2010). But I'm no bigot: How prejudiced White Americans maintain unprejudiced self-images. *Journal of Applied Social Psychology, 40*(4), 917–946.

O'Brien, L. T., & Major, B. (2009). Group status and feelings of personal entitlement: The roles of social comparison and system-justifying beliefs. In J. T. Jost, A. C. Kay, & H. Thorisdottir (Eds.), *Social and psychological bases of ideology and system justification* (pp. 427–443). New York: Oxford University Press.

Oh, D., Buck, E. A., & Todorov, A. (2019). Revealing hidden gender biases in competence impressions of faces. *Psychological Science, 30,* 65–79.

Olcaysoy Okten, I., & Moskowitz, G. B. (2018). Goal vs. trait explanations: Causal attributions beyond the trait-situation dichotomy. *Journal of Personality and Social Psychology, 114*(2), 211–229.

Olcaysoy Okten, I., & Moskowitz, G. B. (2020a). Easy to make, hard to revise: Updating spontaneous trait inferences in the presence of trait-inconsistent information. *Social Cognition, 38*(6), 571–624.

Olcaysoy Okten, I., & Moskowitz, G. B. (2020b). Spontaneous goal versus spontaneous trait inferences: How ideology shapes attributions and explanations. *European Journal of Social Psychology, 50*(1), 177–188.

Olcaysoy Okten, I., Schneid, E., & Moskowitz, G. B. (2019). On the updating of spontaneous impressions. *Journal of Personality and Social Psychology, 117*(1), 1–25.

Oliveira Laux, S. H., Ksenofontov, I., & Becker, J. C. (2015). Explicit but not implicit sexist beliefs predict benevolent and hostile sexist behavior. *European Journal of Social Psychology, 45*(6), 702–715.

Olivola, C. Y., & Todorov, A. (2010). Elected in 100 milliseconds: Appearance-based trait inferences and voting. *Journal of Nonverbal Behavior, 34,* 83–110.

Olson, M. A., & Fazio, R. H. (2001). Implicit attitude formation through classical conditioning. *Psychological Science, 12*(5), 413–417.

Olson, M. A., & Fazio, R. H. (2003). Relations between implicit measures of prejudice: What are we measuring? *Psychological Science, 14*(6), 636–639.

Olson, M. A., & Fazio, R. H. (2004). Reducing the influence of extrapersonal associations on the Implicit Association Test: Personalizing the IAT. *Journal of Personality and Social Psychology, 86*(5), 653–667.

Olson, M. A., & Fazio, R. H. (2006). Reducing automatically activated racial prejudice through implicit evaluative conditioning. *Personality and Social Psychology Bulletin, 32*(4), 421–433.

Oosterhof, N. N., & Todorov, A. (2008). The functional basis of face evaluation. *Proceedings of the National Academy of Sciences, 105,* 11087–11092.

Ostrom, T. M. (1984). The sovereignty of social cognition. In R. S. Wyer, Jr., & T. K. Srull (Eds.), *Handbook of social cognition* (vol. 1, pp. 1–38). Hillsdale, NJ: Erlbaum.

Osgood, C. E., Suci, G. J., & Tannenbaum, P. H. (1957). *The measurement of meaning.* Urbana, IL: University of Illinois Press.

Ostrom, T. M., Carpenter, S. L., Sedikides, C., & Li, F. (1993). Differential processing of ingroup and out-group information. *Journal of Personality and Social Psychology, 64*(1), 21–34.

Ostrom, T. M., Pryor, J. B., & Simpson, D. D. (1981). The organization of social information. In E. T. Higgins, C. P. Herman, & M. P. Zanna (Eds.), *Social cognition: The Ontario symposium* (Vol. 1, pp. 1–38). Hillsdale, NJ: Erlbaum.

O'Sullivan, M., Ekman, P., Friesen, W. V., & Scherer, K. R. (1985). What you say and how you say it: The contribution of speech content and voice quality to judgments of others. *Journal of Personality and Social Psychology, 48*(1), 54–62.

Otten, S. (2016). The minimal group paradigm and its maximal impact in research on social categorization. *Current Opinion in Psychology, 11*, 85–89.

Otten, S., & Moskowitz, G. B. (2000). Evidence for implicit evaluative ingroup bias: Affect-biased spontaneous trait inference in a minimal group paradigm. *Journal of Experimental Social Psychology, 36*, 77–89.

Over, H., & Carpenter, M. (2009). Eighteen-month-old infants show increased helping following priming with affiliation. *Psychological Science, 20*(10), 1189–1193.

Packer, D. J. (2008). On being both with us and against us: A normative conflict model of dissent in social groups. *Personality and Social Psychology Review, 12*, 50–72.

Packer, D. J., & Miners, C. T. (2014). Tough love: The normative conflict model and a goal system approach to dissent decisions. *Social and Personality Psychology Compass, 8*, 354–373.

Packer, D. J., & Ungson, N. D. (2017). Group decision-making: Revisiting Janis' groupthink studies. In J. R. Smith & S. A. Haslam (Eds.), *Social psychology: Revisiting the classic studies* (2nd ed., pp. 182–200). Thousand Oaks, CA: Sage.

Pager, D., & Shepherd, H. (2008). The sociology of discrimination: Racial discrimination in employment, housing, credit, and consumer markets. *Annual Review of Sociology, 34*, 181–209.

Pariser, E. (2011). *The filter bubble: What the Internet is hiding from you.* London: Penguin.

Park, B. (1989). Trait attributes as on-line organizers in person impressions. In J. N. Bassili (Ed.), *On-line cognition in person perception* (pp. 39–60). Hillsdale, NJ: Erlbaum.

Park, B., & Judd, C. M. (1990). Measures and models of perceived group variability. *Journal of Personality and Social Psychology, 59*(2), 173–191.

Parkin, A. (1979). Specifying levels of processing. *Quarterly Journal of Experimental Psychology, 31*, 175–195.

Parks-Stamm, E. J., & Gollwitzer, P. M. (2009). Goal implementation: The benefits and costs of if-then planning. In G. B. Moskowitz & H. Grant (Eds.), *The psychology of goals* (pp. 362–391). New York: Guilford Press.

Paul, P. (2023, March 17). "I pledge allegiance to . . . My conscience." *New York Times*, p. A19.

Paulhus, D. L. (1991). Measurement and control of response bias. In J. P. Robinson, P. R. Shaver, & L. S. Wrightsman (Eds.), *Measures of personality and social psychological attitudes* (pp. 17–59). New York: Academic Press.

Payne, B. K. (2001). Prejudice and perception: The role of automatic and controlled processes in misperceiving a weapon. *Journal of Personality and Social Psychology, 81*(2), 181–192.

Payne, B. K. (2006). Weapon bias: Split-second decisions and unintended stereotyping. *Current Directions in Psychological Science, 15*(6), 287–291.

Payne, B. (2008). What mistakes disclose: A process dissociation approach to automatic and controlled processes in social psychology. *Social and Personality Psychology Compass, 2*, 1073–1092.

Payne, B. K., & Cameron, C. D. (2014). Dual-process theory from a process dissociation perspective. In J. W. Sherman, B. Gawronski, & Y. Trope (Eds.), *Dual-process theories of the social mind* (pp. 107–120). New York: Guilford Press.

Payne, B. K., Cheng, C. M., Govorun, O., & Stewart, B. D. (2005). An inkblot for attitudes: Affect misattribution as implicit measurement. *Journal of Personality and Social Psychology, 89*, 277–293.

Payne, B. K., & Jacoby, L. L. (2006). What should a process model deliver? *Psychological Inquiry, 17*, 194–198.

Payne, B. K., Lambert, A. J., & Jacoby, L. L. (2002). Best laid plans: Effects of goals on accessibility bias and cognitive control in race-based misperceptions of weapons. *Journal of Experimental Social Psychology, 38*(4), 384–396.

Payne, B. K., & Lundberg, K. (2014). The affect misattribution procedure: Ten years of evidence on reliability, validity, and mechanisms. *Social and Personality Psychology Compass, 8*(12), 672–686.

Pearson, A. R., Dovidio, J. F., & Gaertner, S. L. (2009). The nature of contemporary prejudice: Insights from aversive racism. *Social and Personality Psychology Compass, 3*(3), 314–338.

Peck, B. M., & Denney, M. (2012). Disparities in the conduct of the medical encounter: The effects of physician and patient race and gender. *Sage Open, 2*(3), 2158244012459193.

Penner, L. A., Dovidio, J. F., West, T. V., Gaertner, S. L., Albrecht, T. L., Dailey, R. K., et al. (2010). Aversive racism and medical interactions with Black patients: A field study. *Journal of Experimental Social Psychology, 46*(2), 436–440.

Pennycook, G. (2023). A framework for understanding reasoning errors: From fake news to climate change and beyond. *Advances in Experimental Social Psychology, 67,* 131–208.

Pennycook, G., & Rand, D. G. (2021). The psychology of fake news. *Trends in Cognitive Sciences, 25*(5), 388–402.

Pérez, J. A., Falomir, J. M., & Mugny, G. (1995). Internalization of conflict and attitude change. *European Journal of Social Psychology, 25,* 117–124.

Perry, S. P., Murphy, M. C., & Dovidio, J. F. (2015). Modern prejudice: Subtle, but unconscious? The role of bias awareness in Whites' perceptions of personal and others' biases. *Journal of Experimental Social Psychology, 61,* 64–78.

Peters, K. R., & Gawronski, B. (2011). Mutual influences between the implicit and explicit self-concepts: The role of memory activation and motivated reasoning. *Journal of Experimental Social Psychology, 47*(2), 436–442.

Petsko, C. D., & Bodenhausen, G. V. (2019). Racial stereotyping of gay men: Can a minority sexual orientation erase race? *Journal of Experimental Social Psychology, 83,* 37–54.

Petsko, C. D., & Bodenhausen, G. V. (2020). Multifarious person perception: How social perceivers manage the complexity of intersectional targets. *Social and Personality Psychology Compass, 14*(2), e12518.

Pettigrew, T. F. (1979). The ultimate attribution error: Extending Allport's cognitive analysis of prejudice. *Personality and Social Psychology Bulletin, 5*(4), 461–476.

Pettigrew, T. F. (1997). Generalized intergroup contact effects on prejudice. *Personality and Social Psychology Bulletin, 23,* 173–185.

Petty, R. E., & Briñol, P. (2010). Attitude structure and change: Implications for implicit measures. In B. Gawronski & B. K. Payne (Eds.), *Handbook of implicit social cognition: Measurement, theory, and applications* (pp. 335–352). New York: Guilford Press.

Petty, R. E., & Briñol, P. (2014). The elaboration likelihood and metacognitive models of attitudes: Implications for prejudice, the self, and beyond. In J. W. Sherman, B. Gawronski, & Y. Trope (Eds.), *Dual-process theories of the social mind* (pp. 172–187). New York: Guilford Press.

Petty, R. E., Briñol, P., & DeMarree, K. G. (2007). The meta-cognitive model (MCM) of attitudes: Implications for attitude measurement, change, and strength. *Social Cognition, 25*(5), 657–686.

Petty, R. E., & Cacioppo, J. T. (1986). The elaboration likelihood model of persuasion. In L. Berkowitz (Ed.), *Advances in experimental social psychology* (Vol. 19, pp. 123–205). New York: Academic Press.

Petty, R. E., Cacioppo, J. T., & Schumann, D. (1983). Central and peripheral routes to advertising effectiveness: The moderating role of involvement. *Journal of Consumer Research, 10,* 135–146.

Petty, R. E., Tormala, Z. L., Briñol, P., & Jarvis, W. B. G. (2006). Implicit ambivalence from attitude change: An exploration of the PAST model. *Journal of Personality and Social Psychology, 90*(1), 21–41.

Pflugshaupt, T., Mosimann, U., Schmitt, W., Wartburg, R., Wurtz, P., Steinheimer, M. L., et al. (2007). To look or not to look at threat? Scanpath differences within a group of spider phobics. *Journal of Anxiety Disorders, 21,* 353–366.

Pham, M. T., & Avnet, T. (2004). Ideals and oughts and the reliance on affect versus substance in persuasion. *Journal of Consumer Research, 30*(4), 503–518.

Phelan, J. E., Moss-Racusin, C. A., & Rudman, L. A. (2008). Competent yet out in the cold: Shifting criteria for hiring reflect backlash toward agentic women. *Psychology of Women Quarterly, 32*(4), 406–413.

Phillips, J. E., & Olson, M. A. (2014). When implicitly and explicitly measured racial attitudes align: The roles of social desirability and thoughtful responding. *Basic and Applied Social Psychology, 36*(2), 125–132.

Pickett, C. L., & Brewer, M. B. (2001). Assimilation and differentiation needs as motivational determinants of perceived ingroup and outgroup homogeneity. *Journal of Experimental Social Psychology, 37*, 341–348.

Pietri, E. S., Hennes, E. P., Dovidio, J. F., Brescoll, V. L., Bailey, A. H., Moss-Racusin, C. A., et al. (2019). Addressing unintended consequences of gender diversity interventions on women's sense of belonging in STEM. *Sex Roles, 80*(9), 527–547.

Pinkus, R. T., Lockwood, P., Schimmack, U., & Fournier, M. A. (2008). For better and for worse: Everyday social comparisons between romantic partners. *Journal of Personality and Social Psychology, 95*(5), 1180–1201.

Pittman, T. S., & D'Agostino, P. R. (1989). Motivation and cognition: Control deprivation and the nature of subsequent information processing. *Journal of Experimental Social Psychology, 25*, 465–480.

Pittman, T. S., & Pittman, N. L. (1980). Deprivation of control and the attribution process. *Journal of Personality and Social Psychology, 39*, 377–389.

Plaks, J., Levy, S. R., & Dweck, C. (2009). Lay theories of personality: Cornerstones of meaning in social cognition. *Social and Personality Psychology Compass, 3*, 1069–1081.

Plaks, J. E., Shafer, J. L., & Shoda, Y. (2003). Perceiving individuals and groups as coherent: How do perceivers make sense of variable behavior? *Social Cognition, 21*(1), 26–60.

Plant, E. A., & Devine, P. G. (1998). Internal and external motivation to respond without prejudice. *Journal of Personality and Social Psychology, 75*, 811–832.

Plant, E. A., & Devine, P. G. (2003). The antecedents and implications of interracial anxiety. *Personality and Social Psychology Bulletin, 29*(6), 790–801.

Plant, E. A., & Devine, P. G. (2009). The active control of prejudice: Unpacking the intentions guiding control efforts. *Journal of Personality and Social Psychology, 96*, 640–652.

Plaut, V. C. (2010). Diversity science: Why and how difference makes a difference. *Psychological Inquiry, 21*, 77–99.

Plaut, V., Garnett, F., Buffardi, L., & Sanchez-Burks, J. (2011). "What about me?" Perceptions of exclusion and Whites' reactions to multiculturalism. *Journal of Personality and Social Psychology, 101*(2), 337–353.

Plaut, V. C., Thomas, K., Hurd, K., & Romano, C. (2018). Do colorblindness and multiculturalism remedy or foster discrimination and racism? *Current Directions in Psychological Science, 27*(3), 200–206.

Pleskac, T. J., Cesario, J., & Johnson, D. J. (2018). How race affects evidence accumulation during the decision to shoot. *Psychonomic Bulletin and Review, 25*(4), 1301–1330.

Porath, C. L., Overbeck, J. R., & Pearson, C. M. (2008). Picking up the gauntlet: How individuals respond to status challenges. *Journal of Applied Social Psychology, 38*(7), 1945–1980.

Porter, S., ten Brinke, L., & Gustaw, C. (2010). Dangerous decisions: The impact of first impressions of trustworthiness on the evaluation of legal evidence and defendant culpability. *Psychology, Crime & Law, 16*(6), 477–491.

Posner, M. I., & Snyder, C. R. R. (1975). Attention and cognitive control. In R. L. Solso (Ed.), *Information processing and cognition: The Loyola symposium* (pp. 55–85). Hillsdale, NJ: Erlbaum.

Postman, L., Bruner, J. S., & McGinnies, E. (1948). Personal factors as selective factors in perception. *Journal of Abnormal and Social Psychology, 43*, 142–154.

Povinelli, D. J., & Vonk, J. (2003). Chimpanzee minds: Suspiciously human? *Trends in Cognitive Sciences, 7*(4), 157–160.

Pratto, F., & Bargh, J. A. (1991). Stereotyping based on apparently individuating information: Trait and global components of sex stereotypes under attention overload. *Journal of Experimental Social Psychology, 27*, 26–47.

Pratto, F., & John, O. P. (1991). Automatic vigilance: The attention-grabbing power of negative social information. *Journal of Personality and Social Psychology, 61*(3), 380–391.

Pratto, F., Sidanius, J., Stallworth, L. M., & Malle, B. F. (1994). Social dominance orientation: A personality variable predicting social and political attitudes. *Journal of Personality and Social Psychology, 67*, 741–763.

Prentice, D. A. (1990). Familiarity and differences in self- and other-representations. *Journal of Personality and Social Psychology, 59*, 369–383.

Prentice, D. A., & Carranza, E. (2002). What women and men should be, shouldn't be, are allowed to be, and don't have to be: The contents of prescriptive gender stereotypes. *Psychology of Women Quarterly, 26*(4), 269–281.

Prentice, D. A., & Miller, D. T. (1993). Pluralistic ignorance and alcohol use on campus: Some consequences of misperceiving the social norm. *Journal of Personality and Social Psychology, 64*, 243–256.

Prior, M., Sood, G., & Khanna, K. (2015). You cannot be serious: The impact of accuracy incentives on partisan bias in reports of economic perceptions. *Quarterly Journal of Political Science, 10*(4), 489–518.

Pronin, E. (2007). Perception and misperception of bias in human judgment. *Trends in Cognitive Science, 11*, 37–43.

Pronin, E. (2008). How we see ourselves and how we see others. *Science, 320*, 1177–1180.

Pronin, E., Lin, D. Y., & Ross, L. (2002). The bias blind spot: Perceptions of bias in self versus others. *Personality and Social Psychology Bulletin, 28*(3), 369–381.

Prothro, E., & Melikian, L. (1955). Studies in stereotypes: V. Familiarity and the kernel of truth hypothesis. *Journal of Social Psychology, 41*, 3–10.

Pryor, J. B., & Reeder, G. D. (2006). A critique of three dueling models of dual processes. *Psychological Inquiry, 17*(3), 231–236.

Purdie-Vaughns, V., & Eibach, R. P. (2008). Intersectional invisibility: The distinctive advantages and disadvantages of multiple subordinate-group identities. *Sex Roles, 59*, 377–391.

Quattrone, G. A. (1982). Overattribution and unit formation: When behavior engulf the person. *Journal of Personality and Social Psychology, 42*, 593–607.

Ramos, T., Garcia-Marques, L., Hamilton, D. L., Ferreira, M., & Van Acker, K. (2012). What I infer depends on who you are: The influence of stereotypes on trait and situational spontaneous inferences. *Journal of Experimental Social Psychology, 48*(6), 1247–1256.

Rathje, S., Van Bavel, J. J., & van der Linden, S. (2021). Out-group animosity drives engagement on social media. *Proceedings of the National Academy of Sciences of the USA, 118*(26), e2024292118.

Ratner, K. G., & Amodio, D. M. (2013). Seeing "us vs. them": Minimal group effects on the neural encoding of faces. *Journal of Experimental Social Psychology, 49*(2), 298–301.

Ratner, K. G., Dotsch, R., Wigboldus, D. H. J., van Knippenberg, A., & Amodio, D. M. (2014). Visualizing minimal ingroup and outgroup faces: Implications for impressions, attitudes, and behavior. *Journal of Personality and Social Psychology, 106*(6), 897–911.

Read, S. J., Jones, D. K., & Miller, L. C. (1990). Traits as goal-based categories: The importance of goals in the coherence of dispositional categories. *Journal of Personality and Social Psychology, 58*(6), 1048–1061.

Read, S. J., & Miller, L. C. (1989). Interpersonalism: Toward a goal-based theory of persons in relationships. In L. Pervin (Ed.), *Goal concepts in personality and social psychology* (pp. 413–472). Hillsdale, NJ: Erlbaum.

Reber, P. J. (2013). The neural basis of implicit learning and memory: A review of neuropsychological and neuroimaging research. *Neuropsychologia, 51*(10), 2026–2042.

Redford, L., & Ratliff, K. A. (2016). Perceived moral responsibility for attitude-based discrimination. *British Journal of Social Psychology, 55*, 279–296.

Reeder, G. (2009). Mindreading: Judgments about intentionality and motives in dispositional inference. *Psychological Inquiry, 20*(1), 1–18.

Reeder, G. D., & Spores, J. M. (1983). The attribution of morality. *Journal of Personality and Social Psychology, 44*(4), 736–745.

Reeder, G. D., & Trafimow, D. (2005). Attributing Motives to Other People. In B. F. Malle & S. D. Hodges (Eds.), *Other minds: How humans bridge the divide between self and others* (pp. 106–123). New York: Guilford Press.

Reeder, G. D., Vonk, R., Ronk, M. J., Ham, J., & Lawrence, M. (2004). Dispositional attribution: Multiple inferences about motive-related traits. *Journal of Personality and Social Psychology, 86*(4), 530–544.

Rees, L., Rothman, N. B., Lehavy, R., & Sanchez-Burks, J. (2013). The ambivalent mind can be a wise mind: Emotional ambivalence increases judgment accuracy. *Journal of Experimental Social Psychology, 49*, 360–367.

Reich, T., & Wheeler, S. C. (2016). The good and bad of ambivalence: Desiring ambivalence under outcome uncertainty. *Journal of Personality and Social Psychology, 110*, 493–508.

Reyna, C., Henry, P. J., Korfmacher, W., & Tucker, A. (2006). Examining the principles in principled conservatism: The role of responsibility stereotypes as cues for deservingness in racial policy decisions. *Journal of Personality and Social Psychology, 90*(1), 109–128.

Riccio, M., Cole, S., & Balcetis, E. (2013). Seeing the expected, the desired, and the feared: Influences on perceptual interpretation and directed attention. *Social and Personality Psychology Compass, 7*(6), 401–414.

Richeson, J. A., & Ambady, N. (2003). Effects of situational power on automatic racial prejudice. *Journal of Experimental Social Psychology, 39*(2), 177–183.

Richeson, J. A., Baird, A. A., Gordon, H. L., Heatherton, T. F., Wyland, C. L., Trawalter, S., et al. (2003). An fMRI investigation of the impact of interracial contact on executive function. *Nature Neuroscience, 6*(12), 1323–1328.

Richeson, J. A., & Nussbaum, R. J. (2003). The impact of multiculturalism versus colorblindness on racial bias. *Journal of Experimental Social Psychology, 40*, 417–423.

Richeson, J. A., & Shelton, J. N. (2007). Negotiating interracial interactions: Costs, consequences, and possibilities. *Current Directions in Psychological Science, 16*(6), 316–320.

Richeson, J. A., & Trawalter, S. (2008). The threat of appearing prejudiced and race-based attentional biases. *Psychological Science, 19*, 98–102.

Richeson, J. A., Trawalter, S., & Shelton, J. N. (2005). African Americans' implicit racial attitudes and the depletion of executive function after interracial interactions. *Social Cognition, 23*(4), 336–352.

Rim, S., Hansen, J., & Trope, Y. (2013). What happens why? Psychological distance and focusing on causes versus consequences of events. *Journal of Personality and Social Psychology, 104*(3), 457–472.

Rim, S., Uleman, J. S., & Trope, Y. (2009). Spontaneous trait inference and construal level theory: Psychological distance increases nonconscious trait thinking. *Journal of Experimental Social Psychology, 45*(5), 1088–1097.

Rips, L. J., & Collins, A. (1993). Categories and resemblance. *Journal of Experimental Psychology, 122*, 468–486.

Riskind, J. H., Moore, R., & Bowley, L. (1995). The looming of spiders: The fearful perceptual distortion of movement and menace. *Behaviour Research and Therapy, 33*(2), 171–178.

Robins, R. W., & Pals, J. L. (2002). Implicit self-theories in the academic domain: Implications for goal orientation, attributions, affect, and self-esteem change. *Self and Identity, 1*(4), 313–336.

Robinson, R. J., Keltner, D., Ward, A., & Ross, L. (1995). Actual versus assumed differences in construal: "Naïve realism" in intergroup perception and conflict. *Journal of Personality and Social Psychology, 68*, 404–417.

Roese, N. J. (1997). Counterfactual thinking. *Psychological Bulletin, 121*, 133–148.

Roese, N. J., & Epstude, K. (2017). The functional theory of counterfactual thinking: New evidence, new challenges, new insights. In J. M. Olson (Ed.), *Advances in experimental social psychology* (pp. 1–79). Cambridge, MA: Elsevier Academic Press.

Roese, N. J., & Vohs, K. D. (2012). Hindsight Bias. *Perspectives on Psychological Science, 7*(5), 411–426.

Rogers, T. B., Kuiper, N. A., & Kirker, W. S. (1977). Self-reference and the encoding of personal information. *Journal of Personality and Social Psychology, 35*, 677–688.

Rosch, E. (1975). Cognitive representations of semantic categories. *Journal of Experimental Psychology, 104*, 192–233.

Rosen, S., & Tesser, A. (1970). On reluctance to communicate undesirable information: The MUM effect. *Sociometry, 33*, 253–263.

Rosenberg, S., & Sedlak, A. (1972). Structural representations of perceived personality trait relationships. In R. N. Shepard, A. K. Romney, & S. B. Nerlove (Eds.), *Multidimensional scaling: Theory and applications in the behavioral sciences* (Vol. 2, pp. 134–162). New York: Seminar Press.

Rosenthal, R. (1974). *On the social psychology of the self-fulfilling prophecy: Further evidence for Pygmalion effects and their mediating mechanisms.* New York: MSS Modular Publications.

Roskos-Ewoldsen, D. R., & Fazio, R. H. (1992). On the orienting value of attitudes: Attitude accessibility as a determinant of an object's attraction of visual attention. *Journal of Personality and Social Psychology, 63*, 198–211.

Ross, L. (1977). The intuitive psychologist and his shortcomings: Distortions in the attribution process. In L. Berkowitz (Ed.), *Advances in experimental social psychology* (Vol. 10, pp. 174–221). New York: Academic Press.

Ross, L., Amabile, T. M., & Steinmetz, J. L. (1977). Social roles, social control, and biases in social-perception processes. *Journal of Personality and Social Psychology, 35*, 484–494.

Ross, L., Greene, D., & House, P. (1977). The false consensus effect: An egocentric bias in social perception and attribution processes. *Journal of Experimental Social Psychology, 13*(3), 279–301.

Ross, L., Lepper, M. R., & Hubbard, M. (1975). Perseverance in self-perception and social perception: Biased attributional processes in the debriefing paradigm. *Journal of Personality and Social Psychology, 32,* 880–892.

Ross, L., & Nisbett, R. E. (1991). *The person and the situation. Perspectives of social psychology.* New York: McGraw Hill.

Rothbart, M., Evans, M., & Fulero, S. (1979). Recall for confirming events: Memory processes and the maintenance of social stereotypes. *Journal of Experimental Social Psychology, 15,* 343–355.

Rothbart, M., & Park, B. (1986). On the confirmability and disconfirmability of trait concepts. *Journal of Personality and Social Psychology, 50*(1), 131–142.

Rothbart, M., Sriram, N., & Davis Stitt, C. (1996). The retrieval of typical and atypical category members. *Journal of Experimental Social Psychology, 32,* 1–29.

Rothman, N. B., & Melwani, S. (2017). Feeling mixed, ambivalent, and in flux: The social functions of emotional complexity for leaders. *Academy of Management Review, 42*(2), 259–282.

Rothman, N. B., Pratt, M. G., Rees, L., & Vogus, T. J. (2017). Understanding the dual nature of ambivalence: Why and when ambivalence leads to good and bad outcomes. *Academy of Management Annals, 11,* 33–72.

Rothman, N., Vitriol, J., & Moskowitz, G. B. (2022). Internal conflict and prejudice-regulation: Emotional ambivalence buffers against defensive responding to implicit bias feedback. *PLOS One, 17*(3), e0264535.

Rotter, J. B. (1966). Generalized expectancies for internal versus external control of reinforcement. *Psychological Monographs: General and Applied, 80*(1), 1–28.

Rubin, D. C., Stoltzfus, E. R., & Wall, K. L. (1991). The abstraction of form in semantic categories. *Memory and Cognition, 19*(1), 1–7.

Rubin, M., & Badea, C. (2012). They're all the same! . . . but for several different reasons: A review of the multicausal nature of perceived group variability. *Current Directions in Psychological Science, 21*(6), 367–372.

Rubin, M., Hewstone, M., & Voci, A. (2001). Stretching the boundaries: Strategic perceptions of intragroup variability. *European Journal of Social Psychology, 31*(4), 413–429.

Rudman, L. A. (1998). Self-promotion as a risk factor for women: The costs and benefits of counterstereotypical impression management. *Journal of Personality and Social Psychology, 74*(3), 629–645.

Rudman, L. A., & Glick, P. (1999). Feminized management and backlash toward agentic women: The hidden costs to women of a kinder, gentler image of middle managers. *Journal of Personality and Social Psychology, 77*(5), 1004–1010.

Rudman, L. A., & Glick, P. (2001). Prescriptive gender stereotypes and backlash toward agentic women. *Journal of Social Issues, 57*(4), 743–762.

Rudman, L. A., Greenwald, A. G., Mellott, D. S., & Schwartz, J. L. K. (1999). Measuring the automatic components of prejudice: Flexibility and generality of the Implicit Association Test. *Social Cognition, 17,* 437–465.

Rudman, L. A., Moss-Racusin, C. A., Phelan, J. E., & Nauts, S. (2012). Status incongruity and backlash effects: Defending the gender hierarchy motivates prejudice against female leaders. *Journal of Experimental Social Psychology, 48*(1), 165–179.

Rudman, L. A., & Phelan, J. (2008). Backlash effects for disconfirming gender stereotypes in organizations. *Research in Organizational Behavior, 28,* 61–79.

Rule, N. O., Tskhay, K. O., Freeman, J. B., & Ambady, N. (2014). On the interactive influence of facial appearance and explicit knowledge in social categorization. *European Journal of Social Psychology, 44*(6), 529–535.

Ruscher, J. B. (1998). Prejudice and stereotyping in everyday communication. *Advances in Experimental Social Psychology, 30,* 241–307.

Ryan, C. S., Judd, C. M., & Park, B. (1996). Effects of racial stereotypes on judgments of individuals: The moderating role of perceived group variability. *Journal of Experimental Social Psychology, 32*(1), 71–103.

Rydell, R. J., & Gawronski, B. (2009). I like you, I like you not: Understanding the formation of context-dependent automatic attitudes. *Cognition and Emotion, 23*(6), 1118–1152.

Rydell, R. J., & Jones, C. R. M. (2009). Competition between unconditioned stimuli in attitude formation: Negative asymmetry versus spatio-temporal contiguity. *Social Cognition, 27*, 905–916.

Rydell, R. J., & McConnell, A. R. (2006). Understanding implicit and explicit attitude change: A systems of reasoning analysis. *Journal of Personality and Social Psychology, 91*(6), 995–1008.

Rydell, R. J., McConnell, A. R., & Mackie, D. M. (2008). Consequences of discrepant explicit and implicit attitudes: Cognitive dissonance and increased information processing. *Journal of Experimental Social Psychology, 44*(6), 1526–1532.

Rydell, R. J., McConnell, A. R., Mackie, D. M., & Strain, L. M. (2006). Of two minds forming and changing valence-inconsistent implicit and explicit attitudes. *Psychological Science, 17*(11), 954–958.

Rydell, R. J., McConnell, A. R., Strain, L. M., Claypool, H. M., & Hugenberg, K. (2007). Implicit and explicit evaluations respond differently to increasing amounts of counterattitudinal information. *European Journal of Social Psychology, 37*(5), 867–878.

Sabin, J. A., & Greenwald, A. G. (2012). The influence of implicit bias on treatment recommendations for 4 common pediatric conditions: Pain, urinary tract infection, attention deficit hyperactivity disorder, and asthma. *American Journal of Public Health, 102*(5), 988–995.

Sadler, M. S., Correll, J., Park, B., & Judd, C. M. (2012). The world is not black and white: Racial bias in the decision to shoot in a multiethnic context. *Journal of Social Issues, 68*, 286–313.

Sahakyan, L., Delaney, P. F., Foster, N. L., & Abushanab, B. (2013). List-method directed forgetting in cognitive and clinical research: A theoretical and methodological review. In B. H. Ross (Ed.), *Psychology of learning and motivation* (Vol. 59, pp. 131–189). New York: Academic Press.

Said, C. P., & Todorov, A. (2011). A statistical model of facial attractiveness. *Psychological Science, 22*(9), 1183–1190.

Sands, E., & Harris, L. T. (2023). Expressed accuracy: Spontaneous trait production and inference from voice. In E. Balcetis & G. B. Moskowitz (Eds.), *Handbook of impression formation: A social psychological approach* (pp. 34–53). New York: Routledge.

Sanna, L. J., Schwarz, N., & Stocker, S. L. (2002). When debiasing backfires: Accessible content and accessibility experiences in debiasing hindsight. *Journal of Experimental Psychology: Learning, Memory, and Cognition, 28*(3), 497–502.

Sassenberg, K., Jonas, K. J., Shah, J. Y., & Brazy, P. C. (2007). Why some groups just feel better: The regulatory fit of group power. *Journal of Personality and Social Psychology, 92*(2), 249–267.

Sassenberg, K., & Moskowitz, G. B. (2005). Do not stereotype, think different! Overcoming automatic stereotype activation by mindset priming. *Journal of Experimental Social Psychology, 41*(5), 317–413.

Sassenberg, K., Moskowitz, G. B., Fetterman, A., & Kessler, T. (2017). Priming creativity as a strategy to increase creative performance by facilitating the activation and use of remote associations. *Journal of Experimental Social Psychology, 68*, 128–138.

Sassenberg, K., Winter, K., Becker, D., Ditrich, D., Scholl, A., & Moskowitz, G. B. (2022). Flexibility mindsets: Reducing biases that result from spontaneous processing. *European Review of Social Psychology, 33*(1), 171–213.

Savary, J., Kleiman, T., Hassin, R. R., & Dhar, R. (2015). Positive consequences of conflict on decision making: When a conflict mindset facilitates choice. *Journal of Experimental Psychology: General, 144*(1), 1–6.

Savitsky, K., & Gilovich, T. (1998, February). *Speech anxiety and the illusion of transparency.* Paper presented at the meeting of the Eastern Psychological Association, Boston, MA.

Schachter, S., & Singer, J. E. (1962). Cognitive, social, and psychological determinants of emotional state. *Psychological Review, 69*, 379–399.

Schaller, M., & Conway, L. G., III. (2001). From cognition to culture: The origins of stereotypes that really matter. In G. B. Moskowitz (Ed.), *Cognitive social psychology: The Princeton Symposium on the Legacy and Future of Social Cognition* (pp. 163–176). Hillsdale, NJ: Erlbaum.

Schank, R. C. (1982). *Dynamic memory: A theory of reminding and learning in computers and people.* New York: Cambridge University Press.

Schank, R. C., & Abelson, R. P. (1977). *Scripts, plans, goals, and understanding: An inquiry into human knowledge structures.* Hillsdale, NJ: Erlbaum.

Schilpzand, P., De Pater, I. E., & Erez, A. (2016). Workplace incivility: A review of the literature and agenda for future research. *Journal of Organizational Behavior, 37*(Suppl. 1), S57–S88.

Schkade, D. A., & Kahneman, D. (1998). Does living in California make people happy? A focusing illusion in judgments of life satisfaction. *Psychological Science, 9*(5), 340–346.

Schlenker, B. R., & Leary, M. R. (1982). Social anxiety and self-presentation: A conceptual model. *Psychological Bulletin, 92*(3), 641–669.

Schmader, T., Block, K., & Lickel, B. (2015). Social identity threat in response to stereotypic film portrayals: Effects on self-conscious emotion and implicit ingroup attitudes. *Journal of Social Issues, 71*(1), 54–72.

Schmader, T., Dennehy, T. C., & Baron, A. S. (2022). Why antibias interventions (need not) fail. *Perspectives on Psychological Science, 17*(5), 1381–1403.

Schmader, T., & Lickel, B. (2006). The approach and avoidance function of guilt and shame emotions: Comparing reactions to self-caused and other-caused wrongdoing. *Motivation and Emotion, 30*(1), 43–56.

Schmemann, S. (2021, September 11). "I Wrote the Lead Times Article on 9/11. Here's What Still Grips Me." *New York Times*, Section A, p. 23.

Schneider, D. J. (1973). Implicit personality theory: A review. *Psychological Bulletin, 79,* 294–309.

Schneider, D. J., & Blankmeyer, B. L. (1983). Prototype salience and implicit personality theories. *Journal of Personality and Social Psychology, 44*(4), 712–722.

Schock, A., Gruber, F. M., Scherndl, T., & Ortner, T. M. (2019). Tempering agency with communion increases women's leadership emergence in all-women groups: Evidence for role congruity theory in a field setting. *Leadership Quarterly, 30*(2), 189–198.

Schultner, D. T., Lindström, B. R., Cikara, M., & Amodio, D. M. (2024). Transmission of social bias through observational learning. *Science Advances.*

Schwarz, N., Bless, H., Strack, F., Klumpp, G., Rittenauer Schatka, H., & Simons, A. (1991). Ease of retrieval as information: Another look at the availability heuristic. *Journal of Personality and Social Psychology, 61,* 195–202.

Schwarz, N., & Clore, G. L. (1983). Mood, misattribution, and judgments of well-being: Informative and directive functions of affective states. *Journal of Personality and Social Psychology, 45,* 513–523.

Schwarz, N., & Clore, G. L. (1996). Feelings and phenomenal experiences. In E. T. Higgins & A. W. Kruglanski (Eds.), *Social psychology: Handbook of basic principles* (pp. 433–465). New York: Guilford Press.

Schwarz, N., Sanna, L. J., Skurnik, I., & Yoon, C. (2007). Metacognitive experiences and the intricacies of setting people straight: Implications for debiasing and public information campaigns. In M. P. Zanna (Ed.), *Advances in experimental social psychology* (vol. 39, pp. 127–161). Boston: Elsevier Academic Press.

Schwarz, N., Strack, F., Mueller, G., & Chassein, B. (1988). The range of response alternatives may determine the meaning of the question: Further evidence on informative functions of response alternatives, *Social Cognition, 6*(2), 107–117.

Sciara, S., Regalia, C., & Gollwitzer, P. M. (2022). Resolving incompleteness on social media: Online self-symbolizing reduces the orienting effects of incomplete identity goals. *Motivation Science, 8*(3), 268–275.

Scopelliti, I., Morewedge, C. K., McCormick, E., Min, L., Lebrecht, S., & Kassam, K. S. (2015). Bias blind spot: Structure, measurement, and consequences. *Management Science, 61*(10), 2468–2486.

Scully, I. D., & Hupbach, A. (2020). Directed forgetting affects how we remember and judge other people. *Journal of Applied Research in Memory and Cognition, 9*(3), 336–344.

Sears, D. O., & Henry, P. J. (2003). The origins of symbolic racism. *Journal of Personality and Social Psychology, 85*(2), 259–275.

Sedikides, C. (1993). Assessment, enhancement, and verification determinants of the self-evaluation process. *Journal of Personality and Social Psychology, 65,* 317–338.

Sedikides, C., & Anderson, C. A. (1994). Causal perceptions of intertrait relations: The glue that holds person types together. *Personality and Social Psychology Bulletin, 20,* 294–302.

Sedikides, C., Gaertner, L., & Toguchi, Y. (2003). Pancultural self-enhancement. *Journal of Personality and Social Psychology, 84*(1), 60–79.

Sedikides, C., Green, J. D., & Pinter, B. (2004). Self-protective memory. In D. R. Beike, J. M.

Lampinen, & D. A. Behrend (Eds.), *The self and memory* (pp. 161–179). London: Psychology Press.

Sedikides, C., & Hepper, E. G. D. (2009). Self-improvement. *Social and Personality Compass, 3*(6), 899–917.

Sedikides, C., & Strube, M. J. (1997). Self-evaluation: To thine own self be good, to thine own self be sure, to thine own self be true, and to thine own self be better. *Advances in Experimental Social Psychology, 29*, 209–269.

Segall, M. H., Campbell, D. T., & Herskovit, M. J. (1963). Cultural differences in the perception of geometric illusions. *Science, 139*(3556), 769–771.

Seligman, M. E. P. (1975). *Helplessness: On depression, development, and death.* Oxford, UK: Freeman.

Seligman, M. E. P. (1990). *Learned optimism.* New York: Knopf.

Semin, G. R., & Fiedler, K. (1991). The linguistic category model, its bases, applications and range. *European Review of Social Psychology, 2*(1), 1–30.

Sesko, A. K., & Biernat, M. (2010). Prototypes of race and gender: The invisibility of Black women. *Journal of Experimental Social Psychology, 46,* 356–360.

Shafir, E. (1993). Choosing versus rejecting: Why some options are both better and worse than others. *Memory and Cognition, 21,* 546–556.

Shah, J. (2003). Automatic for the people: How representations of significant others implicitly affect goal pursuit. *Journal of Personality and Social Psychology, 84,* 661–681.

Shah, J. Y., Hall, D., & Leander, N. P. (2009). Moments of motivation: Towards a model of regulatory rotation. In G. B. Moskowitz & H. Grant (Eds.), *The psychology of goals* (pp. 234–254). New York: Guilford Press.

Shah, J., Higgins, T., & Friedman, R. S. (1998). Performance incentives and means: How regulatory focus influences goal attainment. *Journal of Personality and Social Psychology, 74,* 285–293.

Shaver, K. G. (1985). *The attribution of blame: Causality, responsibility, and blameworthiness.* New York: Springer-Verlag.

Shelton, J. N. (2000). A reconceptualization of how we study issues of racial prejudice. *Personality and Social Psychology Review, 4*(4), 374–390.

Shelton, J. N., & Richeson, J. A. (2006). Ethnic minorities' racial attitudes and contact experiences with White people. *Cultural Diversity and Ethnic Minority Psychology, 12*(1), 149–164.

Shelton, J. N., Richeson, J. A., & Salvatore, J. (2005). Expecting to be the target of prejudice: Implications for interethnic interactions. *Personality and Social Psychology Bulletin, 31*(9), 1189–1202.

Shen, X., & Ferguson, M. (2023). Are we stuck on the face? New evidence for when and how people update face-based implicit impressions. In E. Balcetis & G. B. Moskowitz (Eds.). *Handbook of impression formation: A social psychological approach* (pp. 393–415). New York: Routledge.

Shepperd, J., Malone, W., & Sweeny, K. (2008). Exploring causes of the self-serving bias. *Social and Personality Psychology Compass, 2*(2), 895–908.

Sherif, M. (1936). *The psychology of social norms.* New York: Harper.

Sherif, M. (1967). *Group conflict and cooperation: Their social psychology.* New York: Routledge & K. Paul.

Sherif, M., & Hovland, C. I. (1961). *Social judgment: Assimilation and contrast effects in communication and attitude change.* New Haven, CT: Yale University Press.

Sherman, D. K., Hogg, M. A., & Maitner, A. T. (2009). Perceived polarization: Reconciling ingroup and intergroup perceptions under uncertainty. *Group Processes and Intergroup Relations, 12,* 95–109.

Sherman, J. W. (1996). Development and mental representation of stereotypes. *Journal of Personality and Social Psychology, 70,* 1126–1141.

Sherman, J. (2001). The dynamic relationship between stereotype efficiency and mental represention. In G. B. Moskowitz (Ed.), *Cognitive social psychology: The Princeton symposium on the legacy and future of social cognition* (pp. 177–190). Mahwah, NJ: Erlbaum.

Sherman, J. W. (2006). On building a better process model: It's not only how many, but which ones and by which means? *Psychological Inquiry, 17,* 173–184.

Sherman, J. W., & Frost, L. A. (2000). On the encoding of stereotype-relevant information under cognitive load. *Personality and Social Psychology Bulletin, 26*(1), 26–34.

Sherman, J. W., Gawronski, B., Gonsalkorale, K., Hugenberg, K., Allen, T. J., & Groom, C. J. (2008). The self-regulation of automatic associations and behavioral impulses. *Psychological Review, 115,* 314–335.

Sherman, J. W., & Klein, S. B. (1994). Development and representation of personality impressions. *Journal of Personality and Social Psychology, 67,* 972–983.

Sherman, J. W., Klein, S. B., Laskey, A., & Wyer, N. A. (1998). Intergroup bias in group judgment processes: The role of behavioral memories. *Journal of Experimental Social Psychology, 34,* 51–65.

Sherman, J. W., Kruschke, J. K., Sherman, S. J., Percy, E. J., Petrocelli, J. V., & Conrey, F. R. (2009). Attentional processes in stereotype formation: A common model for category accentuation and illusory correlation. *Journal of Personality and Social Psychology, 96,* 305–323.

Sherman, J. W., Lee, A. Y., Bessenoff, G. R., & Frost, L. A. (1998). Stereotype efficiency reconsidered: Encoding flexibility under cognitive load. *Journal of Personality and Social Psychology, 75,* 589–606.

Sherman, J. W., Stroessner, S. J., Conrey, F. R., & Azam, O. A. (2005). Prejudice and stereotype maintenance processes: Attention, attribution, and individuation. *Journal of Personality and Social Psychology, 89*(4), 607–622.

Shiffrin, R. M. (1988). Attention. In R. C. Atkinson, R. T. Herrnstein, G. Lindzey, & R. D. Luce (Eds.), *Steven's handbook of experimental psychology* (2nd ed., Vol., 2, pp. 739–811). New York: Wiley.

Shiffrin, R. M., & Schneider, W. (1977). Controlled and automatic human information processing: II. Perceptual learning, automatic attending, and a general theory. *Psychological Review, 84,* 127–190.

Shuell, T. J. (1977). Clustering and organization in free recall. *Psychological Bulletin, 72,* 353–374.

Sicoly, F., & Ross, M. (1977). Facilitation of ego-biased attributions by means of self-serving observer feedback. *Journal of Personality and Social Psychology, 35*(10), 734–741.

Sidanius, J. (1993). The psychology of group conflict and the dynamics of oppression: A social dominance perspective. In W. McGuire & S. Iyengar (Eds.), *Current approaches to political psychology* (pp. 183–219). Durham, NC: Duke University Press.

Sim, J. J., Correll, J., & Sadler, M. S. (2013). Understanding police and expert performance: When training attenuates (vs. exacerbates) stereotypic bias in the decision to shoot. *Personality and Social Psychology Bulletin, 39*(3), 291–304.

Sim, M., Almaraz, S. M., & Hugenberg, K. (2022). Stereotyping at the intersection of race and weight: Diluted threat stereotyping of obese Black men. *Journal of Experimental Social Psychology, 99,* 1–14.

Simon, H. A. (1956). A comparison of game theory and learning theory. *Psychometrika, 21,* 267–272.

Simon, L., Greenberg, J., & Brehm, J. (1995). Trivialization: The forgotten mode of dissonance reduction. *Journal of Personality and Social Psychology, 68*(2), 247–260.

Skitka, L. J., Mullen, E., Griffin, T., Hutchinson, S., & Chamberlin, B. (2002). Dispositions, scripts, or motivated correction? Understanding ideological differences in explanation for social problems. *Journal of Personality and Social Psychology, 83*(2), 470–487.

Skowronski, J. J., & Carlston, D. E. (1987). Social judgment and social memory: The role of cue diagnosticity in negativity, positivity, and extremity biases. *Journal of Personality and Social Psychology, 52,* 689–699.

Skowronski, J. J., & Carlston, D. E. (1989). Negativity and extremity biases in impression formation: A review of explanations. *Psychological Bulletin, 105,* 131–142.

Skowronski, J. J., & Carlston, D. E. (1992). Caught in the act: When impressions based on highly diagnostic behaviours are resistant to contradiction. *European Journal of Social Psychology, 22*(5), 435–452.

Skurnik, I., Moskowitz, G. B., & Johnson, M. (2001). *Biases in remembering true and false information: Illusions of truth and falseness.* Unpublished manuscript, Princeton University, Princeton, NJ.

Skurnik, I., Yoon, C., Park, D. C., & Schwarz, N. (2005). How warnings about false claims become recommendations. *Journal of Consumer Research, 31*(4), 713–724.

Smith, B., & Holmes, D. (2003). Community accountability, minority, threat, and police brutality: An examination of civil rights criminal complaints. *Criminology, 41*(4), 1035–1063.

Smith, E. R., & DeCoster, J. (2000). Dual-process

models in social and cognitive psychology: Conceptual integration and links to underlying memory systems. *Personality and Social Psychology Review, 4*(2), 108–131.

Smith, E. R., & Zarate, M. A. (1992). Exemplar-based model of social judgment. *Psychological Review, 99*, 3–21.

Smith, S. M., Ward, T. B., & Schumacher, J. S. (1993). Constraining effects of examples in a creative generation task. *Memory and Cognition, 21*(6), 837–845.

Sniderman, P., Hagen, M., Tetlock, P., & Brady, H. (1986). Reasoning chains: Causal models of policy reasoning in mass publics. *British Journal of Political Science, 16*(4), 405–430.

Snowden, D. (2002). Complex acts of knowing: Paradox and descriptive self-awareness. *Journal of Knowledge Management, 6*, 100–111.

Snyder, M. L., & Frankel, A. (1976). Observer bias: A stringent test of behavior engulfing the field. *Journal of Personality and Social Psychology, 34*, 857–864.

Snyder, M., & Swann, W. B. (1978). Hypotheses testing processes in social interaction. *Journal of Personality and Social Psychology, 36*, 1202–1212.

Snyder, M., Tanke, E. D., & Berscheid, E. (1977). Social perception and interpersonal behavior: On the self-fulfilling nature of social stereotypes. *Journal of Personality and Social Psychology, 35*(9), 656–666.

Snyder, M., & Uranowitz, S. W. (1978). Reconstructing the past: Some cognitive consequences of person perception. *Journal of Personality and Social Psychology, 36*, 941–950.

Sommers, S. R., & Norton, M. I. (2006). Lay theories about White racists: What constitutes racism (and what doesn't). *Group Processes and Intergroup Relations, 9*(1), 117–138.

Son Hing, L. S., Chung-Yan, G. A., Hamilton, L. K., & Zanna, M. P. (2008). A two-dimensional model that employs explicit and implicit attitudes to characterize prejudice. *Journal of Personality and Social Psychology, 94*(6), 971–987.

Sorrentino, R. M., & Higgins, E. T. (Eds.). (1986). Motivation and cognition: Warming up to synergism. In R. M. Sorrentino & E. T. Higgins (Eds.), *Handbook of motivation and cognition: Foundations of social behavior* (pp. 3–19). New York: Guilford Press.

Sorrentino, R. M., & Short, J. C. (1986). Uncertainty orientation, motivation, and cognition. In R. M. Sorrentino & E. T. Higgins (Eds.), *Handbook of motivation and cognition* (pp. 379–403). New York: Guilford Press.

Spears, R., Doosje, B., & Ellemers, N. (1997). Self-stereotyping in the face of threats to group status and distinctiveness: The role of group identification. *Personality and Social Psychology Bulletin, 23*, 538–553.

Spellman, B. A., & Kincannon, A. (2001). The relation between counterfactual ("but for") and causal reasoning: Experimental findings and implications for jurors' decisions. *Law and Contemporary Problems, 64*(4), 241–264.

Spencer, K. B., Charbonneau, A. K., & Glaser, J. (2016). Implicit bias and policing. *Social and Personality Psychology Compass, 10*(1), 50–63.

Spencer, S. J., Fein, S., Wolfe, C. T., Fong, C., & Dunn, M. A. (1998). Automatic activation of stereotypes: The role of self-image threat. *Personality and Social Psychology Bulletin, 24*, 1139–1152.

Spencer, S. J., Steele, C. M., & Quinn, D. (1999). Stereotype threat and women's math performance. *Journal of Experimental and Social Psychology, 35*, 4–28.

Spencer-Rodgers, J., Hamilton, D. L., & Sherman, S. J. (2007). The central role of entitativity in stereotypes of social categories and task groups. *Journal of Personality and Social Psychology, 92*(3), 369–388.

Spielman, L. A., & Bargh, J. A. (1990). Does the depressive self-schema really exist? In C. D. McCann & N. S. Endler (Eds.), *Depression: New directions in theory, research, and practice* (pp. 111–126). Toronto: Wall & Emerson.

Spruyt, A., Hermans, D., De Houwer, J., Vandromme, H., & Eelen, P. (2007). On the nature of the affective priming effect: Effects of stimulus onset asynchrony and congruency proportion in naming and evaluative categorization. *Memory and Cognition, 35*(1), 95–106.

Srinivasan, A. (2021, September 3). "What's wrong with sex between professors and students? It's not what you think." *New York Times*, Section SR, p. 4.

Srull, T. K. (1981). Person memory: Some tests of associative storage and retrieval models. *Journal of Experimental Psychology: Human Learning and Memory, 7*(6), 440–463.

Srull, T. K. (1983). Organizational and retrieval

processes in person memory: An examination of processing objectives, presentation format, and the possible role of self-generated retrieval cues. *Journal of Personality and Social Psychology, 44,* 1157–1170.

Srull, T. K., & Brand, J. F. (1983). Memory for information about persons: The effect of encoding operations on subsequent retrieval. *Journal of Verbal Learning and Verbal Behavior, 22,* 219–230.

Srull, T. K., & Wyer, R. S., Jr. (1979). The role of category accessibility in the interpretation of information about persons: Some determinants and implications. *Journal of Personality and Social Psychology, 37,* 1660–1672.

Srull, T. K., & Wyer, R. S., Jr. (1980). Category accessibility and social perception: Some implications for the study of person memory and interpersonal judgment. *Journal of Personality and Social Psychology, 38,* 841–856.

Srull, T. K., & Wyer, R. S., Jr. (1989). Person memory and judgment. *Psychological Review, 96,* 58–83.

Stangor, C., Lynch, L., Duan, C., & Glas, B. (1992). Categorization of individuals on the basis of multiple social features. *Journal of Personality and Social Psychology, 62*(2), 207–218.

Stangor, C., & Ruble, D. N. (1989). Strength of expectancies and memory for social information: What we remember depends on how much we know. *Journal of Experimental Social Psychology, 25,* 18–35.

Stangor, C., Sechrist, G. B., & Jost, J. T. (2001). Changing racial beliefs by providing consensus information. *Personality and Social Psychology Bulletin, 27*(4), 486–496.

Stapel, D. A., & Koomen, W. (2001). Let's not forget the past when we go to the future: On our knowledge of knowledge accessibility. In G. B. Moskowitz (Ed.), *Cognitive social psychology: The Princeton symposium on the legacy and future of social cognition* (pp. 229–246). Mahwah, NJ: Erlbaum.

Steele, C. M. (1988). The psychology of self-affirmation: Sustaining the integrity of the self. In L. Berkowitz (Ed.), *Advances in experimental social psychology* (Vol. 21, pp. 261–302). New York: Academic Press.

Steele, C. M. (1997). A threat in the air: How stereotypes shape intellectual identity and performance. *American Psychologist, 52,* 613–629.

Steele, C. M., & Aronson, J. (1995). Stereotype threat and the intellectual test performance of African Americans. *Journal of Personality and Social Psychology, 69,* 797–811.

Steele, C. M., & Liu, T. J. (1983). Dissonance processes as self-affirmation. *Journal of Personality and Social Psychology, 45*(1), 5–19.

Stephan, W. G., & Stephan, C. W. (1985). Intergroup anxiety. *Journal of Social Issues, 41*(3), 157–175.

Stevens, L., & Jones, E. E. (1976). Defensive attribution and the Kelley cube. *Journal of Personality and Social Psychology, 34,* 809–820.

Stewart, B. D., & Payne, B. K. (2008). Bringing automatic stereotyping under control: Implementation intentions as efficient means of thought control. *Personality and Social Psychology Bulletin, 34*(10), 1332–1345.

Stillman, P. E., Shen, X., & Ferguson, M. J. (2018). How mouse-tracking can advance social cognitive theory. *Trends in Cognitive Science, 22*(6), 531–543.

Stone, J. (2001). Behavioral discrepancies and the role of construal processes in cognitive dissonance. In G. B. Moskowitz (Ed.), *Cognitive social psychology: The Princeton symposium on the legacy and future of social cognition* (pp. 41–58). Mahwah, NJ: Erlbaum.

Stone, J., Aronson, E., Crain, A. L., Winslow, M. P., & Fried, C. B. (1994). Inducing hypocrisy as a means of encouraging young adults to use condoms. *Personality and Social Psychology Bulletin, 20*(1), 116–128.

Stone, J., Moskowitz, G. B., Zestcott, C., & Wolsiefer, K. (2020). Testing active learning workshops for reducing implicit stereotyping of Hispanics by majority and minority group medical students. *Stigma and Health, 5*(1), 94–103.

Stone, J., Whitehead, J., Schmader, T., & Focella, E. (2011). Thanks for asking: Self-affirming questions reduce backlash when stigmatized targets confront prejudice. *Journal of Experimental Social Psychology, 47*(3), 589–598.

Stone, J., Wiegand, A. W., Cooper, J., & Aronson, E. (1997). When exemplification fails: Hypocrisy and the motive for self-integrity. *Journal of Personality and Social Psychology, 72*(1), 54–65.

Storms, M. D. (1973). Videotape and the attribution process: Reversing actors' and observers' points of view. *Journal of Personality and Social Psychology, 27*(2), 165–175.

Strack, F., & Deutsch, R. (2004). Reflective and impulsive determinants of social behavior.

Personality and Social Psychology Review, 8(3), 220–247.

Strack, F., & Hannover, B. (1996). Awareness of influence as a precondition for implementing correctional goals. In P. M. Gollwitzer & J. A. Bargh (Eds.), *The psychology of action: Linking cognition and motivation to behavior.* New York: Guilford Press.

Strack, F., Martin, L. L., & Stepper, S. (1988). Inhibiting and facilitating conditions of the human smile: A nonobtrusive test of the facial feedback hypothesis. *Journal of Personality and Social Psychology, 54*(5), 768–777.

Strack, F., Schwarz, N., Bless, H., Kübler, A., & Wänke, M. (1993). Awareness of the influence as a determinant of assimilation versus contrast. *European Journal of Social Psychology, 23,* 53–62.

Strahan, E. J., Spencer, S. J., & Zanna, M. P. (2002). Subliminal priming and persuasion: Striking while the iron is hot. *Journal of Experimental Social Psychology, 38*(6), 556–568.

Strauman, T. J., & Higgins, E. T. (1987). Automatic activation of self-discrepancies and emotional syndromes: When cognitive structures influence affect. *Journal of Personality and Social Psychology, 53*(6), 1004–1014.

Strauman, T. J., & Higgins, E. T. (1988). Self-discrepancies as predictors of vulnerability to distinct syndromes of chronic emotional distress. *Journal of Personality, 56*(4), 685–707.

Stroessner, S. J., & Dweck, C. S. (2015). Inferring group traits and group goals: A unified approach to social perception. In S. J. Stroessner & J. W. Sherman (Eds.), *Social perception from individuals to groups* (pp. 177–196). London: Psychology Press.

Stroessner, S. J., & Heuer, L. B. (1996). Cognitive bias in procedural justice: Formation and implications of illusory correlations in perceived intergroup fairness. *Journal of Personality and Social Psychology, 71,* 717–728.

Stroessner, S. J., & Plaks, J. E. (2001). Illusory correlation and stereotype formation: Tracing the arc of research over a quarter century. In G. B. Moskowitz (Ed.), *Cognitive social psychology: The Princeton symposium on the legacy and future of social cognition* (pp. 247–260). Mahwah, NJ: Erlbaum.

Stroop, J. R. (1935). Studies of interference in serial verbal reactions. *Journal of Experimental Psychology 18,* 643–662.

Sue, D. W. (2010). *Microaggressions in everyday life: Race, gender, and sexual orientation.* New York: Wiley.

Sussman, A. B., Petkova, K., & Todorov, A. (2013). Competence ratings in US predict presidential election outcomes in Bulgaria. *Journal of Experimental Social Psychology, 49*(4), 771–775.

Sutton, R. M., & McClure, J. (2001). Covariational influences on goal-based explanation: An integrative model. *Journal of Personality and Social Psychology, 80,* 222–236.

Swann, W. B. (1983). Self-verification: Bringing social reality into harmony with the self. In J. Suls & A. G. Greenwald (Eds.), *Social psychological perspectives on the self* (Vol. 2, pp. 33–66). New York: Erlbaum.

Swann, W. B., Jr. (1990). To be adored or to be known? The interplay of self-enhancement and self-verification. In E. T. Higgins & R. Sorrentino (Eds.), *Handbook of motivation and cognition: Foundations of social behavior* (Vol. 2, pp. 527–561). New York: Guilford Press.

Swann, W. B., Jr., Pelham, B. W., & Krull, D. S. (1989). Agreeable fancy or disagreeable truth? Reconciling self-enhancement and self-verification. *Journal of Personality and Social Psychology, 57*(5), 782–791.

Swann, W. B., & Read, S. J. (1981). Self-verification processes: How we sustain our self-conceptions. *Journal of Experimental Social Psychology, 17*(4), 351–372.

Swim, J., Borgida, E., Maruyama, G., & Myers, D. G. (1989). Joan McKay versus John McKay: Do gender stereotypes bias evaluations? *Psychological Bulletin, 105*(3), 409–429.

Tajfel, H. (1969). Cognitive aspects of prejudice. *Journal of Social Issues, 25,* 79–97.

Tajfel, H., Billig, M. G., Bundy, R. P., & Flament, C. (1971). Social categorization and intergroup behavior. *European Journal of Social Psychology, 1,* 149–178.

Tajfel, H., & Turner, J. C. (1979). An integrative theory of intergroup conflict. In S. Worchel & W. G. Austin (Eds.), *The social psychology of intergroup relations* (pp. 33–47). Monterey, CA: Brooks/Cole.

Tajfel, H., & Turner, J. C. (1986). An integrative theory of intergroup relations. In S. Worchel & W. G. Austin (Eds.), *Psychology of intergroup relations* (pp. 7–24). Chicago: Nelson-Hall.

Tajfel, H., & Wilkes, A. L. (1963). Classification and quantitative judgment. *British Journal of Psychology, 54,* 101–114.

Tankard, M. E., & Paluck, E. L. (2017). The effect of a Supreme Court decision regarding gay marriage on social norms and personal attitudes. *Psychological Science, 28*(9), 1334–1344.

Taylor, D. M., & Jaggi, V. (1974). Ethnocentrism and causal attribution in a South Indian context. *Journal of Cross-Cultural Psychology, 5,* 162–171.

Taylor, D. M., & Moghaddam, F. M. (1987). *Theories of intergroup relations: International social psychological perspectives.* New York: Praeger.

Taylor, S. E. (1981). The interface of cognitive and social psychology. In J. H. Harvey (Ed.), *Cognition, social behavior, and the environment* (pp. 189–212). Hillsdale, NJ: Erlbaum.

Taylor, S. E., & Brown, J. D. (1988). Illusion and well-being: A social psychological perspective on mental health. *Psychological Bulletin, 103*(2), 193–210.

Taylor, S. E., & Crocker, J. (1981). Schematic bases of social information processing. In E. T. Higgins, P. Herman, & M. Zanna (Eds.), *Social cognition: The Ontario symposium* (Vol. 1, pp. 89–134). Hillsdale, NJ: Erlbaum.

Taylor, S. E., Crocker, J., Fiske, S. T., Sprinzen, M., & Winkler, J. D. (1979). The generalizability of salience effects. *Journal of Personality and Social Psychology, 31,* 357–368.

Taylor, S. E., & Fiske, S. T. (1975). Point-of-view and perceptions of causality. *Journal of Personality and Social Psychology, 32,* 439–445.

Taylor, S. E., & Fiske, S. T. (1978). Salience, attention, and attribution: Top of the head phenomena. In L. Berkowitz (Ed.), *Advances in experimental social psychology* (Vol. 11, pp. 249–288). San Diego, CA: Academic Press.

Taylor, S. E., Fiske, S. T., Etcoff, N., & Ruderman, A. (1978). The categorical and contextual bases of person memory and stereotyping. *Journal of Personality and Social Psychology, 36,* 778–793.

Taylor, V. J., Garcia, R. L., Shelton, J. N., & Yantis, C. (2018). "A threat on the ground": The consequences of witnessing stereotype-confirming ingroup members in interracial interactions. *Cultural Diversity and Ethnic Minority Psychology, 24*(3), 319–333.

Taylor, V. J., Yantis, C., Bonam, C., & Hart, A. (2021). What to do? Predicting coping strategies following ingroup members' stereotypical behaviors in interracial interactions. *Personality and Social Psychology Bulletin, 47*(7), 1084–1100.

Taylor, V. J., Yantis, C., & Valladares, J. V. (in press). "Will they assume I'm racist?" How racial ingroup members' stereotypical behavior impacts White Americans' interracial interaction experiences. *Group Processes and Intergroup Relations.*

Tenney, E., Coll, K., Bain, K., & Kreps, T. (2021). Silenced by incivility: People, especially women, voice less in uncivil groups. *Academy of Management Proceedings, 2021,* 1.

Terrill, W., & Reisig, M. D. (2003). Neighborhood context and police use of force. *Journal of Research in Crime and Delinquency, 40*(3), 291–321.

Tesser, A. (1988). Toward a self-evaluation maintenance model of social behavior. In L. Berkowitz (Ed.), *Advances in experimental social psychology* (Vol. 21, pp. 181–227). San Diego, CA: Academic Press.

Tesser, A. (2001). On the plasticity of self-defense. *Current Directions in Psychological Science, 10,* 66–69.

Tetlock, P. E. (1983). Accountability and complexity of thought. *Journal of Personality and Social Psychology, 45,* 74–83.

Tetlock, P. E. (1985). Accountability: The neglected social context of judgment and choice. *Research in Organizational Behavior, 7,* 297–332.

Tetlock, P. E. (1992). The impact of accountability on judgment and choice: Toward a social contingency model. In M. P. Zanna (Ed.), *Advances in experimental social psychology* (Vol. 25, pp. 331–376). San Diego, CA: Academic Press.

Tetlock, P. E., & Kim, J. I. (1987). Accountability and judgment processes in a personality prediction task. *Journal of Personality and Social Psychology, 52,* 700–709.

Thibodeau, R., & Aronson, E. (1992). Taking a closer look: Reasserting the role of the self-concept in dissonance theory. *Personality and Social Psychology Bulletin, 18*(5), 591–602.

Thomas, E. L., Dovidio, J. F., & West, T. V. (2014). Lost in the categorical shuffle: Evidence for the social non-prototypicality of Black women. *Cultural Diversity and Ethnic Minority Psychology, 20*(3), 370–376.

Thompson, E. P., Roman, R. J., Moskowitz, G. B., Chaiken, S., & Bargh, J. A. (1994). Accuracy motivation attenuates covert priming effects: The systematic reprocessing of social information. *Journal of Personality and Social Psychology, 66,* 259–288.

Thompson, M. M., Naccarato, M. E., Moskow-itz, G. B., & Parker, K. J. (2001). The personal need for structure and personal fear of inva-lidity measures: Historical perspectives, cur-rent applications, and future directions. In G. B. Moskowitz (Ed.), *Cognitive social psychol-ogy: The Princeton symposium on the legacy and future of social cognition* (pp. 19–40). Mahwah, NJ: Erlbaum.

Tipler, C., & Ruscher, J. (2014). Agency's role in dehumanization: Non-human metaphors of out-groups. *Social and Personality Psychology Compass, 8,* 214–228.

Tipples. J. (2010). Time flies when we read taboo words. *Psychonomic Bulletin and Review, 17,* 563–568.

Todd, A. R., Bodenhausen, G. V., & Galinsky, A. D. (2012). Perspective taking combats the denial of intergroup discrimination. *Journal of Experimental Social Psychology, 48*(3), 738–745.

Todd, A. R., Bodenhausen, G. V., Richeson, J. A., & Galinsky, A. D. (2011). Perspective taking combats automatic expressions of racial bias. *Journal of Personality and Social Psychology, 100*(6), 1027–1042.

Todd, A. R., & Burgmer, P. (2013). Perspective taking and automatic intergroup evaluation change: Testing an associative self-anchoring account. *Journal of Personality and Social Psy-chology, 104*(5), 786–802.

Todd, A. R., & Galinsky, A. D. (2014). Perspective-taking as a strategy for improving intergroup relations: Evidence, mechanisms, and quali-fications. *Social and Personality Psychology Compass, 8*(7), 374–387.

Todd, A. R., Molden, D. C., Ham, J., & Vonk, R. (2011). The automatic and co-occurring acti-vation of multiple social inferences. *Journal of Experimental Social Psychology, 47*(1), 37–49.

Todorov, A. (2017). *Face value: The irresistible influ-ence of first impressions.* Princeton, NJ: Prince-ton University Press.

Todorov, A. (2023). From spontaneous trait inferences to spontaneous person impres-sions. In E. Balcetis & G. B. Moskowitz (Eds.), *Handbook of impression formation: A social psy-chological approach* (pp. 20–33). New York: Routledge.

Todorov, A., Dotsch, R., Porter, J. M., Oosterhof, N. N., & Falvello, V. B. (2013). Validation of data-driven computational models of social perception of faces. *Emotion, 13,* 724–738.

Todorov, A., Dotsch, R., Wigboldus, D. H. J., & Said, C. P. (2011). Data-driven methods for modeling social perception: Modeling social perception. *Social and Personality Psychology Compass, 5,* 775–791.

Todorov, A., Gobbini, M. I., Evans, K. K., & Haxby, J. V. (2007). Spontaneous retrieval of affective person knowledge in face percep-tion. *Neuropsychologia, 45*(1), 163–173.

Todorov, A., Loehr, V., & Oosterhof, N. N. (2010). The obligatory nature of holistic processing of faces in social judgments. *Perception, 39,* 514–532.

Todorov, A., Mandisodza, A. N., Goren, A., & Hall, C. C. (2005). Inferences of competence from faces predict election outcomes. *Science, 308,* 1623–1626.

Todorov, A., & Oh, D. (2021). The structure and perceptual basis of social judgments from faces. In B. Gawronski (Ed.), *Advances in exper-imental social psychology* (pp. 189–245). Cam-bridge, MA: Elsevier Academic Press.

Todorov, A., Olivola, C. Y., Dotsch, R., & Mende-Siedlecki, P. (2015). Social attributions from faces: Determinants, consequences, accuracy, and functional significance. *Annual Review of Psychology, 66,* 519–545.

Todorov, A., & Oosterhof, N. (2011). Modeling social perception of faces. *IEEE Signal Process-ing Magazine, 28,* 117–122.

Todorov, A., Pakrashi, M., & Oosterhof, N. N. (2009). Evaluating faces on trustworthiness after minimal time exposure. *Social Cognition, 27,* 813–833.

Todorov, A., Said, C. P., Engell, A. D., & Ooster-hof, N. N. (2008). Understanding evaluation of faces on social dimensions. *Trends in Cogni-tive Sciences, 12*(12), 455–460.

Todorov, A., & Uleman, J. S. (2002). Spontane-ous trait inferences are bound to actors' faces: Evidence from a false recognition paradigm. *Journal of Personality and Social Psychology, 83,* 1051–1065.

Towles-Schwen, T., & Fazio, R. H. (2006). Auto-matically activated racial attitudes as predic-tors of the success of interracial roommate relationships. *Journal of Experimental Social Psychology, 42*(5), 698–705.

Trawalter, S., & Richeson, J. A. (2006). Regula-tory focus and executive function after inter-racial interactions. *Journal of Experimental Social Psychology, 42*(3), 406–412.

Trawalter, S., Richeson, J. A., & Shelton, J. N.

(2009). Predicting behavior during interracial interactions: A stress and coping approach. *Personality and Social Psychology Review, 13*(4), 243–268.

Trawalter, S., Todd, A. R., Baird, A. A., & Richeson, J. A. (2008). Attending to threat: Race-based patterns of selective attention. *Journal of Experimental Social Psychology, 44*(5), 1322–1327.

Treisman, A., & Geffen, G. (1967). Selective attention: Perception or response? *Quarterly Journal of Experimental Psychology, 19*, 1–17.

Trope, Y. (1986a). Identification and inferential processes in dispositional attribution. *Psychological Review, 93*, 239–257.

Trope, Y. (1986b). Self-enhancement and self-assessment in achievement behavior. In R. M. Sorrentino & E. T. Higgins (Eds.), *Handbook of motivation and cognition: Foundations of social behavior* (pp. 350–378). New York: Guilford Press.

Trope, Y., & Alfieri, T. (1997). Effortfulness and flexibility of dispositional judgment processes. *Journal of Personality and Social Psychology, 73*, 662–674.

Trope, Y., & Bassok, M. (1982). Confirmatory and diagnosing strategies in social information gathering. *Journal of Personality and Social Psychology, 43*, 22–34.

Trope, Y., & Bassok, M. (1983). Information-gathering strategies in hypothesis-testing. *Journal of Experimental Social Psychology, 19*(6), 560–576.

Trope, Y., & Liberman, A. (1993). The use of trait conceptions to identify other people's behavior and to draw inferences about their personalities. *Personality and Social Psychology Bulletin, 19*, 553–562.

Trope, Y., & Liberman, N. (2000). Temporal construal and time-dependent changes in preference. *Journal of Personality and Social Psychology, 79*(6), 876–889.

Trope, Y., & Liberman, N. (2003). Temporal construal. *Psychological Review, 110*, 403–421.

Trost, M. R., Maass, A., & Kenrick, D. T. (1992). Minority influence: Personal relevance biases cognitive processes and reverses private acceptance. *Journal of Experimental Social Psychology, 28*, 234–254.

Tulving, E. E., & Thomson, D. M. (1973). Encoding specificity and retrieval processes in episodic memory. *Psychological Bulletin, 30*, 352–373.

Turner, J. C., Hogg, M. A., Oakes, P. J., Reicher, S. D., & Wetherell, M. S. (1987). *Rediscovering the social group: A self-categorization theory.* Oxford, UK: Blackwell.

Turner, J. C., & Reynolds, K. J. (2001). The social identity perspective in intergroup relations: Theories, themes, and controversies. In R. Brown & S. L. Gaertner (Eds.), *Blackwell handbook of social psychology* (pp. 133–152). Blackwell: Intergroup Processes.

Turner, R. N., & Crisp R. J. (2010). Imagining intergroup contact reduces implicit prejudice. *British Journal of Social Psychology, 49*(1), 129–142.

Tversky, A., & Kahneman, D. (1973). Availability: A heuristic for judging frequency and probability. *Cognitive Psychology, 5*, 207–232.

Tversky, A., & Kahneman, D. (1974). Judgment under uncertainty: Heuristics and biases. *Science, 185*, 1124–1131.

Tversky, A., & Kahneman, D. (1981). The framing of decisions and the psychology of choice. *Science, 211*, 453–458.

Uleman, J. S., Hon, A., Roman, R. J., & Moskowitz, G. B. (1996). On-line evidence for spontaneous trait inferences at encoding. *Personality and Social Psychology Bulletin, 22*(4), 377–394.

Uleman, J. S., & Moskowitz, G. B. (1994). Unintended effects of goals on unintended inferences. *Journal of Personality and Social Psychology, 66*, 490–501.

Uleman, J. S., Newman, L. S., & Moskowitz, G. B. (1996). People as flexible interpreters: Evidence and issues from spontaneous trait inference. In M. Zanna (Ed.), *Advances in experimental social psychology* (Vol. 28, pp. 211–280). San Diego, CA: Academic Press.

Uleman, J. S., Rim, S., Saribay, S. A., & Kressel, L. M. (2012). Controversies, questions, and prospects for spontaneous social inferences. *Social and Personality Psychology Compass, 6*(9), 657–673.

Uluğ, Ö. M., & Tropp, L. R. (2021). How witnessing racialized incidents shapes willingness to stand up for racial justice: Enhancing awareness of inequality among members of advantaged racial groups. *Journal of Applied Social Psychology, 51*, 248–261.

U.S. Department of Justice, Office of Public Affairs (2016). *Department of Justice announces new department-wide implicit bias training for personnel.* Press release 16–747. Washington, D.C.: Author.

Vaidis, D. C., & Bran, A. (2019). Respectable challenges to respectable theory: Cognitive dissonance theory requires conceptualization clarification and operational tools. *Frontiers in Psychology, 10,* 1189.

Vallacher, R. R., & Wegner, D. M. (1985). *A theory of action identification.* Hillsdale, NJ: Erlbaum.

Vallacher, R. R., & Wegner, D. M. (1987). What do people think they're doing? Action identification and human behavior. *Psychological Review, 94,* 3–15.

Vallacher, R. R., Wegner, D. M., & Samoza, M. P. (1989). That's easy for you to say: Action identification and speech fluency. *Journal of Personality and Social Psychology, 56*(2), 199–208.

Vallone, R. P., Ross, L., & Lepper, M. R. (1985). The hostile media phenomenon: Biased perception and perceptions of media bias in coverage of the Beirut massacre. *Journal of Personality and Social Psychology, 49,* 577–585.

van Baaren, R. B., Maddux, W. W., Chartrand, T. L., de Bouter, C., & van Knippenberg, A. (2003). It takes two to mimic: Behavioral consequences of self-construals. *Journal of Personality and Social Psychology, 84*(5), 1093–1102.

Van Bavel, J. J., & Cunningham, W. A. (2009). Self-categorization with a novel mixed-race group moderates automatic social and racial biases. *Personality and Social Psychology Bulletin, 35*(3), 321–335.

Van Bavel, J. J., & Packer, D. J. (2021). *The power of us: Harnessing our shared identities to improve performance, increase cooperation, and promote social harmony.* Boston: Little, Brown Spark.

Van Bavel, J. J., Packer, D. J., & Cunningham, W. A. (2008). The neural substrates of in-group bias: A functional magnetic resonance imaging investigation. *Psychological Science, 19*(11), 1131–1139.

Van Bavel, J. J., Packer, D. J., & Cunningham, W. A. (2011). Modulation of the fusiform face area following minimal exposure to motivationally relevant faces: Evidence of in-group enhancement (not out-group disregard). *Journal of Cognitive Neuroscience, 23*(11), 3343–3354.

Van der Cruyssen, L., Van Duynslaeger, M., Cortoos, A., & Van Overwalle, F. (2009). ERP time course and brain areas of spontaneous and intentional goal inferences. *Social Neuroscience, 4*(2), 165–184.

van der Linden, S. (2022). Misinformation: Susceptibility, spread, and interventions to immunize the public. *Nature Medicine, 28,* 460–467.

Van Dessel, P., Ye, Y., & De Houwer, J. (2019). Changing deep-rooted implicit evaluation in the blink of an eye: Negative verbal information shifts automatic liking of Gandhi. *Social Psychological and Personality Science, 10*(2), 266–273.

Van Duynslaeger, M., Van Overwalle, F., & Verstraeten, E. (2007). Electrophysiological time course and brain areas of spontaneous and intentional trait inferences. *Social Cognitive and Affective Neuroscience, 2*(3), 174–188.

van Harreveld, F., van der Pligt, J., & de Liver, Y. N. (2009). The agony of ambivalence and ways to resolve it: Introducing the MAID model. *Personality and Social Psychology Review, 13*(1), 45–61.

Van Overwalle, F. (1997a). A test of the joint model of causal attribution. *European Journal of Social Psychology, 27*(2), 221–236.

Van Overwalle, F. (1997b). Dispositional attributions require the joint application of the methods of difference and agreement. *Personality and Social Psychology Bulletin, 23,* 974–980.

Van Overwalle, F., Van Duynslaeger, M., Coomans, D., & Timmermans, B. (2012). Spontaneous goal inferences are often inferred faster than spontaneous trait inferences. *Journal of Experimental Social Psychology, 48*(1), 13–18.

Vasiljevic, M., & Crisp, R. (2013). Tolerance by surprise: Evidence for a generalized reduction in prejudice and increased egalitarianism through novel category combination. *PLOS One, 8,* e57106.

Vescio, T. K., Sechrist, G. B., & Paolucci, M. P. (2003). Perspective taking and prejudice reduction: The mediational role of empathy arousal and situational attributions. *European Journal of Social Psychology, 33*(4), 455–472.

Vitriol, J. A., Appleby, J., & Borgida, E. (2019). Racial bias increases false identification of Black faces in simultaneous lineups. *Social and Personality Psychological Science, 10*(6), 722–734.

Vitriol, J., & Moskowitz, G. B. (2021). Reducing defensive responding to implicit bias feedback: On the role of perceived moral threat and efficacy to change. *Journal of Experimental Social Psychology, 96,* 1–16.

Vitriol, J. A., O'Shea, B. A., & Calanchini, J. (2023). Less biased yet more defensive: The impact of control processes. *Journal of Experimental Psychology: Applied*. Advance online publication.

Vohs, K. D., & Baumeister, R. F. (Eds.). (2004). Understanding self-regulation: An introduction. In R. F. Baumeister & K. D. Vohs (Eds.), *Handbook of self-regulation: Research, theory, and applications* (pp. 1-9). New York: Guilford Press.

Vohs, K. D., & Heatherton, T. F. (2000). Self-regulatory failure: A resource-depletion approach. *Psychological Science, 11*(3), 249-254.

Vorauer, J. D. (2001). The other side of the story: Transparency estimation in social interaction. In G. B. Moskowitz (Ed.), *Cognitive social psychology: The Princeton symposium on the legacy and future of social cognition* (pp. 261-276). Mahwah, NJ: Erlbaum.

Vorauer, J. D., & Claude, S. (1998). Perceived versus actual transparency of goals in negotiation. *Personality and Social Psychology Bulletin, 24*, 371-385.

Vorauer, J., & Kumhyr, S. M. (2001). Is this about you or me? Self- versus other-directed judgments and feelings in response to intergroup interaction. *Personality and Social Psychology Bulletin, 27*(6), 706-719.

Vorauer, J. D., Main, K. J., & O'Connell, G. B. (1998). How do individuals expect to be viewed by members of lower status groups? Content and implications of meta-stereotypes. *Journal of Personality and Social Psychology, 75*(4), 917-937.

Vorauer, J. D., & Ross, M. (1999). Selfawareness and transparency overestimation: Failing to suppress one's self. *Journal of Experimental Social Psychology, 35*, 415-440.

Wandner, L. D., Heft, M. W., Lok, B. C., Hirsh, A. T., George, S. Z., Horgas, A. L., et al. (2014). The impact of patients' gender, race, and age on health care professionals' pain management decisions: An online survey using virtual human technology. *International Journal of Nursing Studies, 51*(5), 726-733.

Ward, T. B. (1994). Structured imagination: The role of category structure in exemplar generation. *Cognitive Psychology, 27*(1), 1-40.

Warren, C., & McGraw, A. P. (2016). Differentiating what is humorous from what is not. *Journal of Personality and Social Psychology, 110*(3), 407-430.

Warren, E., & Supreme Court of The United States. (1953). *U.S. Reports: Brown v. Board of Education*, 347 U.S. 483. [Periodical] Retrieved from the Library of Congress.

Waytz, A., Hoffman, K. M., & Trawalter, S. (2014). A superhumanization bias in Whites' perceptions of Blacks. *Social Psychological and Personality Science, 6*(3), 352-359.

Wegener, D. T., & Petty, R. E. (1995a). Effects of mood on persuasion processes: Enhancing, reducing, and biasing scrutiny of attitude relevant information. In L. L. Martin & A. Tesser (Eds.), *Striving and feeling: Interactions between goals and affect* (pp. 141-208). Hillsdale, NJ: Erlbaum.

Wegener, D. T., & Petty, R. E. (1995b). Flexible correction processes in social judgment: The role of naïve theories in corrections for perceived bias. *Journal of Personality and Social Psychology, 68*, 36-51.

Wegener, D. T., Petty, R. E., & Dunn, M. (1998). The metacognition of bias correction: Naïve theories of bias and the flexible correction model. In V. Yzerbyt, G. Lories, & B. Dardenne (Eds.), *Metacognition: Cognitive and social dimensions* (pp. 202-227). London: Sage.

Wegner, D. M. (1994). Ironic processes of mental control. *Psychological Review, 101*, 34-52.

Wegner, D. M. (2002). *The illusion of conscious will.* Cambridge, MA: MIT Press.

Wegner, D. M., & Bargh, J. A. (1998). Control and automaticity in social life. In D. T. Gilbert, S. T. Fiske, & G. Lindzey (Eds.), *The handbook of social psychology* (4th ed., Vol. 1, pp. 446-496). New York: Oxford University Press.

Wegner, D. M., & Erber, R. (1992). The hyperaccessibility of suppressed thoughts. *Journal of Personality and Social Psychology, 63*, 903-912.

Wegner, D. M., & Erskine, J. A. K. (2003). Voluntary involuntariness: Thought suppression and the regulation of the experience of will. *Consciousness and Cognition: An International Journal, 12*(4), 684-694.

Wegner, D. M., Schneider, D. J., Carter, S., III, & White, L. (1987). Paradoxical effects of thought suppression. *Journal of Personality and Social Psychology, 58*, 409-418.

Wegner, D. M., & Vallacher, R. R. (1977). *Implicit psychology: An introduction to social cognition.* London: Oxford University Press

Weiner, B. (1985a). An attributional theory of achievement motivation and emotion. *Psychological Review, 92*, 548-573.

Weiner, B. (1985b). "Spontaneous" causal thinking. *Psychological Bulletin, 97*, 74-84.

Weisbuch, M., Pauker, K., & Ambady, N. (2009). The subtle transmission of race bias via televised nonverbal behavior. *Science, 326*(5960), 1711–1714.

Wellman, H. M. (1990). *The child's theory of mind.* Cambridge, MA: MIT Press.

Wells, G. L., & Gavanski, I. (1989). Mental simulation of causality. *Journal of Personality and Social Psychology, 56,* 161–169.

Werth, L., & Foerster, J. (2007). How regulatory focus influences consumer behavior. *European Journal of Social Psychology, 37,* 33–51.

West, H. C., & Sabol, W. J. (2009). *Prison inmates at midyear 2008—statistical tables.* Washington, DC: Bureau of Justice Statistics. Available at *www.ojp.gov/bjs/abstract/pim08st.htm.*

West, T. V., & Kenny, D. A. (2011). The truth and bias model of judgment. *Psychological Review, 118*(2), 357–378.

Whitley, B., & Webster, G. (2019). The relationship of intergroup ideologies to ethnic prejudice: A meta- analysis. *Personality and Social Psychology Review, 23*(3), 207–237.

Whittlesea, B. W. A., & Williams, L. D. (2000). The source of feelings of familiarity: The discrepancy–attribution hypothesis. *Journal of Experimental Psychology: Learning, Memory, and Cognition, 26*(3), 547–565.

Whittlesea, B. W. A., & Williams, L. D. (2001). The discrepancy-attribution hypothesis: II. Expectation, uncertainty, surprise, and feelings of familiarity. *Journal of Experimental Psychology: Learning, Memory, and Cognition, 27*(1), 14–33.

Wicklund. R. A., & Gollwitzer, P. M. (1982). *Symbolic self-completion.* Hillsdale, NJ: Erlbaum.

Wigboldus, D. H. J., Dijksterhuis, A., & Van Knippenberg, A. (2003). When stereotypes get in the way: Stereotypes obstruct stereotype-inconsistent trait inferences. *Journal of Personality and Social Psychology, 84*(3), 470–484.

Wigboldus, D. H. J., Semin, G. R., & Spears, R. (2000). How do we communicate stereotypes? Linguistic bases and inferential consequences. *Journal of Personality and Social Psychology, 78*(1), 5–18.

Wilkes, A. L., & Leatherbarrow, M. (1988). Editing episodic memory following the identification of error. *The Quarterly Journal of Experimental Psychology A: Human Experimental Psychology, 40A*(2), 361–387.

Williams, J. C. (2014, October). Hacking tech's diversity problem. *Harvard Business Review,* 94–100.

Williams, J. M. G., Watts, F. N., MacLeod, C., & Mathews, A. (1988). *Cognitive psychology and emotional disorders.* New York: Wiley.

Williams, L., & Bargh, J. A. (2008). Experiencing physical warmth promotes interpersonal warmth. *Science, 322*(5901), 606–607.

Willis, J., & Todorov, A. (2006). First impressions: Making up your mind after a 100-ms exposure to a face. *Psychological Science, 17*(7), 592–598.

Wilson, J. P., Remedios, J. D., & Rule, N. O. (2017). Interactive effects of obvious and ambiguous social categories on perceptions of leadership: When double-minority status may be beneficial. *Personality and Social Psychology Bulletin, 43*(6), 888–900.

Wilson, J. P., & Rule, N. O. (2015). Facial trustworthiness predicts extreme criminal-sentencing outcomes. *Psychological Science, 26*(8), 1325–1331.

Wilson, J. P., & Rule, N. O. (2016). Hypothetical sentencing decisions are associated with actual capital punishment outcomes: The role of facial trustworthiness. *Social Psychological and Personality Science, 7*(4), 331–338.

Wilson, T. D. (2011). *Redirect: The surprising new science of psychological change.* Little Brown/Hachette Book Group.

Wilson, T. D., & Brekke, N. (1994). Mental contamination and mental correction: Unwanted influences on judgments and evaluations. *Psychological Bulletin, 116,* 117–142.

Wilton, L., Apfelbaum, E., & Good, J. (2019). Valuing differences and reinforcing them: Multiculturalism increases race essentialism. *Social Psychological and Personality Science, 10*(5), 681–689.

Winston, J., Strange, B., O'Doherty, J., & Dolan, R. (2002). Automatic and intentional brain responses during evaluation of trustworthiness of faces. *Nature Neuroscience, 5,* 277–283.

Winter, D. G., John, O. P., Stewart, A. J., Klohnen, E. C., & Duncan, L. E. (1998). Traits and motives: Toward an integration of two traditions in personality research. *Psychological Review, 105*(2), 230–250.

Winter, K., Scholl, A., & Sassenberg, K. (2021). A matter of flexibility: Changing outgroup attitudes through messages with negations. *Journal of Personality and Social Psychology, 120*(4), 956–976.

Winter, L., & Uleman, J. S. (1984). When are social judgments made? Evidence for the spontaneousness of trait inferences. *Journal of Personality and Social Psychology, 47*, 237–252.

Winter, L., Uleman, J. S., & Cunniff, C. (1985). How automatic are social judgments? *Journal of Personality and Social Psychology, 49*(4), 904–917. (Retraction published 1970, *Journal of Experimental Psychology, 86*[2], 255–262)

Wittenbrink, B., Gist, P. L., & Hilton, J. L. (1997). Structural properties of stereotypic knowledge and their influences on the construal of social situations. *Journal of Personality and Social Psychology, 72*, 526–543.

Wittenbrink, B., Judd, C. M., & Park, B. (1997). Evidence for racial prejudice at the implicit level and its relationship with questionnaire measures. *Journal of Personality and Social Psychology, 72*, 262–274.

Wolsiefer, K. J., Mehl, M., Moskowitz, G. B., Cagno, C. K., Zestcott, C. A., Tejeda-Padron, A., et al. (2023). Investigating the relationship between resident physician implicit bias and language use during a clinical encounter with Hispanic patients. *Health Communication, 38*(1), 124–132.

Wolsko, C., Park, B., Judd, C. M., & Wittenbrink, B. (2000). Framing interethnic ideology: Effects of multicultural and color-blind perspectives on judgments of groups and individuals. *Journal of Personality and Social Psychology, 78*, 635–654.

Wood, W., Pool, G. J., Leck, K., & Purvis, D. (1996). Self-definition, defensive processing, and influence: The normative impact of majority and minority groups. *Journal of Personality and Social Psychology, 71*(6), 1181–1193.

Woodhams, C., Lupton, B., & Cowling, M. (2015). The presence of ethnic minority and disabled men in feminised work: Intersectionality, vertical segregation and the glass escalator. *Sex Roles: A Journal of Research, 72*(7–8), 277–293.

Word, C. O., Zanna, M. P., & Cooper, J. (1974). The nonverbal mediation of self-fulfilling prophecies in interracial interaction. *Journal of Experimental Social Psychology, 10*, 109–120.

Wortman, C. B., & Silver, R. C. (1989). The myths of coping with loss. *Journal of Consulting and Clinical Psychology, 57*(3), 349–357.

Wright, J. C., & Baril, G. (2011). The role of cognitive resources in determining our moral intuitions: Are we all liberals at heart? *Journal of Experimental Social Psychology, 47*(5), 1007–1012.

Wright, S. C., Taylor, D. M., & Moghaddam, F. M. (1990). Responding to membership in a disadvantaged group: From acceptance to collective protest. *Journal of Personality and Social Psychology, 58*, 994–1003.

Wundt, W. M. (1862). *Beiträge zur Theorie der Sinneswahrnehmung* [Contributions Toward a Theory of Sense Perception]. Leipzig: C.F. Winter.

Wyer, N. A. (2010). You never get a second chance to make a first (implicit) impression: The role of elaboration in the formation and revision of implicit impressions. *Social Cognition, 28*(1), 1–19.

Wyer, N. A. (2016). Easier done than undone … by some of the people, some of the time: The role of elaboration in explicit and implicit group preferences. *Journal of Experimental Social Psychology, 63*, 77–85.

Wyer, R. S., & Gordon, S. E. (1982). The recall of information about persons and groups. *Journal of Experimental Social Psychology, 18*(2), 128–164.

Wyer, R. S., & Gordon, S. E. (1984). The cognitive representation of social information. In R. S. Wyer & T. K. Srull (Eds.), *Handbook of social cognition* (Vol. 2, pp. 73–150). Hillsdale, NJ: Erlbaum.

Wyer, R. S., Jr., & Srull, T. K. (1989). *Memory and cognition in its social context*. Hillsdale, NJ: Erlbaum.

Xiao, Y. J., & Van Bavel, J. J. (2012). See your friends close, and your enemies closer: Social identity and identity threat shape the representation of physical distance. *Personality and Social Psychology Bulletin, 38*(7), 959–972.

Yan, X., Wang, M., & Zhang, Q. (2012). Effects of gender stereotypes on spontaneous trait inferences and the moderating role of gender schematicity: Evidence from Chinese undergraduates. *Social Cognition, 30*, 220–231.

Yantis, C., & Bonam, C. (2021). Inconceivable middle-class Black space: The architecture and consequences of space-focused stereotypes at the intersection of race and class. *Personality and Social Psychology Bulletin, 47*(7), 1101–1118.

Ybarra, O. (2001). When first impressions don't last: The role of isolation and adaptation processes in the revision of evaluative impressions. *Social Cognition, 19*(5), 491–520.

Yogeeswaran, K., & Dasgupta, N. (2014). The devil is in the details: Abstract versus concrete construals of multiculturalism differentially impact intergroup relations. *Journal of Personality and Social Psychology, 106*(5), 772–789.

Yogeeswaran, K., Verkuyten, M., & Ealam, B. (2021). A way forward? The impact of interculturalism on intergroup relations in culturally diverse nations. *Group Processes and Intergroup Relations, 24*(6), 945–965.

Yoshida, E., Peach, J. M., Zanna, M. P., & Spencer, S. J. (2012). Not all automatic associations are created equal: How implicit normative evaluations are distinct from implicit attitudes and uniquely predict meaningful behavior. *Journal of Experimental Social Psychology, 48*, 694–706.

Young, S. G., & Hugenberg, K. (2010). Mere social categorization modulates identification of facial expressions of emotion. *Journal of Personality and Social Psychology, 99*(6), 964–977.

Yzerbyt, V. R., Corneille, O., Dumont, M., & Hahn, K. (2001). The dispositional inference strikes back: Situational focus and dispositional suppression in causal attribution. *Journal of Personality and Social Psychology, 81*(3), 365–376.

Yzerbyt, V. Y., Rogier, A., & Fiske, S. T. (1998). Group entitativity and social attribution: On translating situational constraints into stereotypes. *Personality and Social Psychology Bulletin, 24*(10), 1089–1103.

Yzerbyt, V. Y., Schadron, G., Leyens, J., & Rocher, S. (1994). Social judgeability: The impact of meta-informational cues on the use of stereotypes. *Journal of Personality and Social Psychology, 66*, 48–55.

Zadny, J. G., & Gerard, H. B. (1974). Attributed intentions and informational selectivity. *Journal of Experimental Social Psychology, 10*(1), 34–52.

Zajonc, R. B. (1980b). Feeling and thinking: Preferences need no inferences. *American Psychologist, 35*, 151–175.

Zanna, M. P., & Cooper, J. (1974). Dissonance and the pill: An attribution approach to studying the arousal properties of dissonance. *Journal of Personality and Social Psychology, 29*, 703–709.

Zebrowitz, L. A. (1997). *Reading faces: Window to the soul?* Boulder, CO: Westview Press.

Zebrowitz, L. A., Andreoletti, C., Collins, M. A., Lee, S. Y., & Blumenthal, J. (1998). Bright, bad, babyfaced boys: Appearance stereotypes do not always yield self-fulfilling prophecy effects. *Journal of Personality and Social Psychology, 75*(5), 1300–1320.

Zebrowitz, L. A., & McDonald, S. M. (1991). The impact of litigants' baby-facedness and attractiveness on adjudications in small claims courts. *Law and Human Behavior, 15*(6), 603–623.

Zeigarnik, B. (1927). Das Behalten erledigter und unerledigter Handlungen [The retention of completed and uncompleted actions]. *Psychologische Forschung, 9*, 1–85.

Zemborian, M. R., & Johar, G. V. (2007). Attitudinal ambivalence and openness to persuasion: A framework for interpersonal influence. *Journal of Consumer Research, 33*, 506–514.

Zhong, C.-B., & Leonardelli, G. J. (2008). Cold and lonely: Does social exclusion literally feel cold *Psychological Science, 19*(9), 838–842.

Zhou, R., & Pham, M. T., Mick, D. G., Iacobucci, D., & Huber, J. (Eds.). (2004). Promotion and prevention across mental accounts: When financial products dictate consumers' investment goals. *Journal of Consumer Research, 31*(1), 125–135.

Zhou, S., Page-Gould, E., Aron, A., Moyer, A., & Hewstone, M. (2019). The extended contact hypothesis: A meta-analysis on 20 years of research. *Personality and Social Psychology Review, 23*(2), 132–160.

Zuckerman, M. (1979). Attribution of success and failure revisited: The motivational bias is alive and well in attribution theory. *Journal of Personality, 47*(2), 245–287.

Author Index

Subject Index